Practical Guide to the
Care of the
Medical Patient

Marianne Ho-Bojoe
229-6675

Fred F. Ferri, M.D.

Department of Medicine

St. Vincent's Medical Center
Bridgeport, Connecticut

St. Joseph's Hospital
Providence, Rhode Island

Rhode Island Hospital
Providence, Rhode Island

with 63 illustrations

The C. V. Mosby Company

St. Louis • Washington, D.C. • Toronto   1987

MOSBY

A TRADITION OF PUBLISHING EXCELLENCE

Editor: Dennis Carson
Assistant Editor: Elizabeth Raven
Project Editor: Teri Merchant
Design: John Rokusek
Production Editors: Mary Stueck and Suzanne Glazer

Printed in the United States of America

The C.V. Mosby Company
11830 Westline Industrial Drive, St. Louis, Missouri 63146

Library of Congress Cataloging-in-Publication Data

Practical guide to the care of the medical patient.

   Includes index.
   1. Internal medicine—Handbooks, manuals, etc.
2. Diagnosis—Handbooks, manuals, etc.   I. Ferri, Fred F.
[DNLM: 1. Diagnosis—handbooks.   2. Therapeutics—
handbooks.   WB 39 P895]
RC55.P84   1987   616   87-7661
ISBN 0-8016-1661-1

C/D/D   9 8 7 6   03/A/328

Contributors

Dennis L. Bordan, M.D., F.A.C.S.

Chapter 4: Preparation of the patient for surgery

Chairman, Department of Surgery, Director, Surgical Residency Program, St. Vincent's Medical Center, Bridgeport, Connecticut; Associate Professor of Surgery, New York Medical College, New York, New York

Robert Burd, M.D., F.A.C.P.

Section 14.1: Approach to the patient with anemia

Chief, Division of Hematology, St. Vincent's Medical Center, Bridgeport, Associate Clinical Professor of Medicine, Yale University School of Medicine, New Haven, Connecticut

Saul Feldman, M.D.

Section 13.1: Acute gastrointestinal bleeding

Chief, Division of Gastroenterology, St. Vincent's Medical Center, Associate Clinical Professor of Medicine Yale University School of Medicine, New Haven, Connecticut

Marvin Garrell, M.D., F.A.C.P.

Section 17.3: Evaluation of the patient with dementia

Director of Medical Education, St. Vincent's Medical Center, Bridgeport Associate Clinical Professor of Medicine, Yale University School of Medicine, New Haven, Medical Director, Jewish Home of Fairfield, Fairfield, Connecticut

James Grant, M.D.

Section 16.1: Renal failure

Chief, Division of Renology, St. Vincent's Medical Center, Bridgeport, Associate Internal Medicine Program Director, Associate Clinical Professor of Medicine, Yale University School of Medicine, New Haven, Connecticut

H. Christina Hanley, M.D.

Section 12.1: Diabetes mellitus

Chief, Division of Endocrinology, St. Vincent's Medical Center, Bridgeport, Assistant Clinical Professor of Medicine, Yale University School of Medicine, New Haven, Connecticut

Joseph Herbin, M.D.

Section 15.1: Nosocomial infections
Chief, Division of Infectious
Diseases, St. Vincent's Medical
Center, Bridgeport, Assistant
Clinical Professor of Medicine,
Yale University School of
Medicine, New Haven, Connecticut

George T. Kiss, M.D.

*Section 18.1: Use and interpretation of
pulmonary function tests*
Chief, Division of Pulmonary
Diseases, St. Vincent's Medical
Center, Bridgeport, Associate
Clinical Professor of Medicine,
Yale University School of
Medicine, New Haven, Connecticut

Iradj Nejad, M.D.

Section 12.4: Hypoglycemia
Endocrinologist, St. Vincent's
Medical Center, Bridgeport,
Assistant Clinical Professor of
Medicine, University of
Connecticut, Farmington,
Connecticut

Kenneth Siegel, M.D.

Section 17.1: Generalized tonic-clonic seizures
Chief, Division of Neurology, St.
Vincent's Medical Center,
Bridgeport, Associate Clinical
Professor of Medicine, Yale
University School of Medicine,
New Haven, Connecticut

Michael S. Weinstock, M.D., F.A.C.E.P.

*Chapter 5: General management of poisoning
and drug overdose*
Chairman, Department of
Emergency Medicine, St. Vincent's
Medical Center, Bridgeport,
Connecticut

CONSULTANTS

Everett B. Cooper, M.D., F.A.C.P.

*Chapters 1, 2, 3, 6, 7, 8, 9, 10, 11, 12, 13,
14, 15, 16, 17, 18, and 19*
Chairman, Department of Medicine,
St. Vincent's Medical Center,
Bridgeport, Associate Clinical
Professor of Medicine, Yale
University School of Medicine,
New Haven, Connecticut

Vincent Spinelli, R.Ph.

Chapter 21
Director Pharmacy Department, St.
Vincent's Medical Center,
Bridgeport, Connecticut

David H. Lobdell, M.D., F.C.A.P.

Chapter 20
Chairman, Pathology and
Laboratory Medicine, St. Vincent's
Medical Center, Bridgeport,
Connecticut

Preface

This manual is a clear and concise reference for the busy clinician in need of immediate medical information. Its purpose is to provide a fast and efficient way to identify important clinical and laboratory information. It is not intended to substitute for the many excellent medical reference texts that form the cornerstone of one's medical education.

To limit the size of the manual to a pocket reference, less emphasis has been placed on pathophysiology and epidemiology and more emphasis on practical clinical information. A conservative approach to the various medical syndromes is followed throughout the book. Elegant but unnecessary words have been eliminated in favor of simple and accurate expositions of the various subjects. Medical tables have been used extensively throughout the manual to simplify difficult topics and to enhance recollection of principal points.

It is hoped that the concise style of this manual will be of help to the reader, particularly during an active clinical service when time to read is severely limited.

The combination of practical clinical information with drug therapeutics and laboratory medicine makes this manual unique and useful not only to medical residents and medical students but also to practicing physicians and allied health professionals.

Fred F. Ferri

Acknowledgments

I wish to acknowledge the many contributors and consultants for their excellent expositions and sage advise. I am particularly indebted to Everett B. Cooper, M.D., F.A.C.P., Chairman of the Department of Medicine at St. Vincent's Medical Center, for his scholarly guidance.

To my family, whose constant
support and encouragement
made this book a reality

Contents

Medical Record
Abbreviations

@ at
a arterial
A₂ aortic second sound
āā of each
AB apical beat
abd abdomen
ABG arterial blood gas
abn abnormal
ac before meals
A/C assist control
acet acetone
ACLS advanced cardiovascular life support
ACT activated clotting time
ACTH adrenocorticotropic hormone
ADL activities of daily living
ad lib as desired, freely
adm admission
AF atrial fibrillation
AFB acid-fast bacilli
A/G albumin globulin
AIDS acquired immune deficiency syndrome
AJ ankle jerk
AKA above-knee amputation
AL arterial line
alb albumin
alk phos alkaline phosphatase
ALL acute lymphocytic leukemia
AM morning
AMA against medical advice
AMI acute myocardial infarction
AML acute myelogenous leukemia
amp ampul
amt amount
amy amylase
ANA antinuclear antibody
AODM adult-onset diabetes mellitus
AP anteroposterior
A & P auscultation and percussion
appt appointment

aq water
ARD acute respiratory distress
ARM arterial rupture of membranes
ART assessment, review, and treatment
AS atriosystolic
asa aspirin
A.S.A. American Society of Anesthesiologists
ASHD arteriosclerotic heart disease
ATC around the clock
at fib atrial fibrillation
AV arteriovenous
B black
ba barium
BBB bundle branch block
BCG bacillus Calmette-Guérin
BCP birth control pill
BE barium enema
bid two times a day
bilat bilateral
bili bilirubin
BKA below-knee amputation
Bl s blood sugar
BM bowel movement
BMR basal metabolic rate
BP blood pressure
BPH benign prostatic hypertrophy
BR bed rest
BRP bathroom privileges
BS or **bs** breath sounds
BSA body surface area
BSO bilateral salpingo-oophorectomy
BTL bilateral tubal ligation
BUN blood urea nitrogen
Bx biopsy
c̄ with
C centigrade
Ca cancer
Ca² calcium, ionized
C/A clinitest and acetone

CAB coronary artery bypass
CABG coronary artery bypass graft
CAD coronary artery disease
cal calorie
cap capsule
CAT computerized axial tomography
cath catheterization
CBC complete blood cell count
CBD common bile duct
cc cubic centimeter
CC chief complaint
CCU coronary care unit
CEA carcinoembryonic antigen
CHF congestive heart failure
cho carbohydrate
CI cardiac index
CK creatine kinase
CKMB creatine kinase/MB
cl clear
Cl chloride
CLL chronic lymphocytic leukemia
cm centimeter
CM costal margin
CML chronic myelogenous leukemia
CMV continuous mechanical ventilation
CMV cytomegalovirus
CNS central nervous system
CO cardiac output
c/o complains of
CO₂ carbon dioxide
COPD chronic obstructive pulmonary disease
CPAP continuous positive airway pressure
CPR cardiopulmonary resuscitation
Cr (lab) creatinine
CR cardiorespiratory
C/S culture and sensitivity
CSF cerebrospinal fluid
C/sec cesarean section
CT scan CAT scan (see also CAT)
CV cardiovascular
cva costovertebral angle
CVA cerebrovascular accident
CVP central venous pressure
CXR chest x-ray
cysto cystoscopy
DAT diet as tolerated
DBIL direct bilirubin
D/C discontinue
D & C dilatation and curettage
Dial dialysis
DIC disseminated intravascular coagulation
dil dilute
DKA diabetic ketoacidosis

DM diabetes mellitus
DOA dead on arrival
DP dorsalis pedis
DPT diphtheria, pertussis, tetanus
DR delivery room
DSD dry sterile dressing
D & S dilation and suction
DTR deep tendon reflex
DTs delirium tremens
DUB dysfunctional uterine bleeding
D/W dextrose in water
Dx diagnosis
EBL estimated blood loss
ECF extended care facility
ECG electrocardiogram
EDC estimated date of confinement
EEG electroencephalogram
EENT eyes, ears, nose, and throat
EF ejection fraction
elect electrolyte
elix elixir
EMG electromyogram
ENT ear, nose, and throat
EOM extraocular movements
EPS extrapyramidal symptoms
ER emergency room
ERCP endoscopic retrograde cholangiopancreatography
ERS evacuation retained secundines
ESRD end-stage renal disease
EST, ECT electroshock therapy
EUA examination under anesthesia
et al and others
ext extract
F Fahrenheit
FBS fasting blood sugar
FEV forced expiratory volume
FF force fluids
FH family history
FHC family health center
FHM fetal heart monitor
FHR fetal heart rate
fl fluid
FS frozen section
FUO fever of undetermined origin
FWB full weight bearing
fx fracture
5FU fluorouracil
g or **gm** gram
G6PD glucose 6-phosphatase deficiency
GA general anesthesia
GB gallbladder
Gc gonococcus
GGT γ-glutamyltransferase
GI gastrointestinal
glu glucose

GN   graduate nurse
gr   grain
GSW   gun shot wound
gtt   drop
GTT   glucose tolerance test
GU   genitourinary
G/W enema   glycerine and water enema
Gyn   gynecology
h   hour
H/A   headache
HA   hyperalimentation
HBP   high blood pressure
hct   hematocrit
HD   hospital discharge
HDL   high-density lipoprotein
HEENT   head, eyes, ears, nose, and throat
HEMPAS   hereditary erythroblastic multinuclearity associated with positive acidified serum
Hg   hemoglobin
H/H   hemoglobin/hematocrit
HIV   human immunodeficiency virus
H & L   heart and lungs
HNP   herniated nucleus pulposus
H$_2$O   water
H$_2$O$_2$ hydrogen peroxide
HORF   high-output renal failure
H & P   history and physical examination
HPI   history of present illness
HR   heart rate
hs   hour of sleep (at bedtime)
ht   height
hx   history
IBC   iron-binding capacity
ICU   intensive care unit
ID   intradermal
IHSS   idiopathic hypertrophic subaortic stenosis
I & D   incision and drainage
IM   intramuscular
Imp   impression
IMV   intermittent mandatory ventilation
I & O   intake and output
IPPB   intermittent positive pressure breathing
IQ   intelligence quotient
ITP   idiopathic thrombocytopenic purpura
IUD   intrauterine device
IV   intravenous
IVP   intravenous pyelogram
JVD   jugular venous distention
JVP   jugular vein pulse

K$^+$ potassium
KJ   knee jerk
kg   kilogram
KUB   kidney, ureter, and bladder
l or **lt**   left
l or **L**   liter
lab   laboratory
lac   laceration
lap   laparotomy
lb   pound
LBP   low back pain
LBBB   left bundle branch block
LDH   lactic dehydrogenase
Lip   lipid
LLL   left lower lobe
LLQ   left lower quadrant
LMD   local medical doctor
LMP   last menstrual period
LNMP   last normal menstrual period
LOC   level of consciousness
LP   lumbar puncture
LPN   licensed practical nurse
LSB   left sternal border
LSK   liver, spleen, and kidney
LUL   left upper lobe
LUQ   left upper quadrant
LVH   left ventricular hypertrophy
L & W   living and well
m   murmur
M   midnight
max   maximum
m or **min**   minute
MCL   midclavicular line
med   medication
MED   medical
mEq   milliequivalent
mets   metastases
mg   milligram
Mg^{2+}   magnesium
MI   myocardial infarction
mixt   mixture
ml   milliliter
mm   millimeter
mmol or **mM**   millimole
mod   moderate
MOM   milk of magnesia
MP   metacarpophalangeal
MS   mental status
MVA   motor vehicle accident
NA   not applicable
Na$^+$ (lab)   sodium
NaHCO$_3$ sodium bicarbonate
NB   newborn
NCP   nursing care plan
neg   negative
NETT   nasal endotracheal tube
Neuro   neurology

ng nanogram
NG nasogastric
NH₃ ammonia
NKDA no known drug allergy
NKA no known allergy
NM neuromuscular
no number
noc night
NPO nothing by mouth
OA oral airway
OB obstetrics
OD overdose
OD right eye
OETT oral endotracheal tube
OOB out of bed
OOP out on pass
OPD outpatient department
opt optimum
ophth ophthalmology
OR operating room
Oral oral surgery
Orth or **ortho** orthopedics
OS left eye
osm osmolality
OT occupational therapy
OU each eye
oz ounce
p after
p̄ pulse
P₂ pulmonic second sound
P & A percussion and auscultation
PAD pulmonary artery diastolic
pap Papanicolaou
PAP pulmonary arterial pressure
para number of pregnancies
pc after meals
Pco₂ carbon dioxide tension
PCWP pulmonary capillary wedge pressure
PE physical exam
PEARL pupils equal and react to light
PEEP positive end-expiratory pressure
ped pediatric
per by
PERRLA pupils equal, round, reactive to light and accommodation
pg picogram
PH past history
phos phosphorus
PHR peak heart rate
PI present illness
PID pelvic inflammatory disease
PIP proximal interphalangeal
PKU phenylketonuria
PM afternoon
PMI point of maximum impulse

PMP previous menstrual period
PM & R physical medicine and rehabilitation
PND paroxysmal nocturnal dyspnea
PO by mouth
postop postoperative
Po₂ oxygen tension
PP postpartum
PPD purified protein derivative
pr per rectum
preop preoperative
prep preparation
PROM premature rupture of membranes
prn as needed
Psych or **psych** psychiatry
PT posterior tibial
PT physical therapy
pt patient
PTA prior to admission
PWP pulmonary wedge pressure
PVC premature ventricular contraction
PVR pulmonary vascular resistance
PX physical
q every
qd every day
qh every hour
qid four times a day
qns quantity not sufficient
qod every other day
qs quantity sufficient
R right
RA right atrial
RAN resident's admission note
RBBB right bundle branch block
RBC red blood cells
RDS respiratory distress syndrome
R & E round and equal
readm readmission
REM rapid eye movement
Rh Rhesus blood factor
RIA radio immunoassay
RL Ringer's lactate
RIND reversible ischemic neurologic deficit
RLL right lower lobe
RLQ right lower quadrant
RML right middle lobe
R/O rule out
ROM range of motion
ROS review of systems
RN registered nurse
rpt repeat
RPT registered physical therapist
RR recovery room
RSR regular sinus rhythm

rt right
R/T related to
RTC return to clinic
RUL right upper lobe
RV right ventricular
RUQ right upper quadrant
Rx therapy, treatment, prescription
s̄ without
S/A sugar and acetone
sat saturated
SB stillbirth
SC subcutaneous
SCP standard care plan
SGA small for gestational age
SGOT serum glutamic oxaloacetic transaminase
SIADH syndrome of inappropriate secretion of antidiuretic hormone
SGPT serum glutamic pyruvate transaminase
SL sublingual
SLE systemic lupus erythematosus
SLR straight leg raising
SNF skilled nursing facility
SO₂ oxygen saturation
SOB short of breath
SOC state of consciousness
sol solution
S/P status post
SRM spontaneous rupture membranes
s̄s̄ half
S/S signs and symptoms
SSE soap suds enema
stat immediately
subcu, SC subcutaneous
supp suppository
Surg surgery
SVR systemic vascular resistance
Sx symptoms
syr syrup
T, tbsp tablespoon
t, tsp teaspoon
T & A tonsillectomy and adenoidectomy
tab tablet
TAH total abdominal hysterectomy
TB, Tbc tuberculosis
TBIL total bilirubin
T/C throat culture
temp temperature
TIA transient ischemic attack
TIBC total iron-binding capacity
tid three times daily
tinc tincture
TM tympanic membrane
TO telephone order

TP total protein
TPN total parenteral nutrition
TPR temperature, pulse, and respiration
TRIG triglycerides
TTP ribothymidine 5'triphosphate
TUR transurethal resection
TURP transurethral resection prostate
TX therapy
U unit
UA umbilical artery
U/A urinalysis
UGI upper gastrointestinal
ung ointment
URAC uric acid
URI upper respiratory tract infection
UTI urinary tract infection
V venous
v mixed venous
vag hyst vaginal hysterectomy
VD veneral disease
VO verbal order
vs visit
VS vital signs
W white
WBC white blood (cell) count
w/c wheel chair
WD well developed
WF white female
WN well nourished
WNL within normal limits
wt weight
y/o years old
X times

SYMBOLS
+ + moderate amount
+ + + large amount
0 zero, none
° degree
♀ female
♂ male
number
↑ increased
↓ decreased
> greater than
< less than
μ micron
+ positive, presence
" minute
' second
∅ absence of
√ check
− negative, absence
△ changes

2

Approach to the Medical Patient

2.1 HISTORY AND PHYSICAL EXAM[1-3]

1. Chief complaint: reason for seeking medical attention; when possible it should be stated in the patient's own words.
2. Present illness: chronologic narrative of the patient's medical problems. The description of the symptoms should include the following: location, quality (deep, sharp, stinging), quantity or severity, timing (onset, duration, frequency), aggravating or relieving factors, associated manifestations, prior investigations, prior treatment, and radiation to another site.
3. Past medical history: general state of health, significant childhood illnesses, prior hospitalizations (medical, surgical), blood transfusions, and traumas.
4. Allergies: foods, drugs; describe the type of allergic reaction.
5. Current medications: dosage, frequency, and duration of present drug regimen; include all nonprescription drugs.
6. Family history: age and health status or age and cause of death of each immediate family member. Inquire about a family history of diabetes, heart disease, hypertension, cancer, arthritis, mental disorders, or any hereditary conditions.
7. Social history
   a. Life style, home situation, significant others
   b. Cigarette smoking (quantity in pack years), alcohol usage (specific as possible)
   c. Occupational history
   d. Religious beliefs relevant to health
8. Review of systems
   a. General: overall state of health, usual weight, recent weight change, fever, night sweats, sleeping habits, appetite
   b. Skin: rashes, pruritus, color change, pigmentation
   c. Head: headaches, trauma
   d. Eyes: vision, visual disturbances, last eye exam
   e. Ears: hearing, tinnitus, vertigo, infections, discharge
   f. Nose and sinuses: epistaxis, nasal stuffiness, sinusitis, sense of smell
   g. Mouth and throat: condition of teeth, last dental exam, presence of sore throat or mouth lesions
   h. Neck: lumps, "swollen glands," pain in neck region
   i. Breasts: pain, history of lumps, bleeding, nipple discharge; if female, inquire if she performs self-exam

    j. Respiratory: cough, wheezing, sputum (quantity, color), shortness of breath, pain associated with breathing

    k. Cardiac: chest pain, palpitations, orthopnea, edema, heart murmurs, history of high blood pressure

    l. Gastrointestinal: nausea, vomiting, change in bowel habits, GI bleeding, constipation, diarrhea, abdominal pain, increased girth

    m. Genitourinary: dysuria, frequency, urgency, nocturia, discharges, venereal diseases, libido, sexual problems, bleeding

    n. Gynecologic/reproductive: age at menarche, last menstrual period, frequency and duration of periods, number and complications of pregnancies, age at menopause, contraception

    o. Musculoskeletal: weakness, arthritis, gout, joint pains, swelling or stiffness, muscle cramps

    p. Peripheral vascular: varicose veins, thrombophlebitis, claudication, Raynaud's phenomenon

    q. Neuropsychiatric: seizures, syncope, weakness, paralysis/paresis, extreme mood changes, insomnia, anxiety, psychiatric care, suicidal ideation

    r. Endocrine: heat or cold intolerance, polydypsia, polyuria, polyphagia

    s. Hematologic: easy bruising, transfusion reactions, excessive bleeding, history of anemia

9. Physical exam (see boxed material on p. 15 for description of normal physical exam)

    a. Vital signs: record pulse, respiration, temperature, and blood pressure (position, measured in both arms)

    b. General description: observe state of health, general appearance, nutritional status, body development, personal hygiene, posture, signs of anxiety, and apparent age

    c. Skin

        (1) Observe texture, color, temperature, turgor, color, and note any lesions

        (2) Note distribution, amount, and texture of hair

        (3) Note color of nail beds and shape of nails

    d. Lymph nodes: note size, consistency, mobility, and tenderness of lymph nodes

    e. Head: note size, shape, symmetry, and any unusual lesions

    f. Eyes: note position and alignment of eyes; inspect lacrimal glands, eyelids, cornea, sclera, and pupils; test visual fields and pupillary reactions; closely examine the fundi; observe range of eye movements (see Fig. 2-1)

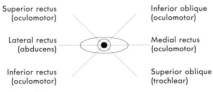

Figure 2-1
Muscles that control eye movements.

g. Ears: inspect auricles, canals, and tympanic membranes; check auditory acuity by whispering in the patient's ear or by placing watch against the patient's ear
h. Nose and sinuses: inspect the external nose, nasal mucosa, and septum; palpate frontal and maxillary sinuses for evidence of tenderness
i. Mouth and throat: inspect lips, gums, teeth, tongue, palate, and pharynx
j. Neck
    (1) Palpate thyroid gland, inspect and palpate cervical nodes, and examine trachea

Table 2-1 Response of selected murmurs to physiologic intervention

Cardiac Murmurs	Accentuation of Murmur
Systolic	
Aortic stenosis (AS)	Valsalva release
	Sudden squatting
	Passive leg raising
Idiopathic hypertrophic subaortic stenosis (IHSS)	Valsalva strain
	Standing
Mitral regurgitation	Sudden squatting
	Isometric handgrip
Pulmonic stenosis	Valsalva release
Tricuspid regurgitation	Inspiration
	Passive leg raising
Diastolic	
Aortic regurgitation	Sudden squatting
	Isometric handgrip
Mitral stenosis	Exercise
	Left lateral position
	Isometric handgrip
	Coughing
Tricuspid stenosis	Inspiration
	Passive leg raising

Table 2-2 Grading of cardiac murmurs

Grade	Description
I	Faintest audible murmur
	Can be heard only with special effort
II	Faint, but easily audible
III	Moderately loud
IV	Loud; associated with a thrill
V	Very loud; associated with a thrill
	May be heard with a stethoscope off chest
VI	Maximum loudness; associated with a thrill
	Heard without a stethoscope

    (2) Auscultate carotids for pulses, upstroke, and presence of bruits

    (3) Note presence of jugular venous distention and angle of distention

    (4) Note range of neck movements and any nuchal rigidity

k. Back: Inspect and palpate spine and muscles of back; note any kyphosis or scoliosis

l. Chest

    (1) Inspect, palpate, and percuss lungs and heart

    (2) Observe respiratory movements and use of respiratory muscles

    (3) Listen to quality and intensity of breath sounds

    (4) Listen for e to a change, whispered pectoriloquy (99)

m. Heart

    (1) Inspect and palpate precordium; locate apical impulse

    (2) Using both bell and diaphragm, auscultate for S_1, S_2 (intensity, splitting), abnormal heart sounds (S_3, S_4 clicks, rubs, hums, snaps), murmurs (note timing, intensity, pitch, location, radiation, quality)

    (3) Use special maneuvers or positions to accentuate abnormal heart sounds (Table 2-1); refer to Table 2-2 for grading of murmurs and to Fig. 2-2 for description of murmurs

n. Breast:

    (1) Inspect breasts with patient's arms relaxed, elevated, and then with patient's hands pressed against hips

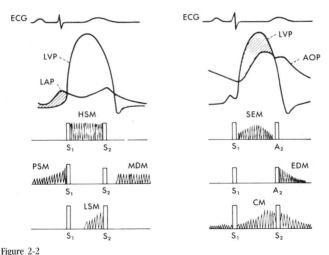

Figure 2-2
Simultaneous recording of ECG, aortic pressure (AOP), left ventricular pressure (LVP), and left atrial pressure (LAP). *HSM,* Holosystolic murmur; *PSM,* presystolic murmur; *MDM,* middiastolic murmur; *MSM,* midsystolic murmur; *EDM,* early diastolic murmur; *LSM,* late systolic murmur; *CM,* continuous murmur. From O'Rourke, R.A., and Braunwauld, E.: Physical examination of the heart. In Petersdorf, R.G., et al.: Harrison's principles of internal medicine, ed. 10, New York, 1983, McGraw-Hill Book Co.

      (2) Note symmetry, contour, abnormal shapes, skin color, retraction, thickening, edema, venous pattern

      (3) Inspect nipples for size, shape, inversion, rashes, ulceration, discharge

      (4) Palpate for presence of masses and tenderness; feel for the presence of axillary adenopathy

o. Abdomen

      (1) Observe skin color, contour, scars, masses, obesity, rigidity, ascites, venous pattern, and pulsatile masses

      (2) Auscultate for bowel sounds and abdominal bruits

      (3) Percuss abdomen and note tympany, shifting dullness, and size of liver and spleen

      (4) Note size, shape, consistency, and tenderness

p. Rectal examination

      (1) Examine anus and rectal wall for lesions, inflammation, and sphincter tone; note any nodules or other abnormalities

      (2) Test any fecal material for occult blood

      (3) In male patients, palpate prostate and identify lateral lobes (note size, shape, and consistency of prostate)

q. Genitalia

      (1) Male

          (a) Inspect distribution of pubic hair

          (b) Examine penis (note any ulcers, nodules, scars, signs of inflammation); gently compress glans and note any discharge or tenderness

          (c) Inspect scrotum (note any lumps, swelling, nodules, ulcers, size and shape of both testicles); transilluminate any swelling

          (d) Inspect inguinal and femoral areas for bulges; examine patient for presence of hernias

      (2) Female

          (a) Inspect external genitalia (labia, clitoris, urethral orifice, vaginal opening) and note distribution of pubic hair; note any nodules, discharges, bulges, and swelling

          (b) Perform internal examination (if indicated): insert speculum and note vaginal wall and cervical os; obtain specimen for cervical cytology; perform bimanual exam with index and middle finger (placing the other hand above abdomen); identify position and mobility of cervix; note any uterine and ovarian masses, enlargement, or tenderness

          (c) Perform rectovaginal exam; note any nodules or other lesions

r. Inguinal area: palpate for inguinal nodes; palpate femoral arteries (describe pulses, note any bruits)

s. Neurologic

      (1) Mental status and speech: check orientation, memory, expression, quality, quantity, and organization of speech (see Table 2-3 for description of Glasgow coma scale, useful in patients with neurologic abnormalities)

      (2) Cranial nerves: see Table 2-4 for testing of cranial nerves

      (3) Sensory: pinprick, light touch, joint position, temperature, vibration (see Fig. 2-3 and 2-4 for peripheral nerve distribution in the skin)

Table 2-3 Glasgow coma scale*

Eye Opening	Best Motor Response	Best Verbal Response	Score
No response	No response	No response	1
Opens eyes with painful stimulus	Extensor response (decerebrate rigidity) with painful stimulus	Makes unintelligible sounds	2
Opens eyes with verbal command	Flexor response (decorticate rigidity) with painful stimulus	Uses inappropriate words	3
Opens eyes spontaneously	Withdraws from noxious stimulus	Carries on a confused, disoriented conversation	4
	Localizes pain and pushes away noxious stimulus	Oriented, carries on a conversation	5
	Obeys simple verbal commands	Alert and oriented	6

*Total score is determined by adding the best score from each category (eye opening, best motor response, best verbal response), for example:

Open eyes with verbal command	3
Obeys simple verbal commands	6
Uses inappropriate words	3
Total score	12

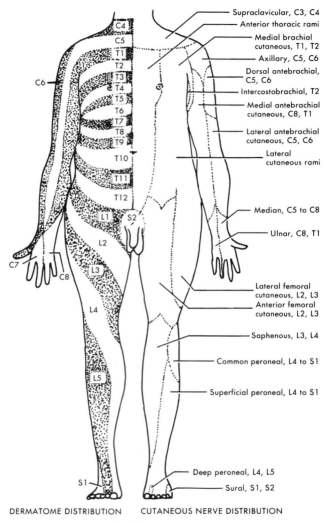

Supraclavicular, C3, C4
Anterior thoracic rami
Medial brachial cutaneous, T1, T2
Axillary, C5, C6
Dorsal antebrachial, C5, C6
Intercostobrachial, T2
Medial antebrachial cutaneous, C8, T1
Lateral antebrachial cutaneous, C5, C6
Lateral cutaneous rami
Median, C5 to C8
Ulnar, C8, T1
Lateral femoral cutaneous, L2, L3
Anterior femoral cutaneous, L2, L3
Saphenous, L3, L4
Common peroneal, L4 to S1
Superficial peroneal, L4 to S1
Deep peroneal, L4, L5
Sural, S1, S2

DERMATOME DISTRIBUTION   CUTANEOUS NERVE DISTRIBUTION

Anterior

Figure 2-3
Cutaneous sensation in anterior aspect of body. From DeGowin, E.L., and DeGowin, R.L.: Bedside diagnostic examination, ed. 4, New York, 1981, MacMillan Publishing Co.

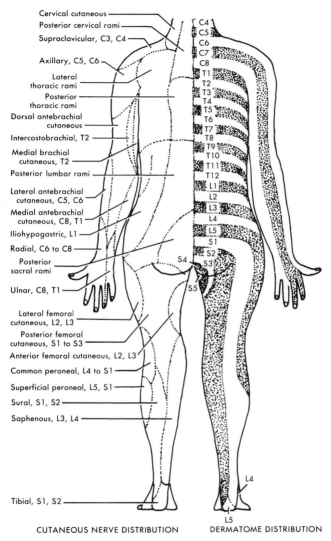

Cervical cutaneous
Posterior cervical rami
Supraclavicular, C3, C4
Axillary, C5, C6
Lateral thoracic rami
Posterior thoracic rami
Dorsal antebrachial cutaneous
Intercostobrachial, T2
Medial brachial cutaneous, T2
Posterior lumbar rami
Lateral antebrachial cutaneous, C5, C6
Medial antebrachial cutaneous, C8, T1
Iliohypogastric, L1
Radial, C6 to C8
Posterior sacral rami
Ulnar, C8, T1
Lateral femoral cutaneous, L2, L3
Posterior femoral cutaneous, S1 to S3
Anterior femoral cutaneous, L2, L3
Common peroneal, L4 to S1
Superficial peroneal, L5, S1
Sural, S1, S2
Saphenous, L3, L4
Tibial, S1, S2

C4
C5
C6
C7
C8
T1
T2
T3
T4
T5
T6
T7
T8
T9
T10
T11
T12
L1
L2
L3
L4
L5
S1
S2
S3
S4
S5
L4
L5

CUTANEOUS NERVE DISTRIBUTION   DERMATOME DISTRIBUTION

Posterior

Figure 2-4

Cutaneous sensation in posterior aspect of body. From DeGowin, E.L., and DeGowin, R.L.: Bedside diagnostic examination, ed. 4, New York, 1981, MacMillan Publishing Co.

      (4) Cerebellar functions: evaluate rapid alternating hand movements, heel-to-shin, finger-to-nose, and gait

      (5) Motor: check muscle strength (see Table 2-5 for grading muscle strength), muscle tone, coordination; check Romberg's sign, reflexes (see Table 2-6 for grading of deep tendon reflexes), plantar responses, note any abnormal reflexes

Table 2-4   Testing of cranial nerves

I Olfactory	Sense of smell
II Optic	Vision (visual acuity, visual fields, color)
III Oculomotor IV Trochlear VI Abducens	Extraocular movements (Fig. 2-1), pupillary constriction (oculomotor), elevation of upper lids
V Trigeminal	Mastication, sensory of forehead, face, and jaw
VII Facial	Facial expression, taste in anterior two thirds of tongue
VIII Acoustic	Hearing and balance
IX Glossopharyngeal X Vagus	Sensory and motor functions of pharynx and larynx (gag reflex, position of uvula, swallowing)
XI Accessory	Shrugging of shoulders, movement of head
XII Hypoglossal	Motor control of tongue

Table 2-5   Grading of muscle strength

0	Absent muscular contraction
1	Minimal contraction
2	Active movement with gravity eliminated
3	Active movement against gravity only
4	Active movement against gravity and some resistance
5	Normal muscle strength

Table 2-6   Grading of deep tendon reflexes

0	Absent
+	Hypoactive
+ +	Normal
+ + +	Brisker than average
+ + + +	Hyperactive, often indicative of disease

Normal Physical Exam

1. Vital signs
   a. Blood pressure: 124/70
   b. Pulse: 74
   c. Respirations: 16
   d. Temperature: 37° C
2. General description: the patient is a 45-year-old white female who looks her stated age; she is pleasant, well nourished, and appears to be in a good state of health.
3. Skin: the skin is warm and dry; turgor is adequate; color is normal. There is no icterus, purpura, rash, or unusual pigmentation noted. Hair is normal in appearance, distribution, and texture.
4. Lymph nodes: there is no cervical, supraclavicular, axillary, epitrochlear, or inguinal adenopathy.
5. HEENT:
   a. Head: normocephalic and atraumatic; no lesions noted.
   b. Eyes: cornea is without lesions, conjunctiva is clear, sclera is white. Pupils are equal, measuring approximately 3 mm in diameter, round, and reactive to light and accommodation. Extraocular movements are within normal limits without any nystagmus or strasbismus. Fundi appear benign. Disks are well delineated. There are no hemorrhages or exudates. Visual acuity is 20/20 bilaterally, and visual fields are within normal limits.
   c. Ears: normal in appearance. Auditory canal appears clean and without lesions. The tympanic membranes are intact. Hearing is intact.
   d. Nose: septum appears to be within normal limits and without deviation. Nasal mucosa appears pink and without any nasal discharge. No nasal polyps or other lesions are noted. Frontal and maxillary sinuses are nontender.
   e. Mouth and throat: lips are without cyanosis or pallor. Buccal mucosa is normal in appearance. Teeth appear to be in good condition. Tongue shows no lesions or tremor. Pharyngeal mucosa is pink and does not reveal any lesions, exudates, erythema, or evidence of inflammation. Gag reflex is intact.
6. Neck: neck is supple. Full range of motion is present. There is no evidence of tracheal deviation, jugular venous distention, or lymphadenopathy. Carotid pulses are 2+, equal bilaterally, and without any bruits. Carotid upstroke is within normal limits. Thyroid gland is normal in size; its palpation does not reveal any nodules or masses.
7. Back: spinal curvature is normal; there is no scoliosis or kyphosis present.
8. Chest: thorax is symmetric. Full expansion is noted bilaterally. AP diameter is within normal limits.
9. Lungs: fremitus is equal bilaterally. Lung fields are resonant throughout. Breath sounds and voice sounds are normal. There are no rales or rhonchi.

Continued.

Normal Physical Exam—cont'd

10. Heart: palpation reveals no heaves or thrills. The point of maximum impulse (PMI) is medial to the midclavicular line, fourth intercostal space. Auscultation reveals S_1, S_2 of normal intensity. There are no S_3, S_4 rubs, clicks, or other abnormal heart sounds. Heart rate is approximately 70 beats/min and rhythm is regular.

11. Breasts: breasts are symmetric and have a normal contour. Skin is of normal color and appearance; there is no edema, ulceration, or erythema. Nipples are of normal size and shape; there is no nipple retraction, ulceration, or discharge. Palpation does not reveal any tenderness or masses.

12. Abdomen: abdomen is of normal size and contour. There are no capillary dilatations, skin lesions, or surgical scars noted. Auscultation reveals normoactive bowel sounds and no abdominal bruits. Palpation reveals no abdominal tenderness, guarding, or masses. The liver edge is felt approximately 1 inch below the right costal margin; it is firm, sharp, and smooth. The liver percusses to approximately 8 to 10 cm in total span. The spleen is not palpable.

13. Rectal exam: rectal exam reveals no external anal lesions. Sphincter tone is normal. There are no internal or external hemorrhoids. Rectal mucosa appears normal, and there are no nodules or masses present. Stool is brown and negative for occult blood.

14. Genitalia: inspection reveals normal distribution of pubic hair. Clitoris and labia are without lesions. Internal examination with speculum reveals normal vaginal wall. The cervical os is well visualized. No lesions or discharges are noted. A specimen was obtained for cervical cytology. Bimanual exam reveals no cervical tenderness or masses. Uterus and ovaries are nontender and of normal size.

15. Inguinal area: there is no lymphadenopathy noted. Femoral pulses are 2+ and equal bilaterally. Auscultation reveals no femoral bruits.

16. Extremities: there is no clubbing, cyanosis, or edema. Brachial, radial, popliteal, dorsalis pedis, and posterior tibialis pulses are 2+ and equal bilaterally. Musculoskeletal exam reveals no joint deformities and full range of motion. There is no bone, joint, or muscle tenderness noted.

17. Neurologic: patient is alert and oriented to time, person, and place. Cranial nerves 2 to 12 are within normal limits. Speech, memory, and expression are within normal limits. Muscle strength is 5/5 in both upper and lower extremities. There is no muscle atrophy or involuntary movement noted. Testing of cerebellar function reveals normal gait, negative Romberg test, and good coordination in finger-to-nose, heel-to-shin, and alternate motion testing. Sensory is intact to light touch, pain, and vibratory sense. There are no focal motor sensory deficits present. Deep tendon reflexes are 2+ and equal bilaterally.

| 2.2 | ADMISSION ORDERS

Use the mnemonic: ABC-DAVID

A (admit to): indicate ward where patient is being admitted and attending physician (e.g., admit to CCU, Dr. Smith's service)

B (because): indicate admitting diagnosis (e.g., diagnosis: R/O MI)

C (condition): patient's general condition (stable, fair, poor, critical)

D (diet) specify whether regular, clear liquids, no added sodium (see boxed material below for description of various diets)

A (allergies): indicate medications and specific food products to which the patient has experienced an allergic reaction
(activity): specify bed rest, ad lib, bathroom privileges

V (vital signs): specify frequency (e.g., qid, q4h); also indicate any special nursing orders (e.g., vital signs and neurologic signs qh × 24h, then q4h if stable)

I (IV fluids): specify any IV solutions and rate of infusion (refer to Table 2-7 for description of commonly used IV solutions)

D (diagnostic tests): laboratory tests, x-rays, ECG, special tests
(drugs): indicate medication, dose, frequency, special restrictions (e.g., digoxin 0.25 mg PO qd; if heart rate <55 beats/min hold digoxin and notify house officer)

Common Hospital Diets

Bland: eliminates gastric irritants such as pepper, alcohol, caffeine, coffee, tea, soda, cocoa, and foods not tolerated by patient

Calorie control: physician determines calorie level; sugar and sweets are generally eliminated

Low-cholesterol: restricts food high in cholesterol, decreases saturated fat, provides approximately 300 mg of cholesterol daily

Diabetic (ADA): physician indicates calorie level

Low-fat: eliminates high-fat foods, fried foods, and whole milk; designed to limit the total amount of fat to 40-45 g/day

Gluten-free: eliminates products and by-products of wheat, oats, rye and barley

High-fiber: increases volume of indigestible carbohydrates

High-protein, high-calorie: no restriction, 3000+ calories, 120 g protein

Hypoglycemic: no sugar or sweets; six small meals containing protein

Lactose-free: eliminates milk, milk products, and foods containing lactose, milk, or milk solids

Lactose-restricted: provides foods that contain only minimum lactose, based on the individual's tolerance

Low-residue: limits volume of indigestible carbohydrates, milk, and dairy products

Clear liquid: clear broth and juice, gelatin, water, ice, coffee, tea, soda, sugar and salt; 600 calories; 10 g protein

Continued.

Common Hospital Diets—cont'd

Sodium restriction: 4 g-NAS (no added salt)—no salt or highly salted foods: *2 g* —no salt or highly salted foods, limited milk, meat, bread, butter; *1 g*—more limited milk, meat, bread, butter; *500 mg*—no salt or salty foods, extremely limited milk, meat, bread and butter (unpalatable for most)

Full liquid: clear liquid items plus strained cream soups, juices, cooked cereal, ice cream, sherbet, custard, pudding, milk, and milk beverages; calorie and protein content adequate

High-protein, clear liquid: clear liquid items, Citrotein, and high-protein gelatin supplements; 1500 calories; 75 g protein

Mechanical soft: minimizes the amount of chewing necessary for the ingestion of food; ground meats are provided along with a soft diet

Potassium-restricted: physician should specify level: *2 g*—moderate restriction, eliminates high-potassium foods; *1.5 g or less*—strict restriction, eliminates high-potassium foods, limits quantity of acceptable foods; achieving adequate calories may be a problem

Postgastrectomy: six small feedings, simple sugars kept to a minimum, no fluids served with meals

Protein-restricted: physician should specify level: *60 g*— liberal, approaches regular diet with some limit on quantities; *40 gm*—moderate restriction, severely limits quantity of milk, meat or substitute and egg; *20 gm*— severe restriction, eliminates milk, limits meat, egg, or substitute to 2 oz daily and starch to 3 servings daily, fruit, sugars, and fat are given ad lib, caloric intake is inadequate (very unpalatable)

Regular: no restriction

Soft: texture of food is soft; NOTE: if modification of texture is desired, physician should order mechanical soft (ground)

2.3   PROGRESS NOTES

Use the "SOAP" outline:

S (subjective): observations, patient's complaints

    S: "My chest hurts when I take a deep breath"

O (objective): description of physical findings and record of lab, x-ray, or ECG data

    O: Blood pressure: 140/90; pulse: 84; respirations: 20; temperature: 38°C

       Skin: warm, dry, no petechiae

       HEENT: pharyngeal erythema

       Lungs: ↓ BS in rt base, no rubs, rales, or wheezing

       Heart: S_1, S_2, tachycardic, s̄ murmurs

       Abd: soft, bowel sounds active, s̄ tenderness

Table 2-7 Composition of selected IV solutions

IV Solution	Na (mEq/L)	K (mEq/L)	Cl (mEq/L)	Lactate (mEq/L)	Ca (mEq/L)	Calories/L	mOsm/L
0.9% NaCl (NS)	154	0	154	0	0	0	308
5% Dextrose (D_5W)	0	0	0	0	0	170	252
5% Dextrose + 0.9% NaCl (D_5NS)	154	0	154	0	0	170	560
5% Dextrose + 0.45% NaCl ($D_5\frac{1}{2}NS$)	77	0	77	0	0	170	406
5% Dextrose + 0.33% NaCl ($D_5\frac{1}{3}NS$)	56	0	77	0	0	170	365
Lactated Ringer's solution	130	4	109	28	3	9	273

Ext: no clubbing, cyanosis, or edema
Lab
    WBC: 15,900 c̄ shift to left (12 stabs, 65 segs)
    ABG: P_{O_2}—55, P_{CO_2}—30, pH—7.50
CXR: RLL infiltrate
ECG: normal sinus rhythm without evidence of ischemia
A (assessment): analysis of data and tentative diagnosis
    A: RLL pneumonia
P (plan): diagnostic studies and therapeutic regimen
    P: 1. Nasal O_2—2L
        2. Sputum Gram stain and cultures, blood cultures
        3. Antibiotic therapy based on results of Gram stain

| 2.4 | DISCHARGE SUMMARY

The discharge summary should contain only essential information regarding the investigation and treatment of the patient's illness. It should briefly describe the following:

1. Why the patient entered the hospital: a brief clinical statement of the chief complaint, admission diagnosis, and history of the present illness
2. The pertinent laboratory, x-ray, and physical findings, negative findings may be as pertinent as positive ones
3. The medical and/or surgical treatment, including the patient's response, any complications, and consultations; give a rationale for what was or was not done.
4. The patient's condition when discharged (ambulation, self-care, ability to work)
5. Instructions given on continuing care, such as medication by name and specific dosage, diet, type and amount of physical activity, other therapeutic measures, referrals, and appointments
6. The principal diagnosis and additional or secondary diagnoses

Definitions

Principal diagnosis: the diagnosis that best explains the reason for admission to the hospital; this may not be the same as the most serious event.

Complication: a significant event that either prolongs the stay or requires alteration of treatment, such as a pulmonary embolus after a hip fracture.

References

1. Bates, B.: A guide to physical examination, ed. 3, Philadelphia, 1983, J.B. Lippincott Co.
2. DeGowin E.L., and DeGowin, R.L.: Bedside diagnostic examination, ed. 4, New York, 1981, Macmillan Publishing Co., Inc.
3. Sherman, J.L., and Fields, S.K.: Guide to patient evaluation, ed. 3, New York, 1978, Medical Examination Publishing Co., Inc.

Data Evaluation

3

GRAM STAIN PROCEDURE

1. Briefly heat-fix air-dried smear by passing it gently through a Bunsen flame
2. Flood slide with crystal violet for 1 min
3. Wash off slide lightly with water and then flood with Gram's iodine for 1 min
4. Wash off slide and add 95% ethyl alcohol to decolorize for 15 sec
5. Wash off slide and add counterstain (safranin) for 1 min
6. Wash off safranin and blot slide dry
7. Examine smear under oil immersion (a properly stained area will show pink PMN nuclei):

    Gm + organism: (purple)

    Gm − organism: (red)

3.2 **ACID-FAST STAIN PROCEDURE**

1. Briefly heat-fix air-dried smear by passing it gently through a Bunsen flame
2. Flood slide with carbol-fuchsin for 2½ min
3. Wash off slide with water and completely decolorize the slide with acid alcohol
4. Wash off slide and flood it with methylene blue for 30 sec
5. Wash off methylene blue and blot slide dry
6. Examine smear under oil immersion:

    Acid-fast organisms: (red)

    Non–acid-fast organisms: (blue)

3.3 **EVALUATION OF URINE SEDIMENT**

Fig. 3-1 illustrates various abnormalities frequently observed in urine sediment.

3.4 **EVALUATION OF CHEST X-RAY FILM**

Fig 3-2 illustrates the location of various pulmonary and cardiac structures seen on a chest x-ray film (posteroanterior view).

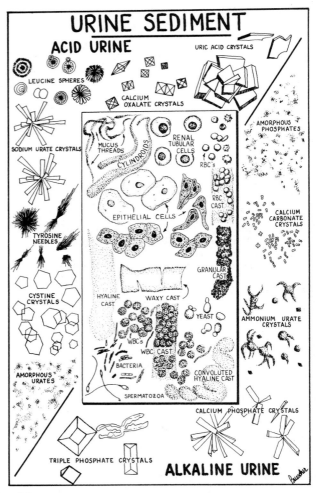

Figure 3-1
Microscopic examination of urine sediment. From Biller, J.A., and Yeager, A.M.,
(editors): The Harriet Lane handbook: a manual for pediatric house officers, ed. 9,
Chicago, 1981, Year Book Medical Publishers, Inc. Reproduced with permission from
Johns Hopkins Hospital and Yearbook Medical Publishers, Inc.

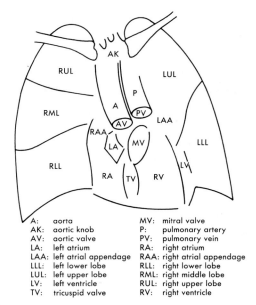

A:	aorta	MV:	mitral valve
AK:	aortic knob	P:	pulmonary artery
AV:	aortic valve	PV:	pulmonary vein
LA:	left atrium	RA:	right atrium
LAA:	left atrial appendage	RAA:	right atrial appendage
LLL:	left lower lobe	RLL:	right lower lobe
LUL:	left upper lobe	RML:	right middle lobe
LV:	left ventricle	RUL:	right upper lobe
TV:	tricuspid valve	RV:	right ventricle

Figure 3-2
Chest x-ray film: recognition of pulmonary lobes, heart chambers, and heart valves (posteroanterior view).

3.5 ELECTROCARDIOGRAM

Fig. 3-3 illustrates a normal 12-lead ECG. Note the normal QRS configuration in the various leads and the R wave progression in the precordial leads.

3.6 USE AND INTERPRETATION OF SWAN-GANZ CATHETER DATA

1. Description: the Swan-Ganz catheter is a flexible quadruple-lumen tube 110 cm long and scored in 10 cm increments (Fig. 3-4). Its four lumens are as follows:
   a. Distal (PA) lumen: used to record PAP, PCWP, and to obtain mixed venous blood for oxygen content analysis.
   b. Proximal (RA) lumen: used to record RA or CVP.
   c. Balloon lumen: terminates 1 cm from the tip of the catheter. When the balloon is inflated, it moves in the direction of the blood flow, guiding the cathether through the right atrium, right ventricle, and into the pulmonary artery wedging into one of the smaller vessels. In this position it records downstream pressure (PCWP), which is normally about equal to left atrial pressure.
   d. Thermistor lumen: contains temperature-sensitive wires. It is used to calculate cardiac output by thermodilution technique.

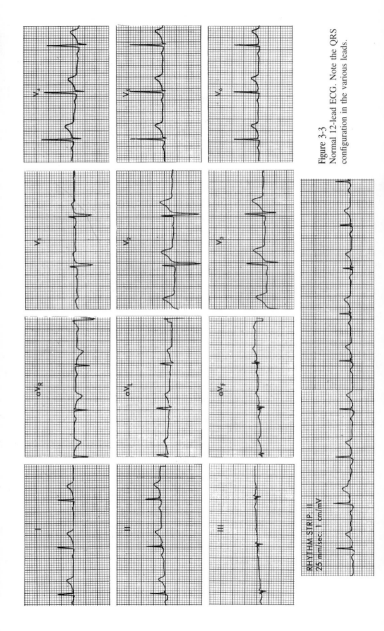

Figure 3-3
Normal 12-lead ECG. Note the QRS configuration in the various leads.

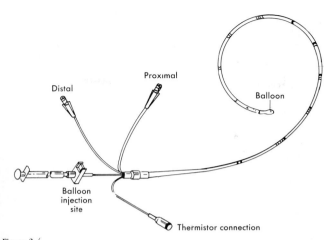

Figure 3-4
Swan-Ganz catheter. From Quaal, S.J.: Comprehensive intraaortic balloon pumping, St. Louis, 1984, The C.V. Mosby Co.

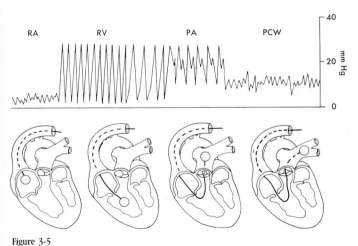

Figure 3-5
Swan-Ganz pressure waveforms in relation to catheter position. From Rosen, P., et al., (editors): Emergency medicine: concepts and clinical practice, St. Louis, 1983, The C.V. Mosby Co.

2. Catheter insertion: percutaneous insertion via the internal jugular (central or anterior) approach appears to be the safest. Complications (sepsis, thrombophlebitis, deep venous thrombosis) occur more often when the catheter is placed through antecubital cutdown.[4]
3. Verification of catheter tip location: the location of the catheter tip is determined by recognition of the characteristic pressure waveform morphology of each heart chamber (Fig. 3-5)
4. Risks of right heart catheterization[3]:
   a. Cardiac dysrhythmias: 77.5%
   b. Thrombosis: 2.6%
   c. Sepsis: 1.7%
   d. Pulmonary infarction: 1.7%
   e. Pulmonary valve perforation: 0.8%
5. Indications for hemodynamic monitoring: pulmonary artery flow-directed catheters should be used only in situations where there is a high probability that the data collected will result in more effective patient management.[5] It is generally agreed that Swan-Ganz catheterization is indicated in severely ill, hemodynamically unstable patients who do not respond to therapy that is deemed appropriate after a careful clinical evaluation.[2] Additional indications for hemodynamic monitoring in the medical setting are as follows[5]:

Table 3-1   Effects of therapeutic measures on hemodynamic measurements

Therapeutic Measure	CO	SVR	PCWP
IV fluids	N/ ↑	N/ ↑	↑
Diuretics	N/ ↓ ↓	↓ /Secondary ↑	↓
Nitrates	N/ ↑ / ↓	↓	↓
Nitroprusside	↑	↓ ↓	N/ ↓
Catecholamines	N/ ↑ ↑	↑ ↑ ↑	N/ ↑
Dopamine	N/ ↑	↑ ↑	N/ ↑ ↑
Dobutamine	↑ ↑	↓	N/ ↓

KEY: N, no effect; ↑, increases; ↓, decreases.

Table 3-2   Hemodynamic measurements in specific disease states

Septic shock
   Early: ↓ PCWP, ↓ SVR, ↑ CO
   Late: ↓ PCWP, ↑ SVR, ↓ CO
Neurogenic shock: ↓ PCWP, ↓ SVR, N/ ↓ CO
Cardiac tamponade: ↑ PCWP, ↑ SVR, ↓ CO, ↓ CI, CVP
   = PADP = PCWP
Pulmonary embolism: Normal PCWP, ↑ PAD ↓ CI
Cardiogenic shock: ↑ PCWP, ↑ PAD, ↓ CO, ↓ CI, ↑ SVR
Hypovolemic shock: ↓ PCWP, ↓ CO, ↑ SVR, ↓ CI
Right ventricular infarct: RA/PCWP ≥ 0.8

KEY: ↑, Increases; ↓, decreases.

Table 3-3 Data collection and interpretation

Hemodynamic Measurement	Normal Value	Clinical Significance	Abnormalities
Right atrial pressure (RA)	0-8 mm Hg	Equivalent to central venous pressure (CVP)	↑ Right ventricular failure, pulmonary embolism, tricuspid valve abnormalities, pericardial tamponade, right ventricular infarction ↓ Hypovolemia
Pulmonary arterial pressure (PAP)	Systolic 15-30 mm Hg; Diastolic 5-12 mm Hg; Mean 10-20 mm Hg	PAP is equal to RV pressure during systole while the pulmonary valve is open. If the pulmonary vascular resistance is normal, the pulmonary artery diastolic (PAD) pressure is 1-4 mm Hg greater than PCWP and can be substituted for it in following the patient's hemodynamic measurements.	↑ Pulmonary embolism, chronic lung disease, VSD, cardiogenic shock, right ventricular infarction If the PAD is 5 mm Hg > PCWP consider: ARDS, pulmonary emboli, or COPD

Continued.

Table 3-3 Data collection and interpretation—cont'd

Hemodynamic Measurement	Normal Value	Clinical Significance	Abnormalities

Pulmonary capillary wedge pressure (PCWP)	5-12 mm Hg	PCWP is normally equal to left atrial pressure; it is therefore a sensitive indicator of the presence of pulmonary congestion and left-sided CHF. PCWP is not equal to left ventricular end diastolic pressure (LVEDP) in the following situations:
		PCWP > LVEDP:
		  Mitral stenosis
		  Patient receiving PEEP
		  Left atrial myxoma
		  Pulmonary venous obstruction
		PCWP < LVEDP:
		  "Stiff" left ventricle
		  ↑ LVEDP (> 25 mm Hg)
			↑ Left ventricular failure with resultant pulmonary congestion, acute mitral insufficiency, tamponade, decreased left ventricular compliance (hypertrophy, infarction)

Cardiac output (CO)	3.5-7 L/min	CO = stroke volume multiplied by heart rate	↓ Cardiac dysrhythmias, ↓ contracting muscle mass (myocardial ischemia, MI), mitral insufficiency, VSD

Parameter	Normal range	Description/Formula	Clinical conditions
Cardiac index (CI)	2.5–4.0 L/min^2	CI relates CO to body surface area (BSA), CI = CO/BSA	↑ High output failure secondary to fluid overload, hepatocellular failure, renal disease, septic shock ↓ Hypovolemia, cardiogenic shock, pulmonary embolism, hypothyroidism, CHF with failing ventricle
Systemic vascular resistance (SVR)	900–1300 dyne/sec/cm^{-5}	Resistance against which the left ventricle must work to eject its stroke volume. $$SVR = \frac{(\overline{MAP} - RA) \times 80}{CO}$$	↑ Hypervolemic vasoconstrictive states (hypertension, cardiogenic shock, traumatic shock) ↓ Septic shock, acute renal failure, pregnancy
Pulmonary vascular resistance (PVR)	155–255 dyne/sec/cm^{-5}	$$PVR = \frac{(\overline{PA} - PAWP) \times 80}{CO}$$	↑ Cor pulmonale, pulmonary embolism, valvular heart disease, CHF ↓ Hypervolemic states, pregnancy

a. Acute cardiac conditions (complicated MI, right ventricular infarction, perforated ventricular septum, and mitral regurgitation)
b. Postinfarction angina
c. Chronic cardiac insufficiency (constrictive pericarditis, congestive cardiomyopathy, and therapy of end-stage cardiac failure)
d. Miscellaneous (acute non–myocardial infarction pulmonary edema, severe non–cardiac hypotension)
6. Data interpretation: see Tables 3-1, 3-2, and 3-3.

3.7 INTRAAORTIC BALLOON PUMP (IABP)

1. Description: the intraaortic balloon pump is a polyurethane balloon inserted percutaneously in the femoral artery and positioned in the descending aorta.
2. Mechanism of action: it provides left ventricular support using the following mechanisms[1]:
   a. Systolic unloading: its deflation immediately before the onset of systole creates a low pressure which results in:
      (1) ↓ Left ventricular work for ejection
      (2) ↓ Myocardial O_2 requirements
      (3) ↓ LVEDP
      (4) ↑ Stroke volume
   b. Diastolic augmentation: its inflation at end of systole results in:
      (1) ↑ Diastolic pressure
      (2) ↑ Coronary perfusion pressure
      (3) Potential ↑ in coronary blood flow
3. Major indications:
   a. Low-output state (cardiogenic shock, gram-negative septic shock)
   b. Angina refractory to medical management
   c. Postinfarction VSD and MR
   d. Surgery in high-risk cardiac patients
4. Major contraindications:
   a. Dissecting aortic aneurysm
   b. Severe aortic regurgitation
   c. Severe peripheral vascular disease

References

1. Chatterjee, K., and Don, H., (editors): Intraaortic balloon pump, In Don, H: Decisions in critical care, Toronto, B.C. Decker, Inc., St. Louis, 1985, The C.V. Mosby Co.
2. Connors, A.F., et al.: Evaluation of right heart catheterization in the critically ill patient without acute myocardial infarction, N. Engl. J. Med. **308**(5):263, 1983.
3. Elliot, C.G., et al.: Complications of pulmonary artery catheterization in the care of critically ill patients: a prospective study, Chest **76**:647, 1979.
4. Moza, S.K., and DelGuercio, L.R.M.: The Swan-Ganz catheter: its clinical versatility, Hosp. Pract. **18**:239, 1983.
5. Robin, E.D.: The cult of the Swan-Ganz catheter, Ann. Int. Med. **103**:445, 1985.
6. Swan, H.J.C., and Ganz, W.: Measurement of right arterial and pulmonary arterial pressures and cardiac output: clinical applications of hemodynamic monitoring. In Stollerman, G.H., et al. (editors): Advances in internal medicine, vol. 27, Chicago, 1982, Year Book Medical Publishers, Inc.

Preparing the Patient
For Surgery

Dennis L. Bordan

Much has been written with regard to preparing a patient for surgery, but most of the literature generated has been written by surgeons and has generally appeared in surgical texts or in the surgical literature. This section is a synopsis of the areas of concern to the surgical consultant when dealing with a patient on the medical service.

4.1 NUTRITION

There is a close relationship between the patient's nutritional status and potential morbidity or mortality for any specific surgical procedure.

1. Nutritional assessment (methods)
   a. Fat stores: ideal weight for height, triceps skin-fold thickness
   b. Protein stores: midarm muscle circumference, creatinine/height index
   c. Visceral protein: serum proteins, immune response proteins (total lymphocyte counts and skin testing)
   d. Prognostic nutritional index (PNI): % risk = 15.8-16.6 (Alb)- 0.78 (TSF)- 0.20 (TFN)- 5.8 (DH)
      (1) where Alb = Serum albumin

              TFN = Serum transferrin

              TSF = Triceps skin-fold thickness

              DH = Delayed hypersensitivity (0- nonreactive; 1- <5 mm; 2- >5 mm)
2. Nutritional requirements
   a. Calculate caloric needs; a patient's basal energy expenditure (BEE) can be determined by using the following Harris-Benedict formulas[2]:
      BEE (men): 66 + (13.7 × weight in kg) + (5 × height in cm) − (6.8 × age in years)
      BEE (women): 65.5 + (9.6 × weight in kg) + (1.7 × height in cm) − (4.7 × age in years)
      The patient's caloric needs may vary with severity of illness, medications, and other factors.
   b. Calculate protein requirements; the normal adult protein requirement is about 0.6-0.8 g/kg/day[1]

3. Nutritional support
   a. Determine route (enteral, parenteral)
   b. Special considerations based on route
      (1) Enteral
         (a) Oral versus tube feeding
         (b) Types of formulas, (see Appendix I)
         (c) Specific complications, considerations in special situations, (i.e., liver or renal disease)
      (2) Parenteral
         (a) Nature of fluids
         (b) Inclusion of minerals, vitamins, and trace elements
         (c) Technical complications
         (d) Metabolic complications
         (e) Special considerations such as renal or hepatic disease

4.2   FLUID, ELECTROLYTE, BLOOD, AND VOLUME REQUIREMENTS

1. Blood
   a. Correct circulating red cell volume to levels adequate to provide oxygen delivery to the tissues without inappropriately increasing viscosity (Hct $\geq 30\%$)
   b. Allow at least 24 hours for equilibration of blood replacement before accepting validity of measured hematocrit
   c. Available blood replacement must be appropriate for a given surgical procedure (type and crossmatch a sufficient number of units of packed RBC) (This is extremely important for patients requiring large blood volume replacement)
2. Volume
   a. Avoid hypovolemia; almost all surgical patients undergo marked fluid shifts during induction of anesthesia as well as surgery itself. All available criteria must be used to ascertain hypovolemia preoperatively (urinary output, body weight, serum/urine osmolarity, skin turgor, hypernatremia, orthostatic vital signs changes)
   b. Correct any existing volume deficit with Ringer's lactate (most physiologic solution)
   c. Avoid excessive (in some cases—any) use of colloid solutions such as SPA or plasmanate as a volume expander (can result in CHF)
   d. Closely monitor fluid status (Foley catheter, CVP, or Swan Ganz catheter in selected high-risk patients)
   e. Have IV lines in place that are appropriate for the patient's disease process, fluid requirements, or potential for fluid replacement (no "scalp vein needles")
3. Electrolytes: correct any alterations of the following:
   a. Serum sodium (see Chapter 16, section 16.2)
   b. Serum potassium (see Chapter 16, section 16.3)
   c. Serum calcium (see Chapter 12, section 12.10)
   d. Serum magnesium (see Chapter 16, section 16.4)
   e. Serum phosphorus
   f. Acid-base balance (see Chapter 8)

Alterations in any of the above mentioned electrolytes may seriously and adversely affect the outcome of any surgical procedure. Scrupulous correction of significant disturbances in these areas is indicated.

4.3 HEMATOLOGIC PROBLEMS

1. Anemia: a hematocrit below 30% (or Hb <10g/dl) significantly increases potential morbidity and mortality of any proposed surgical procedure (impaired cardiac function and reserve). Existing anemia, particularly acute anemia, should be corrected preoperatively if possible.

2. Erythrocytosis: a marked increase in hematocrit (>60%) results in elevated blood viscosity, increasing the rate of clinically evident thrombosis. Secondarily, there may also be a marked depression of cardiac function.

3. Platelet disorders: Abnormalities in platelet number (above 1 million or below 50,000) or function may result in excessive intraoperative bleeding problems as well as an increased risk of thrombosis. Bleeding time is the best parameter to measure platelet function. Injudicious use of platelet transfusions must be avoided because the half-life of transfused platelets is extremely short. Transfusions of platelets are more appropriately employed when bleeding becomes clinically evident.

4. Common bleeding problems that require recognition and correction preoperatively are:

   a. Liver disease: it results in abnormalities of factors II, VII, IX, and X (vitamin K dependent), and factor V; correct with fresh frozen plasma (FFP)

   b. Warfarin therapy: it should be stopped 2-3 days before surgery, and prothrombin time (PT) should be monitored; may use FFP or vitamin K if necessary to normalize PT

Table 4-1 Dosage of factor VIII$_{AHF}$

Bleeding Risk	Desired Factor VIII Level (%)	Initial Dose (units/kg)
Mild	5-10	12.5
Moderate	20-30	25
Severe	50 or greater	50

Standard Calculation

1. Patients plasma volume (50 ml/kg × weight in kg) × (Desired level of factor VIII in percent) − (Present level of factor VIII in percent) = Number of units for initial dose

2. In emergency therapy, the present level of factor VIII is assumed to be zero.

3. One unit is the activity of the coagulation factor present in 1 ml of normal human male plasma.

4. Because the half-life of factor VIII is 8 to 12 hours, the desired level is maintained by giving half the initial dose every 8 to 12 hours.

5. Cryoprecipitate is assumed to have 70 to 80 units of factor VIII per bag; factor VIII concentrates list the units per bottle on the label.

From Rosen, P., et al. (editors): Emergency medicine: concepts and clinical practice, St. Louis, 1983, The C.V. Mosby Co.

c. Aspirin: patient should stop taking it at least 1 week before surgery
d. Hemophilia A or B: use factor VIII for hemophilia A or prothrombin complex concentrates prn for hemophilia B to control significant bleeding abnormalities (refer to Table 4-1 for correct dosage of factor VIII_{AHF})
e. Von Willebrand's disease: correct significant abnormalities with cryoprecipitate or fresh frozen plasma
f. Circulating anticoagulants: plasmapheresis may be useful in selected patients to reduce circulating anticoagulant levels
5. Massive preoperative blood transfusions: the following are some possible complications:
   a. Excessive bleeding (low platelets, decreased factor VIII)
   b. Citrate intoxication: danger is cardiac dysrhythmias
   c. Use of cold blood: dysrhythmias
   d. Low red blood cell 2, 3 DPG levels
   e. Microaggregates (170 P filter may be used)

4.4 **DRUGS**

The list of drugs that may alter a patient's response to the stress of planned or emergent surgery is almost endless; categories include the following:

Analgesics	Antineoplastic drugs
Antiarthritics	Bronchodilators
Anticholinergics	Cardiovascular drugs
Anticoagulants	Diuretics
Anticonvulsants	Gastric acid inhibitors
Antidiabetic agents	Hormones
Antihistamines	Psychotropic drugs
Antihypertensive agents	Steroids
Antimicrobials	

It is obviously beyond the scope of this discussion to review each of these categories or the many agents within each group. For our purposes, it is sufficient to state that there is a wide range of agents that can potentially alter a patient's surgical risk. Some of these agents must be specifically removed, reduced, or even increased (e.g., steroids) preoperatively.

4.5 **SYSTEM-ORIENTED PREOPERATIVE EVALUATION**

1. Cardiac system
   a. Clinical assessment and history
   b. Routine lab including chest x-ray film, ECG, and serum electrolytes
   c. Determine need for specialized cardiac studies, including stress test, Holter monitor, echocardiogram, and nuclear noninvasive studies (e.g., MUGA scan)
   d. Determine need for preoperative maximization of cardiac reserve
2. Endocrine system
   a. Preoperative evaluation and optimization of diabetic patients
      (1) For type II (NIDDM) patients well controlled by diet alone, monitor blood glucose preoperatively and q6h during the surgical and early postoperative period. If blood glucose is >250-300 mg/dl, use short-acting (regular) insulin q6h to control the glucose level.

      (2) For patients on sulfonylureas, do not administer the oral hypogly-
cemic agent on the day of surgery, control glucose with regular
insulin as described above. Patients taking long-acting sulfonylureas (e.g., chlorpropamide) may require discontinuation 3-4 days
before surgery.

      (3) For type I (IDDM) patients, determine the fasting blood glucose
level on the day of surgery and administer ½-⅔ of the total AM
insulin dose as NPH insulin. Start an IV containing glucose and
monitor blood glucose frequently. Use regular insulin to maintain
blood glucose 150-250 mg/dl. A continuous intravenous infusion
with low-dose insulin may be necessary in selected patients.

    b. Preoperative evaluation and management of hyperthyroid and hypothy-
roid states to minimize surgical risk (check TSH, T₄).

    c. Correction of adrenal insufficiency. Anticipate need for increased ste-
roid replacement in patients receiving chronic steroid therapy.

    d. Assessment of specific preoperative status including hyperadenocorti-
cism and pheochromocytoma.

3. Gastrointestinal system

    a. Correct any volume and coagulation defects associated with upper and
lower GI bleeding

    b. Correct volume and electrolyte disturbances associated with diarrhea,
emesis, or prolonged GI suctioning

4. Hepatobiliary system

    a. Check liver function studies to exclude underlying liver disease; eval-
uate degree of functional impairment

    b. Evaluate risks associated with and timing of surgery related to specific
liver problems including hepatitis, fatty liver, portal hypertension, and
cirrhosis

5. Vascular system: evaluate extremities for evidence of peripheral occlusive
disease and deep vein thrombosis; check for evidence of aortic aneurysms
(pulsatile abdominal mass, widened mediastinum on CXR)

6. Respiratory system

    a. Perform preoperative evaluation of pulmonary function and reserve in-
cluding pulmonary function tests and arterial blood gases when appropriate

    b. Aggressive pulmonary toilet preoperatively is indicated particularly in
patients with COPD

References

1. Munro, H.N.: Nutritional requirements in health, Crit. Care Med. 8:2-8, 1979.
2. Rutten, P., Blackburn, G.L., et al.: Determination of optimal hyperalimentation infusion rate, J. Surg. Res. 18:477-83, 1975.

General Management
of Poisoning and
Drug Overdose

Michael S. Weinstock

Over the last two decades there has been an alarming increase in drug overdose and poisoning throughout the United States. Patients who come to the emergency department as victims of poisoning or overdose, whether accidental or intentional, can be diagnostic dilemmas for the clinician. The physician should consider the possibility of poisoning in patients who are comatose or have psychotic/combative behavior, unusual cardiac dysrhythmias, unexplained acidosis, or after traumatic suicide attempts. Individuals who use street drugs may not be aware of the ingredients or adulteration of such substances and may have a confusing presentation as a result of polydrug ingestion.

For the purpose of this chapter, the terms poisoning and drug overdose are used interchangeably.

According to Haddad,[2] the general management of poisoned patients can be divided into the following phases:
1. Emergency management and stabilization
2. History and physical examination
3. Clinical evaluation of major toxic signs
4. Elimination of the poison from the GI tract, skin, and eyes
5. Administration of an antidote, if available
6. Elimination of adsorbed substances
7. Supportive therapy

5.1 GENERAL APPROACH TO MANAGEMENT

1. Emergency stabilization
   a. Ensure adequate ventilation and examine the airway for patency and intact gag reflex. In comatose patients, suction excessive secretions and provide an oral airway. Patients who are obtunded, comatose, or who have a depressed respiratory effort should be ventilated by endotracheal intubation. If the patient is awake and resistance is too great, proceed with treatment. Oxygen therapy should be liberal (100% in "young lungs") in the initial phases of management. After intubation, listen to the chest to ensure adequate and symmetric ventilation.
   b. Establish intravenous access using a large-bore angiocath, and simultaneously draw adequate samples for appropriate lab studies, including electrolytes, glucose PT, PTT, and toxicologic screening; evaluation of arterial blood gases may also be indicated at this time. CAUTION: Carbon monoxide levels may require a separate order. A balanced salt

solution is preferred for initial resuscitation. If the patient is hypotensive, a fluid challenge based on weight should be administered. Ensure adequate perfusion. Note that some poisons can enhance or promote pulmonary edema, and large volumes of fluids are to be administered with caution.

c. All comatose patients should receive an intravenous bolus of 50 g of glucose followed by 1 to 2 mg of Narcan intravenously. The patient is then reevaluated for response.

d. Foley catheterization should be considered in patients who are comatose. Urine should be sent for toxicologic studies.

e. If the patient has generalized seizures, these should be controlled with appropriate dosages of diazepam. NOTE: Withdrawal may be heralded by seizures, and the clinician should be alert to that possibility.

2. History and physical exam
   a. When the patient is unable to communicate, identification of the poison or any antecedent medical history is sometimes available from police, emergency medical service personnel, family, or friends. Good detective work can save time and decrease morbidity and mortality.
   b. Careful examination can provide reliable information as to the type of poisoning (Table 5-1). Unusual odors on the patient's breath should be noted along with any bruising (suspect trauma), skin markings, diaphoresis, variation in pupil size, or dysrhythmias, especially in young patients.

3. Clinical evaluation
   a. A 12-lead ECG should be taken. Even in the absence of any dysrhythmia, the ECG can provide clues as to what was ingested, such as a prolonged QT interval in phenothiazine overdose or a widened QRS complex in tricyclic overdose. Several substances may cause dysrhythmias (Table 5-2).
   b. Laboratory evaluation can help identify toxic agents or an underlying disease. The many causes of high anion gap metabolic acidosis are summarized in the following list:*

Uremia	Methanol poisoning
Diabetic ketoacidosis	Ethylene glycol poisoning
Lactic acidosis	Nondiabetic alcoholic ketoacidosis
Salicylate toxicity	Paraldehyde toxicity

4. Elimination of ingested poisons from the GI tract: An attempt should be made to remove the substances from the GI tract in either an antegrade or retrograde fashion. Whether vomiting should be induced with syrup of ipecac or the gastric contents emptied with a large-bore tube and irrigation depends on what was ingested and the level of consciousness.
   a. Syrup of ipecac: for an awake child or adult, 15 ml or 30 ml respectively is given PO and followed by large amounts of fluids such as water. Exceptions to this include: patients who are comatose or obtunded, and those who have ingested caustics, petroleum products of low volatility and surface tension, or phenothiazines. Haddad[2] notes that most authorities agree that the use of syrup of ipecac with petroleum distillates is justified when this product is a carrier for a more toxic substance.

*From Haddad L.M., Winchester, J.: Clinical management of poisoning and drug overdose, Philadelphia, 1983, W.B. Saunders Co.

Table 5-1 Examples of symptom complexes or toxidromes

Level of Consciousness	Respirations	Pupils	Other	Possible Toxic Agent
Coma	⇕	Pinpoint	Fasciculations	Organophosphate insecticides
Coma	→	Pinpoint	Tracks	Opiates
Coma	Apneustic	Pinpoint	Decerebrate posturing	Pontine (brainstem) structural lesion
Awake			Torsion head neck	Phenothiazines, haloperidol
Coma	→	Pinpoint	Cardiac dysrhythmia	Phenothiazines
Coma	→	Dilated	Cardiac dysrhythmia Convulsions	Tricyclic antidepressants
Coma	←→		Uremic frost	(Uremia)
Coma	←→←	Dilated	Hypothermia	Sedatives, barbiturates
Semicoma	←		Diaphoresis Tinnitus Fever	Salicylates
Agitated, hallucinating	↑	Dilated	Fever Flushing Dry skin and mucous membranes	Anticholinergics

From Haddad, L.M., and Winchester, J.: Clinical management of poisoning and drug overdose, Philadelphia, 1983, W.B. Saunders Co.

Table 5-2 Examples of cardiac dysrhythmias secondary to drug toxicity

Drug	Common Dysrhythmias
Amphetamines	Sinus tachycardia, SVT
β-Blockers	Bradycardia, AV block
Digitalis	Bradycardia, AV block, PAT with block, PVC, junctional tachycardia
Ethylene glycol	Narrow QRS (from hypocalcemia)
Phencyclidine (PCP)	Tachycardia, PVC
Phenothiazines	Q and T wave distortions
Quinidine	Prolonged QT, AV block, widened QRS complex
Sympathomimetics	Tachycardia, ventricular dysrhythmias
Theophylline	Tachycardia, MAT, ventricular dysrhythmias
Tricyclic antidepressants	SVT, wide QRS

 b. Gastric lavage: to recover pill fragments, a large-bore No. 36 French Ewald tube should be used, keeping in mind that the airway should be cautiously guarded. Intubation is especially appropriate in the obtunded patient or when removing petroleum distillates.

 c. Activated charcoal is a standard treatment for poisoned patients. Adults should receive 50 to 100 g of activated charcoal in a slurry or instilled down a gastric or nasogastric tube. The pediatric dose is 30 to 50 g. This dose maybe repeated in the initial 24 hours of management. Following is a partial list of common substances known to be adsorbed by activated charcoal:

Atropine	Morphine
Barbiturates	Phenytoin
Chlorpromazine	Quinidine
Cocaine	Salicylates
Colchicine	Theophylline
Dextroamphetamine	Tolbutamide
Digitalis	Tricyclic antidepressants
Meprobamate	

 d. Cathartics increase transit time and therefore hasten elimination of the bound toxic substance. Either magnesium sulfate or magnesium citrate is usually employed. However, Krenzelok, Keller, and Stewart[3] demonstrated a mean transient time of 0.9 hours using Sorbitol in a slurry with activated charcoal (50 g of charcoal in a 70% Sorbitol solution), compared with 4.4 hours with magnesium citrate.

5. Elimination of adsorbed substances: the clinician essentially has four modalities, depending on the type of poisoning.[2]

 a. Forced diuresis (caution: some poisons enhance pulmonary edema)

 b. Alkalinization by adding sodium bicarbonate to the solution (e.g., 0.5-1 mEq/kg/L)

  (1) Dysrhythmias secondary to tricyclic poisoning

  (2) Salicylates

  (3) Barbiturates

  (4) Phenylbutazone

  (5) Isoniazid

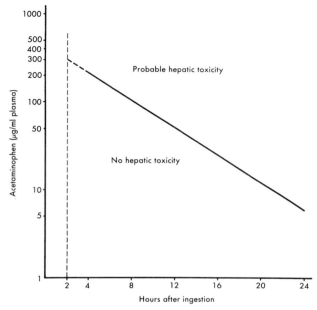

Figure 5-1
Semialgorithmic plot of plasma acetaminophen levels versus time. Reproduced with permission from Rumack, B.H., and Matthew, H.: Pediatrics 55:871, 1975.

   c. Acidification by administering ammonium chloride or ascorbic acid
     (1) Phencyclidine
     (2) Amphetamines
     (3) Quinine
     (4) Fenfluramine
   d. Sorbent hemoperfusion and dialysis
6. The pharmacokinetics of salicylates[1] and acetaminophen[5] has been well studied. Using standardized nomograms, the clinician can predict toxicity (Figs. 5-1 and 5-2). It is emphasized that the time from ingestion to the time of serum sample is critical in the interpretation of the nomogram.
   a. Management of salicylate overdose should include the following[4]:
     (1) Gastric lavage
     (2) Administration of activated charcoal
     (3) Forced alkaline diuresis (e.g., $D_5\frac{1}{2}NS$ IV with 44 mEq bicarbonate/L at 300 ml/h)
     (4) Consider dialysis if serum salicylate level is greater than 70 mg/dl
     (5) Vitamin K 10 mg IM or IV (salicylate inhibition of vitamin K may lead to GI bleeding)

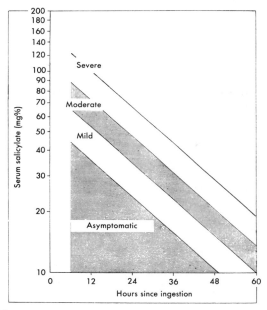

Figure 5-2
The Done nomogram correlates the serum salicylate level with the severity of ingestion at a given time after ingestion of a single dose of salicylate. Reproduced with permission from Done, A.K.: Salicylate intoxication: significance of salicylate in blood in cases of acute ingestion, Pediatrics **26**:805, 1960.

    (6) Monitor ABG (respiratory alkalosis initially, followed by meta-
        bolic acidosis)
    (7) Monitor serum K^+ (tendency to hypokalemia)
  b. Acetaminophen overdose requires the following[4]
    (1) Gastric lavage (activated charcoal should not be used since it may
        impair absorption)
    (2) Determine blood level; if in toxic range, start N-acetylcysteine
        (Mucomyst) 140 mg/kg PO loading dose followed by 70 mg/kg
        PO q4h for 68 hours (N-acetylcysteine therapy must be started
        within 16 hours of acetaminophen overdose)
    (3) Monitor acetaminophen level, use graph to plot possible hepatic
        toxicity
    (4) Provide adequate IV hydration (e.g., $D_5\frac{1}{2}NS$ at 150 ml/h)
    (5) Monitor liver function studies, ABGs, serum glucose, electrolytes,
        BUN, and creatinine

Table 5-3 Emergency antidotes

Poison	Antidote	Adult Dosage*	Comments
Acetaminophen	N-Acetylcysteine	140 mg/kg initial dose	Most effective within 16 hrs
Arsenic	See Mercury		
Atropine	Physostigmine	Initial dose 0.5-2 mg IV	Can produce convulsions or bradycardia
Carbon monoxide	Oxygen		
Cyanide	Amyl nitrite	Pearls every 2 min	Methemoglobin-cyanide complex
	then		
	Sodium nitrite	10 ml of 3% solution over 3 min IV	Causes hypotension; dosage assumes normal hemoglobin
		0.33 ml (10 mg of 3% sol) kg initially for children	
	Sodium thiosulfate	25% solution: 50 ml IV over 10 min; 1.65 ml/kg for children	Forms harmless sodium thiocyanate
Ethylene glycol	See Methyl alcohol		
Gold	See Mercury		
Iron	Deferoxamine	Initial dose: 40-90 mg/kg IM not to exceed 1 g	Deferoxamine mesylate—forms excretable ferrioxamine complex
Lead	Calcium disodium versenate	1 ampul/250 ml D_5W over 1 hr	5 ml ampul IV 20% solution; dilute to less than 3% solution—calcium displaced by lead

Mercury (arsenic, gold)	BAL (British anti-lewisite)	5 mg/kg IM as soon as possible	Each ml BAL in oil has dimercaprol, 100 mg in 210 mg (21%) benzyl benzoate and 680 mg peanut oil—forms stable nontoxic excretable cyclic compound
Methyl alcohol (ethylene glycol)	Ethyl alcohol In conjunction with dialysis	1 ml/kg of 100% ethanol initially in glucose solution: maintain blood level of 100 mg/dl	Competes for alcohol dehydrogenase; prevents formation of formic acid; oxalates
Nitrites	Methylene blue	0.2 ml/kg of 1% solution IV over 5 min	Often exchange transfusion is needed for severe methemoglobinemia
Opiates, Darvon, Lomotil	Naloxone	0.4-0.8 mg IV 0.01 mg/kg IV for children	Naloxone—no respiratory depression (0.4 mg/1 ml ampul)
Organophosphates	Atropine	Initial dose: 0.5-2 mg IV 0.05 mg/kg IV initially for children	Physiologically blocks acetylcholine; up to 5 mg IV every 15 min may be necessary in the critical adult patient
	Pralidoxime (2 PAM-chloride) (Protopam)	Initial dose: 1 g IV children: 25-50 mg/kg IV	Specific: breaks alkyl phosphate-cholinesterase bond; up to 500 mg every hr may be necessary in the critical adult patient

Adapted from the American College of Emergency Physicians poster on poisoning, Dallas, Texas 1980. From Haddad, L.M., and Winchester, J.: Clinical management of poisoning and drug overdose, Philadelphia, 1983, W. B. Saunders Co.

*Dosages listed may require modification according to specific clinical conditions.

SPECIFIC ANTIDOTES

Few antidotes are available for specific therapy of drug overdose or toxic exposure. The number of pharmaceutical, industrial, and naturally occurring products or substances that are potentially lethal is almost infinite. Examples of specific antidotes appear in Table 5-3.

5.3 SUPPORTIVE THERAPY

Throughout the treatment process, supportive therapy is the mainstay of patient care. Continual monitoring, maintaining the airway, and ensuring adequate ventilation and perfusion will influence patient outcome.

References

1. Done, A.K.: Salicylate intoxication, Pediatrics **26**(5):800, 1960.
2. Haddad, L.M.: General approach to the emergency management of poisoning. In Haddad, L.M., and Winchester, J.F., (editors): Clinical management of poisoning and drug overdose, Philadelphia, 1983, W.B. Saunders Co.
3. Krenzelok, E.P., Keller, R., and Stewart, R.D.: Gastrointestinal transit times of cathartics combined with charcoal, Ann. Emerg. Med. **14**:1152, 1985.
4. Nicholson, D.P.: The immediate management of overdose, Med. Clin. North Am. **67**:1285, 1983.
5. Rumack, B.H., and Peterson, R.G.: Acetaminophen overdose: incidence, diagnosis, and management in 416 patients, Pediatrics (suppl) **62**:(5)898, 1978.

Management of Alcohol Withdrawal

6

Alcohol withdrawal syndrome occurs when a person stops ingesting alcohol after prolonged consumption. It can result in four possible clinical patterns, depending on the severity of the patient's alcohol abuse and the time interval from the patient's previous alcohol ingestion. Although discussed separately, these alcohol withdrawal states blend together in real life.

1. Tremulous state (early alcohol withdrawal, ''impending DT's,'' ''shakes,'' ''jitters'')

   a. Time interval: usually occurs 12-48 hours after reduction of alcohol intake

   b. Manifestation: tremors, mild agitation, insomnia, tachycardia; symptoms are relieved by alcohol

   c. Treatment

      (1) Admit to medical floor (private room); monitor vital signs q4h; institute seizure precautions; maintain adequate sedation

      (2) Administer chlordiazepoxide as follows:
      Day 1: 50 mg PO q4h while awake and not lethargic
      Day 2: 25 mg PO q4h while awake and not lethargic
      Day 3: 10 mg PO q4h while awake and not lethargic

      (3) In the presence of jaundice or known liver disease, lorazepam may be substituted as follows:
      Day 1: 2 mg PO q4h while awake and not lethargic
      Day 2: 1 mg PO q4h while awake and not lethargic
      Day 3: 0.5 mg PO q4h while awake and not lethargic
      NOTE: Hold sedation for drowsiness or abnormal vital or neurologic signs. The above doses are only guidelines; it is best to titrate the dose case by case.

      (4) β-adrenergic blockers: atenolol 50-100 mg PO qd reportedly normalizes vital signs rapidly and significantly reduces the mean length of hospital stay in patients with alcohol withdrawal.[1] However, further studies are needed to clarify the role (if any) of β-adrenergic blockers in the treatment of alcohol withdrawal. β blockers should be avoided in patients with contraindications to their use (e.g., bronchospasm, bradycardia, or CHF).

      (5) Hydration PO or IV (high-caloric solution); if IV: glucose with Na^+, K^+, Mg^{2+}, and PO_4 replacement prn

      (6) Vitamin replacement: thiamine 100 mg IM or PO qd; plus multivitamins

(7) Laboratory studies
   (a) CBC and differential, platelet count, PT, PTT
   (b) Electrolytes, glucose, BUN, creatinine
   (c) Amylase, liver profile
   (d) Phosphorus and magnesium
   (e) Routine urinalysis
   (f) 2-hour urine amylase and serum lipase (if pancreatitis is suspected)
   (g) Blood cultures (if febrile or if infection is suspected)
   (h) Serum B_{12} and folic acid (if megaloblastic features in blood smear)
   (i) Lumbar puncture (if meningitis is suspected)
(8) X-ray studies; if subdural hematoma is suspected, CT scan should be ordered
(9) Social rehabilitation: group therapy such as Alcoholics Anonymous; identification and treatment of social and family problems should be initiated during the patient's hospital stay

2. Hallucinosis
   a. Manifestations: usually hallucinations are auditory, but occasionally hallucinations are visual, tactile, or olfactory; usually there is no clouding of sensorium as in delirum (clinical presentation may be mistaken for an acute schizophrenic episode)
   b. Treatment: same as for delirium tremens (see below)

3. Withdrawal seizures (rum fits)
   a. Time interval: usually occur 12-48 hours after cessation of drinking, with a peak incidence between 13-24 hours
   b. Manifestations: generalized convulsions with loss of consciousness; focal signs are usually absent; consider further investigation with CT scan of head and EEG if indicated (e.g., presence of neurologic deficits)
   c. Treatment
      (1) Diazepam 2.5 mg/min IV until seizure is controlled (check for respiratory depression or hypotension); a single loading dose of Dilantin (1000 mg at 50 mg/min IV) can also be given to prevent immediate recurrence of seizure, but its need and efficacy have been questioned (chronic anticonvulsant therapy is not indicated)
      (2) Thiamine 100 mg IM, followed by IV dextrose should also be administered
      (3) Correct electrolyte imbalances ($\downarrow$ Mg, $\downarrow$ K, $\downarrow$ PO_4) that may exacerbate seizures

4. Delirium tremens (DTs)
   a. Time interval: variable; usually occurs within 1 week after reduction or cessation of heavy alcohol intake
   b. Manifestations: confusion, tremors, vivid visual and tactile hallucinations, autonomic hyperactivity; this is the most serious clinical presentation of alcohol withdrawal (mortality is approximately 15% in untreated patients)

c. Treatment
   (1) Admit to ICU or to unit where patient can be observed closely
   (2) Vital signs q30min (neurologic signs, if necessary)
   (3) Restrain in lateral decubitus or prone position if restraints are necessary
   (4) NPO: NG tube for abdominal distention may be necessary
   (5) Lab studies: same as for early alcohol withdrawal
   (6) Hydration: IV with glucose (Na^+, K^+, PO_4, and Mg^{2+} replacement)
   (7) Vitamins: thiamine, 100 mg IM qd; multivitamins (may be added to the hydrating solution)
   (8) Sedation
       (a) Initially: chlordiazepoxide 12.5 mg/min IV or diazepam 5-10 mg q5-10 min until patient is calm
       (b) Maintenance (individualize dosage): chlordiazepoxide, 50-100 mg PO q4-6h, lorazepam 2 mg PO q4h, or diazepam 5-10 mg PO tid
   (9) Treatment of seizures (as previously described)
   (10) Diagnosis and treatment of any associated illness (pancreatitis pneumonia, sepsis, meningitis, or hepatic failure)

References

1. Kraus, M.L., Gottlieb, L.D., et al.: Randomized clinic trial of atenolol in patients with alcohol withdrawal, N. Engl. J. Med. 313:905, 1985.

Disorders of Thermoregulation

7

ACCIDENTAL HYPOTHERMIA

Definitions

Hypothermia: rectal temperature $<35°$ C (95.8° F)

Accidental hypothermia: unintentionally induced decrease in core temperature in absence of preoptic anterior hypothalamic conditions[9]

Clinical presentation

1. Varies with the severity of hypothermia
2. Always measure rectal temperature with a low-reading rectal thermometer
3. Hypothermia may masquerade as CVA (ataxia, slurred speech) or the patient may appear comatose or clinically dead; there are various reports in the medical literature[5] of cyanotic, rigid patients with fixed pupils and no audible heart sounds who have been successfully resuscitated, therefore "no one is dead until warm and dead"[6]

Physiologic stages of hypothermia[3]

1. Mild hypothermia: 33° to 35° C (91.4° to 95° F)
   a. Dysarthria, ataxia
2. Moderate hypothermia: 27° to 32° C (80.6° to 89.6° F)
   a. Progressive decrease in level of consciousness, pulse, CO, and respiration
   b. Atrial fibrillation and other dysrhythmias (increased susceptibility to ventricular tachycardia)
   c. Elimination of shivering mechanism for thermogenesis
3. Severe hypothermia: $\leq 26°$ C (78.8° F)
   a. Absence of reflexes or response to pain
   b. $\downarrow$ Cerebral blood flow, $\downarrow\downarrow$ CO
   c. $\uparrow$ risk of ventricular fibrillation or asystole

Lab evaluation

1. Metabolic and respiratory acidosis are usually present
   a. ABGs must be corrected for temperature; correction factors as follows[15]:
      (1) pH $\downarrow$ 0.008 units/° F $\downarrow$ in temperature
      (2) Pao_2 $\uparrow$ 3.3%/° F $\downarrow$ in temperature
      (3) $Paco_2$ $\downarrow$ 2.4%/° F $\downarrow$ in temperature

2. ↓ K⁺ initially, then ↑ K⁺ with increasing hypothermia
3. ↑ Hct (secondary to hemoconcentration), ↓ leukocytes, ↓ platelets (secondary to splenic sequestration)
4. ↑ Blood viscosity, ↑ clotting time

ECG[10]

1. Prolonged PR, QT, and QRS segments
2. Depressed ST segment
3. Inverted T waves
4. AV block
5. Hypothermic J waves (Osborn waves) may appear at 25° to 30° C; these waves are characterized by a notching at the junction of the QRS complex and ST segment (Fig. 7-1)

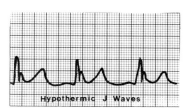

Figure 7-1
Hypothermic J waves.

Therapy

1. Treatment of hypothermia varies with the following:
   a. Degree of hypothermia
   b. Existence of concomitant diseases (e.g., cardiovascular insufficiency)
   c. Patient's age and medical condition (e.g., elderly debilitated patient vs young healthy patient)
2. General measures
   a. Secure an airway before rewarming in all unconscious patients; precede endotracheal intubation with oxygenation (if possible) to minimize the risk of dysrhythmias during the procedure
   b. Correct acidosis and electrolyte abnormalities
   c. Monitor patients, treat dysrhythmias
3. Specific treatment
   a. Mild hypothermia
      (1) Passive external rewarming is indicated. The patient should be placed in a warm room >21° C (69.8° F) and covered with insulating material. Recommended rewarming rates vary between 0.5° to 2.0° C/hr, but should not exceed 0.55° C/hr in elderly patients[3]
   b. Moderate to severe hypothermia
      (1) Active core rewarming
         (a) Delivery of heat via fluids, such as the following:
            • Warm GI irrigation (with saline enemas and via NG tube)
            • Warm IV fluids[2]

- Peritoneal dialysis with dialysate heated to 40.5° to 42.5° C[7, 13]
- Hemodialysis, extracorporeal blood rewarming
  - (b) Inhalation of heated humidified oxygen[8]
- (2) Active external rewarming
  - (a) Immersion in a bath of warm water (40° to 41° C). Active external rewarming may produce shock because of excessive peripheral vasodilation. Ideal candidates are previously healthy young patients with acute immersion hypothermia.[4]

| 7.2 | HEAT STROKE

Clinical presentation

1. Exposure to heat load (environmental or internally generated)
2. Elevated body temperature (usually >40° C [104° F])
3. Major form of CNS dysfunction (confusion, delirium, seizures, coma)
4. Marked elevation of SGOT, SGPT, LDH

Predisposing factors[14]

1. Exogenous heat gain (↑ ambient temperature)
2. ↑ Heat production (exercise, infection, hyperthyroidism, drugs)
3. Impaired heat dissipation (high humidity, heavy clothing, neonates or elderly patients, drugs: phenothiazines, anticholinergics, diuretics, propranolol)

Differential diagnosis

1. CNS pathology
   a. Infections (meningitis, encephalitis)
   b. Head trauma
   c. Epilepsy
2. Thyroid storm
3. Heat exhaustion
   a. Generalized malaise, weakness, headache, muscle cramps, nausea, vomiting, hypotension, and tachycardia
   b. Rectal temperature is usually normal
   c. Sweating is usually present
   d. Differentiated from heat stroke by the following:
      (1) Essentially intact mental functions and lack of significant fever
      (2) Mild or absent increases in CPK, SGOT, LDH, SGPT
   e. Treatment consists of the following[1]:
      (1) Rest in a well-ventilated, cool environment
      (2) Fluid replacement. If young athlete, give NS IV (3 to 4 L over 6-8 hours). If elderly patient, consider D_5 ½ NS IV with rate titrated to cardiovascular status
4. Heat cramps[11]
   a. Severe muscle cramps, often involving the lower extremities
   b. Rectal temperature is usually normal
   c. Sweating is usually present
   d. History often reveals profuse sweating and fluid replacement with hypotonic solutions (e.g., water)

e. Lack of acclimatization and recent use of ethanol are often contributory factors
f. Treatment consists of the following[1]:
  (1) Rest in a cool environment
  (2) Salt replacement
    (a) PO: ¼ tsp of salt or two 10 gr salt tablets dissolved in 1L of H_2O
    (b) IV: NS, 1 L infused over 1 to 4 hours depending on the patient's cardiovascular status

Clinical presentation of heat stroke

1. Neurologic manifestations (seizures, tremor, hemiplegia, coma, psychosis, and other bizarre behavior)
2. Evidence of dehydration (poor skin turgor, sunken eyeballs)
3. Tachycardia, hyperventilation
4. Skin is hot, red, and flushed
5. Sweating is often (not always) absent, particularly in elderly patients[12]
6. Lab studies reveal:
  a. ↑ BUN, ↑ creatinine, ↑ Hct, ↑/↓ Na^+, ↑/↓ K
  b. ↑ LDH, ↑ SGOT, ↑ SGPT, ↑ CPK, ↑ bilirubin, ↓ calcium
  c. Lactic acidosis, respiratory alkalosis
  d. Myoglobinuria, hypofibrinogenemia, fibrinolysis

Treatment of heat stroke[1]

1. Immediate cooling: remove clothes, place patient in a cool and well-ventilated room, apply ice packs to axillae, groin, and neck, or immerse in ice water
2. Intubate comatose patients, insert Foley catheter, start nasal O_2 and continuous ECG monitoring
3. Begin IV hydration with NS or Ringer's lactate
4. Draw initial lab studies: electrolytes, CBC, BUN, creatinine, SGOT, SGPT, CPK, LDH, glucose, PT, PTT, platelet count, FDP, Ca, uric acid, lactic acid, ABGs
5. Treat complications
  a. Hypotension: vigorous hydration with normal saline or Ringer's lactate
  b. Convulsions: diazepam 5-10 mg IV (slowly)
  c. Shivering: chlorpromazine 25-50 mg IV
  d. Acidosis if pH < 7.2 give sodium bicarbonate
6. Observe for evidence of hepatic, renal, or cardiac failure and treat accordingly

References

1. Callaham, M.: Heat illness. In Rosen, P., et al. (editors): Emergency medicine: concepts and clinical practice, St. Louis, 1983, The C.V. Mosby Co.
2. Chinard, F.P.: Accidental hypothermia: a brief review, J. Med. Soc., N.J., **75**:610, 1978.
3. Danzl, D.F.: Accidental hypothermia. In Rosen, P., and others, (editors): Emergency medicine: concepts and clinical practice, St. Louis, 1983, The C.V. Mosby Co.
4. Golden, F.: Recognition and treatment of immersion hypothermia, Proc. Royal. Soc. Med. **66**:1058, 1973.

5. Gregory, R.T., and Doolittle, W.H.: Accidental hypothermia II: clinical implications of experimental studies, Alaska Med. **15**:48, 1973.
6. Gregory, R.T., and Patton, J.F.: Treatment after exposure to cold, Lancet **1**:377, 1972.
7. Klarskov, P., and Amter, F.: Hypothermia after submersion: correction with peritoneal dialysis, Ugeskr. Laeger, **138**:1937, 1976.
8. Lloyd, E.L.: Accidental hypothermia treated by central rewarming through the airway, Br. J. Anaesth. **45**:41, 1973.
9. MacLean, D., and Emslie-Smith, D.: Accidental hypothermia, Philadelphia, 1977, J.B. Lippincott.
10. Popvic, V., and Popvic, P.: Hypothermia in biology and in medicine, 1974, Grune and Statton.
11. Proulx, R.P.: Heat stress disease. In Schwartz, G.R., et al. (editors): Principles and practice of emergency medicine, Philadelphia, 1978, W.B. Saunders, Co.
12. Schoenfield, Y., and Udassin, R.: Age and sex difference in response to short exposure to extreme heat, J. Appl. Physiol. **44**:1, 1978.
13. Soung, L.S., et al.: Treatment of accidental hypothermia with peritoneal dialysis, J.A.C.E.P. **6**:556, 1977.
14. Stine, R.: Heat illness, J.A.C.E.P. **8**:154, 1978.
15. Wears, R.L.: Blood gases in hypothermia, J.A.C.E.P. **8**:247, 1979.

Acid-Base
Disturbances

Definitions

The suffix -osis does not correspond to blood acidity but is used only to refer to the primary process generating OH^- or H^+

Acidosis: primary process that generates H^+

Alkalosis: primary process that generates OH^-

The suffix -emia refers to blood acidity.

Acidemia: blood pH <7.36

Alkalemia: blood pH >7.44

8.1   APPROACH TO THE PATIENT WITH ACID-BASE DISTURBANCES

1. Draw ABG and electrolytes concomitantly; evaluate the following[2]:
   a. Plasma HCO_3
      (1) Increased in metabolic alkalosis or respiratory acidosis (compensated)
      (2) Decreased in metabolic acidosis or respiratory alkalosis (compensated)
   b. Serum K^+ (ΔpH 0.1 = ΔK^+ 0.6)
      (1) Increased in acidemia
      (2) Decreased in alkalemia
   c. Serum Cl^-: compare with plasma sodium concentration; they should be proportionally increased or decreased if the change in Cl^- concentration is the result of a change in the hydration of the patient.
      (1) If the Cl^- is disproportionately increased, think of metabolic acidosis or respiratory alkalosis
      (2) If the Cl^- is disproportionately decreased think of metabolic alkalosis or respiratory acidosis
2. Calculate anion gap (AG)

$$AG = Na^+ - (Cl^- + HCO^-_3)$$
$$normal = 8\text{-}16 \text{ mEq/L}$$

The anion gap represents unmeasured anions in the plasma (negative charges on plasma proteins and negative charges contributed by organic and inorganic anions normally present in the plasma but not routinely measured). This measurement is important because it enables us to divide the causes of metabolic acidosis into two main categories:
1. Normal anion gap acidosis (hyperchloremic acidosis)
2. Elevated anion gap acidosis (AG acidosis)

Table 8-1 Primary abnormality and compensatory responses in simple acid-base disorders[2]

Disorder	Primary Abnormality	Secondary Response	pH	$Paco^2$	HCO_3^-
Metabolic acidosis	Gain of H^+ or loss of HCO_3^-	↑ Ventilation (and chemical buffering)	↓	↓	↓
Respiratory acidosis	Hypoventilation	HCO_3^- generation	↓	↑	↑
Metabolic alkalosis	Gain of HCO_3^- or loss of H^+	↓ Ventilation (and chemical buffering)	↑	↑	↑
Respiratory alkalosis	Hyperventilation	HCO_3^- consumption	↑	↓	↓

An elevated anion gap is the result of the presence of acid ions (e.g., lactic acid) in the extracellular fluid.

3. Evaluate ABGs to determine the type of disturbance present (see Table 8-1)
4. Calculate if the degree of compensation is adequate:
   a. Metabolic acidosis
      (1) If adequate compensation $Paco_2 = (1.5 \times HCO_3^-) + 8.4$[1]
      (2) If actual $Paco_2$ is less than calculated, then metabolic and respiratory acidosis is present
      (3) If actual $Paco_2$ is greater than calculated, then metabolic acidosis and respiratory alkalosis are present
   b. Respiratory acidosis
      (1) Acute: an increase in $Paco_2$ by 10 will decrease pH by 0.8 and increase HCO_3^- by 1.0
      (2) Chronic: an increase in $Paco_2$ by 10 will increase HCO_3^- by 0.4
   c. Metabolic alkalosis
      (1) An increase in HCO_3^- by 1.0 will increase pH by 0.015 and increase $Paco_2$ by 0.7
      (2) Limitations: the compensatory response (↑ $Paco_2$) is usually limited to a maximum $Paco_2$ of 55
      (3) There is an impaired compensatory response in patients with COPD, heart failure, and hepatic coma
   d. Respiratory alkalosis
      (1) Acute: A decrease in $Paco_2$ by 10 will decrease pH by 0.8 and decrease HCO_3^- by 2
      (2) Chronic: A decrease in $Paco_2$ by 10 will decrease pH by 0.8 and decrease HCO_3^- by 5

If the degree of compensation is inadequate, consider the simultaneous presence of two or more primary abnormalities (mixed acid-base disturbances). Fig. 8-1 demonstrates the acid-base nomogram constructed from arterial pH, $Paco_2$, and HCO_3^-. The normal values are labeled N. The specific acid-base disturbance present can be determined by plotting the pH, $Paco_2$, and HCO_3^-.

The boxed material on p. 56 describes common causes of mixed acid-base disturbances.

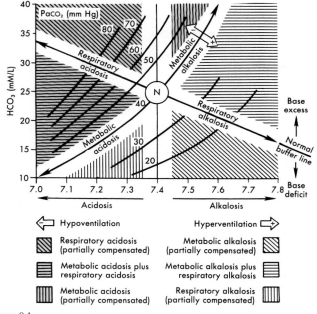

Figure 8-1
Graphic representation of Henderson-Hasselbach equation of acid-base relationships.
From Rosen, P., et al., (editors): Emergency medicine: concepts and clinical practice,
St. Louis, 1983, The C.V. Mosby Co.

8.2   COMMON CAUSES OF ACID-BASE DISTURBANCES

Metabolic acidosis

1. Metabolic acidosis with increased anion gap (AG acidosis)
   a. Lactic acidosis (see the boxed material on p. 57 for causes of lactic acidosis)
   b. Ketoacidosis (diabetes mellitus, ethanol intoxication, starvation)
   c. Uremia (chronic renal failure)
   d. Ingestion of toxins (paraldehyde, methanol, salicylate, ethylene glycol)
2. Metabolic acidosis with normal anion gap (hyperchloremic acidosis)
   a. Renal tubular acidosis (including acidosis of aldosterone deficiency)
   b. Intestinal loss of bicarbonate (diarrhea, pancreatic fistula)
   c. Carbonic anhydrase inhibitors (e.g., acetazolamide)
   d. Dilutional acidosis (as a result of rapid infusion of bicarbonate-free isotonic saline)

Common Causes of Mixed Disturbances Associated With Metabolic Acidosis

Mixed Anion Gap Acidosis

Ketoacidosis and lactic acidosis
Methanol or ethylene glycol intoxication and lactic acidosis
Uremic acidosis and ketoacidosis

Mixed Anion Gap and Hyperchloremic Acidosis

Diarrhea and lactic acidosis or ketoacidosis
Progressive renal failure
Type IV renal tubular acidosis and diabetic ketoacidosis
Diabetic ketoacidosis during treatment

Mixed Hyperchloremic Acidosis

Diarrhea and renal tubular acidosis
Diarrhea and hyperalimentation
Diarrhea and acetazolamide or mafenide (Sulfamylon)

Anion Gap Acidosis or Hyperchloremic Acidosis and Metabolic Alkalosis

Ketoacidosis and protracted vomiting or nasogastric suction
Chronic renal failure and vomiting or nasogastric suction
Diarrhea and vomiting or nasogastric suction
Renal tubular acidosis and vomiting
Lactic or ketoacidosis plus $NaHCO_3$ therapy

Anion Gap Acidosis or Hyperchloremic Acidosis and Respiratory Alkalosis

Respiratory alkalosis
Lactic acidosis
Salicylate poisoning
Hepatic disease
Gram-negative sepsis
Pulmonary edema

Anion Gap Acidosis or Hyperchloremic Acidosis and Respiratory Acidosis

Cardiopulmonary arrest
Pulmonary edema
Respiratory failure in chronic lung disease
Phosphate depletion
Drug overdose and poisoning

From DuBose, T.D., Jr.: Clinical approach to patients with acid-base disorders, Med. Clin. North Am. **67:** (4)807, 1983.

Etiology of Lactic Acidosis[3,5]

Tissue hypoxia

Shock (hypovolemic, cardiogenic, endotoxic
Respiratory failure (asphyxia)
Severe CHF
Severe anemia
Carbon monoxide or cyanide poisoning

Associated with systemic disorders

Neoplastic diseases (e.g., leukemia, lymphoma)
Liver or renal failure
Sepsis
Diabetes mellitus
Seizure activity
Abnormal intestinal flora (D-lactic acidosis)
Alkalosis

Secondary to drugs or toxins

Salicylates
Ethanol, methanol, ethylene glycol
Fructose and sorbitol
Biguanides (e.g., phenphormin)
Isoniazid
Streptozocin

Hereditary disorders

Glucose-6-phosphatase deficiency and others

    e. Ingestion of exogenous acids (ammonium chloride, methionine, cystine, calcium chloride)
    f. Ileostomy
    g. Ureterosigmoidostomy

Respiratory acidosis

1. Pulmonary disease (COPD, severe pneumonia, pulmonary edema, interstitial fibrosis)
2. Airway obstruction (foreign body, severe bronchospasm, laryngospasm)
3. Thoracic cage disorders (pneumothorax, flail chest, kyphoscoliosis)
4. Defects in muscles of respiration (myasthenia gravis, hypokalemia, muscular dystrophy)
5. Defects in peripheral nervous system (amyotrophic lateral sclerosis, poliomyelitis, Guillain-Barré syndrome, botulism, tetanus, organophosphate poisoning, spinal cord injury)
6. Depression of respiratory center (anesthesia, narcotics, sedatives, vertebral artery embolism or thrombosis, increased intracranial pressure)
7. Failure of mechanical ventilator

Metabolic alkalosis

1. Vomiting
2. Nasogastric suction
3. Severe potassium depletion
4. Excessive alkali intake (e.g., milk-alkali syndrome)
5. Diuretics
6. Hyperreninemic states (volume contraction, Bartter's syndrome)
7. Hyperadrenocorticoid states (Cushing's syndrome, primary hyperaldosteronism)
8. Hypomagnesemia, hypercalcemia
9. Posthypercapnic alkalosis

Respiratory alkalosis

1. Hypoxemia (pneumonia, pulmonary embolism, atelectasis, high-altitude living)
2. Drugs (salicylates, xanthines, progesterone, epinephrine, thyroxine, nicotine)
3. CNS disorders (tumor, CVA, trauma, infections)
4. Psychogenic hyperventilation (anxiety, hysteria)
5. Hepatic encephalopathy
6. Gram-negative sepsis
7. Hyponatremia
8. Sudden recovery from metabolic acidosis
9. Assisted ventilation

References

1. Albert, M.D., Dell, R.B., and Winters, R.W.: Quantitative displacement of acid-base equilibrium in metabolic acidosis, Ann. Intern. Med. **66**:312, 1964.
2. Bia, M., and Thier, S.: Mixed acid base disturbances: a clinical approach, Med. Clin. North Am. **65**:347, 1981.
3. Cohen, R.D., and Woods, H.F.: Clinical and biochemical aspects of lactic acidosis, London, 1976, Blackwell Scientific Publications.
4. Dubose, T.D., Jr.: Clinical approach to patients with acid base disorders, Med. Clin. North Am. **67**:799, 1983.
5. Narins, R.G., Jones, E.R., et al.: Metabolic acid-base disorders: pathophysiology, classification and treatment. In Arieff, A.I., and DeFranzo, R.A., et al.: Fluid electrolyte and acid-base disorders, vol. 1, New York, 1985, Churchill Livingstone.

Procedures
and Interpretation
of Results

9.1 LUMBAR PUNCTURE

Indications

1. Suspected meningitis
2. Suspected encephalitis
3. Diagnosis of meningeal carcinomatosis and meningeal leukemia
4. Diagnosis of tertiary syphilis
5. Follow-up of therapy for meningitis
6. Evaluation for Guillain-Barré syndrome
7. Evaluation for multiple sclerosis
8. Staging of lymphomas
9. Evaluation of dementia (only when clearly indicated)
10. Treatment of pseudotumor cerebri
11. Suspected subarachnoid hemorrhage
12. Introduction of drugs, anesthetics, or radiographic media in the CNS

Contraindications

1. Infection at the site of lumbar puncture
2. Increased intracranial pressure
3. Severe hemorrhagic diathesis

Procedure[1-3,11]

1. Perform a careful ophthalmoscopic exam; if increased intracranial pressure and/or a CNS space occupying lesion is suspected, CT scan of the head should be done before LP
2. Place the patient in a lateral decubitus position with spine flexed (draw shoulders forward and bring thighs toward the abdomen, Fig. 9-1)
3. Identify the L4-5 interspace (imaginary line connecting the iliac crests)
4. Clean area with povidone-iodine solution
5. Anesthetize skin and subcutaneous tissues with 1%-2% lidocaine
6. Gently introduce the spinal needle (with bevel turned upward) in the L4-5 interspace in a horizontal direction and with a slight cephalad inclination (Fig. 9-2)
7. Measure opening pressure (normal is 100 to 200 mm H_2)
   a. If the pressure is elevated, instruct the patient to relax and ensure that there is no abdominal compression or breath holding (straining and pressure on the abdominal wall will increase the CSF pressure) (Fig. 9-3); if the pressure is markedly elevated, remove only 5 ml of spinal fluid and remove the needle immediately

59

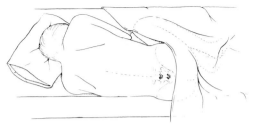

Figure 9-1
Lateral decubitus position. From Surratt, P.M., and Gibson, R.S.: Manual of medical procedures, St. Louis, 1982, The C.V. Mosby Co.

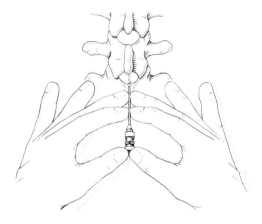

Figure 9-2
Insert spinal needle into subcutaneous tissue and slowly advance needle into subarachnoid space. From Surratt, P.M., and Gibson, R.S.: Manual of medical procedures, St. Louis, 1982, The C.V. Mosby Co.

  b. If the pressure is markedly elevated, remove only 5 ml of spinal fluid and remove the spinal needle immediately

8. Collect 5-10 ml of spinal fluid in four collection tubes (2 ml/tube) (Fig. 9-4)

9. Measure closing pressure, then remove manometer and stopcock, and replace stylet before removing the spinal needle; apply pressure to the puncture site with sterile gauze for a few minutes

10. Instruct the patient to remain in a horizontal position for approximately 4 hours to minimize post–lumbar puncture headache (caused by CSF fluid leakage through the puncture site)

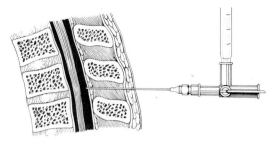

Figure 9-3
Measure opening pressure. Note position of stopcock. From Surratt, P.M., and Gibson, R.S.: Manual of medical procedures, St. Louis, 1982, The C.V. Mosby Co.

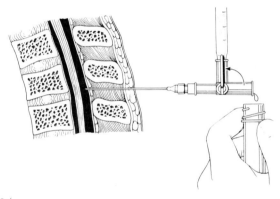

Figure 9-4
Collect cerebrospinal fluid. From Surratt, P.M., and Gibson, R.S.: Manual of medical procedures, St. Louis, 1982, The C.V. Mosby Co.

11. Process the CSF fluid
    a. Tube 1: protein, glucose
    b. Tube 2: Gram stain
    c. Tube 3: save fluid until further notice
    d. Tube 4: cell count (total and differential)
12. Consider additional tests (if indicated)
    a. Bacterial cultures in suspected bacterial meningitis
    b. Assay for cryptococcal antigen in immunocompromised patients
    c. Countercurrent immunoelectrophoresis (CIE): to detect specific polysaccharide bacterial antigens (*N. meningitidis, H. influenzae, S. pneumoniae*) in the CSF of patients with inconclusive Gram staining (e.g., patients with partially treated meningitis)

    d. Oligoclonal banding and assay for myelin basic protein are useful to diagnose multiple sclerosis

    e. VDRL, AFB stain, Wright stain of sediment, India ink preparation, fungal or viral cultures, and cytologic exam should not be routinely ordered, but only when specifically indicated

Interpretation of results[4]

1. Appearance of the fluid
   a. Clear: normal
   b. Yellow color (xanthochromia) in the supernatant of centrifuged CSF within 1 hour or less after collection is usually the result of previous bleeding (subarachnoid hemorrhage); it may also be caused by increased CSF protein, melanin from meningeal melosarcomas, or carotenoids
   c. Pinkish color is usually the result of a bloody tap; the color generally clears progressing from tubes 1 to 4 (the supernatant is usually crystal clear in traumatic taps)
   d. Turbidity usually indicates the presence of leukocytes (bleeding introduces approximately 1 WBC/500 RBC) in the CSF
2. CSF pressure: elevated pressure can be seen with meningitis, meningoencephalitis, pseudotumor cerebri, mass lesions, and intracerebral bleeding
3. Cell count: in the adult, the CSF is normally free of cells (although up to 5 mononuclear cells/mm^3 is considered normal); the presence of granulocytes is never normal
   a. Neutrophils: seen in bacterial meningitis, early viral meningoencephalitis and early TB meningitis
   b. Increased lymphocytes: TB meningitis, viral meningoencephalitis, syphilitic meningoencephalitis, fungal meningitis
4. Protein: serum proteins are generally too large to cross the normal blood/CSF barrier; however, increased CSF protein is seen with meningeal inflammation, traumatic tap, increased CNS synthesis, tissue degeneration, obstruction to CSF circulation, and Guillain-Barré syndrome
5. Glucose
   a. Decreased glucose is seen with bacterial meningitis, TB meningitis, fungal meningitis, subarachnoid hemorrhage, and some cases of viral meningitis
   b. A mild increase in CSF glucose can be seen in patients with very elevated serum glucose levels

NOTE: Table 9-1 describes CSF abnormalities found in various CNS conditions.

| 9.2 | **THORACENTESIS**[8]

Major indications

1. Presence of any pleural effusion of unknown cause
2. Relief of dyspnea caused by large pleural effusion

Contraindications

1. Clotting abnormalities
2. Thrombocytopenia
3. Uncooperative patient, or patient with severe cough or hiccups

Table 9-1 CSF abnormalities in various CNS conditions

	Appearance	Glucose mg/dl	Protein mg/dl	Cell Count (cells/mm³) and Cell Type	Pressure mm H₂O
Normal	Clear	50-80	20-45	<6 Lymphocytes	100-200
Acute bacterial meningitis	Cloudy	↓↓*	↑↑	↑↑ PMN†	↑↑
Aseptic (viral) meningitis	Clear/cloudy	N	↑	↑, Usually mononuclear cells May be PMN in early stages	N/↑
Hemorrhage	Bloody/xanthochromic	N/↓	↑	↑↑ RBC	↑
Neoplasm	Clear/xanthochromic	N/↓	N/↑	N/↑ Lymphocytes	↑↑
Tuberculous meningitis	Cloudy	↓	↑	↑ PMN (early) ↑ Lymphocytes (later)	↑
Fungal meningitis	Clear/cloudy	↓	↑	↑ Monocytes	↑
Neurosyphilis	Clear/cloudy	N	N/↑	↑ Monocytes	N/↑
Guillain-Barré syndrome	Clear/cloudy	N	↑	N/↑ Lymphocytes	N

*↑, Increased; ↑↑, markedly increased; ↓, decreased; ↓↓, markedly decreased; N, normal.
†PMN, polymorphonucleocytes; RBC, red blood cells.

Localization of pleural effusion

1. Physical exam: dullness to percussion
2. Chest x-ray film: posteroanterior view is usually sufficient in identifying the fluid collection, but in case of equivocal effusions, a lateral decubitus chest x-ray film can demonstrate layering out of the pleural fluid
3. Fluoroscopy or ultrasound[9]: useful before thoracentesis if the fluid collection is
   a. <10 mm thick
   b. Not freely moveable on the lateral decubitus x-ray view

Procedure[11]

1. Position patient in a sitting position with arms and head resting supported on a bedside adjustable table (Fig. 9-5)
2. Identify the area of effusion by gentle percussion
3. Clean the area with povidone-iodine solution, and maintain strict aseptic technique
4. Insert the needle in the posterior chest (approximately 5-10 cm lateral to the spine) in an interspace below the point of dullness to percussion
5. Anesthetize the skin and subcutaneous tissues with 1%-2% lidocaine
6. Make sure that the needle is positioned and advanced above the superior margin of the rib (the intercostal nerve and the blood supply are located near the inferior margin)

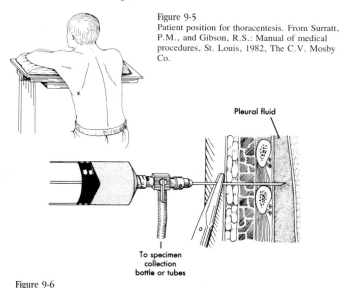

Figure 9-5
Patient position for thoracentesis. From Surratt, P.M., and Gibson, R.S.: Manual of medical procedures, St. Louis, 1982, The C.V. Mosby Co.

Pleural fluid

To specimen
collection
bottle or tubes

Figure 9-6
Fluid removal through thoracentesis needle and a three-way stopcock. From Surratt, P.M., and Gibson, R.S.: Manual of medical procedures, St. Louis, 1982, The C.V. Mosby Co.

7. Gently advance a 20-gauge needle; anesthetize the pleura and gently aspirate until pleural fluid is noted in the syringe, then remove the needle and note the depth of insertion needed for the thoracentesis needle
8. In the previous puncture site, insert a 17-gauge needle (flat bevel) attached to a 30 ml syringe via a 3-way stopcock connected to a drainage tube (Fig. 9-6)
9. Slowly advance the needle (above the superior margin of the rib), and gently aspirate while advancing
10. When pleural fluid is noted, place a snap-on clip or a hemostat on the needle to prevent it from inadvertently advancing forward
11. Remove the necessary amount of pleural fluid (usually 100 ml for diagnostic studies), but do not remove more than 1500 ml of fluid at any one time because of increased risk of pulmonary edema or hypotension[5] (pneumothorax from needle laceration of the visceral pleura is also much more likely to occur if an effusion is completely drained[6])
12. Gently remove the needle
13. Obtain serum LDH, glucose levels, and total protein level
14. Process the pleural fluid; the *initial* lab studies should be aimed only at distinguishing an exudate from a transudate
    a. Tube 1: protein, LDH
    b. Tubes 2, 3, 4: save fluid until further notice
    NOTE: Do not order further tests until the presence of an exudate is confirmed on the basis of protein and LDH determinations[7] (Table 9-2); however, if the results of protein and LDH determinations cannot be obtained within a reasonable time (resulting in unnecessary delay), additional lab tests should be ordered at the time of thoracentesis

Evaluation of results

1. For differential diagnosis of pleural effusions refer to Chapter 10
2. If transudate, consider CHF, cirrhosis, chronic renal failure, and other hypoproteinemic states and perform direct subsequent work-up accordingly
3. If exudate, consider ordering the following tests on the pleural fluid:
    a. Cytologic exam for malignant cells (for suspected neoplasm)
    b. Gram stain, cultures (aerobic and anaerobic) and sensitivities (for suspected infectious process)
    c. AFB stain and cultures (for suspected TB)
    d. pH: a value <7.0 suggests a parapneumonic effusion[9] or empyema
    e. Glucose: low glucose levels suggest parapneumonic effusions and rheumatoid arthritis
    f. Amylase: a high amylase level suggests pancreatitis or ruptured esophagus

Table 9-2 Evaluation of pleural and peritoneal effusions

Test	Exudate	Transudate
Fluid LDH	>200 IU/dl	<200 IU/dl
Fluid protein	>3 g	<3 g
Fluid/serum LDH ratio	>0.6	<0.6
Fluid/serum protein ratio	>0.5	<0.5

Complications of thoracentesis[3]

1. Pneumothorax
2. Hemorrhage
3. Vasovagal episode
4. Infection
5. Unilateral pulmonary edema
6. Puncture of liver or spleen
7. Subcutaneous emphysema
8. Air embolism

| 9.3 | PARACENTESIS

Indications

1. Ascites of undetermined etiology
2. Evaluation for possible peritonitis
3. Relief of abdominal pain and discomfort caused by tense ascites
4. Relief of dyspnea caused by elevated diaphragm (from ascites)
5. Evaluation of possible intraabdominal hemorrhage in a patient with blunt abdominal trauma
6. Institution of peritoneal dialysis

Contraindications

1. Bleeding disorders
2. Bowel distention
3. Infection or surgical scars at the site of needle entry

Procedure[3,11]

1. Have patient empty bladder (insertion of a Foley catheter is not recommended but may be necessary in certain patients)
2. To identify the site of paracentesis, first locate the rectus muscle; a good site is approximately 2-3 cm lateral to the rectus muscle border in the lower abdominal quadrants (Fig. 9-7). Avoid the following:
   a. Rectus muscles (increased risk of hemorrhage from epigastric vessels)

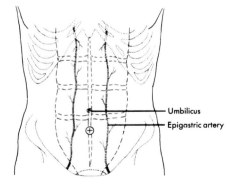

Figure 9-7
Anatomic landmarks for paracentesis. From Surratt, P.M., and Gibson, R.S.: Manual of medical procedures, St. Louis, 1982, The C.V. Mosby Co.

    b. Surgical scars (increased risk of perforation caused by adhesion of bowel to the wall of the peritoneum)

    c. Areas of skin infection (increased risk of intraperitoneal infection)

    NOTE: An alternate site is on the linea alba 3-4 cm below the umbilicus

3. Cleanse the area with povidone-iodine and drape the abdomen
4. Anesthetize the puncture site with 1%-2% lidocaine
5. Cautiously insert the needle (attached to a syringe) perpendicular to the skin; a small pop is felt as the needle advances through the anterior and posterior muscular fascia, and entrance into the peritoneal cavity is evidenced as a sudden "give" (use caution to avoid the sudden forward thrust of the needle)
6. Remove the necessary amount of fluid (do not remove more than 1 L of fluid, particularly in cirrhotic patients)
7. If diagnostic paracentesis, process the fluid as follows:

    a. Tube 1: LDH, glucose

    b. Tube 2: protein, specific gravity

    c. Tube 3: cell count and differential

    d. Tube 4: save until further notice

8. Draw serum LDH, protein
9. Gram stain, AFB stain, bacterial and fungal cultures, amylase, and triglycerides should be ordered only when indicated
10. If malignant ascites is suspected, consider a carcinoembryonic antigen (CEA) level on the paracentesis fluid

Interpretation of results

1. Peritoneal effusion can be classified as exudative or transudative based on its characteristics (Table 9-2)
2. For the differential diagnosis of ascites refer to Chapter 10
3. Table 9-3 describes the characteristics of ascitic fluid in various conditions

Complications

1. Persistent leakage of ascitic fluid
2. Hypotension and shock
3. Bleeding
4. Perforated bowel
5. Abscess formation in area of puncture site
6. Peritonitis

9.4 ARTHROCENTESIS

Indications

1. Presence of effusion of unexplained etiology
2. Steroid injection
3. Decompression of a hemorrhagic effusion in traumatized joints
4. Evaluation of antibiotic response in patients with infectious arthritis
5. Removal of purulent fluid in distended infected joints

Contraindication

1. Infection at the arthrocentesis site

Table 9-3 Characteristics of ascitic fluid in various conditions[1-5]

Etiology	Appearance	Total Protein (g/dl)	LDH (IU)	Specific Gravity	Glucose (mg/dl)	WBC/mm³	RBC/mm³	Amylase
Neoplasm	Bloody	>2.0	>200	Variable	<60	↑ *	↑ ↑	
	Clear							
	Chylous							
Cirrhosis	Straw-colored	<2.5	<200	<1.016	<60	→	→	
Nephrosis	Straw-colored	<2.5	<200	<1.016	>60	→	→	
CHF	Straw-colored	<2.5	<200	<1.016	>60	→	→	
Pyogenic	Turbid	>2.5	>200	>1.016	>60	↑ ↑ PMN†		
Pancreatic	Clear	>2.5	>200	Variable	>60	Variable	Variable	↑ ↑
	Hemorrhagic							
	Turbid							
	Chylous							

*↑, High; ↑ ↑, markedly high; ↓, low.
†PMN, Polymorphonuclear leukocytes.

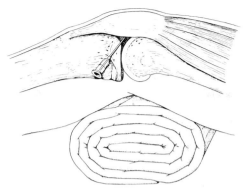

Figure 9-8
Arthrocentesis of knee joint, anteromedial approach. Flex knee and insert needle
approximately 1 cm below patella. From Surratt, P.M., and Gibson, R.S.: Manual of
medical procedures, St. Louis, 1982, The C.V. Mosby Co.

Procedure[11]

1. Palpate the joint and identify the extensor surface (vessels and nerves are
   less commonly found here)
2. With firm pressure, use a ballpoint pen that has the writing portion re-
   tracted to mark the specific area of the joint to be aspirated
3. Clean the skin with an antiseptic solution
4. Use a 25-gauge needle to infiltrate the skin with 1%-2% lidocaine
5. Gently insert an 18- or 20-gauge needle connected to a 20-30 ml syringe;
   a slight "pop" may be felt as the needle penetrates through the capsule
   (Fig. 9-8 shows arthrocentesis of knee joint)
6. Apply gentle suction to the syringe to aspirate the fluid
7. Gently remove the needle and apply slight pressure to the puncture site
8. Process the aspirated synovial fluid:
   a. Tube 1 (no heparin): viscosity, mucin clot
   b. Tube 2 (containing heparin): glucose
   c. Tube 3 (containing heparin): Gram stain, culture and sensitivity, cy-
      tology, cell count and differential
   d. Glass slide: place a drop of fluid and examine under polarized light
   e. Plate with Thayer-Martin medium: used in cases of suspected gono-
      coccal arthritis; cultures for anaerobes, *Mycobacterium tuberculosis*,
      and fungi should be ordered only when clearly indicated
9. Draw serum glucose

Interpretation of results[3,4,10]

1. Color: normally it is clear or pale yellow; cloudiness indicates inflammatory process or presence of crystals, cell debris, fibrin, or triglycerides
2. Viscosity: normally it has a high viscosity because of hyaluronate; when
   fluid is placed on a slide it can be stretched to a string >2 cm in length
   before separating (low viscosity indicates breakdown of hyaluronate [ly-
   sosomal enzymes from leukocytes] or the presence of edema fluid)

Table 9-4 Classification and interpretation of synovial fluid analysis[3,4,10]

Group	Diseases	Appearance	Viscosity	Mucin Clot	WBC/mm³	% PMN*	Glucose (mg/dl) (Blood-Synovial Fluid)
Normal	—	Clear		Firm	<200	<25	<10
I (Noninflammatory)	Osteoarthritis, aseptic necrosis, traumatic arthritis, erythema nodosum, osteochondritis dissecans	Clear, yellow (may be xanthochromic if traumatic arthritis)	↑† ↑	Firm	↑ Up to 10,000	<25	<10
II (Inflammatory)	Crystal-induced arthritis, rheumatoid arthritis Reiter's syndrome, collagen vascular disease, psoriatic arthritis, serum sickness, rheumatic fever	Clear, yellow Turbid	↓	Friable	↑↑ Up to 100,000	40-90	<40
III (Septic)	Bacterial (staphylococcal, gonococcal, TB)	Turbid	↓ / ↑	Friable	↑↑↑ Up to 5,000,000	40-100	20-100

*PMN = polymorphonucleocytes
↑↑, Elevated; ↑↑, markedly high; ↓, decreased.

3. Mucin clot: add 1 ml of fluid to 5 ml of a 5% acetic acid solution and allow 1 minute for the clot to form; a firm clot (does not fragment on shaking) is normal and indicates the presence of large molecules of hyaluronic acid (this test is nonspecific and infrequently done)
4. Glucose: normally it approximately equals serum glucose, a difference of more than 40 mg/dl is suggestive of infection
5. Microscopic examination for crystals
   a. Gout: monosodium urate crystals (MSU)
   b. Pseudogout: calcium pyrophosphate dihydrate crystals (CPPD)

NOTE: Synovial fluid is classified into three major groups based on its characteristics (Table 9-4)

Complications

1. Infection
2. Hemorrhage
3. Tendon rupture
4. Nerve palsies

References

1. Bauer, J.D.: Clinical laboratory methods, ed. 9, St. Louis, 1982, The C.V. Mosby Co.
2. Bennington, J.L.: Saunders' dictionary and encylopedia of laboratory medicine and technology, Philadelphia, 1984, W.B. Saunders Co.
3. Eknoyan, G.: Medical procedures manual, Chicago, 1982, Year Book Medical Publishers, Inc.
4. Henry, J.B.: Todd, Sanford, Davidsohn clinical diagnosis and management by laboratory methods, Philadelphia, 1984, W.B. Saunders Co.
5. Light, R.W.: Management of parapneumonic effusions, Arch Int. Med. **141:**1339, 1981.
6. Light, R.W.: Pleural diseases, Philadelphia, 1983, Lea and Febiger.
7. Light, R.W., Jenkinson, S.G., Mihn, V.D., and George, R.B.: Observation on pleural fluid pressures as fluid is withdrawn during thoracentesis, Am. Rev. Resp. Dis. **121:**799, 1980.
8. Hall, W.J., and Mayewski, R.J.: Diagnostic thoracentesis and pleural biopsy in pleural effusions, Ann. Int. Med. **103:**798, 1985.
9. Peterman, T.A., and Speicher, C.E.: Evaluating pleural effusions: a two-stage laboratory approach, JAMA, **252:**1051, 1984.
10. Schumacher, H.R.: Synovial fluid analysis. In Kelley, W. N., Harris, E.D., Jr., Ruddy, S., and Sledge C.B., (editors): Textbook of rheumatology, ed. 2, vol. 1, Philadelphia, 1985, W.B. Saunders Co.
11. Surratt, P.M., and Gibson R.S.: Manual of medical procedures, St. Louis, 1982, The C.V. Mosby Co.

10

Differential Diagnosis

This chapter covers the differential diagnoses of the following disorders:

Abdominal pain
Amenorrhea
Ascites
Ataxia
Back pain
Cardiac murmurs
Chest pain (nonpleuritic)
Chest pain (pleuritic)
Coma
Constipation
Dysphagia
Edema of lower extremities
Fever and rash
GI bleeding
Headache
Hematuria

Hemoptysis
Hepatomegaly
Hirsutism
Jaundice
Lymphadenopathy
Mediastinal masses or widening
Metastatic neoplasms
Paraplegia
Pleural effusions
Polyuria
Popliteal swelling
Proteinuria
Shoulder pain
Splenomegaly
Vertigo
Vomiting

The differential diagnoses of many other medical conditions (e.g., delirium, dementia, diarrhea, hypoglycemia, hypocalcemia/hypercalcemia, hyponatremia/hypernatremia, syncope) are discussed in more detail in other chapters.

10.1 ABDOMINAL PAIN

Diffuse

Early appendicitis
Aortic aneurysm
Gastroenteritis
Intestinal obstruction
Diverticulitis
Peritonitis
Mesenteric insufficiency or
 infarction
Pancreatitis
Inflammatory bowel disease
Irritable bowel
Mesenteric adenitis

Metabolic: toxins, lead poisoning,
 uremia, drug overdose, DKA,
 heavy metal poisoning
Sickle cell crisis
Pneumonia (rare)
Trauma
Urinary tract infection, PID
OTHER: Acute intermittent
 prophyria, tabes dorsalis,
 periarteritis nodosa, Henoch-
 Schöenlein purpura, adrenal
 insufficiency

Epigastric

Gastric: PUD, gastric outlet obstruction, gastric ulcer
Duodenal: PUD, duodenitis
Biliary: cholecystitis, cholangitis
Hepatic: hepatitis
Pancreatic: pancreatitis
Intestinal: high small bowel obstruction, early appendicitis
Cardiac: angina, MI, pericarditis
Pulmonary: pneumonia, pleurisy, pneumothorax
Subphrenic abscess

Suprapubic

Intestinal: colon obstruction or gangrene, diverticulitis, right-sided appendicitis
Reproductive system: ectopic pregnancy, mittelschmerz torsion of ovarian cyst, PID, salpingitis, endometriosis
Cystitis

Right upper quadrant (RUQ)

Biliary: calculi, infection, inflammation, neoplasm
Hepatic: hepatitis, abscess, hepatic congestion, neoplasm, trauma
Gastric: PUD, pyloric stenosis, neoplasm, alcoholic gastritis, hiatal hernia
Pancreatic: pancreatitis, neoplasm, stone in pancreatic duct or ampulla
Renal: calculi, infection, inflammation neoplasm
Pulmonary: pneumonia, pulmonary infarction
Intestinal: retrocecal appendicitis, intestinal obstruction, high fecal impaction
Cardiac: myocardial ischemia (particularly involving the inferior wall), pericarditis
Cutaneous: herpes zoster
Trauma
Fitz-Hugh-Curtis syndrome: (perihepatitis)

Left upper quadrant (LUQ)

Gastric: PUD, gastritis, pyloric stenosis, hiatal hernia
Pancreatic: pancreatitis, neoplasm, stone in pancreatic duct or ampulla
Cardiac: MI, angina pectoris
Splenic: splenomegaly, ruptured spleen, splenic abscess, splenic infarction
Renal: calculi, pyelonephritis, neoplasm
Pulmonary: pneumonia, empyema, pulmonary infarction
Vascular: ruptured aortic aneurysm
Cutaneous: herpes zoster
Trauma
Intestinal: high fecal impaction, perforated colon

Periumbilical

Intestinal: small bowel obstruction or gangrene, early appendicitis
Vascular: mesenteric thrombosis, dissecting aortic aneurysm
Pancreatic: pancreatitis
Metabolic: uremia, DKA
Trauma

Right lower quadrant (RLQ)

Intestinal: acute appendicitis, regional enteritis, incarcerated hernia, cecal diverticulitis, intestinal obstruction, perforated ulcer, perforated cecum, Meckel diverticulitis
Reproductive: ectopic pregnancy, ovarian cyst, torsion of ovarian cyst, salpingitis, tubo-ovarian abscess, mittelschmerz, endometriosis, seminal vesiculitis
Renal: renal and ureteral calculi, neoplasms, pyelonephritis
Vascular: leaking aortic aneurysm
Psoas abscess
Trauma
Cholecystitis

Left lower quadrant (LLQ)

Intestinal: diverticulitis, intestinal obstruction, perforated ulcer, inflammatory bowel disease, perforated descending colon, inguinal hernia, neoplasm, appendicitis

Reproductive: ectopic pregnancy, ovarian cyst, torsion of ovarian cyst, tubo-ovarian abscess, mittelschmerz, endometriosis; seminal vesiculitis

Renal: renal or ureteral calculi, pyelonephritis, neoplasm

Vascular: leaking aortic aneurysm

Psoas abscess

Trauma

10.2   AMENORRHEA

Hypothalamic dysfunction: defective synthesis or release of LRH, anorexia nervosa, stress, exercise

Pituitary dysfunction: neoplasm, postpartum hemorrhage, surgery, radiotherapy

Ovarian dysfunction: gonadal dysgenesis, 17-α-hydroxylase deficiency, premature ovarian failure, polycystic ovarian disease, gonadal stromal tumors

Uterovaginal abnormalities
  * Congenital: imperforate hymen, imperforate cervix, imperforate or absent vagina, müllerian agenesis
  * Acquired: destruction of endometrium with curettage (Asherman's syndrome), closure of cervix or vagina caused by traumatic injury

Other: metabolic diseases (liver, kidney), malnutrition, rapid weight loss, exogenous obesity, endocrine abnormalities (Cushing's syndrome, Graves' disease, hypothyroidism)

10.3   ASCITES

Hypoalbuminemia: nephrotic syndrome, protein-losing gastroenteropathy, starvation

Cirrhosis

Hepatic congestion: CHF, constrictive pericarditis, tricuspid insufficiency, hepatic vein obstruction (Budd-Chiari syndrome), inferior vena cava or portal vein obstruction

Peritoneal infections: TB and other bacterial infections, fungal diseases, parasites

Neoplasms: primary hepatic neoplasms, metastases to liver or peritoneum, lymphomas, leukemias, myeloid metaplasia

Lymphatic obstruction: mediastinal tumors, trauma to the thoracic duct, filariasis

Ovarian disease: Meigs' syndrome, struma ovarii

Chronic pancreatitis or pseudocyst: pancreatic ascites

Leakage of bile: bile ascites

Urinary obstruction or trauma: urine ascites

Myxedema

Chylous ascites

ATAXIA

Vertebral—basilar artery ischemia
Diabetic neuropathy
Tabes dorsalis
Vitamin B_{12} deficiency
Multiple sclerosis and other demyelinating diseases
Meningomyelopathy
Cerebellar neoplasms, hemorrhage, abscess, infarct
Nutritional (Wernicke's encephalopathy)
Paraneoplastic syndromes
Parainfectious: Guillain-Barré syndrome, acute ataxia of childhood and
    young adults
Toxins: phenytoin, alcohol, sedatives, organophosphates
Wilson's disease (hepatolenticular degeneration)
Hypothyroidism
Myopathy
Cerebellar and spinocerebellar degeneration: ataxia telengiectasia, Fried-
    reich's ataxia
Frontal lobe lesions: tumors, thrombosis of anterior cerebral artery, hydro-
    cephalus
Labyrinthine   destruction: neoplasm,   injury,   inflammation,   compres-
    sion
Hysteria

10.5   **BACK PAIN**

Trauma: injury to bone, joint, or ligament
Mechanical: pregnancy, obesity, fatigue, scoliosis
Degenerative: osteoarthritis
Infections: osteomyelitis, subarachnoid or spinal abscess, TB, meningitis
Metabolic: osteoporosis, osteomalacia
Vascular: leaking aortic aneurysm, subarachnoid or spinal hemorrhage/in-
    farction
Neoplastic: myeloma, Hodgkin's disease, carcinoma of pancreas, metastatic
    neoplasm from breast, prostate, lung
GI: penetrating ulcer, pancreatitis, cholelithiasis, inflammatory bowel disease
Renal: hydronephrosis, calculus, neoplasm
Hematologic: sickle cell crisis, acute hemolysis
Gynecologic: neoplasm of uterus, ovary, dysmenorrhea, salpingitis, uterine
    prolapse
Inflammatory: ankylosing spondylitis, psoriatic arthritis, Reiter's syndrome
Lumbosacral strain
Psychogenic: malingering, hysteria, anxiety

10.6   **CARDIAC MURMURS**

Systolic
Mitral regurgitation (MR)
Tricuspid regurgitation (TR)
Ventricular septal defect (VSD)
Aortic stenosis (AS)

Idiopathic hypertrophic subaortic stenosis (IHSS)
Pulmonic stenosis (PS)
Innocent murmur of childhood
Coarctation of aorta

Diastolic

Aortic regurgitation (AR)
Atrial myxoma
Mitral stenosis (MS)
Pulmonary artery branch stenosis
Tricuspid stenosis (TS)
Graham-Steel murmur (diastolic decrescendo murmur heard in severe pulmonary hypertension)
Pulmonary regurgitation (PR)
Severe mitral regurgitation (MR)
Austin Flint murmur (diastolic rumble heard in severe AR)
Severe VSD and patent ductus arteriosus

Continuous

Patent ductus arteriosus
Pulmonary AV fistula

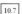 **CHEST PAIN (NONPLEURITIC)**

Cardiac: myocardial ischemia/infarction, myocarditis
Esophageal: spasm, rupture, esophagitis, ulceration, neoplasm, achalasia, diverticula, foreign body
Referred pain from subdiaphragmatic GI structures
- Gastric and duodenal: hiatal hernia, alcoholic gastritis, neoplasm, PUD
- Gallbladder and biliary: cholecystitis, cholelithiasis, impacted stone, neoplasm
- Pancreatic: pancreatitis, neoplasm
Dissecting aortic aneurysm
Pain originating from skin, breasts, and musculoskeletal structures: herpes zoster, mastitis, cervical spondylosis
Mediastinal tumors: lymphoma, thymoma
Pulmonary: neoplasm, pneumonia, pulmonary embolism/infarction
Psychoneurosis
Chest pain associated with mitral valve prolapse

10.8   **CHEST PAIN (PLEURITIC)**

Cardiac: peridarditis, postpericardiotomy/Dressler syndrome
Pulmonary: pneumothorax, hemothorax embolism/infarction, pneumonia, empyema, neoplasm, bronchiectasis, TB, carcinomatous effusion
GI: liver abscess, pancreatitis, Whipple's disease with associated pericarditis
Subdiaphragmatic abscess
Pain originating from skin and musculoskeletal tissues: costochondritis, chest wall trauma, fractured rib, interstinial fibrositis, myositis, strain of pectoralis muscle, herpes zoster, soft tissue and bone tumors
Collagen-vascular diseases with pleuritis
Psychoneurosis
Familial mediterranean fever (FMF)

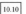 **COMA**

Vascular: hemorrhage, thrombosis, embolism
CNS infections: meningitis, encephalitis, cerebral abscess
Cerebral neoplasms with herniation
Head injury: subdural hematoma, cerebral concussion, cerebral contusion
Drugs: narcotics, sedatives, hypnotics
Ingestion or inhalation of toxins: CO, alcohol, lead
Metabolic disturbances:
- Hypoxia
- Hypoglycemia, hyperglycemia
- Electrolyte disorders

- Acid-base disorders
- Hepatic failure
- Uremia

Hypothyroidism
Hypothermia, hyperthermia
Hypotension, malignant hypertension
Postictal

10.10 **CONSTIPATION**

Intestinal obstruction
- Fecal impaction
- GI neoplasm
- Gallstone ileus
- Adhesions
- Volvulus
- Intussusception

- Inflammatory bowel disease
- Diverticular disease
- Strangulated femoral hernia
- Tuberculous stricture
- Ameboma
- Hematoma bowel wall secondary to trauma or anticoagulants

Poor dietary habits: insufficient bulk in diet, inadequate fluid intake
Change from daily routine: travel, hospital admission, physical inactivity
Acute abdominal conditions: renal colic, salpingitis, biliary colic, appendicitis
Hypercalcemia or hypokalemia
Irritable bowel syndrome
Painful anal conditions: hemorrhoids, rectal fissure
Decreased intestinal peristalsis: old age, spinal cord injuries, myxedema, diabetes, multiple sclerosis, and other neurologic diseases
Drugs: codeine, morphine, probanthine
Hirschsprung's disease, meconium ileus, congenital atresia in infants

10.11 **DYSPHAGIA**

Esophageal obstruction: neoplasm, foreign body, achalasia, stricture, spasm, esophageal web, diverticulum
Peptic esophagitis with stricture
External esophageal compression: neoplasms (thyroid neoplasm, lymphoma, mediastinal tumors), aortic aneurysm, vertebral spurs, aberrant right subclavian artery (dysphagia lusoria)
Hiatal hernia
Oropharyngeal lesions: pharyngitis, glossitis, stomatitis, neoplasms
Hysteria: globus hystericus
Neurologic and/or neuromuscular disturbances: bulbar paralysis, myasthenia gravis

Toxins: poisoning, botulism, tetanus, postdiphtheric dysphagia
Systemic diseases: scleroderma, amyloidosis, dermatomyositis
Candida and herpes esophagitis
Presby esophagus

| 10.12 | **DYSPNEA**

Upper airway obstruction: trauma, neoplasm. epiglottitis, laryngeal edema,
   tongue retraction, laryngospasm, abductor paralysis of vocal cords, aspi-
   ration of foreign body
Lower airway obstruction: neoplasm, COPD, asthma, aspiration of foreign
   body
Pulmonary infection: pneumonia, abscess, empyema, TB, bronchiectasis
Pulmonary hypertension
Pulmonary embolism/infarction
Parenchymal lung disease
Pulmonary vascular congestion
Cardiac disease: ASHD, valvular lesions, cardiac dysrhythmias, cardiomy-
   opathy
Space-occupying lesions: neoplasm, large hiatal hernia, pleural effusions
Disease of chest wall: severe kyphoscoliosis, fractured ribs, sternal compres-
   sion, morbid obesity
Neurologic dysfunction: Guillain-Barré syndrome, botulism, polio, spinal
   cord injury
Interstitial pulmonary disease: sarcoidosis, collagen vascular diseases, DIP,
   Hamman-Rich pneumonitis
Pneumoconioses: silicosis, berylliosis
Mesothelioma
Pneumothorax, hemothorax, pleural effusion
Inhalation of toxins
Cholinergic drug intoxication
Carcinoid syndrome
Anemia
Hyperthyroidism
Diaphragmatic compression caused by abdominal distention, subphrenic ab-
   scess
Excessive lung resection
Metabolic abnormalities
Sepsis
Atelectasis
Psychoneurosis
Diaphragmatic paralysis

| 10.13 | **EDEMA OF LOWER EXTREMITIES**

CHF
Hepatic cirrhosis
Nephrosis
Myxedema
Lymphedema
Pregnancy
Abdominal mass: neoplasm, cyst

Venous compression from abdominal aneurysm
Varicose veins
Bilateral cellulitis
Bilateral thrombophlebitis
Venous thrombosis
Retroperitoneal fibrosis

| 10.14 | FEVER AND RASH

Drug hypersensitivity: penicillin, sulfonamides, thiazides, anticonvulsants, etc.
Viral infection: measles, rubella, varicella, erythema infectiosum, roseola, enterovirus infection, viral hepatitis, infectious mononucleosis
Bacterial infection: meningococcemia, staphylococcemia, scarlet fever, typhoid fever, *Pseudomonas* bacteremia, Rocky Mountain spotted fever, Lyme disease, secondary syphilis, bacterial endocarditis
Serum sickness
Erythema multiforme
Erythema marginatum
Erythema nodosum
SLE
Dermatomyositis
Allergic vasculitis
Pityriasis rosea
Herpes zoster

| 10.15 | GASTROINTESTINAL BLEEDING

Upper GI bleeding (GI bleeding originating above the ligament of Treitz)

Oral or pharyngeal lesions: swallowed blood from nose or oropharynx
Swallowed hemoptysis
Esophageal: varices, ulceration, esophagitis, Mallory-Weiss tear, carcinoma, trauma
Gastric: peptic ulcer (including Cushing and Curling's, ulcers), gastritis, angiodysplasia, gastric neoplasms, hiatal hernia, gastric diverticulum, pseudoxanthoma elasticum
Duodenal: peptic ulcer, duodenitis, angiodysplasia, aortoduodenal fistula, duodenal diverticulum, duodenal tumors, carcinoma of ampulla of Vater
Biliary: hematobilia

Lower GI bleeding (GI bleeding originating below the ligament of Treitz

Small intestine
Ischemic bowel disease
Small bowel neoplasm: leiomyomas, carcinoids
Hereditary hemorrhagic telangiectasia (Osler-Webber-Rendu syndrome)
Meckel's diverticulum and other small intestine diverticula
Aortoenteric fistula
Intestinal hemangiomas: blue rubber-bleb nevi, intestinal hemangiomas, cutaneous vascular nevi

Hamarthomatous polyps: Peutz-Jeghers syndrome (intestinal polyps, muco-
cutaneous pigmentation)
Infections of small bowel: tuberculous enteritis, enteritis necroticans
Volvulus
Intussusception
Lymphoma of small bowel
Irradiation ileitis
AV malformation of small intestine
Inflammatory bowel disease
Polyarteritis nodosa
OTHERS: Pancreatoenteric fistulas, Schöenlein-Henoch purpura, Ehler-Danlos
syndrome, SLE, amyloidosis
Colon
Carcinoma (particularly left colon)
Diverticular disease
Inflammatory bowel disease
Ischemic colitis
Colonic polyps
Vascular abnormalities: angiodysplasia, vascular ectasia
Radiation colitis
Infectious colitis
Aortoenteric fistula
Lymphoma of large bowel
Hemorrhoids
Anal fissure
Trauma, foreign body
Solitary rectal/cecal ulcers

10.16   HEADACHE

Vascular: migraine, cluster headaches, temporal arteritis, hypertension, cav-
ernous sinus thrombosis
Musculoskeletal: neck and shoulder muscle contraction, strain of extraocular
and/or intraocular muscles, cervical spondylosis, temporomandibular ar-
thritis
Infections: meningitis,   encephalitis,   brain   abscess,   sepsis,   sinus-
itis, osteomyelitis, parotitis
Cerebral neoplasm
Subdural hematoma
Cerebral hemorrhage/infarct
Pseudotumor cerebri
Normal pressure hydrocephalus (NPH)
Postlumbar puncture
Cerebral aneurysm, arteriovenous malformations
Posttrauma
Dental problems: abscess, periodontitis, poorly fitting dentures
Trigeminal neuralgia, glossopharyngeal neuralgia
Otitis and other ear diseases
Glaucoma and other eye diseases
Metabolic: uremia, carbon monoxide inhalation, hypoxia
Pheochromocytoma

Paget's disease of skull
Emotional, psychiatric

| 10.17 | HEMATURIA

Use the mnemonic: TICS
T (trauma): blow to kidney, insertion of Foley catheter or foreign body in urethra, prolonged and severe exercise, very rapid emptying of overdistended bladder
(tumor): hypernephroma, Wilms tumor, papillary carcinoma of the bladder, prostatic and urethral neoplasms
(toxins): turpentine, phenols, sulfonamides, cyclophosphamide
I (infections): glomerulonephritis, TB, cystitis, prostatitis, urethritis, schistosoma hemobotium, yellow fever, blackwater fever
(inflammatory process): Goodpasture's syndrome, periarteritis, postirradiation
C (calculi): renal, ureteral, bladder, urethra
(cysts): simple cysts, polycystic disease
(congenital anomalies): hemangiomas, aneurysms, AVM
S (surgery): invasive procedures, prostatic resection, cystoscopy
(sickle cell disease and other hematologic disturbances): hemophilia, thrombocytopenia, anticoagulants
(somewhere else): bleeding genitals, factitious (drug addicts)

| 10.18 | HEMOPTYSIS

Cardiovascular

Pulmonary embolism/infarction
Left ventricular failure
Mitral stenosis
AV fistula
Severe hypertension
Erosion of aortic aneurysm

Pulmonary

Neoplasm (primary or metastatic)
Infection
* Pneumonia: *Streptococcus pneumoniae* (pneumococcal), *Klebsiella pneumoniae* (Friedländer bacillus)
* Bronchiectasis
* Abscess
* TB
* Bronchitis
* Fungal and parasitic infections
Wegener's granulomatosis
Goodpasture's syndrome
Trauma (needle biopsy, foreign body, right heart catheterization, prolonged and severe cough)
Cystic fibrosis
Pulmonary sequestration

Other

Epistaxis
Laryngeal bleeding (laryngitis, laryngeal neoplasm)
Hematologic disorders (clottings abnormalities, thrombocytopenia)

| 10.19 | HEPATOMEGALY

Frequent jaundice

Infectious hepatitis
Toxic hepatitis
Carcinoma: liver, pancreas, bile ducts, metastatic neoplasm to liver
Cirrhosis
Obstruction of common bile duct
Alcoholic hepatitis
Biliary cirrhosis
Cholangitis
Hemochromatosis with cirrhosis

Infrequent jaundice

CHF
Amyloidosis
Liver abscess
Sarcoidosis
Infectious mononucleosis
Alcoholic fatty infiltration
Lymphoma
Leukemia
Budd-Chiari syndrome
Myelofibrosis with myeloid metaplasia
Familial hyperlipoproteinemia type 1
OTHER: amebiasis, hydatid disease of liver, schistosomiasis, kala-azar (*Leishmania donovani*), Hurler's syndrome, Gaucher's disease, kwashiorkor

| 10.20 | HIRSUTISM

Idiopathic: familial, possibly increased sensitivity to androgens
Menopause
Polycystic ovarian syndrome
Drugs: androgens, anabolic steroids, methyltestosterone, minoxidil diazoxide, phenytoin, glucocorticoids, cyclosporine
Congenital adrenal hyperplasia
Adrenal virilizing tumor
Ovarian virilizing tumor: arrhenoblastoma, hilus cell tumor
Pituitary adenoma
Cushing's syndrome
Hypothyroidism (congenital and juvenile)
Acromegaly
Testicular feminization

| 10.21 | JAUNDICE |

Predominance of direct (conjugated) bilirubin

Extrahepatic obstruction:
- Common duct abnormalities: calculi, neoplasm, stricture, cyst, sclerosing cholangitis
- Metastatic carcinoma
- Pancreatic carcinoma, pseudocyst
- Ampullary carcinoma

Hepatocellular disease: hepatitis, cirrhosis
Drugs: estrogens, phenothiazines, captopril, methyltestosterone
Cholestatic jaundice of pregnancy
Hereditary disorders: Dubin-Johnson's syndrome, Rotor's syndrome
Recurrent benign intrahepatic cholestasis

Predominance of indirect (unconjugated) bilirubin

Hemolysis: hereditary and acquired hemolytic anemias
Inefficient marrow production
Impaired hepatic conjugation: chloramphenicol, pregnanediol
Neonatal jaundice
Hereditary disorders: Gilbert's syndrome, Crigler-Najjar's syndrome
Hepatic congestion secondary to right sided heart failure

| 10.22 | LYMPHADENOPATHY |

Generalized

AIDS, ARC
Lymphoma: Hodgkin's disease, non–Hodgkin's lymphoma
Leukemias
Infectious mononucleosis
Rheumatoid arthritis (more common in chronic juvenile arthritis)
Diffuse skin infection: generalized furunculosis, multiple thick bites
Parasitic infections: toxoplasmosis, filariasis, leishmaniosis
Serum sickness
Collagen vascular diseases
Dengue (arbovirus infection)
Sarcoidosis
Drugs: INH, hydantoin derivatives, antithyroid and antileprosy drugs
Secondary syphilis

Localized

Any of the causes of generalized lymphadenopathy
Draining lymphatics from local infection: infected furuncle, throat infection, dental abscess, lymphogranuloma venereum, brucellosis, parasitic infections, cat-scratch disease
Neoplasm
TB (scrofula)

| 10.23 | MEDIASTINAL MASSES OR WIDENING ON CHEST X-RAY FILM |

Lymphoma: Hodgkin disease and non-Hodgkin lymphoma
Sarcoidosis
Vascular: aortic aneurysm, ectasia or tortuosity of aorta or bronchocephalic
vessels
Carcinoma: lungs, esophagus
Esophageal diverticula
Hiatal hernia
Prominent pulmonary outflow tract: pulmonary hypertension, pulmonary em-
bolism, right-to-left shunts
Trauma: mediastinal hemorrhage
Pneumomediastinum
Lymphodenopathy caused by silicosis, pneumoconiosis
Leukemias
Infections: TB, viral, mycoplasma, fungal
Substernal thyroid
Thymoma
Teratoma
Bronchogenic cyst
Pericardial cyst
Neurofibroma, neurosarcoma, ganglioneuroma

| 10.24 | METASTATIC NEOPLASMS |

Bone	**Brain**	**Liver**	**Lung**
Breast	Lung	Colon	Breast
Lung	Breast	Stomach	Colon
Prostate	Melanoma	Pancreas	Kidney
Thyroid	GU tract	Breast	Testis
Kidney	Colon	Lymphomas	Stomach
Bladder	Sinuses	Bronchus	Thyroid
Endometrium	Sarcoma	Lung	Melanoma
Cervix	Skin		Sarcoma

| 10.25 | PARAPLEGIA |

Trauma: penetrating wounds to the motor cortex, fracture-dislocation of the
vertebral column with compression of spinal cord or cauda equina, pro-
lapsed disk, electrical injuries
Neoplasm: parasagittal region, vertebrae, meninges, spinal cord, cauda
equina, Hodgkin's disease, NHL, leukemic deposits, pelvic neoplasms
Multiple sclerosis and other demyelinating disorders
Mechanical compression of spinal cord, cauda equina, or lumbosacral plexus:
Paget's disease, kyphoscoliosis, herniation of intervertebral disc, spondy-
losis, ankylosing spondylitis, rheumatoid arthritis, aortic aneurysm
Infections: spinal abscess, syphilis, TB, poliomyelitis, leprosy
Thrombosis of superior sagittal sinus
Polyneuritis: Gullain-Barré syndrome, diabetes, alcohol, beri-beri, heavy
metals

Heredofamilial muscular dystrophies
Amyotrophic lateral sclerosis
Congenital and familial conditions: syringomyelia, meningomyelocele, myelodysplasia
Hysteria

| 10.26 | PLEURAL EFFUSIONS

Exudative

Neoplasm: bronchogenic carcinoma, breast carcinoma, mesothelioma, lymphoma, ovarian carcinoma, multiple myeloma, leukemia
Infections: viral pneumonia, bacterial pneumonia, mycoplasma, TB, fungal and parasitic diseases
Trauma
Collagen-vascular diseases: SLE, RA, scleroderma, polyarteritis, Wegener's granulomatosis
Pulmonary infarction
Pancreatitis
Postcardiotomy/Dressler's syndrome
Drug-induced lupus erythematosus (hydralazine, procainamide)
Postabdominal surgery
Ruptured esophagus
Chronic effusion secondary to congestive failure

Transudative

CHF
Hepatic cirrhosis
Nephrotic syndrome
Hypoproteinemia from any cause
Meig's syndrome

| 10.27 | POLYURIA

Diabetes mellitus
Diabetes insipidus
Primary polydipsia (compulsive waterdrinking)
Hypercalcemia
Hypokalemia
Postobstructive uropathy
Diuretic phase of renal failure
Drugs: diuretics, caffeine, lithium
Sickle cell trait or disease, chronic pyelonephritis (failure to concentrate urine)
Anxiety, cold weather

| 10.28 | POPLITEAL SWELLING

Phlebitis (superficial)
Lymphadenitis
Trauma: fractured tibia or fibula, contusion, traumatic neuroma
Deep vein thrombosis
Ruptured varicose vein

Baker's cyst
Popliteal abscess
Osteomyelitis
Ruptured tendon
Aneurysm of popliteal artery
Neoplasm: lipoma, osteogenic sarcoma, neurofibroma, fibrosarcoma

| 10.29 | PROTEINURIA

Nephrotic syndrome as a result of primary renal diseases
Malignant hypertension
Multiple myeloma
CHF
Diabetes mellitus
SLE
Sickle cell disease
Goodpasture's syndrome
Malaria
Amyloidosis
Tubular lesions: cystinosis
Functional (after heavy exercise)
Pyelonephritis
Constrictive pericarditis
Renal vein thrombosis
Toxic nephropathies: heavy metals, drugs
Radiation nephritis
Orthostatic (postural) proteinuria

| 10.30 | SHOULDER PAIN

With local findings in shoulder

Trauma: contusion, fracture, muscle strain, trauma to spinal cord
Arthrosis, arthritis, rheumatoid arthritis, ankylosing spondylitis
Bursitis, synovitis, tendinitis, tenosynovitis
Aseptic (avascular) necrosis
Local infection: septic arthritis, ostoemyelitis, abscess, herpes zoster, TB

Without local findings in shoulder

Cardiovascular disorders: ischemic heart disease, pericarditis, aortic aneurysm
Subdiaphragmatic abscess, liver abscess
Cholelithiasis, cholecystitis
Pulmonary lesions: apical bronchial carcinoma, pleurisy, pneumothorax, pneumonia
GI lesions: PUD, gastric neoplasm, peptic esophagitis
Pancreatic lesions: carcinoma, calculi, pancreatitis
CNS abnormalities: neoplasm, vascular abnormalities
Multiple sclerosis
Syringomyelia
Polymyositis/dermatomyositis
Psychogenic
Polymyalgia rheumatica

| 10.31 | SPLENOMEGALY |

Hepatic cirrhosis
Neoplastic involvement: CML, CLL, lymphoma, polycythemia vera, myeloid metaplasia, multiple myeloma
Bacterial infections: TB, SBE, typhoid fever, splenic abscess
Viral infections: infectious mononucleosis, viral hepatitis
Gaucher disease and other lipid storage diseases
Sarcoidosis
Parasitic infections (malaria, kala-azar, histoplasmosis)
Hereditary and acquired hemolytic anemias
Idiopathic thrombocytopenic purpura (ITP)
Collagen-vascular disorders: SLE, rheumatoid arthritis (Felty's syndrome), polyarteritis nodosa
Serum sickness, drug hypersensitivity reaction
Splenic cysts and benign tumors: hemangioma, lymphangioma
Thrombosis of splenic or portal vein

| 10.32 | VERTIGO |

Peripheral

Otitis media
Acute labyrinthitis
Vestibular neuronitis
Benign positional vertigo
Ménierè's disease
Ototoxic drugs: streptomycin, gentamycin
Lesions of the eighth nerve: acoustic neuroma, meningioma, mononeuropathy, metastatic carcinoma
Mastoiditis

CNS or systemic

Vertebrobasilar artery insufficiency
Posterior fossa tumor or other brain tumors
Infarction/hemorrhage of cerebral cortex, cerebellum, or brainstem
Basilar migraine
Metabolic: drugs, hypoxia, anemia, fever
Hypotension/severe hypertension
Multiple sclerosis
CNS infections: viral, bacterial
Temporal lobe epilepsy
Arnold-Chiari malformation, syringobulbia

| 10.33 | VOMITING |

GI disturbances:
- Obstruction: esophageal, pyloric, intestinal
- Infections: viral or bacterial enteritis, viral hepatitis, food poisoning
- Pancreatitis
- Appendicitis
- Biliary colic
- Peritonitis

- Perforated bowel
- Diabetic gastroparesis
- OTHER: Gastritis, PUD, IBD, GI tract neoplasms

Drugs: morphine, digitalis, cytotoxic agents, bromocriptine

Severe pain: MI, renal colic

Metabolic disorders: uremia, acidosis/alkalosis, hyperglycemia, DKA, thyrotoxicosis

Trauma: blows to the testicles, epigastrium

Vertigo

Reye's syndrome

Increased intracranial pressure

CNS disturbances: trauma, hemorrhage, infarction, neoplasm, infection, hypertensive encephalopathy, migraine

Radiation sickness

Vomiting associated with pregnancy

Motion sickness

Bulimia, anorexia nervosa

Psychogenic: emotional disturbances, offensive sights or smells

Irritation of the fauces

Severe coughing

Cardiovascular Diseases

11

11.1 ANGINA PECTORIS

Definition

Angina pectoris is characterized by discomfort that occurs when the myocardium's demand for oxygen exceeds its supply. It can be classified into the following types:

1. Chronic (stable) angina: angina that usually follows a precipitating event, such as climbing stairs, sexual intercourse, heavy meal, or cold weather. It is usually of the same severity as previous attacks and is relieved by the usual dose of nitroglycerin. Stable angina is caused by a fixed coronary artery obstruction secondary to atherosclerosis.
2. Unstable angina
   a. Angina of recent onset
   b. Increasing severity, duration, or frequency of chronic angina
   c. Angina at rest or with minimal exertion
3. Variant angina (Prinzmetal's angina): angina that occurs when the patient is at rest and that manifests itself electrocardiographically with episodic ST segment elevations. It is caused by coronary artery spasms with or without superimposed coronary artery disease. These patients are also more likely to develop ventricular dysrhythmias.

Risk[9,45]

1. Uncontrollable factors
   a. Age
   b. Male sex
   c. Genetic predisposition
2. Preventable factors
   a. Smoking (risk is almost doubled)
   b. Hypertension (risk is doubled if systolic BP is >180 mm Hg)
   c. Hyperlipidemia
   d. Glucose intolerance
   e. Obesity
   f. Hypothyroidism

Mechanisms contributing to myocardial ischemia[14]

1. Progression of atherosclerosis
2. Acute coronary thrombosis
3. Coronary artery spasm
4. Platelet aggregation

89

Clinical presentation

Although there is significant individual variation, the patient usually has substernal pain (pressure, tightness, heaviness, sharp pain, sensation similar to intestinal gas or dysphagia). The pain is usually of short duration (30 seconds to 30 minutes) and is often accompanied by shortness of breath, nausea, diaphoresis, and numbness or pain in the left arm or shoulder.

Differential diagnosis

Noncardiac pain mimicking angina may be caused by:
1. Pulmonary diseases such as pulmonary hypertension, pulmonary embolism, pleurisy, pneumothorax, or pneumonia
2. GI disorders such as peptic ulcer disease, pancreatitis, esophageal spasm, esophageal reflux, cholecystitis, or cholelithiasis
3. Musculoskeletal conditions such as costochondritis, chest wall trauma, cervical arthritis with radiculopathy, muscle strain, or myositis
4. Acute aortic dissection
5. Herpes zoster

Diagnostic studies

1. The most important diagnostic factor is the history
2. The physical exam is of little diagnostic help and may be totally normal in many patients
   a. Listen for the presence of heart murmurs to exclude a valvular cause for the chest pain (i.e., MVP, AS, IHSS, MS)
   b. Look for evidence of hyperlipidemia, hypertension, or evidence of cardiac decompensation
3. An ECG taken during the acute episode may show transient T wave inversion or ST segment depression/elevation, but some patients may have a normal tracing
4. Chest x-ray films may show cardiomegaly or pulmonary vascular congestion
5. Echocardiogram is indicated for patients with suspected valvular abnormalities
6. Multiple gated acquisition (MUGA) scan to determine left ventricular ejection fraction in selected patients
7. Exercise tolerance test to evaluate patients with angina
   a. Indications
      (1) Evaluation of chest pain syndromes
          (a) Typical angina or effort-induced angina
          (b) Atypical chest pain
      (2) Evaluation of exercise tolerance
          (a) Post MI (modified exercise tolerance test)
          (b) Post-CABG, postangioplasty
          (c) Evaluate effectiveness of medical therapy
      (3) Evaluation of dysrhythmias
          (a) Sick sinus syndrome
          (b) PVCs (benign PVCs usually disappear with exercise)
   b. Contraindications
      (1) Aortic stenosis
      (2) Idiopathic hypertrophic subaortic stenosis (IHSS)
      (3) Unstable angina

    (4) Poorly controlled dysrhythmias, malignant PVCs

    (5) ECG suggestive of ischemia

    (6) Severe COPD

    (7) Clinically manifested CHF

  c. Choice of protocols[10]

    (1) Bruce protocol is preferred for patients with minimum symptomatic limitation; it entails a higher initial workload and greater work increments

    (2) Naughton protocol is preferred for post-MI, post-CABG, and for more debilitated patients; it entails a lower initial workload and smaller increments than the Bruce protocol

  d. Interpretation: both protocols aim at eliciting a diagnostic response within 6 to 15 minutes; a stress test is generally considered positive for ischemia if:

    (1) ST segment depression

      (a) ≥ 1 mm flat or downsloping ST segment depression at 0.08 seconds after the J point[10]

      (b) Early onset (within 3 minutes of exercise)

      (c) Persists beyond 6 minutes of recovery phase

    (2) Patient develops chest pain

    (3) Patient develops hypotension (normally in exercise there is an increase in systolic BP because of an increase in stroke volume)

    (4) Patient develops significant dysrhythmias

    (5) ST segment elevation during exercise, although uncommon, provides reliable information about the location of the underlying coronary lesion (e.g., anterior ST segment elevation generally indicates left anterior descending coronary disease, whereas inferior ST segment elevation is suggestive of a lesion in or proximal to the posterior descending artery)[37]

8. Thallium stress test: viable myocardial cells extract thallium 201 from the blood

  a. An absent thallium uptake (cold spot on thallium scan) is an indicator of an absence of blood flow to an area of the myocardium

  b. A fixed defect on thallium scanning indicates MI at that site, whereas a defect that reperfuses suggests myocardial ischemia

  c. The following are indications for thallium 201 scintigraphy:

    (1) Evaluation of patients whose resting ECG may cause false positive results on conventional stress test:

      (a) Patients with left bundle branch block (LBBB)

      (b) Patients with left ventricular hypertrophy (LVH)

      (c) Patients with sloping of ST segment secondary to digitalis administration

    (2) Evaluation of chest pain in patients with Wolff-Parkinson-White (WPW) syndrome

    (3) Evaluation of young female patients with chest pain (high rates of false positives with conventional stress test)

9. Ambulatory (Holter) electrocardiographic monitoring can detect silent ischemia (ischemic ECG changes without accompanying symptoms), which occurs in more than 50% of patients with unstable angina, despite intensive medical therapy, and identifies a subset of patients at risk for early unfavorable outcomes[22]

Table 11-1   Common nitrate preparations[1,31,40]

Drug	Dosage	Onset of Action	Duration of Action
Nitroglycerin			
Sublingual	0.3-0.6 mg prn	1-3 min	30-60 min
2% Ointment	2.5-12.5 cm q4-6h	15 min	3-6 hr
Transdermal	5, 10, 15, 20, 30 cm^2 q24h	30-60 min	Up to 24 hr
Sustained release (SR)	Cap: 2.5, 6.5, 9 mg q8-12h Tab: 1.3, 2.6, 6.5 mg q8-12h	Hours	8-12 hr
Intravenous (IV)	50 mg/500 ml, start at 5 μg/min	Immediate	Minutes
Isosorbide dinitrate	Tab: 10-60 mg q4-6h	30 min	3-6 hr
	Chewable tab: 10-40 mg q4-6h	15-30 min	3-6 hr

Medical therapy

Medical therapy consists of aggressive modification of the preventable risk factors (weight reduction in obese patients, regular exercise program, diet low in cholesterol and sodium, cessation of cigarette smoking) and combination drug therapy with nitrates, β-adrenergic blockers, and calcium channel blockers.

1. Nitrates cause venodilatation and relaxation of vascular smooth muscle; the decreased venous return caused by venodilatation decreases diastolic ventricular wall tension (preload) and thereby reduces the mechanical activity (and myocardial O_2 consumption) during systole (Table 11-1 describes common nitrate preparations).

2. β-adrenergic blocking agents achieve their major antianginal effect by reducing heart rate and systolic blood pressure (Table 11-2 describes commonly used β-adrenergic blockers in patients with angina).

3. Calcium channel blockers play a major role in preventing and terminating myocardial ischemia induced by coronary artery spasm. They all reduce the influx of calcium into the myocardial and vascular smooth muscle cells through slow channels, but they differ in their mode of action. Nifedipine exerts its antianginal effect through arterial vasodilation (both coronary and peripheral), thereby lowering left ventricular systolic wall tension and increasing coronary blood flow. Both diltiazem and verapamil produce coronary vasodilation and decrease heart rate. However, verapamil has more pronounced vasodilatory and AV nodal activity than diltiazem (Table 11-3).

Table 11-2 Commonly used β-blockers in patients with angina[21,31,54]

Drug	Initial Dosage (PO)	Usual Maintenance Dosage	Cardioselectivity	Lipid Solubility
Atenolol (Tenormin)	50 mg qd	50-100 mg qd	(up to 100 mg)	+
Metoprolol (Lopressor)	50 mg bid or 100 mg qd	50-100 mg bid	(up to 100 mg)	++
Nadolol (Corgard)	40 mg qd	80-240 mg qd	No	+
Pindolol (Visken)	10 mg bid	5-10 mg bid	No	++
Propranolol (Inderal)	10-20 mg bid	40-320 mg bid	No	+++
Timolol (Blocadren)	10 mg bid	10-20 mg bid	No	++

KEY: +, Mild; ++, moderate; +++, significant.

Table 11-3 Calcium channel antagonists[3,6,21]

	Verapamil (Calan, Isoptin)	Diltiazem (Cardizem)	Nifedipine (Procardia, Adalat)
Dosage (PO)	80-160 mg q8h	30-90 mg q6-8h	10-40 mg q6-8h
Coronary vasodilatation	↑	↑	↑
Cardiac output	↑/→	N	↑↑
Peripheral vasodilatation	↑↑	↑	↑↑
Hypotension	↑	N	N
AV nodal conduction	↑↑	↑	↑
Peripheral edema	↑	→	↑
Use with β blockers	Caution	Yes	Yes
Major side effects	AV block, left ventricular failure, constipation	Sinus bradycardia, headache, flushing	Hypotension, edema, headache, flushing

KEY: ↑, Increases; ↓, decreases; N, no significant effect.

Experts also advocate daily aspirin for patients with unstable angina; dosage varies from 325 mg qd to qid. In a 2-year Canadian multicenter trial[8] the incidence of cardiac death and nonfatal MI in patients with unstable angina was 8.6% in patients given aspirin (325 mg qid) versus 17% in patients given placebos. However, the risks of chronic salicylate use (e.g., GI bleeding, bronchospasm in susceptible patients) must be considered before starting any patient on daily aspirin.

Although the efficacy of heparin in patients with unstable angina has been reported,[53] further studies are needed to fully define its role.

Surgical therapy

If the stress test indicates myocardial ischemia and the patient is a candidate for surgery or angioplasty, the patient should undergo cardiac catheterization to determine the extent of the disease. The Framingham study[9] showed that overall mortality for angina in medically treated patients is 4%. Mortality drops to 1.5% if angina is based on one- or two-vessel disease and rises to 9% if the patient has three-vessel disease and poor exercise tolerance.

Coronary artery bypass graft (CABG) surgery is recommended for patients with left main coronary disease or symptomatic three-vessel disease since the survival rate is significantly improved in these patients.[15] When CABG is done for relief of severe angina, it brings complete relief of angina in about 70% of patients and partial relief in another 20%.[27]

Percutaneous transluminal coronary angioplasty (PTCA) should be considered for patients with one- or two-vessel disease. Patients selected for PTCA must also be candidates for CABG. The type of lesions best suited for angioplasty are proximal lesions, noncalcified, concentric, and preferably shorter than 5 mm in length (should not exceed 10 mm).[27] Approximately 80% of patients will show immediate benefit after PTCA. Restenosis with recurrence of angina occurs in approximately 20% of patients, usually within the first 3 months after PTCA. In these patients PTCA can be repeated.[21]

11.2   MYOCARDIAL INFARCTION

Definition

Myocardial infarction (MI) is characterized by necrosis resulting from an insufficient supply of oxygenated blood to an area of the heart.
1. Subendocardial infarct: the area of ischemic necrosis is limited to the inner third to half of the myocardial wall
2. Transmural infarct: the area of ischemic necrosis penetrates the entire thickness of the ventricular wall

Etiology
1. Coronary atherosclerosis
2. Coronary artery spasm
3. Coronary embolism (caused by SBE, rheumatic heart disease, intracavity thrombus)
4. Periarteritis and other coronary artery inflammatory diseases
5. Dissection into the coronary arteries (aneurysmal or iatrogenic)

Contributing factors
1. Tachycardia (increased O_2 consumption, decreased diastolic filling time)
2. Left ventricular hypertrophy (increased O_2 demand)

3. Anemia (decreased O_2-carrying capacity)
4. Increased platelet aggregation (increased risk of thrombosis, coronary artery spasm via production of thromboxane A_2)

Clinical presentation

1. Crushing substernal chest pain, usually lasting longer than 30 minutes
2. The pain is unrelieved by rest or sublingual nitroglycerin or it rapidly recurs
3. The pain may radiate to the left or right arm, neck, jaw, back, shoulders, or abdomen
4. The pain may be associated with dyspnea, diaphoresis, nausea, or vomiting
5. Approximately 20% of infarctions are painless (usually in diabetic or elderly patients)

Physical findings

1. Skin may be diaphoretic, cool, with pallor (because of decreased O_2)
2. Lungs may reveal rales at the bases (indicative of CHF)
3. Heart may have an apical systolic murmur caused by mitral regurgitation secondary to papillary muscle dysfunction; an S_3 or S_4 may also be present
4. The physical exam may be completely normal

Diagnostic studies

1. ECG
   a. In transmural (Q wave) infarction there is the development of:
      (1) Inverted T waves, which indicate an area of ischemia
      (2) Elevated ST segments, which indicate an area of injury
      (3) Q waves, which indicate the area of infarction; they usually develop over 12-36 hours (Table 11-4 describes location of transmural infarction based on ECG abnormalities)
   b. In non–Q wave infarction, Q waves are absent but:
      (1) History and myocardial enzyme elevations are compatible with MI
      (2) ECG shows ST segment elevation, depression, or no change followed by T wave inversion
2. Serum enzyme studies: damaged, necrotic heart muscle releases cardiac enzymes (CK, LDH) into the bloodstream in amounts that correlate with

Table 11-4   ECG location of Q wave infarct

Area of Infarction	ECG Abnormality
Anterior wall	Q waves in V_1 - V_4
Anteroseptal	Q waves in V_1 - V_2
Anteroapical	Q waves in V_2 - V_3
Anterolateral	Q waves in V_4 - V_6, I, aV_L
Lateral wall	Q waves in I, aV_L
Inferior wall	Q waves in II, III, aV_F
Posterior wall	R > S in V_1
	Q wave in V_6

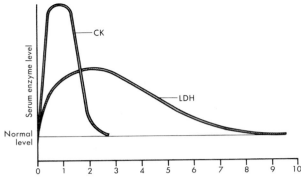

Figure 11-1
Time course of serum enzyme activity following acute MI. *CK*, Creatine kinase; *LDH*, lactic dehydrogenase.

Table 11-5   Serum enzyme concentration changes following acute MI

Enzyme	Rise	Peak	Return to Normal
CK	2-8 hr	12-36 hr	3-4 days
LDH	12-48 hr	3-6 days	8-14 days

the size of the infarct (Fig. 11-1 and Table 11-5). Other parts of the body also have these enzymes (CK in skeletal muscle and brain; LDH in RBC, liver, skeletal muscle, kidneys, and lungs) so their presence could indicate damage to extracardiac tissue. However, electrophoretic fractionation of the enzymes can pinpoint certain isoenzymes (CK-MB and LDH$_1$) that are more sensitive indicators of MI than total CK or LDH.

Therapy

Patients with acute MI can be categorized in four subsets based on their clinical presentation and hemodynamic measurements[16] (see Table 11-6). The therapeutic approach to each patient varies with the subset.
1. Subset I: uncomplicated MI
    a. IV nitroglycerin may be useful for pain control; mix 100 mg/500 ml of D$_5$W, start at 6 µg/min (2 ml/hr) and increase the dose by 6 µg/minute q5 min until:
        (1) The patient is free of chest pain
        (2) Maximum dose of 500 µg/min is reached
        (3) Blood pressure decreases below 100 mm Hg systolic
    b. Nasal O$_2$: administer at 2-4 L/min

Table 11-6 Clinical and hemodynamic subsets after acute MI

Subset	CI	PCWP
I: no pulmonary congestion or peripheral hypoperfusion	2.7 ± 0.5	12 ± 7
II: isolated pulmonary congestion	2.3 ± 0.4	23 ± 5
III: isolated peripheral hypoperfusion	1.9 ± 0.4	12 ± 5
IV: both pulmonary congestion and hypoperfusion	1.6 ± 0.6	27 ± 8

From Forrester, J.S., Diamond, G.A., Swan, H.J.C.: Am. J. Cardiol. **39**:137, 1977.
KEY: CI, Cardiac index; PCWP; pulmonary capillary wedge pressure.

   c. Morphine sulfate: 2 mg IV q5min prn for severe pain unrelieved by IV nitroglycerin
     (1) Hypotension secondary to morphine can be treated with careful IV hydration
     (2) Respiratory depression caused by morphine can be reversed with naloxone (Narcan) 0.8 mg IV
   d. Lidocaine: 1 mg/kg IV bolus followed by infusion at 1-4 mg/min is indicated if frequent, multifocal, or symptomatic PVCs are noted (prophylactic lidocaine therapy in the initial 24 hours of MI may be indicated in any patient less than 70 years old)
   e. Diet: NPO until stable, then no added salt, low-cholesterol diet
   f. Stool softener: dioctyl sulfosuccinate (Colace) 100 mg PO qd; for constipation, may use milk of magnesia 30 ml PO qhs prn (do not use in patients with renal failure)
   g. Anticoagulant therapy: minidose herapin (5000 U SC q8-12h) is particularly indicated (barring specific contraindications) in patients with anterior wall MI (30% risk for developing mural thrombosis) and in patients with very high peak creatinine kinase levels
   h. Strict bed rest: for the initial 24 hours; if the patient remains stable, gradually increase the activity and stop the minidose heparin
   i. Sedation: use short-acting benzodiazepine (e.g., oxazepam 10 mg PO q6h)
2. Subset II: these patients have left ventricular dysfunction (manifested by pulmonary congestion), but can still maintain an adequate cardiac index; therapy consists of IV nitroglycerin, diuretics (to decrease PCWP), and morphine
3. Subset III: these patients often have right ventricular and inferior wall infarcts
   a. Therapy consists of careful IV hydration with normal saline until the PCWP increases to approximately 18 mm Hg
   b. The increased PCWP should increase the cardiac output unless the patient has an extremely poor ventricular function
4. Subset IV: these patients have severe left ventricular dysfunction; therapy consists of the combined use of dobutamine and dopamine to provide inotropic stimulation

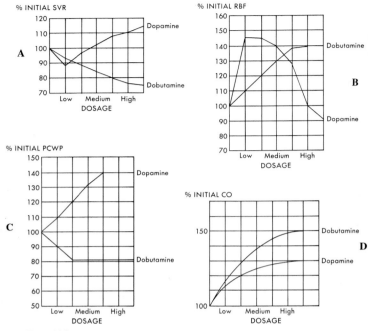

Figure 11-2
Comparison of hemodynamic responses to dobutamine and dopamine. **A,** Systemic vascular resistance. **B,** Renal blood flow. **C,** Pulmonary capillary wedge pressure. **D,** Cardiac output. Reproduced with permission from Eli Lilly and Co.

a. Dopamine also stimulates renal vasodilatation when used at low doses (Fig. 11-2)
b. An intraaortic balloon pump may be necessary to maintain cardiac output and coronary perfusion

Reduction of infarct size

If the duration of the patient's pain has been short (<4 hours, ideally <2 hours) and the hospital is equipped with a cardiac catheterization lab and adequately trained personnel, recanalization of the occluded coronary arteries may be attempted with intracoronary streptokinase, emergency percutaneous transluminal coronary angioplasty (PTCA), or both. Peripheral IV streptokinase can also be used: however, its effectiveness is less certain than intracoronary streptokinase and timing is crucial since thrombolytic therapy with IV streptokinase is most effective if given within the first 1½ hours after the onset of symptoms of acute MI.[32] The role of recombinant tissue-type plas-

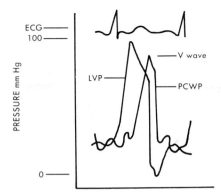

Figure 11-3
Mitral regurgitation. Note the V wave caused by regurgitation of blood in the left atrium. *LVP*, Left ventricular pressure.

minogen activator (rt-PA) in recanalizing occluded coronary arteries during acute MI remains to be fully defined.[51] Early thrombolytic therapy may leave residual ischemia in the salvaged myocardium, resulting in an increased incidence of ischemic manifestation in the post-MI recovery period, particularly if the degree of residual coronary artery stenosis is more than 60%. These patients may benefit from PTCA of the stenosed artery during the early recovery period.[33]

Complications

1. Dysrhythmias: see section 11.9 for recognition and therapy
2. Mitral regurgitation: characterized by the sudden appearance of an apical systolic murmur with radiation to the axilla; a loud first heart sound is often associated with the murmur
   a. Etiology: papillary muscle dysfunction or left ventricular aneurysm (it occurs primarily in inferior, lateral, and subendocardial infarcts)
   b. Diagnostic studies: at cardiac catheterization, the pulmonary wedge tracing shows giant V waves (Fig. 11-3)
   c. Therapy[6]
      (1) IV nitroprusside to decrease PCWP
      (2) If hypotensive, will need dopamine or dobutamine combined with nitroprusside (combined use of inotropic and vasodilator agents)
      (3) Intraaortic balloon counterpulsation (IABC) provides lifesaving physiologic support by facilitating ventricular emptying during systole and increasing retrograde coronary perfusion during diastole
      (4) Surgical repair after stabilization of the patient
      NOTE: Despite the above measures, the mortality for these patients remains extremely high

3. Right ventricular infarct: characterized by jugular venous distention, Kussmaul's sign, and hypotension without pulmonary congestion
   a. Diagnostic studies: hemodynamic monitoring shows right atrial pressure/PCWP ≥ 0.8
   b. Therapy: vigorous IV hydration
4. Ventricular septal defect (VSD): characterized by a systolic murmur at the lower left sternal border; VSD usually occurs within 2 weeks after acute MI
   a. Diagnostic studies: there is an increase in oxygen content in blood samples from the pulmonary artery when compared with blood samples from right atrium
   b. Therapy: same as for acute mitral regurgitation (see above)
5. Myocardial rupture: usually seen in elderly patients 2-4 days after MI; it is characterized by sudden hypotension and loss of consciousness, followed by electromechanical dissociation, and finally ending in death
6. Systemic embolism: characterized by sudden onset of neurologic deficit or pain in the involved area (e.g., CVA tenderness in renal artery embolism)
   a. Etiology: mural thrombi; occur most frequently with anterior wall MI
   b. Diagnostic studies:
      (1) Echocardiogram may reveal the presence of mural thrombi
      (2) Perform arteriography if peripheral embolism is suspected
      (3) Perform renal scintiscan if renal embolism is suspected
   c. Therapy: IV heparinization; embolectomy if the clot is accessible
7. Pericarditis: see section 11.8
8. Dressler's syndrome: characterized by fever, pleurisy, pericarditis, friction rub, pericardial and pleural effusions, and joint pains; usually occurs between 1 week to 6 months after MI
   a. Etiology: autoimmune disorder secondary to previous damage to the myocardium and pericardium
   b. Therapy: indomethacin 50 mg PO q6h or other nonsteroidal antiinflammatory agents; if no improvement, consider prednisone 30 mg PO bid initially, tapered off over several weeks
9. Left ventricular aneurysm
   a. Diagnostic studies: echocardiogram; ECG shows persistent ST elevations 3-4 weeks after MI
   b. Therapy: surgical excision if the aneurysm is associated with recurrent ventricular tachycardia, intractable CHF, recurrent embolization, or persistent angina despite intensive medical treatment[21]
10. Pulmonary embolism: characterized by sudden onset of tachypnea, tachycardia, and chest pain
    a. Prevention: minidose heparin (5000 U SC q12h) and early ambulation after MI
    b. Diagnostic studies: ventilation/perfusion scan; if inconclusive, follow with arteriogram
    c. Therapy: IV heparinization

Hospital mortality during acute MI

Various attempts have been made to identify patients with an increased risk of mortality during an acute MI. The classification developed by Killip and Kimball[30] categorizes patients into four major classes (Table 11-7).

Table 11-7 Killip classification during acute MI

Clinical Class	Description	Hospital Mortality
I	No heart failure (absent rales, absent S_3 gallop)	<10%
II	Heart failure (rales over ≤50% of lung fields or S_3 gallop and venous hypertension)	10-20%
III	Severe heart failure (rales over >50% of lung fields, pulmonary edema)	35-50%
IV	Cardiogenic shock	>80%

Adapted from Killip, P.T., and Kimball, J.T.: Am. J. Cardiol. **20**:457, 1967.

Evaluation of post-MI patients before discharge

1. Submaximal (low-level) treadmill test (done 1-3 weeks after MI)
   a. To assess the patient's functional capacity and formulate an at-home exercise program
   b. To determine the patient's prognosis
2. Radionuclide angiography
   a. To evaluate the patient's left ventricular ejection fraction
   b. To evaluate ventricular size and segmental wall motion
3. 24-hour Holter monitor: to evaluate patients who demonstrated significant dysrhythmias during their hospital stay
4. Echocardiogram is indicated in patients with anterior wall infarction to rule out the presence of mural thrombi

Use of β-adrenergic blocking agents after MI

The beneficial effect of β-blockers following MI has been clearly documented by several studies.[5,28,44] The timing of initiation of β-blocker therapy varies with the particular β-blocker chosen (Table 11-8).

Table 11-8 Use of β-blockers after MI[5,18,28,44]

Drug	Initiation of Therapy	Dosage
Propranolol (Inderal)	5-21 days after MI	40 mg PO tid initially, increasing gradually to 180-240 mg/day in 2-3 divided doses
Timolol (Blocadren)	7-28 days after MI	5 mg PO bid initially, increasing gradually to 10 mg PO bid
Metoprolol (Lopressor)	Within 24 hours in stabilized patients with acute MI	5 mg IV q2min up to 15 mg (if tolerated), followed by 50 mg PO q6h for 48 hours, followed by 100 mg PO bid

Before using β-blockers, the contraindications and side effects (i.e., exacerbation of CHF, exacerbation of asthma, CNS side effects) must be carefully considered. It has been estimated that up to 20% of MI survivors have absolute or relative contraindications to β-adrenergic blockade.[17]

Prognosis after MI

The prognosis following MI depends on multiple factors:

1. Use of β-blockers: the mortality of patients on a regular regimen of β-blockers shows a significant decrease when compared with that of control groups[5,28,44]
2. Presence of dysrhythmias: frequent ventricular ectopic beats ($\geq$10/hr) or repetitive forms of ventricular ectopic beats (couplets, triplets) indicate an increased risk (two to three times greater) of sudden cardiac death[46]
3. Size of infarct: the larger the infarct, the higher the post-MI mortality rate; there is a close correlation between the peak plasma CK values and survival over a 4-year period[56]
4. Site of infarct: inferior wall MI carries a better prognosis than anterior wall MI, because in anterior wall MI the damage is confined exclusively to the left ventricle (resulting in severe left ventricular dysfunction), whereas in inferior wall MI the damage is shared by both ventricles and thus the hemodynamic impact on either ventricle is lessened[47]
5. Type of infarct: although the in-hospital mortality is higher for patients with Q wave infarcts, the long-term prognosis for non-Q wave MI may be worse because these patients have a higher incidence of sudden cardiac death after hospital discharge[29]; diltiazem (30 mg initially, followed by 60 mg after 6 hours, and then 90 mg q6h if tolerated) may prevent early re-infarction and severe angina after non-Q wave infarction[20]
6. Ejection fraction after MI: the lower the left ventricular ejection fraction, the higher the mortality after MI; in one series,[48] the probability of survival was highest in patients with an ejection fraction $\geq$50% and lowest in patients with an ejection fraction $\leq$20% (a low ejection fraction associated with ventricular premature beats signifies a particularly poor prognosis)[49]
7. Presence of post-MI angina: indicates a higher mortality, particularly when angina is accompanied by new ECG changes distant from the acute infarct[50]
8. Performance on low-level exercise test: the presence of ST segment changes during the test is a predictor of higher mortality during the first year,[55] patients with a positive test after MI should undergo coronary artery catheterization to determine if angioplasty or coronary artery bypass is indicated

| 11.3 |

VALVULAR HEART DISEASE

MITRAL STENOSIS

Etiology

1. Progressive fibrosis, scarring, and calcification of the valve
2. Rheumatic fever (still a common cause in underdeveloped countries)
3. Congenital defect (parachute valve)

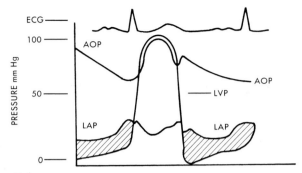

Figure 11-4
Mitral stenosis. Note the pressure gradient between the left atrial pressure, *LAP*, and the left ventricular pressure, *LVP*, during diastole.

Pathophysiology

The cross-section of a normal orifice measures 4-6 cm². Narrowing of the valve orifice causes a pressure gradient across the valve (Fig. 11-4). A murmur becomes audible when the valve orifice becomes smaller than 2 cm². When the orifice approaches 1 cm², the condition becomes critical and symptoms appear.[7]

Symptoms

1. Exertional dyspnea initially, followed by orthopnea and paroxysmal nocturnal dyspnea (PND)
2. Acute pulmonary edema may develop following exertion
3. Systemic emboli (caused by stagnation of blood in the left atrium) may be seen in patients with associated atrial fibrillation
4. Hemoptysis may be present due to persistent pulmonary hypertension

Physical findings

1. Prominent jugular A waves (in patients with NSR)
2. Opening snap occurring in early diastole; a short (<0.07 second) A_2 to opening snap interval indicates severe mitral stenosis
3. Apical middiastolic or presystolic rumble (Fig. 11-5)

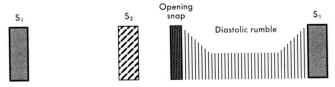

Figure 11-5
Graphic representation of mitral stenosis murmur.

4. Accentuated S_1 (because of delayed and forceful closure of the valve)
5. If pulmonary hypertension is present, there may be a soft, early-diastolic, decrescendo murmur (Graham-Steell murmur) caused by pulmonic regurgitation (it is best heard along the left sternal border and may be confused with aortic regurgitation)

Diagnostic studies

1. Echocardiogram: the characteristic finding on an echocardiogram is a markedly diminished E to F slope of the anterior mitral valve leaflet during diastole; there is also fusion of the commissures resulting in anterior movement of the posterior mitral valve leaflet during diastole (calcification in the valve may also be noted)
2. Chest x-ray film
   a. Straightening of the left cardiac border caused by dilated left atrial appendage
   b. Left atrial enlargement on lateral chest x-ray (appearing as double density on a PA chest x-ray)
   c. Prominence of pulmonary arteries
   d. Possible pulmonary congestion and edema (Kerley-B lines)
   e. Possible elevation of left main bronchus as a result of left atrial enlargement
3. ECG
   a. Right ventricular hypertrophy, right axis deviation caused by pulmonary HTN
   b. Left atrial enlargement (broad, notched P waves)
   c. Atrial fibrillation

Therapy

1. Medical
   a. Decrease level of activity
   b. If the patient is in atrial fibrillation, control the rate response with digitalis
   c. If patient has persistent atrial fibrillation (because of large left atrium) permanent anticoagulation is indicated to decrease the risk of serious thromboembolism
   d. Treat CHF with diuretics and sodium restriction
   e. Antibiotic prophylaxis for dental and surgical procedures
2. Surgical: valve replacement is indicated when symptoms persist despite optimum medical therapy; commissurotomy may be possible if the mitral valve is not calcified and if there is pure mitral stenosis without significant subvalvular disease

MITRAL REGURGITATION

Etiology

1. Papillary muscle dysfunction (as a result of ischemic heart disease)
2. Ruptured chordae tendineae
3. Bacterial endocarditis
4. Calcified mitral valve annulus
5. Left ventricular dilatation
6. Rheumatic heart disease

7. Hypertrophic cardiomyopathy
8. Idiopathic myxomatous degeneration of the mitral valve

Pathophysiology

A large portion of the left ventricular stroke volume is ejected in the left atrium (low-pressure chamber). Eventually there is an increase in left atrial and pulmonary pressures with subsequent right ventricular failure

Symptoms

1. Fatigue, dyspnea, orthopnea, frank CHF
2. Hemoptysis (caused by pulmonary hypertension)
3. Systemic emboli may occur in patients with left atrial mural thrombi associated with atrial fibrillation

Physical findings

1. Hyperdynamic apex often with palpable left ventricular lift and apical thrill
2. Holosystolic murmur at apex with radiation to axilla (Fig. 11-6); there is poor correlation between the intensity of the systolic murmur and the degree of regurgitation
3. Apical early-to-middiastolic rumble (rare)

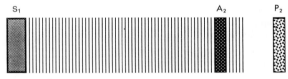

Figure 11-6
Graphic representation of mitral regurgitation murmur.

Diagnostic studies

1. Echocardiogram: enlarged left atrium, hyperdynamic left ventricle (erratic motion of the leaflet is seen in patients with ruptured chordae tendinae)[7]; Doppler electrocardiogram will show evidence of mitral regurgitation
2. Chest x-ray film
   a. Left atrial enlargement (usually more pronounced than mitral stenosis)
   b. Left ventricular enlargement
   c. Possible pulmonary congestion
3. ECG
   a. Left atrial enlargement
   b. Left ventricular hypertrophy
   c. Atrial fibrillation

Therapy

1. Medical
   a. Salt restriction, diuretics
   b. Digitalis (for inotropic effect and to control ventricular response if atrial fibrillation with fast ventricular response is present)

c. Afterload reduction (to decrease the regurgitant fraction and to increase cardiac output) may be accomplished with nifedipine, hydralazine, or captopril

d. Anticoagulants, if persistent atrial fibrillation

e. Antibiotic prophylaxis before dental and surgical procedures

2. Surgical: not recommended unless the patient is severely limited by the disease despite optimum medical therapy; surgery should be considered earlier in patients with moderate to severe mitral regurgitation and minimal symptoms if there is echocardiographic evidence of rapidly progressive increase in left ventricular end-diastolic dimension

MITRAL VALVE PROLAPSE

Incidence

1. Can be found by two-dimensional echo in 5%-10% of the general population

2. Increased incidence is seen with autoimmune thyroid disorders, Ehlers-Danlos syndrome, Marfan's syndrome, pseudoxanthoma elasticum, pectus excavatum, anorexia nervosa, and bulimia

Symptoms (if present)

1. Chest pain

2. Palpitations

3. TIA or stroke

Physical findings

1. Usually young female patient with narrow AP chest diameter

2. Mid-to-late click, heard best at the apex (Fig. 11-7)

3. Crescendo mid-to-late systolic murmur

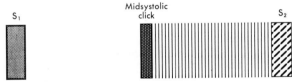

Figure 11-7
Graphic representation of mitral valve prolapse murmur.

Echocardiogram

Echocardiogram shows the anterior and posterior leaflets bulging posteriorly in systole

Complications

1. Bacterial endocarditis

2. TIA or stroke secondary to embolic phenomena

3. Cardiac dysrhythmias

4. Sudden death

5. Mitral regurgitation

NOTE: The incidence of complications is very low (less than 1% per year) and generally associated with an increase in mitral leaflet thickness to ≥ 5 mm[43]

Therapy

1. β-blockers (e.g., propranolol 40-320 mg/day) decrease the heart rate, thus decreasing the stretch on the prolapsing valve leaflets
2. Antibiotic prophylaxis for SBE when having dental, GI, or GU procedures is indicated in patients with MVP and a systolic murmur but controversial in patients with MVP manifested only by an isolated click
3. Reassure patient that the prognosis of this condition is excellent and activity should not be limited

AORTIC STENOSIS

Etiology

1. Rheumatic inflammation of aortic valve
2. Progressive stenosis of congenital bicuspid valve
3. Idiopathic calcification of aortic valve

Pathophysiology

The obstruction to the left ventricular outflow leads to increased left ventricular pressure (Fig. 11-8). This results in concentric hypertrophy and the subsequent decrease in contractile performance and in ejection fraction. Symptoms appear when the valve orifice decreases to less than 1 cm^2 (normal orifice is 3 cm^2). The stenosis is considered severe when the orifice is less than 0.5 cm^2/m^2 or the pressure gradient is 50 mm Hg or higher.[25]

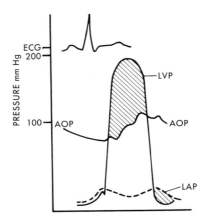

Figure 11-8
Valvular aortic stenosis. Note the pressure gradient between the left ventricular pressure, *LVP*, and the aortic pressure, *AOP*. *LAP*, Left atrial pressure.

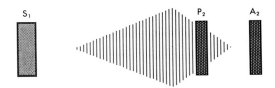

Figure 11-9
Graphic representation of aortic stenosis murmur.

Symptoms

1. Angina: caused by increased O_2 demand secondary to hypertrophy and decreased O_2 supply secondary to decreased coronary artery filling
2. Syncope (particularly with exertion) occurs when vasodilation in muscles during exercise causes insufficient cerebral blood flow as a result of fixed cardiac output
3. CHF: caused by left ventricular failure

NOTE: The average duration of symptoms before death is: angina, 36 months; syncope, 36 months; CHF, 18 months

Physical findings

1. Loud, rough systolic diamond-shaped murmur, best heard at base of heart and transmitted into neck vessels (Fig. 11-9); it is often associated with a thrill or ejection click
2. Absence or diminished intensity of the sound of aortic valve closure (in severe aortic stenosis)
3. Late, slow-rising carotid upstroke with decreased amplitude
4. Strong apical impulse
5. Narrowing of pulse pressure in later stages of aortic stenosis

Diagnostic studies

1. Chest x-ray film
   a. Poststenotic dilation of ascending aorta
   b. Calcification of aortic cusps
   c. Pulmonary congestion (in advanced stages of aortic stenosis)
2. ECG
   a. Left ventricular hypertrophy
   b. ST-T wave changes
3. Echocardiogram: thickening of the left ventricular wall; if the patient has valvular calcifications, multiple echoes may be seen from within the aortic root and there is poor separation of the aortic cusps during systole[7]
4. Cardiac catheterization: confirms the diagnosis and estimates the severity of the disease by measuring the gradient across the valve, allowing calculation of the valve area

Therapy

1. Medical
   a. Strenuous activity should be avoided
   b. Diuretics and sodium restriction if CHF is present
   c. Antibiotic prophylaxis for surgical and dental procedures

2. Surgical: valve replacement is the treatment of choice in symptomatic patients because the 5-year mortality after onset of symptoms is extremely high even with optimum medical therapy; valve replacement is indicated if cardiac catheterization establishes a pressure gradient >50 mm Hg and a valve area <1.0 cm^2

AORTIC REGURGITATION

Etiology

1. Infective endocarditis
2. Rheumatic fibrosis
3. Trauma with valvular rupture
4. Congenital bicuspid aortic valve
5. Myxomatous degeneration
6. Syphilitic aortitis
7. Rheumatoid spondylitis

Pathophysiology

The regurgitation of blood in the left ventricle increases the left ventricular filling pressure, thereby causing left ventricular diastolic volume overload. This results in dilation and hypertrophy of the left ventricle with subsequent decompensation.

Symptoms

Aortic regurgitation (except when secondary to infective endocarditis) is generally well tolerated and patients remain asymptomatic for years. The following are common symptoms after significant deterioration of left ventricular function:

1. Dyspnea on exertion
2. Syncope
3. Chest pain
4. CHF

Physical findings

1. Widened pulse pressure (markedly increased systolic blood pressure, decreased diastolic blood pressure)
2. Bounding pulses, head ''bobbing'' with each systole; ''water hammer'' pulse (Corrigan's pulse) can be palpated at the wrist and is caused by rapid rise and sudden collapse of the arterial pressure during late systole; capillary pulsations (Quincke's pulse) may be seen at the base of the nail beds
3. A to-and-fro ''double Duroziez'' murmur may be heard over the femoral arteries
4. Cardiac auscultation reveals:
   a. Displacement of the cardiac impulse downward and to the patient's left
   b. S$_3$ heard over the apex
   c. Low-pitched, apical diastolic rumble (Austin-Flint murmur) caused by aortic regurgitation impinging on the anterior mitral leaflet
   d. Early systolic apical ejection murmur

Diagnostic studies

1. Chest x-ray film
   a. Left ventricular hypertrophy
   b. Aortic dilation
2. ECG: left ventricular hypertrophy
3. Echocardiogram: coarse diastolic fluttering of the anterior mitral leaflet

Therapy

1. Medical
   a. Digitalis, diuretics, and sodium restriction
   b. Bacterial endocarditis prophylaxis for surgical and dental procedures
2. Surgical: reserved for
   a. Symptomatic patients with chronic aortic regurgitation despite optimum medical therapy
   b. Patients with acute aortic regurgitation (i.e., bacterial endocarditis) producing left ventricular failure
   c. Patients with increased cardiac enlargement, decreased fractional shortening on echocardiogram, decreasing ejection fraction

---

| 11.4 | CONGESTIVE HEART FAILURE

Definition

Congestive heart failure (CHF) is a pathophysiologic state characterized by congestion in the pulmonary or systemic circulation. It is caused by the heart's inability to pump sufficient oxygenated blood to meet the metabolic needs of the tissues.

Etiology

Left ventricular failure	**Right ventricular failure**
Systemic hypertension	Valvular heart disease (mitral stenosis)
Valvular heart disease (AS, AR, MR)	Pulmonary hypertension
Cardiomyopathy	Bacterial endocarditis (right sided)
Bacterial endocarditis	Right ventricular infarction
MI	

Biventricular failure	
Left ventricular failure	Anemia
Cardiomyopathy	Thyrotoxicosis
Myocarditis	AV fistula
Dysrhythmias	Paget's disease

Clinical manifestations

1. Dyspnea: initially on exertion, then with progressively less strenuous activity, and eventually manifesting when patient is at rest; it is caused by increasing pulmonary congestion
2. Orthopnea: caused by increased venous return in the recumbent position
3. Paroxysmal nocturnal dyspnea (PND): results from multiple factors (increased venous return in the recumbent position, decreased PaO_2, decreased adrenergic stimulation of myocardial function)

4. Nocturnal angina: results from increased cardiac work (secondary to increased venous return)
5. Cheyne-Stokes respiration: alternating phases of apnea and hyperventilation caused by prolonged circulation time from lungs to brain
6. Fatigue, lethargy: results from low cardiac output

Physical exam

Left heart failure	**Right heart failure**
Pulmonary rales	Jugular venous distention
Tachypnea	Peripheral edema
S_3 gallop	Perioral and peripheral cyanosis
Cardiac murmurs (AS, AR, MR)	Congestive hepatomegaly
Paradoxical splitting of S_2	Ascites
	Hepatojugular reflux

Chest x-ray film

1. Pulmonary venous congestion
2. Cardiomegaly with dilation of the involved heart chamber
3. Pleural effusions

Functional classification

I   Symptomatic only with greater than ordinary activity
II Symptomatic during ordinary activity
III Symptomatic with minimum activity
IV Symptomatic at rest

Therapy

1. Identify and correct precipitating factors (i.e., anemia, thyrotoxicosis, hypertension, infections, β-blockers or other cardiac depressants, increased sodium load, medical noncompliance)
2. Decrease cardiac workload: restrict patient to bed rest; the risk of thromboembolism during this period can be minimized by using elastic antiembolic stockings and/or heparin 5000 U SC q12h; fluid restriction may be indicated in selected patients
3. Sodium restriction: 2-6 g/day, no added salt diet at home
4. Diuretics
   a. Furosemide: 20-80 mg/day produces prompt venodilation and diuresis; when changing from an IV to oral furosemide, a doubling of the dose is usually necessary to achieve an equal effect
   b. Thiazides are not as powerful as furosemide, but are well tolerated and useful in mild to moderate CHF
5. Digitalis is useful because of its positive inotropic and vagotonic effect
   a. When digoxin is used, the loading dose is 0.5 mg IV/PO, followed by 0.25 mg q4-6h for 4 doses, then 0.125-0.25 mg PO qd; the dosage should be reduced in elderly patients and in patients with renal insufficiency
   b. The serum digoxin level should be checked periodically (therapeutic level is 0.9-2.0 ng/ml)
   c. Major factors predisposing to digitalis toxicity are: quinidine (can cause doubling of digitalis level), hypokalemia, hypomagnesemia,

Table 11-9   Vasodilators used in heart failure[2,31]

Drug	Dosage	Major Site of Action
Nitroprusside	0.5-3 µg/kg/min IV	Arteriolar and venous
Nitrates		
Isosorbide dinitrate	10-60 mg PO q4-6h 2.5-20 mg SL q4h	Venous, minor arteriolar action
2% Nitroglycerin ointment	0.5-2 inches q4-6h	Venous, minor arteriolar action
Transdermal nitroglycerin	5-20 cm^2 q24h	Venous, minor arteriolar action
IV nitroglycerin	Start at 6 µg/min	Venous, minor arteriolar action
Hydralazine	25-100 mg PO q6-8h	Arteriolar
Prazosin	2-7 mg PO q6-8h	Arteriolar and venous
Captopril	6.25-50 mg PO q8-12h	Arteriolar
Nifedipine	10-30 mg PO q6-8h	Arteriolar

    verapamil (can increase digitalis level by 50%), renal insufficiency, and advanced age
6. Vasodilator therapy decreases afterload and SVR (both commonly increased in patients with severe myocardial dysfunction and a dilated heart), improves cardiac output, and increases efficiency of left ventricular emptying (various vasodilators used in patients with CHF are listed in Table 11-9)

CARDIOGENIC PULMONARY EDEMA

Definition
Cardiogenic pulmonary edema is a life-threatening condition caused by severe left ventricular decompensation.

Physical exam
1. Dyspnea with rapid, shallow breathing
2. Diaphoresis, perioral and peripheral cyanosis
3. Pink, frothy sputum
4. Moist, bilateral pulmonary rales
5. Increased pulmonary second sound, S_3 gallop (in association with tachycardia)
6. Bulging neck veins

Diagnostic studies
1. Chest x-ray films
   a. Pulmonary congestion with Kerley-B lines; fluffy perihilar infiltrates may be seen in the early stages
   b. Pleural effusions

2. Arterial blood gases
   a. Respiratory and metabolic acidosis: decreased Pao_2, increased Pco_2, lowered pH
   NOTE: The patient may initially show respiratory alkalosis secondary to hyperventilation
3. Cardiac pressures: increased PAD and PCWP

Therapy[7,21]

All of the following steps can be performed concomitantly:
  1. 100% O_2 by face mask; check ABG, if marked hypoxemia or severe respiratory acidosis, then intubate patient and place on ventilator
  2. Furosemide: 40-100 mg IV bolus to rapidly establish a diuresis and decrease venous return through its venodilator action; may double the dose in 30 minutes if no effect
  3. Vasodilator therapy
     a. Nitrates: particularly useful if the patient has concomitant chest pain
        (1) Nitroglycerin: 150-600 μg SL prn may be given immediately on arrival
        (2) 2% Nitroglycerin ointment: 1-3 inches may be applied cutaneously, but absorption may be erratic
        (3) IV nitroglycerin: 100 mg/500 ml of D_5W, start at 6 μg/min (2 ml/hr)
     b. Nitroprusside: useful in hypertensive patients with decreased cardiac index (CI)
        (1) It increases the CI and decreases left ventricular filling pressure
        (2) The use of nitroprusside in patients with acute MI is controversial because it may intensify ischemia by decreasing the blood flow to the ischemic left ventricular myocardium[6]
  4. Morphine: 3-10 mg IV/SC/IM, may repeat q15min prn; it decreases venous return, anxiety, and systemic vascular resistance (naloxone should be available at bedside to reverse the effects of morphine if respiratory depression occurs)
  5. Place patient in sitting position to decrease venous return
  6. Dobutamine: parenteral inotropic agent of choice in severe cases of cardiogenic pulmonary edema
  7. Rotating tourniquets to the extremities helps decrease venous return
     a. Compress only three extremities at one time and every 15 minutes release one of the tourniquets and apply it to the free extremity
     b. The inflating pressure should exceed venous pressure (to decrease venous return), but should be lower than the arteriolar pressure
  8. Aminophylline: useful *only if* the patient has concomitant severe bronchospasm
  9. Digitalis: has limited value in acute pulmonary edema caused by MI; but it is useful in pulmonary edema resulting from atrial fibrillation or flutter with a fast ventricular response
 10. Identify and treat any precipitating factors, such as MI or dysrhythmias
 11. Phlebotomy is indicated only when all other measures have failed

CARDIOMYOPATHIES

Cardiomyopathies are a group of diseases (three major types) primarily involving the myocardium and characterized by myocardial dysfunction that is not the result of hypertension, coronary atherosclerosis, valvular dysfunction, or pericardial abnormalities.

CONGESTIVE CARDIOMYOPATHY

Definition

In congestive (dilated) cardiomyopathy, the heart is enlarged and both ventricles are dilated.

Etiology

1. Idiopathic
2. Alcoholic
3. Collagen-vascular disease (SLE, rheumatoid arthritis, polyarteritis)
4. Postmyocarditis
5. Peripartum
6. Heredofamiliar neuromuscular
7. Toxins (cobalt, doxorubicin)
8. Nutritional (beri-beri)

Symptoms

1. Dyspnea on exertion, orthopnea, PND
2. Palpitations
3. Systemic and pulmonary embolism

Physical findings

1. Increased jugular venous pressure
2. Small pulse pressure
3. Pulmonary rales, hepatomegaly, peripheral edema
4. S_3, S_4
5. Mitral regurgitation, tricuspid regurgitation (less common)

Diagnostic studies

1. Chest x-ray film
   a. Massive cardiac enlargement
   b. Interstitial pulmonary edema
2. ECG
   a. Left ventricular hypertrophy with ST-T wave changes
   b. RBBB or LBBB
   c. Dysrhythmias (atrial fibrillation, PVC, PAC)
3. MUGA: low ejection fraction with global akinesia

Therapy

1. Treat underlying disease (SLE, alcoholism)
2. Treat CHF (cause of death in 70% of patients) with sodium restriction, diuretics, and digitalis
3. Bed rest when CHF is present

4. Vasodilators (combined use of nitrates and hydralazine or captopril is effective)
5. Prevent thromboembolism with oral anticoagulants
6. Consider heart transplant for young patients who are no longer responsive to medical therapy

RESTRICTIVE CARDIOMYOPATHY

Definition

Restrictive cardiomyopathy is characterized by decreased ventricular compliance, usually secondary to infiltration of the myocardium.

Etiology

1. Infiltrative disorders (glycogen storage disease, amyloidosis sarcoidosis, hemochromatosis)
2. Scleroderma
3. Radiation
4. Endocardial fibroelastosis
5. Endomyocardial fibrosis

Symptoms and physical findings

1. Edema, ascites, hepatomegaly, distended neck veins
2. Fatigue, weakness (secondary to low output)

Diagnostic studies

1. Chest x-ray film
   a. Moderate cardiomegaly
   b. Possible evidence of CHF (pulmonary vascular congestion, pleural effusions)
2. ECG
   a. Low voltage with ST-T wave changes
   b. Frequent dysrhythmias
3. Cardiac catheterization: to distinguish restrictive cardiomyopathy from constrictive pericarditis
   a. Constrictive pericarditis: usually involves both ventricles and produces a plateau of elevated filling pressures
      (1) PCWP is equal to right atrial pressure (RAP)
      (2) Pulmonary artery systolic pressure (PASP) <50 mm Hg
      (3) Right ventricular end-diastolic pressure is greater than one third the right ventricular systolic pressure
   b. Restrictive cardiomyopathy: impairs the left ventricle more than the right
      (1) PCWP > RAP
      (2) PASP >50 mm Hg

Therapy

Cardiomyopathy caused by hemochromatosis may respond to repeated phlebotomies. There is no effective therapy for other causes of restrictive cardiomyopathy. Death usually results from CHF or dysrhythmias, and therefore therapy should be aimed at controlling CHF by restricting salt, administering diuretics and treating potentially lethal dysrhythmias.

HYPERTROPHIC CARDIOMYOPATHY

Pathophysiology

1. There is marked hypertrophy of the myocardium and disproportionately greater thickening of the interventricular septum than that of the free wall of the left ventricle—asymmetric septal hypertrophy (ASH)
2. During midsystole, the apposition of the anterior mitral valve leaflet against the hypertrophied septum can cause a narrowing of the subaortic area and result in left ventricular outflow obstruction; because of this, the disease has been termed idiopathic hypertrophic subaortic stenosis (IHSS) or hypertrophic obstructive cardiomyopathy (HOCM)

Factors influencing obstruction[11]

Increase obstruction

Drugs: digitalis, β-adrenergic stimulators (isoproterenol, epinephrine) nitroglycerin, vasodilators, and diuretics

Hypovolemia

Tachycardia

Valsalva maneuver

Standing position

Decrease obstruction

Drugs: β-adrenergic blockers, calcium channel blockers, α-adrenergic stimulators (phenylephrine)

Volume expansion

Bradycardia

Handgrip exercise

Squatting position

Symptoms

1. Dyspnea
2. Syncope (usually seen with exercise)
3. Angina (decreased angina in recumbent position)
4. Palpitations
5. Sudden death may be the only manifestation (usually seen in young adults during physical exercise)

Physical findings

1. Harsh, systolic, diamond-shaped murmur at the left sternal border or apex that increases with Valsalva maneuver and decreases with squatting
2. Paradoxic splitting of S_2 (if left ventricular obstruction is present)
3. S_4
4. Double or triple apical impulse

Diagnostic studies

1. Chest x-ray film: cardiomegaly
2. ECG
   a. Left ventricular hypertrophy
   b. Abnormal Q waves may be seen in anterolateral and inferior leads
3. Echocardiogram
   a. Ventricular hypertrophy

   b. Ratio of septum thickness: left ventricular wall thickness is greater than 1.3:1
4. MUGA: increased ejection fraction

Treatment[11]

1. Propranolol 160-240 mg/day
2. Verapamil also decreases left ventricular outflow obstruction; however, adverse reactions have been reported
3. 24-hour Holter monitoring to screen for potentially lethal dysrhythmias (dysrhythmias are the principal cause of syncope or sudden death in obstructive cardiomyopathy)
   a. Electrophysiologic study may be used to select prophylactic therapy[34]
   b. Disopyramide is a useful antidysryhthmic agent
4. Surgical myectomy is used only when optimum medical therapy fails to relieve symptomatic patients
5. Antibiotic prophylaxis for surgical procedures
6. Screening of family members may be indicated

| 11.6 | HYPERTENSION

Definition

The WHO defines hypertension as a systolic blood pressure greater than 160 mm Hg and/or a diastolic blood pressure greater than 95 mm Hg. However, stricter control of blood pressure is desirable, especially in young and middle-aged patients. A more reasonable definition of hypertension in these patients is a systolic blood pressure greater than 140 mm Hg and/or a diastolic blood pressure greater than 90 mm Hg.

Etiology*

1. Essential (primary) hypertension (90%)
2. Renal hypertension (5%)
   a. Renal parenchymal disease (3%)
   b. Renovascular hypertension (2%)
3. Endocrine (4%-5%)
   a. Oral contraceptives (4%)
   b. Primary aldosteronism (0.5%)
   c. Pheochromocytoma (0.2%)
   d. Cushing's syndrome (0.2%)
4. Coarctation of aorta (0.2%)

Approach to the hypertensive patient

1. Obtain pertinent history
   a. Age of onset of hypertension
   b. Family history of hypertension
   c. Diet and salt intake, drugs (e.g., oral contraceptives)
   d. Occupation and life-style
   e. Symptoms of secondary hypertension
      (1) Headache, palpitations, excessive perspiration (possible pheochromocytoma)

*Estimates are based on various literature reports.

    (2) Weakness, polyuria (consider hyperaldosteronism)
    (3) Claudication of lower extremities (seen with coarctation of aorta)
2. Physical exam
    a. Evaluate skin for presence of cafe-au-lait spots (neurofibromatosis), uremic appearance (chronic renal failure), striae (Cushing's syndrome)
    b. Perform careful fundoscopic exam: check for papilledema, retinal exudates, hemorrhages
    c. Perform extensive cardiopulmonary exam: check for loud aortic component of S_2, S_4, left ventricular lift
    d. Check abdomen for masses (pheochromocytoma) and presence of bruits over the renal arteries (renal artery stenosis)
    e. Measure blood pressure in both upper and lower extremities (blood pressure is greater in upper extremities in aortic coarctation)
3. Lab evaluation
    a. Urinalysis: examine sediment for evidence of renal disease
    b. BUN, creatinine: to rule out renal disease
    c. Serum potassium level: low potassium is suggestive of primary aldosteronism
    d. CBC: for a baseline value before starting therapy
    e. Screen for coexisting diseases that may adversely effect prognosis
        (1) Fasting serum glucose
        (2) Serum cholesterol
        (3) Serum triglycerides
4. ECG: check for presence of left ventricular hypertrophy (LVH) with strain pattern
5. Chest x-ray film: evaluate cardiac size, presence of LVH, and rib notching (aortic coarctation)
6. Additional tests if particular causes of hypertension are suspected
    a. 24-hour urine collection for VMA and metanephrine levels if pheochromocytoma is suspected
    b. Renal angiography if renal artery stenosis is suspected; findings diagnostic of renal artery stenosis are: stenosis >60%, presence of collateral renal arteries, or poststenotic dilation
    c. Measurement of plasma renin activity from each renal vein is also necessary
        (1) A ratio >1.6:1 of affected to unaffected side is suggestive of renovascular hypertension
        (2) Renin response to captopril is useful for identifying patients with renovascular disease; these patients exhibit greater depressor responses to captopril and also greater reactive increases in plasma renin[42]
7. Factors adversely effecting prognosis[60]
    a. Preventable factors: smoking, obesity, hypercholesterolemia, poorly controlled DM
    b. Uncontrollable factors: early age of onset, male sex, black race
    c. Evidence of end organ damage
        (1) Heart (LVH, MI, CHF)
        (2) Eyes (exudates, papilledema, hemorrhages)
        (3) Kidney (renal insufficiency)
        (4) CNS (CVA)

Initial therapy

1. Borderline hypertension with no risk factors for cardiovascular disease
   a. Initial treatment
      (1) Sodium restriction (2-6 g/day)
      (2) Weight loss if the patient is obese
      (3) Regular aerobic exercise
      (4) Behavior modification to decrease stress
   b. Reevaluate in 4 to 6 weeks, if still hypertensive, prescribe drug therapy (Table 11-10 and Table 11-11)
   c. Patient education is essential for any therapeutic approach
2. Mild to moderate hypertension or risk factors for cardiovascular disease
   a. Stepped-care approach: in this method, each drug is initially started at less than full dosage and then is gradually increased if the blood pressure is still not controlled; proponents state that since hypertension is a multifactorial disease with components that indicate improper sodium handling by the kidney and overactivity of the sympathetic or vasodilator hormones, a stepped-care approach is effective because it modifies each of the above factors.[41] There are four basic steps in this method:[13,19]

Table 11-10   Diuretics commonly used in hypertension[31]

Drug	Dosage	Comments
Amiloride (Midamor)	5-20 mg/day	Potassium-sparing diuretic
Chlorothiazide (Diuril)	500-200 mg/day	Thiazide diuretic
Chlorthalidone (Hygroton)	25-50 mg/day	Thiazide diuretic
Hydrochlorothiazide (various)	50 mg/day	Thiazide diuretic
Indapamide (Lozol)	2.5-5 mg/day	Indoline diuretic
Methyclothiazide (Enduron)	2.5-5 mg/day	Thiazide diuretic
Metolazone (Diulo, Zaroxolyn)	2.5-5 mg/day	Thiazide diuretic
Polythiazide (Renese)	1-4 mg/day	Thiazide diuretic
Spironolactone (Aldactone)	50-100 mg/day	Potassium-sparing diuretic
Triamterene (Dyrenium)	100-300 mg/day	Potassium-sparing diuretic
Bumetanide (Bumex)	0.5-2 mg/day	Loop diuretic
Ethacrynic acid (Edecrin)	50-200 mg/day	Loop diuretic
Furosemide (Lasix)	40-160 mg/day	Loop diuretic
Triamterene and hydrochlorothiazide (Dyazide)	1-2 cap bid	Combination diuretic
Amiloride and hydrochlorothiazide (Moduretic)	1-2 tab qd	Combination diuretic

Table 11-11 Common nondiuretic agents used to manage hypertension

Drug	Dosage	Comments
β-blockers		
Atenolol (Tenormin)	50-100 mg/day	β-Adrenergic blocker
Metoprolol (Lopressor)	50-200 mg/day	β-Adrenergic blocker
Nadolol (Corgard)	40-320 mg/day	β-Adrenergic blocker
Pindolol (Visken)	10-60 mg/day	β-Adrenergic blocker
Propranolol (Inderal)	80-240 mg/day	β-Adrenergic blocker
Timolol (Blocadren)	10-40 mg/day	β-Adrenergic blocker
Captopril (Capoten)	25-150 mg/day	Angiotensin-converting enzyme inhibitor
Clonidine (Catapres)	0.2-2.4 mg/day	α-Adrenergic blocker
Enapril (Vasotec)	5-20 mg/day	Angiotensin-converting enzyme inhibitor
Guanabenz (Wytensin)	8-16 mg/day	α-Adrenergic blocker
Guanethidine (Ismelin)	25-50 mg/day	Ganglionic blocking agent
Hydralazine (Apresoline)	50-200 mg/day	Arterial vasodilator
Labetalol (Trandate, Normodyne)	200-800 mg/day	β-Blocker and α-1 vasodilator
Methyldopa (Aldomet)	500-2000 mg/day	α-Adrenergic blocker
Minoxidil (Loniten)	10-40 mg/day	Arterial vasodilator
Nifedipine (Procardia)	30-120 mg/day	Calcium channel blocker
Prazosin (Minipress)	2-20 mg/day	α-Adrenergic blocker
Reserpine (various)	0.1-0.25 mg/day	α-Adrenergic blocker
Verapamil (Calan, Isoptin)	240 mg/day	Calcium channel blocker

   (1) The patient is initially started on a thiazide diuretic or a β-adrenergic blocker
      (a) A diuretic is preferred in elderly patients with primary systolic hypertension, black hypertensive patients, CHF, and hypertensive patients with COPD or diabetes mellitus
      (b) A β-blocker is indicated in young hypertensive patients with elevated resting heart rate, hypertensive patients with angina, and patients with history of prior MI

    (2) Add a second agent (thiazide, β-blocker, ACE inhibitor, or adrenergic inhibitor)

    (3) Add a vasodilator (hydralazine, prazosin, calcium channel blocker)

    (4) Add ACE inhibitor, guanethidine, or guanadrel

  b. Monotherapy: proponents of this method advocate "individualization" of antihypertensive therapy

    (1) Captopril can be used as a first-line agent in white patients with relatively mild hypertension and high baseline renin levels.[39]

    (2) Calcium channel blockers have also received much attention as first-line agents[38] in hypertension because of the considerable advantage they offer in hypertensive patients with coexisting coronary artery disease, variant angina, or supraventricular dysrhythmias.

    (3) In patients with elevated triglyceride levels and hypercholesterolemia, some experts consider prazosin as a first-line agent for hypertension because it also increases HDL, and decreases cholesterol and triglyceride levels[57] however, its effect on lipids is mild

HYPERTENSIVE EMERGENCIES

Definition

Hypertensive emergencies are potentially life-threatening situations that are secondary to elevated blood pressure. The rate of blood pressure rise is a critical factor. Clinical manifestations consist of grade IV hypertensive retinopathy (exudates, hemorrhages, and papilledema) and/or cardiovascular compromise.

Therapy

Hypertensive emergencies should be treated immediately. The choice of therapeutic agent varies with the cause of the hypertensive crisis. Table 11-12 lists medications commonly used in hypertensive emergencies. All of the drugs require close monitoring of the patient's blood pressure (preferably with an arterial line in an ICU).

    The following are three important points to consider when treating hypertensive emergencies:

  1. A plan for long-term therapy should be introduced at the time of initial emergency treatment

  2. Agents that reduce arterial pressure can cause the kidneys to retain sodium and water, therefore, the judicious administration of diuretics should accompany their use.[19]

  3. Cerebral hypoperfusion may occur if the mean blood pressure is lowered ≥40% in the initial 24 hours[12]

| 11.7 | MYOCARDITIS

Definition

Myocarditis is characterized by inflammation of the myocardial wall.

Table 11-12   Drug therapy of hypertensive emergencies[21,23,60]

Drug	Onset of Action	Duration	Dosage	Mechanism of Action
Nitroprusside (Nipride)	Immediate	<3 min	IV infusion 50 mg/500 ml of D_5W at a rate of 0.5-0.8 μg/kg/min Titrate to blood pressure	Vasodilation
Diazoxide (Hyperstat)	Immediate	4-24 hr	IV injection 25-150 mg over 5 min or IV infusion at 30 mg/min until desired effect	Vasodilation
Hydralazine (Apresoline)	15-20 min	20-30 min	IM/IV 10-50 mg q4-6h prn	Vasodilation
Trimethaphan (Arfonad)	Immediate	10-15 min	IV infusion 500 mg/500 ml D_5W at 1 mg/ml Titrate to blood pressure	Ganglionic blockade
Nifedipine (Procardia)	1-5 min	3-5 hr	10 mg capsule SL*	Vasodilation
Labetalol (Trandate)	1-5 min	16-18 hr	20 mg by slow IV injection over 2 min (may repeat with 40-80 mg q10min, do not exceed 300 mg total)	β-blocker, α-1-vasodilator
Methyldopa (Aldomet)	4-6 hr	10-16 hr	250-500 mg IV q6h prn Maximum dosage is 1 g IV q6h	Depression of sympathetic control or arterial blood pressure

*Perforate capsule (5-10 holes with small needle) and ask patient to chew the capsule and expel material contained within.[23]

Etiology

1. Infection
   a. Viral (coxsackie B virus, echovirus, poliovirus, adenovirus, mumps)
   b. Bacterial *(Staphylococcus aureus, Clostridium perfringens)*
   c. Mycoplasma
   d. Mycotic *(Candida, Mucor, Aspergillus)*
   e. Parasitic *(Trypanosoma cruzi, Echinococcus,* amebic)
   f. Rickettsial *(Rickettsia rickettsii)*
2. Rheumatic fever
3. Secondary to drugs (emetine, doxoribicin)
4. Toxins (carbon monoxide, diphtheria toxin)
5. Collagen–vascular disease (SLE, scleroderma)
6. Sarcoidosis
7. Lyme carditis (caused by circulating immune complexes)
8. Radiation carditis (radiotherapy to mediastinum for lymphoma, lung and breast carcinoma)

Indications	Contraindications	Side Effects
Drug of choice in: Hypertensive encephalopathy Hypertension and intracranial bleed Malignant hypertension Hypertension and heart failure Dissecting aortic aneurysm (used in combination with propranolol)	Hypersensitivity to nitroprusside	Nausea, apprehension, thiocyanate toxicity
Second drug of choice in: Hypertensive encephalopathy Malignant hypertension	Ischemic heart disease Intracranial hemorrhage	Tachycardia, nausea, hyperglycemia, sodium retention, cardiac ischemia
Drug of choice in eclampsia	Hypertension with heart failure	Tachycardia, cardiac ischemia
Drug of choice in dissecting aortic aneurysm (if propranolol cannot be used with nitroprusside)	Hypertension and renal failure	Urinary retention, paralytic ileus, tachyphylaxis
Severe hypertension (Not FDA approved)	Hypersensitivity to nifedipine	Headache, palpitations, fluid retention
Severe hypertension	Bronchial asthma, CHF, bradycardia, second- or third-degree heart block, cardiogenic shock	Postural hypotension, dizziness, fatigue, nausea
Treatment of hypertensive crisis	Hypersensitivity to methyldopa, active hepatic disease	Drowsiness, positive Coombs' test, bradycardia, nausea, vomiting

Symptoms

1. Fatigue, palpitations, dyspnea
2. Precordial discomfort
3. Myalgias

Physical exam

1. May be normal
2. Persistent tachycardia out of proportion to fever
3. Faint S_1
4. Murmur of mitral regurgitation
5. Pericardial friction rub if associated with pericarditis
6. Signs of biventricular failure (hypotension, hepatomegaly, peripheral edema, distention of neck veins)

Diagnostic studies

1. Chest x-ray: enlargement of cardiac silhouette
2. ECG: sinus tachycardia with nonspecific ST-T wave changes
3. Lab results
   a. Increased CK, LDH, SGOT secondary to myocardial necrosis may be seen
   b. Increased erythrocyte sedimentation rate (nonspecific, but may be of value in following the progress of the disease and the response to therapy)
   c. Increased WBC, increased eosinophils if parasitic infection
   d. Viral titers (acute and convalescent)
   e. Cold agglutinins' titer, ASLO titer, blood cultures
4. Cardiac catheterization and angiography
   a. To rule out coronary artery and valvular disease
   b. A right ventricular endomyocardial biopsy can confirm the diagnosis, although a negative biopsy does not exclude myocarditis

Therapy

1. Treat underlying cause (e.g., specific IV antibiotics for bacterial infection)
2. Supportive care
3. Restrict physical activity (to decrease cardiac work)
4. Treat CHF (if present) with digitalis, diuretics, and salt restriction
5. If dysrhythmias are present, treat with quinidine or procainamide
6. Anticoagulation to prevent thromboembolism
7. Preload and afterload reducing agents for treating cardiac decompensation
8. Corticosteroids are contraindicated in early infectious myocarditis; their use is justified only in selected patients with intractable CHF, severe systemic toxicity, and severe life-threatening dysrhythmias
9. Corticosteroids and azathioprine (immunosuppressive therapy) may be beneficial in selected patients with inflammatory infiltrates[59]

11.8   PERICARDITIS

Definition

Pericarditis is characterized by inflammation of the pericardium.

Etiology

1. Idiopathic (possibly postviral)
2. Infectious (viral, bacterial, tuberculous, fungal, amebic, toxoplasmosis)
3. Collagen-vascular disease (SLE, rheumatoid arthritis, scleroderma)
4. Drug-induced lupus syndrome (procainamide, hydralazine)
5. Acute MI
6. Trauma
7. After MI
8. After pericardiotomy
9. After mediastinal radiation (e.g., patients with Hodgkin's disease)
10. Uremia
11. Sarcoidosis

12. Neoplasm (primary or metastatic)
13. Leakage of aortic aneurysm in pericardial sac
14. Familial Mediterranean Fever

Symptoms

1. Severe, constant pain that localizes over the anterior chest and may radiate to arms and back; it can easily be mistaken for myocardial ischemia. Characteristically, however, the pain intensifies with inspiration and is relieved by sitting up and leaning forward.
2. Pericardial friction rub is best heard with the patient upright and leaning forward and by pressing the stethoscope firmly against the chest; it classically consists of three short, scratchy sounds:
   a. Systolic component
   b. Diastolic component
   c. Late diastolic component (associated with atrial contraction)

Diagnostic studies

1. ECG: varies with the evolutionary stage of pericarditis
   a. Acute phase: there are diffuse ST segment elevations (particularly evident in the precordial leads); this can be distinguished from acute MI by:
      (1) Absence of reciprocal ST segment depression in oppositely oriented leads (reciprocal ST segment depression may be seen in aV_r and V_1)
      (2) The elevated ST segments are concave upward
      (3) Absence of Q waves
   b. Intermediate phase: the ST segment returns to baseline and T wave inversion is seen in leads previously showing ST segment elevation
   c. Latent phase: there is resolution of the T wave changes
2. Lab tests (in the absence of an obvious cause):
   a. CBC with differential
   b. Viral titers (acute and convalescent)
   c. Erythrocyte sedimentation rate (nonspecific, but may be of value in following the course of the disease and the response to therapy)
   d. ANA, rheumatoid factor (RF)
   e. Purified protein derivative (PPD), ASLO titers
   f. BUN, creatinine
   g. Blood cultures
3. Echocardiogram is indicated if pericardial effusion is suspected

Treatment

1. Antiinflammatory therapy (salicylates 3-5 g/day or indomethacin 25-50 mg qid)
2. Prednisone 30 mg bid for severe forms of acute pericarditis (before using prednisone, tuberculous pericarditis must be excluded)
3. Codeine 15-60 mg PO qid for pain refractory to salicylates or indomethacin
4. Observe the patient closely for signs of pericardial effusion or cardiac tamponade

5. Treat underlying cause
   a. Bacterial pericarditis
      (1) Commonly caused by streptococci, meningococci, staphylococci, *Haemophilus,* gram-negative bacteria, anaerobic bacteria
      (2) Therapy: systemic antibiotics and surgical drainage of pericardium
   b. Fungal pericarditis
      (1) Caused by histoplasmosis, coccidioidomycosis, candidiasis, blastomycosis, or aspergillosis
      (2) Therapy: IV amphotericin B and drainage of pericardial space (if indicated)
   c. Tuberculous pericarditis
      (1) Therapy: antituberculous drugs
      (2) Corticosteroids may be indicated once antituberculous drugs have been started

Complications

1. Pericardial effusion: the time required for a pericardial effusion (fluid within the pericardial space) to develop is of critical importance; if the rate of fluid accumulation is slow, the pericardium can gradually stretch and accommodate a large effusion (up to 1000 ml), whereas a rapid accumulation (e.g., traumatic hemopericardium) can cause tamponade even with 200 ml of fluid
2. Chronic constrictive pericarditis
   a. Pathophysiology: fibrous scarring and adhesions of the two pericardial layers obliterate the pericardial cavity and cause the pericardium to become rigid and thickened; this prevents the ventricles from adequately filling during diastole and causes increased venous pressures and decreased stroke volume
   b. Etiology
      (1) Idiopathic
      (2) After pericardiotomy
      (3) After radiation therapy
      (4) Uremia
      (5) Tuberculous pericarditis
      (6) After idiopathic pericarditis
   c. Physical exam
      (1) Jugular venous distention, Kussmaul's sign (increase in jugular venous distention during inspiration due to increased venous pulse)
      (2) Pericardial knock (early diastolic filling sound heard 0.06-0.10 seconds after S_2)
      (3) Clear lungs
      (4) Tender hepatomegaly
      (5) Pedal edema, ascites
      (6) ± Pulsus paradoxus
   d. Diagnostic studies
      (1) Chest x-ray film: clear lung fields, normal or slightly enlarged heart
      (2) ECG: low-voltage QRS complexes
      (3) Echocardiogram: may show pericardial thickening or may be normal

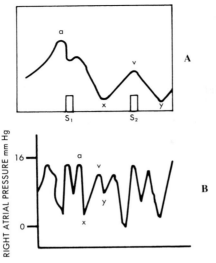

Figure 11-10
Atrial pressure curves in normal patients, **A**, and in patients with constrictive pericarditis, **B**. A wave, increased pressure with atrial contraction; X descent, fall in right atrial pressure seen at the beginning of ventricular systole; V wave, increased pressure in the right atrium due to continuous venous return; Y descent, fall in right atrial pressure seen with the beginning of diastole.

        (4) Cardiac catheterization: there is an **M** or **W** contour of the central venous pattern (Fig. 11-10) caused by both systolic *(X)* and diastolic *(Y)* dips (this differs from cardiac tamponade, which does not display a prominent diastolic *(Y)* descent); in chronic constrictive pericarditis there are also increased right ventricular and pulmonary arterial pressures (for differentiation of constrictive pericarditis from restrictive cardiomyopathy refer to section 11.5)

  e. Therapy: surgical stripping and removal of both layers of the constricting pericardium

3. Cardiac tamponade
  a. Definition: pericardial effusion that significantly impairs diastolic filling of the heart
  b. Symptoms
    (1) Dyspnea, orthopnea
    (2) Interscapular pain
  c. Physical exam
    (1) Distended neck veins
    (2) Distant heart sounds, decreased apical impulse
    (3) Diaphoresis, tachypnea
    (4) Tachycardia (compensatory to maintain cardiac output)

(5) Ewart's sign: an area of dullness at the angle of the left scapula; it is caused by compression of the lung by the pericardial effusion

(6) Pulse paradoxus (decrease in systolic blood pressure >10 mm Hg during inspiration)

(7) Hypotension

(8) Narrowed pulse pressure

d. Diagnostic studies

(1) Chest x-ray film: cardiomegaly (water bottle configuration of the cardiac silhouette) with *clear* lung fields; the chest x-ray film may be normal when acute tamponade occurs rapidly in absence of prior pericardial effusion

(2) ECG

(a) Decreased amplitude of the QRS complex

(b) Variation of the R wave amplitude from beat to beat (electrical alternans); this results from the heart oscillating in the pericardial sac from beat to beat and is frequently seen with neoplastic effusions

(3) Echocardiogram: detects effusions as small as 30 ml (they are seen as an echo-free space), paradoxical wall motion can also be seen

(a) Two-dimensional echocardiography may reveal prolonged diastolic collapse or inversion of the right atrial free wall

(b) Early diastolic collapse of the right ventricular wall is also suggestive of cardiac tamponade

(4) Cardiac catheterization

(a) Equalization of pressures within the chambers of the heart

(b) Elevation of right atrial pressure with a prominent X but no significant Y descent

e. Therapy

(1) Immediate pericardiocentesis

(2) Send aspirated fluid for analysis and cultures (protein, LDH, cytology, cell count, gram stain, AFB stain, cultures and sensitivity)

11.9   DYSRHYTHMIAS

SUPRAVENTRICULAR DYSRHYTHMIAS

Paroxysmal supraventricular tachycardia (SVT)

1. Definition: group of dysrhythmias that generally originate as reentrant rhythm from the AV node and are characterized by sudden onset and abrupt termination

2. Etiology

a. Young patients without evidence of cardiac disease

b. Preexcitation syndromes (e.g., Wolff-Parkinson-White syndrome)

c. Atrial septal defect

d. Acute MI

3. ECG

a. Absolutely regular rhythm at a rate between 150-220 beats/minute (Fig. 11-11)

b. P waves may or may not be seen (the presence of P waves depends on the relationship of atrial to ventricular depolarization)

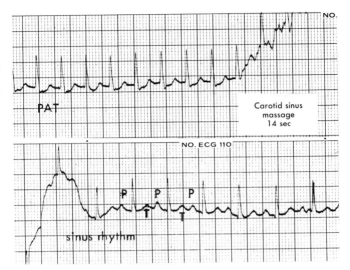

Fig. 11-11
Supraventricular tachycardia *(PAT)*. The upper and lower rows are part of one continuous strip. In the upper row no definite P waves are visible. The diagnosis of this ECG is therefore merely "supraventricular tachydysrhythmia." The ventricular rate is approximately 185/minute. In the lower strip, taken at the end of the carotid sinus massage, sinus rhythm has appeared. However, the heart rate is still rapid (approximately 135/minute). From Goldberger, E.: Treatment of cardiac emergencies, ed. 4, St. Louis, 1985, The C.V. Mosby Co.

Table 11-13 Differentiation of PAT from sinus tachycardia[21]

Rhythm	Ventricular Rate	Effect of Deep Inspiration	Onset and Disappearance	Comparison of P Waves Before and After Tachycardia
Sinus tachycardia	Usually <140/min	Momentary slowing of heart rate	Gradual	P waves remain unchanged
PAT	Usually >160/min	No response	Abrupt	Usually there is aberration of P wave and PR interval

    c. Wide QRS complex (>0.12 second) with initial slurring (delta wave) during sinus rhythm and short PR interval (≤0.12 second) are characteristic of WPW syndrome
    d. See Table 11-13 for differentiation of PAT from sinus tachycardia
4. Symptoms
    a. Usually asymptomatic; the patient may be aware of "fast heart beat"
    b. May precipitate CHF or hypotension during acute MI

5. Therapy
   a. Carotid sinus massage (perform only after excluding occlusive carotid disease); gentle massage of the carotid sinus on one side for a few seconds will elicit vagal efferent impulses
   b. Synchronized DC shock if patient shows signs of cardiogenic shock, angina, or CHF
   c. Verapamil 5-10 mg IV over 5 minutes; if no effect, may repeat in 30 minutes
      (1) Verapamil should be used cautiously in patients with SVT associated with hypotension
      (2) Slow injection of calcium chloride (10 ml of a 10% solution given over 5-8 minutes) before verapamil administration decreases the hypotensive effect without compromising its antidysrhythmic effect[24]
   d. Repeat carotid massage
   e. IV digitalization (0.75-1 mg slow IV loading)
      (1) Repeat carotid sinus massage 30 minutes later; if not successful, give additional 0.25 mg IV digoxin and repeat carotid sinus massage 1 hour later
      (2) Digoxin should be avoided in patients with WPW syndrome and narrow QRS tachycardia (increased risk of atrial fibrillation during AV reentrant tachycardia)
   f. Edrophonium (Tensilon) 5 mg IV bolus over 60 seconds
      (1) If no response in 5 minutes, may give additional 5 mg IV bolus over 60 seconds
      (2) Hypotension may occur with edrophonium
   g. Propranolol 1-3 mg IV at a rate of ≤ 1 mg/minute; stop injection as soon as the heart rate slows down (may use atropine for excessive bradycardia) or when blood pressure decreases significantly (if tachycardia continues, may repeat IV propranolol after 5 minutes, but do not exceed a total dose of 5 mg)
   h. Procainamide is useful in the treatment of WPW syndrome

Multifocal atrial tachycardia (MAT)

1. Definition: chaotic, irregular atrial activity at rates between 100-180 beats/minute
2. Etiology
   a. Chronic obstructive pulmonary disease
   b. Metabolic disturbances (hypoxemia, hypokalemia)
   c. Sepsis
   d. Theophylline toxicity
3. ECG
   a. Variable P-P intervals
   b. Morphology of the P wave varies from beat to beat (Fig. 11-12)
   c. Each QRS complex is preceded by a P wave
4. Therapy
   a. Treat the underlying cause (e.g., improve oxygenation)
   b. Verapamil 5 mg IV (may repeat after 20 minutes); if effective, give 80 mg PO qid[35]

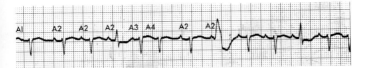

Figure 11-12
Multifocal atrial tachycardia *(MAT)*. A1, A2, A3, and A4 show premature atrial
contractions from varying foci. Notice that the fourth, eighth, and eleventh QRS
complexes are aberrant. From Goldberger, E.: Treatment of cardiac emergencies,
ed. 4, St. Louis, 1985, The C.V. Mosby Co.

Atrial fibrillation

1. Definition: totally chaotic atrial activity caused by simultaneous discharge
   of multiple atrial foci
2. Etiology
   a. CAD
   b. Mitral stenosis
   c. Thyrotoxicosis
   d. Pulmonary embolism
   e. Pericarditis
   f. Myocarditis
   g. Tachycardia-bradycardia syndrome
   h. Alcohol abuse
   i. MI
   j. Wolff-Parkinson-White syndrome
   k. Rarer causes (left atrial myxoma, atrial septal defect, carbon monoxide
      poisoning, pheochromocytoma)
3. Diagnostic studies of new-onset atrial fibrillation should include an echocardiogram to evaluate left atrial size and thyroid function studies to rule
   out thyrotoxicosis
   a. ECG
      (1) Irregular, nonperiodic wave forms (best seen in V_1) reflecting con-
          tinuous atrial reentry
      (2) Absence of P waves
      (3) The conducted QRS complexes show no periodicity (Fig. 11-13)

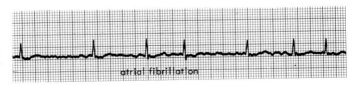

Figure 11-13
Atrial fibrillation with slow ventricular response. From Goldberger, E.: Treatment of
cardiac emergencies, ed. 4, St. Louis, 1985, The C.V. Mosby Co.

4. Therapy (of new-onset atrial fibrillation)
   a. Digoxin 0.5 mg IV loading dose (slow), then 0.25 mg IV q2h until the ventricular rate is controlled; daily dosage varies from 0.125-0.25 mg PO qd (decrease dosage in patients with renal insufficiency and elderly patients)
   b. Conversion to normal sinus rhythm with initial digitalization is successful in only 15%-20% of patients; in the remainder quinidine sulfate 300 mg q6h should be added to help convert the patient to normal sinus rhythm
   c. In acute atrial fibrillation when the rate is not controlled by digoxin, propranolol 0.5 mg IV (slowly) may be given followed by IV boluses of 1 mg q5min to a total of 5 mg
   d. Cardioversion is indicated if the ventricular rate is >140 beats/minute and the patient is symptomatic (particularly in acute MI, chest pain, dyspnea, CHF), or when there is no conversion to normal sinus rhythm after 3 days of therapy with digoxin and quinidine
      (1) Cardioversion will restore sinus rhythm in 90% of patients[36]
      (2) Points to remember when preparing the patient for cardioversion:
         (a) Start quinidine at least 24 hours before cardioversion to help maintain normal sinus rhythm once it is achieved
         (b) If the left atrial size is 4.5 cm, there is little chance of achieving or maintaining normal sinus rhythm
         (c) Hold digoxin and check serum digoxin level on the morning of cardioversion
         (d) The patient should be NPO for 8 hours before cardioversion
         (e) Anticoagulation is advisable for 3 weeks before and 3 weeks after cardioversion, particularly in patients with mitral valve disease or a history of thromboembolism

---

Cardioversion Procedure

1. Use short-acting barbiturate or IV diazepam to induce amnesia and have anesthesiologist in attendence at the procedure.

2. Have adequate IV line in place and continuous ECG monitoring

3. Select energy levels:

Dysrhythmia	Initial energy level	Subsequent shocks (if necessary)
Atrial fibrillation	100 Joules (J)	200 J, 300 J, 360 J
Atrial flutter	20-25 J	50 J, 100 J, 200 J

4. Synchronize the defibrillator to prevent the electrical shock from being applied during repolarization of the ventricles (T wave) and causing ventricular fibrillation.

5. Complications
   a. Ventricular fibrillation (if shock applied on T waves)
   b. Thromboembolism (seen mainly in nonanticoagulated patients with long-standing atrial fibrillation)
   c. Myocardial damage secondary to the current (rare)
   d. Erythema on the chest wall
   e. Recurrence rate of prior dysrhythmia is ≥50% over 12 months[36]

Atrial flutter

1. Definition: rapid atrial rate of 280-340 beats/minute with varying degrees of atrioventricular block
2. Etiology
   a. Atherosclerotic heart disease
   b. MI
   c. Thyrotoxicosis
   d. Pulmonary embolism
   e. Mitral valve disease
   f. Cardiac surgery
   g. COPD
3. ECG
   a. Regular "saw tooth" or "F waves" pattern best seen in II, III, aV$_F$ secondary to atrial depolarization (Fig. 11-14)

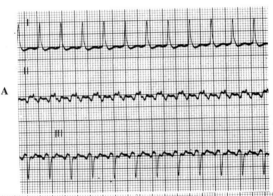

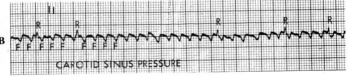

Figure 11-14
Atrial flutter. *F*, Flutter waves. **A,** The flutter waves are not apparent in Lead I but are obvious in Leads II and III; **B,** carotid sinus pressure slowed the ventricular rate but did not change the atrial flutter rate. From Goldberger, E.: Treatment of cardiac emergencies, ed. 4, St. Louis, 1985, The C.V. Mosby Co.

   b. AV conduction block (2:1, 3:1, or varying)
   c. Valsalva maneuver or carotid sinus massage usually slows the ventricular rate (increases the grade of AV block) and may make the flutter waves more evident
4. Therapy[26]
   a. Electrical cardioversion at low energy levels (20-25 J)
   b. In the absence of cardioversion, IV digitalization may be tried to slow the ventricular rate and convert flutter to fibrillation
   c. Atrial pacing may also terminate atrial flutter

AV CONDUCTION DEFECTS
First-degree AV block
1. Definition: prolongation of the PR interval >0.20 seconds (at a rate of 70 beats/minute) the prolongation is constant from beat to beat (Fig. 11-15)
2. Etiology
   a. Vagal stimulation
   b. Degenerative changes in the AV conduction system
   c. Ischemia at the AV nodes (seen particularily in inferior wall MI)
   d. Drugs (digitalis, quinidine, procainamide)
   e. Cardiomyopathies
   f. Aortic regurgitation
3. Therapy: none

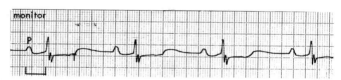

Figure 11-15
First-degree AV block. The PR interval is 0.32 seconds. From Goldberger, E.:
Treatment of cardiac emergencies, ed. 4, St. Louis, 1985, The C.V. Mosby Co.

Second-degree AV block
1. Definition: blockage of some (but not all) impulses from the atria to the ventricles
2. Mobitz type I (Wenkebach)
   a. Definition
      (1) Progressive prolongation of the PR interval before an impulse is completely blocked; the cycle repeats periodically
      (2) Cycle with dropped beat is less than 2 times the previous cycle
   b. Site of block: usually AV nodal (proximal to the bundle of His)
   c. Etiology: same as for first-degree AV block
   d. ECG
      (1) Gradual prolongation of PR interval leading to blocked beat (Fig. 11-16)
      (2) Shortened PR interval after the dropped beat

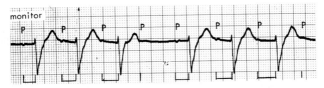

Figure 11-16
Mobitz I second-degree AV block (Wenckebach). From Goldberger, E.: Treatment of cardiac emergencies, ed. 4, St. Louis, 1985, The C.V. Mosby Co.

 e. Therapy
  (1) Usually transient and no treatment is necessary
  (2) If symptomatic, (e.g., dizziness), atropine 1 mg (may repeat once after 5 minutes) may be tried to increase AV conduction; if no response, insert temporary pacemaker
  (3) If block is secondary to drugs (e.g., digitalis), discontinue the drug
  (4) If associated with anterior wall MI, insert pacemaker
3. Mobitz type II
 a. Definition: sudden interruption of AV conduction without prior prolongation of the PR interval
 b. Site of block: infranodal
 c. Etiology
  (1) Degenerative changes in His-Purkinje system
  (2) Acute anterior wall MI
  (3) Calcific aortic stenosis
 d. ECG
  (1) Fixed duration of PR interval
  (2) Sudden appearance of blocked beats (Fig. 11-17)
 e. Therapy: pacemaker insertion, since this type of block is usually permanent and often progresses to complete AV block

Third-degree AV block (complete AV block)

1. Definition: all AV conduction is completely blocked and the atria and ventricles have separate and independent rhythms

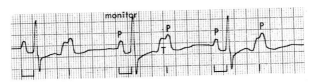

Figure 11-17
Mobitz II second-degree AV block. Notice that every alternate P wave is blocked. From Goldberger, E.: Treatment of cardiac emergencies, ed. 4, St. Louis, 1985, The C.V. Mosby Co

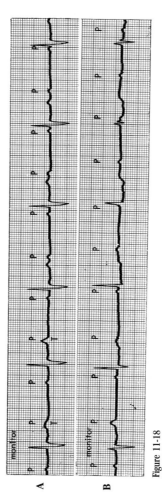

Figure 11-18
Third-degree block. **A** and **B** taken several hours apart. **A**, Atrial rate of 75 beats/minute. The ventricles are beating independently at a slow rate of approximately 40 beats/minute. **B**, A few hours later, same patient; variations in the shape of the QRS complex from beat to beat. From Goldberger, E.: Treatment of cardiac emergencies, ed. 4, St. Louis, 1985, The C.V. Mosby Co.

2. Etiology
   a. Same as for Mobitz II
   b. Cardiomyopathy
   c. Trauma
   d. Cardiovascular surgery
   e. Congenital
3. ECG
   a. The P waves constantly change their relationship to the QRS complexes (Fig. 11-18)
   b. The ventricular rate is usually <50 beats/minute (may be higher in the congenital forms)
   c. Ventricular rate is generally lower than the atrial rate
   d. QRS is wide
4. Symptoms
   a. Dizziness, palpitations
   b. Stokes-Adams syncopal attacks
   c. CHF
   d. Angina
5. Therapy: immediate pacemaker insertion unless the patient has congenital third-degree AV block and is completely asymptomatic

VENTRICULAR DYSRHYTHMIAS

Ventricular tachycardia

1. Definition: three or more consecutive beats of ventricular origin (wide QRS) at a rate between 100-200 beats/minute (Fig. 11-19)

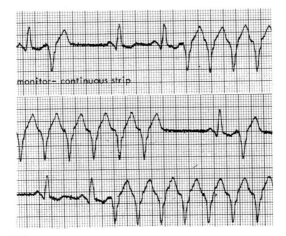

Figure 11-19
Ventricular tachycardia. From Goldberger, E.: Treatment of cardiac emergencies, ed. 4, St. Louis, 1985, The C.V. Mosby Co.

Table 11-14 IV agents used in ventricular dysrhythmias[4,26]

Drug	Indications	Dosage	Onset of Action	Therapeutic Plasma Level
Lidocaine (Xylocaine)	Ventricular tachydys-rhythmias	Loading 1 mg/kg bolus followed by infusion at 1-4 mg/min	Immediate	2-5 µg/ml
Bretylium (Bretylol)	Life-threatening refractory ventricular fibrillation or tachycardia	5 mg/kg slow bolus followed by infusion at 2 mg/min	5 minutes for significant antifibrillatory effect; may be delayed up to 2 hr for prevention of ventricular dysrhythmias	1.33 µg/ml
Procainamide (Pronestyl)	Ventricular tachydys-rhythmias	100 mg slow IV bolus followed by infusion at 1-4 mg/min	Immediate	3-10 µg/ml
Phenytoin (Dilantin)	Digitalis-induced ventricular dysrhythmias	125-250 mg slow bolus q15min prn to maximum of 750 mg/hr	Immediate	5-20 µg/ml

2. The differentiation between ventricular beats and supraventricular tachycardia with aberrant ventricular conduction may be very difficult
   a. Factors favoring ventricular tachycardia
      (1) Similar morphology to premature ventricular contraction (PVC)
      (2) Initiating event is a PVC
      (3) There is usually no response to vagal maneuvers
   b. Factors favoring supraventricular rhythm
      (1) Similar morphology to baseline rhythm
      (2) Initiating event is a premature atrial contraction (PAC)
      (3) The rhythm can slow or break with vagal stimuli
      (4) Physical exam demonstrating ventriculoatrial dissociation (e.g., variation in loudness of S_1 and systolic blood pressure on successive beats)
      (5) ECG may reveal biphasic or monophasic QRS in V_1 with a right bundle branch block (RBBB), QRS >0.14 second, left axis deviation

Table 11-15 Oral agents used in ventricular dysrhythmias[26]

Drug	PO Dosage	Elimination Half-life (T½)
Quinidine sulfate	200-400 mg q6h	6-11 hr
Disopyramide (Norpace)	100-200 mg q6h	4-8 hr; 8-12 hr for sustained release form
Tocainide (Tonocard)	400-600 mg q8h	12 hr
Procainamide (Pronestyl)	250-750 mg q3-4h	3-4 hr; 6 hr for sustained release form
Flecainide (Tambocor)	100-200 mg q12h	12-26 hr
Mexiletine (Mexitil)	200-400 mg q8h	8-10 hr

Table 11-16 Electrophysiologic effects of common antidysrhythmic agents[26]

	Interval			Sinus	
Drug	PR	QRS	QT	Rate	Class
Lidocaine	N	N	N	N	Ib
Procainamide	N/ ↑	↑	↑	N	Ia
Bretylium	N	N	N	N	III
Quinidine	N/ ↑	↑	↑	N/ ↓	Ia
Disopyramide	N/ ↑	↑	↑	N/ ↑	Ia
Digitalis	N/ ↑	N	N/ ↓	N/ ↓	—
Propranolol	N/ ↑	N	N/ ↓	↓	II
Verapamil	↑	N	N	↓	IV

KEY: ↑, Increase; ↓, decrease; N, no change.

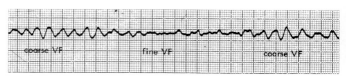

Figure 11-20
Ventricular fibrillation. Coarse and fine fibrillatory waves are shown. From
Goldberger, E.: Treatment of cardiac emergencies, ed. 4, St. Louis, 1985, The C.V.
Mosby Co.

> NOTE: The erroneous administration of verapamil in ventricular tachycar-
> dia often results in a poor outcome; when in doubt, IV procainamide is
> preferred because it is effective in slowing and terminating ventricular
> tachycardia and also tachycardia originating in the atrium, AV node, or
> tachycardia via an accessory pathway[58]

3. Therapy: Table 11-14 lists the major IV agents useful in ventricular dysrhythmias, Table 11-15 lists the commonly used PO agents, and Table
   11-16 describes the major clinical electrophysiologic effects of commonly
   used antidysrhythmic agents

Ventricular fibrillation

Ventricular fibrillation is characterized by a chaotic ventricular rhythm with
disorganized spread of impulses throughout the ventricles (Fig. 11-20).

| 11.10 | CARDIAC PACEMAKERS

Indications for temporary pacemaker in the acute MI setting

1. Complete heart block
2. Alternating bundle branch block
3. Bifascicular block (new RBBB with LAHB or LPHB)
4. Mobitz II
5. Mobitz I with anterior wall MI or inferior wall MI with wide QRS escape
   rhythm
6. Symptomatic sinus bradycardia unresponsive to atropine or isoproterenol
7. New RBBB
8. New LBBB

Indications for permanent pacemaker

1. Sick sinus syndrome
2. Third-degree heart block
3. Mobitz II heart block
4. Symptomatic block at any site of the conduction system
5. Bifascicular block and recurrent syncope

Classifications

Pacemakers are best classified using a three-letter code. The first letter indicates the chamber(s) paced, the second letter the chamber(s) sensed, and the
third letter the mode of response (Table 11-17).

Table 11-17 Classification of pacemakers (Intersociety Commission
for Heart Disease)[52]

Chamber(s) Paced	Chamber(s) Sensed	Modes of Response
V (ventricle)	V	+ (triggered)
A (atrium)	A	I (inhibited)
D (double)	D	D*; 0 (none)
S (single)	0 (none)	R (reverse)

*Double, triggered and inhibited.

Common types of pacemakers

1. VVI (ventricular inhibited): it paces the ventricle at a set rate, senses the
   ventricle, and is inhibited by the patient's own QRS complex. It is indicated in complete AV block, slow ventricular rate associated with atrial
   fibrillation or flutter, sick sinus syndrome, and sinus arrest.
2. DDD (universal pacemaker): most technologically advanced pacemaker;
   it paces both chambers, senses both chambers, and may trigger or inhibit
   output depending on the chamber sensed and paced. It is contraindicated
   in the presence of atrial fibrillation.

References

1. Abrams, J.: Nitroglycerin and long-acting nitrates, N. Engl. J. Med. **302**:1234, 1980.
2. Abrams, J.: Vasodilator therapy for chronic congestive heart failure, JAMA **254**:3070, 1985.
3. Antem, E.M., et al.: Calcium channel blocking agents in the treatment of cardio-vascular disorders. Part II: Hemodynamic effects and clinical implications, Ann. Intern. Med. **93**:886, 1980.
4. Baker, F.J., II, Strauss, R., and Walter, J.J.: Cardiac arrest. In Rosen, P., et al. (editors): Emergency Medicine, St. Louis, 1983, The C.V. Mosby Co.
5. Beta blocker heart attack trial research group: A randomized trial of propranolol in patients with acute myocardial infarction. Part I: Mortality results, JAMA, **247**:1707, 1982.
6. Boden, W.E., and Capone, R.J.: Coronary care, Philadelphia, 1984, W.B. Saunders Co.
7. Braunwauld, E.: In Peterdorf, R.G., et al. (editors): Harrison's principles of internal medicine, ed. 10, New York, 1983, McGraw-Hill Book Co.
8. Cairns, J.A., et al.: Aspirin, sulfinpyrazone, or both in unstable angina: results of a Canadian multicenter trial, N. Engl. J. Med. **313**:1369, 1985.
9. Dawber, T.R.: The Framingham study: the epidemiology of atherosclerotic disease, Cambridge, MA, 1980, Harvard University Press.
10. DeBusk, R.F.: Techniques of exercise testing In Hurst, J.W., et al., (editors): The heart, vol. 2, ed. 6, New York, 1985, McGraw-Hill Book Co.
11. DeSanctis, R.W.: Cardiomyopathies. In Rubenstein, E., and Federman, D.D., (editors): New York, 1985, Scientific American, Inc.
12. Dinsdale, H.B.: Hypertensive encephalopathy, Neurol. Clin. **1**:3, 1983.
13. Dustan, H., et al.: Joint National Committee Report on Detection: evaluation and treatment of high blood pressure, Arch. Intern. Med. **144**:1045, 1984.

14. Epstein, S.E., Palmieri, S.T.: Mechanisms contributing to precipitation of unstable angina and acute myocardial infarction: implications regarding therapy, Am. J. Cardiol, **54**:1245, 1984.

15. European Coronary Surgery Group: Prospective randomized study of coronary artery bypass in stable angina pectoris: second interim report, Lancet **2**:491, 1980.

16. Forrester, J.S., et al.: Medical therapy of acute myocardial infarction by application of hemodynamic subsets, N. Engl. J. Med. **295**:1404, 1976.

17. Friedman, L.M.: How do the various beta blockers compare in type, frequency and severity of their adverse effects? Circulation, **67**(2):189, 1983.

18. Frishman, W.H., Ruggio, J., and Furberg, C.: Use of beta-adrenergic blocking agents after myocardial infarction, Postgrad. Med. **78**:40, 1985.

19. Frohlich, E.D.: Practical management of hypertension, Curr. Probl. Cardiol. **10**(7):1, 1985.

20. Gibson, R.S., et al.: Diltiazem and reinfarction in patients with non–Q wave myocardial infarction, N. Engl. J. Med. **315**:423, 1986.

21. Goldberger, E.: Treatment of cardiac emergencies, ed. 4, St. Louis, 1985, The C.V. Mosby Co.

22. Gottlieb, S.O., et al.: Silent ischemia as a marker for early unfavorable outcomes in patients with unstable angina, N. Engl. J. Med. **314**:1214, 1986.

23. Haft, J.I., and Litterer, W.E., III: Chewing nifedipine to rapidly treat hypertension, Arch. Intern. Med. **144**:2357, 1984.

24. Haft, J.I., and Habbab, M.A.: Treatment of atrial arrhythmias: effectiveness of verapamil when preceded by calcium infusion, Arch. Intern. Med. **146**:1085, 1986.

25. Hancock, E.W.: Valvular heart disease. In Rubenstein, E., and Federman, D.D., (editors): New York, 1985, Scientific American Medicine, Inc.

26. Heger, J.J.: Diagnosis and management of cardiac arrhythmias, Curr. Probl. Cardiol. **10**(12): , 1985.

27. Hutter, A.M., Jr.: Angina pectoris. In Rubenstein, E., and Federman, D.D., (editors): New York, 1985, Scientific American, Inc.

28. Hyjalmarson, A., et al.: Effect on mortality of metoprolol in acute myocardial infarction: a double-blind randomized trial, Lancet, **2**(8251):823, 1981.

29. Kannom, D.S., Levy, W., and Cohen, L.S.: The short-and-long term prognosis of patients with transmural and non-transmural myocardial infarction, Am. J. Med. **61**:452, 1976.

30. Killip, T., and Kimball, J.T.: Treatment of myocardial infarction in a coronary care unit, Am. J. Cardiol. **20**:457, 1967.

31. Knoben, J.E., and Anderson, P.O.: Handbook of clinical drug data, ed. 5, Hamilton, Ill., 1983, Drug Intelligence Publications.

32. Koren, G., et al.: Prevention of myocardial damage in acute myocardial ischemia by early treatment with intravenous streptokinase, N. Engl. J. Med. **313**:1384, 1985.

33. Koren, G., et al.: Early treatment of acute myocardial infarction with intravenous streptokinase, Arch. Intern. Med. **147**:237, 1985.

34. Kowey, P.R., Eisenberg, R., and Engel, T.R.: Sustained arrhythmias in hypertropic obstructive cardiomyopathy, N. Engl. J. Med. **310**:1566, 1984.

35. Levine, J.H., Michael, J.R., and Guarnieri, T.: Treatment of multifocal atrial tachycardia with verapamil, N. Engl. J. Med. **312**:21, 1985.

36. Mancini, G.B.J., and Goldberger, A.L.: Cardioversion of atrial fibrillation: consideration of embolization, anticoagulation, prophylactic pacemakers and long-term success, Am. Heart. J. **104**:617, 1982.

37. Mark, D.B., et al.: Localizing coronary obstruction with the exercise treadmill test, Am. Intern. Med. **106**:53, 1987.

38. Massie, B.M., et al.: Calcium channel blockers as anti-hypertensive agents, New concepts in hypertension therapy symposium, Am. J. Med., Oct. 5, 1984.

39. Materson, B.J.: Monotherapy of hypertension with angiotensin-converting enzyme inhibitors, New concepts in hypertension therapy symposium, Am. J. Med., Oct. 5, 1984.

40. Medical Letter (The), Nitroglycerin patches, vol. 26, June 22, 1984.

41. Moser, M.: Stepped-up approach to hypertension: is it still useful? Primary Cardiol. **10**:186, 1985.

42. Muller, R.B., et al.: The captopril test for identifying renovascular disease in hypertensive patients, Am. J. Med. **80**:633, 1986.

43. Nishimura, R.A., et al.: Echocardiographically documented mitral valve prolapse: long-term follow-up of 237 patients, N. Engl. J. Med. **313**:1305, 1985.

44. Norwegian Multicenter Study Group: Timolol-induced reduction in mortality and re-infarction in patients surviving acute myocardial infarction. Part I: Mortality results, JAMA, **247**:1701, 1982.

45. Pooling Project Research Group: Relationship of blood pressure, serum cholesterol, smoking habits, relative weight and ECG abnormalities to incidence of major coronary events: final report of the pooling project, J. Chron. Dis. **31**:201, 1978.

46. Pratt, C.M., Seals, A.A., and Luck, J.C.: The clinical significance of ventricular arrhythmias after myocardial infarction: symposium on prognosis after MI, Cardiol. Clin. **2**(1):3, 1984.

47. Roberts, R., and Pratt, C.M.: The influence of the site and locus of myocardial damage on prognosis: symposium on prognosis after MI, Cardiol. Clin. **2**(1):21, 1984.

48. Sanz, G., et al.: Determinants of prognosis in survivors of myocardial infarction: a prospective clinical angiographic study, N. Engl. J. Med. **306**:1065, 1982.

49. Schulze, R.A., Schulze, R.A., Jr., Strauss, H.W., and Pitt, B.: Sudden death in the year following myocardial infarction: relation to ventricular premature contractions in the late hospital phase and left ventricular ejection fraction, Am. J. Med. **62**:182, 1977.

50. Schuster, E.H., and Buckley, B.H.: Early post-infarction angina: ischemia at a distance and ischemia in the infarct zone, N. Engl. J. Med. **305**:1101, 1981.

51. Sherry, S.: Tissue plasminogen activator (t-Pa), will it fulfill its promise? N. Engl. J. Med. **313**(16):1014, 1985.

52. Shively, B., and Goldsch, N.: Progress in cardiac pacing: Part II, Arch. Intern. Med. **145**:2238, 1985.

53. Telford, A.M., and Wilson, C.: Trial of heparin vs. atenolol in prevention of myocardial infarction in intermediate coronary syndrome, Lancet, **1**:1225, 1981.

54. Thadani, U., et al.: Comparison of the immediate effects of five beta adrenoreceptor blocking drugs with different ancillary properties in angina pectoris, N. Engl. J. Med. **300**:750, 1979.

55. Theroux, P., et al.: Exercise testing in the early period after myocardial infarction in the evaluation of prognosis: symposium on prognosis after myocardial infarction, Cardiol. Clin. **2**(1):71, 1984.

56. Thompson, P.L., Fletcher, E.E., and Katavatis, V.: Enzymatic indices of myocardial necrosis: influence on short- and long-term prognosis after myocardial infarction, Circulation, **59**:113, 1979.

57. Weinberger, M.H.: Antihypertensive therapy and lipids: evidence, mechanisms, and implications, Arch. Intern. Med. **145**:1102, 1985.

58. Wellens, H.J.: The wide QRS tachycardia, Ann. Intern. Med. **104**:879, 1986.

59. Wenger, N.K., Abelmann, W.H., and Roberts, W.W.C.: Myocarditis. In Hurst J.W., Longe, R.B., et al. (editors): The heart, New York, 1985, McGraw Hill Book Co.

60. Williams, G.H., and Braunwauld, E.: Hypertensive vascular disease. In Petersdorf, R.G., et al. (editors): Harrison's Principles of Internal Medicine, ed. 10, New York, 1983, McGraw Hill Book Co.

DIABETES MELLITUS

H. Christina Hanley

Diabetes mellitus (DM) effects approximately 5% of the American population. It is characterized by an imbalance between the factors that elevate and the counterregulatory factors that lower the blood glucose level:

Increased glucose	**Decreased glucose**
Food intake	Insulin
Glucagon	Exercise
Cortisol	Cellular glucose uptake
Growth hormone	
Catecholamines	
Hepatic gluconeogenesis	

Classification

Table 12-1 gives a recent classification of DM based on newer insights into the causes and conditions associated with diabetes.

Diagnosis

Table 12-2 gives the criteria used by the National Diabetes Data Group and the WHO for blood glucose limits on an oral glucose tolerance test.[20,47] Because of the disagreement on criteria, the nonstandardization of the test (many patients have not eaten 300 g carbohydrate/day diet for 3 days preceding the test), and the day-to-day blood glucose level variation within the same individual, many physicians measure the *glycosylated hemoglobin* (HbA_{1c}) to determine glucose intolerance and to diagnose DM.[25] However, the use of HbA_{1c} to screen for DM has been questioned by many endocrinologists.

Treatment of the patient with nonacute DM

The goal of treatment is to normalize the serum glucose level. This can be achieved with the following modalities:

1. Diet
   a. Calories
      (1) The diabetic patient can be started on 15 calories/lb of ideal body weight; this number can be increased to 20 calories/lb for an active person and 25 calories/lb if the patient does heavy physical labor

Table 12-1   Classification of diabetes mellitus

Type	Associated Factors
Idiopathic diabetes	
Type I: insulin-dependent diabetes mellitus (IDDM)	Hereditary factors: Islet cell antibodies (found in 90% of patients within the first year of diagnosis) Higher incidence of HLA types DR3, DR4 50% concordance in identical twins Environmental factors: viral infection (possibly coxsackie virus, mumps virus)
Type II: non-insulin-dependent diabetes mellitus (NIDDM)	Hereditary factor: 90% concordance in identical twins Environmental factor: obesity
Diabetes secondary to:	
Hormonal excess	Cushing's syndrome, acromegaly, glucagonoma, pheochromocytoma
Drugs	Glucocorticoids, diuretics, oral contraceptives
Insulin receptor unavailability	With or without circulating antibodies
Pancreatic disease	Pancreatitis, pancreatectomy, hemochromatosis
Genetic syndromes	Hyperlipidemias, myotonic dystrophy, lipoatrophy
Gestational diabetes	

Table 12-2   Diagnostic criteria for diabetes mellitus

Lab Test	National Diabetes Data Group	WHO
Fasting blood sugar (FBS)	≥140 mg/dl	≥140 mg/dl
Glucose level 30 or 60 minutes after a 75 g glucose load (Glucola)	≥200 mg/dl	
Glucose level 2 hours after 75 g glucose load (Glucola)	≥200 mg/dl	≥200 mg/dl

(2) The calories should be distributed as 55%-60% carbohydrates, 25%-35% fat, and 15%-20% protein

(3) The emphasis should be on complex carbohydrates rather than simple and refined starches, and on polyunsaturated instead of saturated fats in a ratio of 2:1

b. Seven food groups

(1) The exchange diet of the American Diabetes Association includes: protein, bread, fruit, milk, fat, and low and intermediate carbohydrate vegetables

(2) The diet should be well balanced and may include one or more foods from each of these groups, unless otherwise contraindicated (e.g., milk in a patient with lactose intolerance)

(3) The name of each exchange is meant to be all inclusive (e.g., cereal, muffins, spaghetti, potatoes, rice are in the bread group; meats, fish, eggs, cheese, peanut butter are in the protein group)

c. The *glycemic index*[16] compares the rise in blood sugar after the ingestion of simple sugars and complex carbohydrates with the rise that occurs after the absorption of glucose; equal amounts of starches do not give the same rise in plasma glucose (pasta equal in calories to a baked potato causes less of a rise than the potato), thus it is helpful to know the glycemic index of a particular food product

d. Fiber: insoluble fiber (bran, celery) and soluble globular fiber (pectin in fruit) delay glucose absorption and attenuate the postprandial serum glucose peak; they also appear to lower the elevated triglyceride level often present in uncontrolled diabetics

2. Exercise increases the cellular glucose uptake by increasing the number of cell receptors;[77] the following points must be considered:

a. Exercise programs must be individualized and built up slowly

b. Insulin is more rapidly absorbed when injected into a limb that is then exercised, and this can result in hypoglycemia (patients who have experienced hypoglycemia during exercise should eat a snack before the activity and, if necessary, reduce the insulin dose that peaks at that time of day)

3. Weight loss: to ideal weight if the patient is overweight

4. Oral hypoglycemic agents

a. When the above measures fail to normalize the serum glucose, a sulfonylurea should be added to the regimen (Table 12-3 lists the commonly used sulfonylureas)

b. Oral hypoglycemic agents work best when given before meals (e.g., 15 minutes before breakfast) because they increase the postprandial output of insulin from the pancreas

c. All sulfonylureas are contraindicated in patients allergic to sulfa

d. Second-generation sulfonylureas offer several advantages:

(1) Less interaction with other drugs: the first-generation drugs bind to plasma proteins and can be displaced by other drugs (e.g., warfarin, phenytoin, sulfa) resulting in an intensified hypoglycemic effect; the sulfonylureas can in turn displace these other drugs from plasma proteins and intensify their effect (increased prothrombin time, increased phenytoin level)

(2) Fewer side effects than some first-generation sulfonylureas: chlorpropamide may cause edema secondary to inappropriate antidi-

Table 12-3 Commonly used sulfonylureas

Drug	Starting Dose	Maximum Daily Dose	Frequency	Duration of Action (hr)
First generation				
Tolbutamide (Orinase)	500 mg	1.5 g	qd, bid	6-12
Tolazamide (Tolinase)	100 mg	1.0 g	qd, bid	12-14
Chlorpropamide (Diabinese)	250 mg	750 mg	qd	≥36
Second generation				
Glyburide* (Diabeta, Micronase)	2.5 mg	20 mg	qd, bid	Up to 24
Glipizide (Glucotrol)	5.0 mg	40 mg	qd, bid	12-24

*Useful in patients with renal disease because of dual excretion routes (urine and bile).

    uretic hormone secretion (SIADH); concomitant alcohol ingestion can also result in an antabuse-like flush

    (3) Alternative excretion routes: their excretion in bile permits a safer use in patients with renal impairment

  e. Indications

    (1) Because of these various advantages, second-generation sulfonylureas are indicated in the treatment of new non-insulin-dependent diabetics who are not adequately controlled by diet and exercise, and in diabetic patients who experience significant side effects or who are poorly controlled with first-generation sulfonylureas

    (2) Second-generation sulfonylureas are not indicated in diabetics well controlled on first-generation drugs and who are not experiencing significant side effects

5. Insulin is indicated for the treatment of DM type I (insulin dependent) and DM type II who cannot be adequately controlled with diet and sulfonylureas

  a. Insulin treatment progresses from the administration of once-a-day, intermediate acting insulin (NPH, lente) to twice-a-day insulin, then bid doses of NPH or lente plus regular insulin, to basal insulin with multiple doses of regular[62]

  b. Table 12-4 describes the various types of insulin preparations; human insulin (Humulin) is recommended for first-time diabetic patients to avoid inducing antiinsulin antibodies, and it is now available at prices comparable with pork or beef insulin

  c. Insulin therapy should start with the simplest regimen and advance to the next step only when adequate glucose control cannot be otherwise achieved

  d. Patients receiving insulin should initially monitor their glucose in the morning (before breakfast), before lunch, before dinner, and before bedtime; insulin dosage should be adjusted accordingly

Table 12-4   Insulin preparations[1]

Preparation	Onset of Action*	Duration of Action*	Peak Effect*
Rapid-acting			
Regular (crystalline zinc)	30-60 min	5-7 hr	2-4 hr
Semilente	30 min-3 hr	12-16 hr	4-8 hr
Intermediate-acting			
NPH	2 hr	18-28 hr	6-12 hr
Lente	2-4 hr	24-28 hr	6-12 hr
Long-acting			
Protamine zinc insulin (PZI)	4-6 hr	24-36 hr	8-14 hr
Ultralente	4-6 hr	36+ hr	12-16 hr

*After subcutaneous injection. The onset, duration of action, and peak effect vary with each patient; it is influenced by site and depth of injection, in addition to the concentration and volume of injection.

Determination of the NPH Insulin Dosage

1. Measure blood or urine glucose qid (before meals and before bed); in diabetic patients, glycosuria occurs when the renal threshold is exceeded (serum glucose level of approximately 180-200 mg/dl), but this level varies from person to person and may be higher in certain patients. Blood glucose is much more accurate and is the method of choice for determining glucose levels; however, patient compliance may be a problem.
2. For testing urine glucose, use "second voided" urine samples (discard initial urine sample and test urine sample obtained within 30 minutes of prior voiding).
3. Cover the blood glucose or the glycosuria qid with regular insulin:
   Example: 5% glycosuria   10 U
            3% glycosuria   8 U
            2% glycosuria   5 U
            1% glycosuria   2 U
4. Determine the total amount of regular insulin given and give ⅔ of this dosage as NPH insulin qAM before breakfast.
5. An alternate method is to arbitrarily give 20 U NPH qAM (0.3 U/kg body weight) before breakfast and adjust this amount by 2, 5 or 10 U every 3 days depending on the serum glucose levels (a change in insulin dosage takes about 3 days to stabilize, therefore the dosage should not be changed before then).

Example:

Time	AM	Before Lunch	Before Dinner	Before Bedtime	Insulin adjustment
Glucose level	Normal	↑	Normal	Normal	Add 4 U of regular insulin to AM NPH dose
	↑	Normal	Normal	Normal	Change to bid NPH insulin (prebreakfast and bedtime)

As noted in the above example, bid insulin is necessary when the plasma glucose is inadequately controlled with only one NPH insulin injection; regular insulin may be added to the NPH doses as needed

e. One of the complications of bid NPH insulin is the *Somogyi effect*, which is characterized by early morning (3 AM) hypoglycemia followed by rebound hyperglycemia in the AM. The hypoglycemia is caused by an excessive evening NPH insulin dose (peak effect seen at approximately 3 AM). The rebound hyperglycemia is secondary to the effects of counterregulatory hormones. If the Somogyi effect is suspected (sweating, tremors, tachycardia during the night and increased FBS or awakening in AM with headache and wet clothing), the diagnosis can be confirmed by checking a 3 AM plasma glucose level (markedly decreased).

The treatment is to reduce the evening NPH insulin dose. If a patient requires three insulin injections/day (and the patient is compliant), best control of the hyperglycemia can be achieved by dividing the total insulin dosage in the following manner:

(1) ⅔ of the total daily dosage before breakfast, subdivided in:
   (a) ⅔ intermediate-acting insulin
   (b) ⅓ short-acting insulin

Table 12-5 Correction of insulin dosage

Time	Plasma Glucose	Insulin Adjustment
AM	↑	↓ Evening NPH insulin initially, ↑ NPH insulin when the Somogyi effect has been ruled out
	↓	↓ Evening NPH insulin
Lunch	↑	↑ AM regular insulin
	↓	↓ AM regular insulin
Dinner	↑	↑ AM NPH insulin
	↓	↓ AM NPH insulin
Bedtime	↑	↑ Predinner regular insulin
	↓	↓ Predinner regular insulin

   (2) ⅙ of the dosage before dinner (regular insulin)
   (3) ⅙ of the dosage at bedtime (intermediate-acting insulin)
   For example, if the total daily insulin dosage is 36 U:
   (1) 24 U given before breakfast
      (a) 16 U NPH insulin
      (b) 8 U regular insulin
   (2) 6 U regular insulin given before dinner
   (3) 6 U NPH insulin given at bedtime
   Table 12-5 lists insulin dosage corrections based on the time of the abnormal glucose levels

Monitoring adequacy of glucose control

Since normalization of serum glucose is the ultimate goal, the patient should have a mechanism to measure the degree of control (this will act as a motivator).
1. Urine testing can be done on a qid basis (before meals and at bedtime) on double-voided specimens until the urine is consistently negative, indicating a serum glucose level below 180-200 mg/dl.
2. Blood glucose monitoring is started when the majority of the urine samples demonstrate no glycosuria. Glucose oxidase strips can be compared with the color chart on the container, or they can be used in conjunction with a meter to give a digital reading. The testing can be done once a day, but vary the time each day so that over a period of time the serum glucose level before meals and at bedtime can frequently be assessed without pricking the patient's fingers qid.
3. Glycosylated hemoglobin (HbA_{1c}): nondiabetic patients normally have 2%-7% of their hemoglobin glycosylated (sugar attached to the hemoglobin molecule); this depends on the ambient sugar concentration over the preceding 4-8 weeks, and therefore the higher the average serum glucose the higher the glycohemoglobin level. HbA_{1c} levels greater than 8%-9% indicate poor glycemic control over the previous 4-8 weeks. This test can be obtained at any time of the day and requires no fasting. Factors (other than serum glucose) that can alter HbA_{1c} are:

Decreased HbA_{1c}	**Increased HbA_{1c}**
Chronic blood loss	Increased HbF
Anemia (hemolytic)	Chronic renal failure
Presence of abnormal	Splenectomy
Hb (S,C,D)	Dialysis
	Thalassemia
	Increased triglycerides

Complications

Retinopathy is found in approximately 15% of type I diabetics and in 6% of type II diabetics after 15 years.
1. Nonproliferative retinopathy
   a. Initially: microaneurysms, capillary dilation, waxy or hard exudates, dot and flame hemorrhages, AV shunts
   b. Advanced stage: microinfarcts with macular edema, cotton wool exudates

2. Proliferative retinopathy: formation of new vessels
3. Complications of retinopathy: vitreal hemorrhages, fibrous scarring, retinal detachment
4. Diagnosis: diabetic patients should have a yearly examination by an ophthalmologist
5. Therapy: photocoagulation treatment (laser beam therapy) can greatly improve the prognosis in diabetic retinopathy
6. Cataracts and glaucoma occur with increased frequency in diabetics

• • •

Neuropathy is common in diabetics, its frequency in type II diabetes approaches 70%-80%
1. Peripheral neuropathy
   a. Manifestations
      (1) Paresthesias of extremities (feet more than hands); the symptoms are symmetric, bilateral, and associated with intense burning pain (particularly during the night)
      (2) Mononeuropathies involving cranial nerves III, IV, VI, intercostal nerves, and femoral nerve are also common
   b. Physical exam
      (1) Decreased pinprick sensation, sensation to light touch, and pain sensation
      (2) Decreased vibration sense
      (3) Loss of proprioception (leading to ataxia)
      (4) Motor disturbances (decreased DTR, weakness and atrophy of interossei muscles); when the hands are affected, the patient has trouble picking up small objects, with dressing, and with turning pages in a book
      (5) Diplopia, abnormalities of visual fields
   c. Therapy
      (1) Use mild analgesics (avoid narcotics)
      (2) Additional modalities include amitriptyline (25-75 mg at hs), dilantin (100-200 mg at hs), clonazepam, tegretol
      (3) Mononeuropathies usually resolve spontaneously within 3 months and require no treatment (an eye patch may be helpful in patients with diplopia)
2. Autonomic neuropathy
   a. GI disturbances
      (1) Manifestations
         (a) Disturbances of esophageal motility
         (b) Gastroparesis with delayed gastric emptying
         (c) Diarrhea (usually nocturnal)
      (2) Treatment
         (a) Metoclopramide (Reglan) 10 gm qid or bethanechol 5-10 mg tid-qid to treat impaired esophageal and gastric motility
         (b) H_2 blockers (cimetidine, ranitidine) to decrease gastric acidity
         (c) Clonidine (α-2 adrenergic agonist) to control diarrhea resulting from autonomic neuropathy; initial dosage is 0.1 mg q12h and may be increased to 0.5 mg q12h over 3 days

b. GU disturbances
   (1) Neurogenic bladder is characterized by hesitancy, weak stream, and dribbling
      (a) Treatment consists of frequent voidings (q4h), manual pressure suprapubically to facilitate voiding, and bethanecol 10-50 mg PO tid or qid to increase the tone of the detrusor urinae muscle
      (b) In severe cases, transurethral resection may be indicated
   (2) Impotence occurs frequently in diabetic men
      (a) Sexual desire is normal and ejaculation is preserved, but erection is affected; other causes of impotence should also be ruled out
      (b) Treatment is disappointing, but many patients have been helped by a penile prosthesis implant
c. Orthostatic hypotension
   (1) Manifestations: syncope, dizziness, lightheadedness
   (2) Treatment
      (a) Ensure adequate hydration, liberalize salt intake if indicated
      (b) Fludrocortisone 0.05-0.1 mg qd or bid is helpful in some patients
      (c) Antiembolic stockings to prevent pooling of blood in the lower extremities
      (d) Have patient avoid sudden movement from recumbent to erect position

•   •   •

Nephropathy occurs in 10%-15% of diabetics (higher prevalence in type I diabetics)
1. Manifestations: proteinuria occurs approximately 3 years before a marked reduction in creatinine clearance is evident and approximately 5 years before renal failure
2. Treatment
   a. Rigidly controlling the plasma glucose level from the onset of diabetes may prevent or delay the onset of neuropathy
   b. Dietary restriction in protein and phosphates and maintenance of fluid balance is also essential in patients with renal insufficiency
   c. Hypertension, if present, should be treated aggressively
   d. Contrast material (IVP, CT scan dye) should be avoided (particularly if the serum creatinine is > 2.0 mg/dl)
   e. Urinary tract infections should be treated aggressively
   f. When renal failure has occurred, chronic dialysis or kidney transplant may be possible, depending on whether other complications are present

•   •   •

Infections are generally more common in diabetics because of multiple factors, such as impaired leukocyte function, decreased tissue perfusion secondary to vascular disease, repeated trauma, and urinary retention secondary to neuropathy, Table 12-6 lists infections that have an increased incidence in diabetics.

Table 12-6   Infections with increased prevalence in diabetics

Site of Infection	Organism
Skin and connective tissue	*Candida albicans* and other dermatophytes *Staphylococcus* sp. Anaerobes (e.g., *B. fragilis*)
Nasal mucosa	Fungi of genera *Mucor, Rhizopus,* and *Absidia* (rhinocerebral mucormycosis)
Ears	*Pseudomonas aeruginosa* (malignant external otitis)
Lungs	*Staphylococcus* sp. *Klebsiella* sp. *Mycobacterium tuberculosis*
Gallbladder	*Clostridium* sp. and other anaerobic and aerobic organisms (emphysematous cholecystitis)
Urinary tract	*Escherichia coli* *Torulopsis glabrata*
Vagina	*Candida albicans* (vaginal moniliasis)

•   •   •

The following are other complications seen in diabetic patients:

1. Foot ulcers occur frequently and are usually secondary to poor circulation and repeated trauma (unrecognized because of the sensory loss); treatment includes the following measures:
   a. Have patient eliminate weight bearing on the area of the ulcer
   b. Have patient avoid tight-fitting shoes and keep feet clean; whirlpool therapy may be helpful
   c. Apply povidone-iodine (betadine) solution to the area and cover with a sterile dressing (change dressing two or three times per day)
   d. If the ulcer is significant, surgical debridement will be necessary; IV antibiotics are indicated if there is evidence of infection
   e. Evaluate the adequacy of the vasculature
2. Neuropathic arthropathy (Charcot joints): bone or joint deformities from repeated trauma (secondary to peripheral neuropathy)
3. Osteoporosis has an increased incidence in diabetics
4. Necrobiosis lipoidica diabeticorum: plaquelike reddened areas with a central area that fades to white-yellow found on the anterior surfaces of the legs; in these areas, the skin becomes very thin and can ulcerate readily; the patient should avoid any trauma to the affected area

12.2   DIABETIC KETOACIDOSIS

Definition

Diabetic ketoacidosis (DKA) results from severe insulin deficiency. It is manifested clinically by severe dehydration and alterations in the sensorium. The various pathophysiologic events leading to DKA are described in Fig. 12-1.

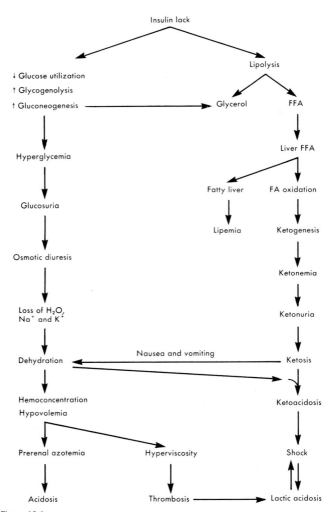

Figure 12-1
Pathophysiologic events leading to diabetic ketoacidosis. From Felts, P.W.:
Ketoacidosis: symposium on acid-base disorders, Med. Clin. North Am. **67**(4):836,
1983.

Symptoms

1. Anorexia, nausea, vomiting
2. Polyuria, polydipsia, generalized malaise
3. Abdominal pain
4. Drowsiness, stupor, coma

Physical exam

1. Evidence of dehydration (tachycardia, hypotension, dry mucous membranes, sunken eyeballs, poor skin turgor)
2. Clouding of mental status
3. Tachypnea with air hunger (Kussmaul respiration)
4. Fruity breath odor (caused by acetone)
5. Lipemia retinalis may be noted in some patients
6. Evidence of precipitating factors may be present (infected wound, pneumonia)

Lab results

1. Hyperglycemia (serum glucose is generally >300 mg/dl)
2. Serum bicarbonate usually <15 mEq/L
3. Arterial pH below 7.3 with a PCO_2 <40 mm Hg (usually)
4. Ketosis

Diagnostic studies

1. Check the initial potassium level; there is always significant total body potassium depletion regardless of the initial level
2. Check the sodium level for hyponatremia as a result of lipemia and hyperglycemia; calculate the corrected sodium level (each 100 mg/dl increase in serum glucose over normal will decrease the serum sodium level by 1.6 mEq/L)
3. Calculate the anion gap ($AG = Na^+ - (Cl^- + HCO_3^-)$); in DKA the anion gap is increased
4. Check for evidence of precipitating factors (e.g., infection, MI)
   a. Obtain blood cultures, urinalysis, and urine culture and sensitivity (catheterize patient only if unconscious)
   b. The CBC with differential is of limited use since the WBC is usually increased and a mild shift to the left may be present
5. Obtain chest x-ray; if negative and pulmonary infection is strongly suspected, may repeat chest x-ray after the patient has been well hydrated
6. Obtain admission serum Ca, Mg, PO_4; the plasma phosphate and magnesium levels may be significantly depressed and should be checked again within 24 hours because they will decrease further with the correction of DKA
7. Obtain admission BUN (↑), creatinine (↑), serum osmolarity (↑)
8. The admission ECG is extremely valuable for the immediate diagnosis of electrolyte abnormalities and can serve as a useful guide to the rate of potassium administration, the following ECG changes may be noted[15]:
   a. Hypokalemia: ST segment depression, decreased amplitude of the T wave (or inverted T waves), increased amplitude of the U wave, apparent prolongation of the QT and PR interval
   b. Hyperkalemia: tall, narrow or tent-shaped T waves, decreased or absent P waves, short QT intervals, widening of the QRS complex

    c. Hypocalcemia: QT interval prolongation, flat or inverted T waves
    d. Hypercalcemia: short or absent ST segment, decreased QT_c interval
    e. Magnesium deficiency: ventricular and supraventricular dysrhythmias

Differential diagnosis

1. Alcoholic ketoacidosis: usually seen in poorly nourished alcoholics with vomiting, abdominal pain, and only minimal food intake over several days
    a. Lab values
      (1) Increased AG metabolic acidosis (due to increased hydroxybutyric acid > acetoacetic acid)
      (2) Low or absent serum ethanol level
      (3) Positive nitroprusside test
      (4) Normal to low serum glucose
    b. Therapy mainly consists of glucose infusion
2. Uremic acidosis: absent ketosis, markedly elevated BUN
3. Metabolic acidosis secondary to methyl alcohol, ethylene glycol
    a. Lab shows an increased osmolar gap (measured serum osmolarity − calculated osmolarity)

$$\text{Calculated osmolarity} = 2(Na^+ + K^+) + \left(\frac{glucose}{18}\right) + \left(\frac{BUN}{2.8}\right)$$

    b. In methyl alcohol poisoning, the patient complains of blindness or decreased visual acuity
    c. In ethylene glycol poisoning, the urine contains Ca oxalate crystals
    d. Ketosis is absent
4. Salicylate poisoning: history of aspirin ingestion

Therapy

1. Fluid replacement: the usual fluid deficit is 6-8 L
    a. Do not delay fluid replacement until lab results have been received
    b. Use 0.45% saline infusion in elderly patients or patients with a history of CHF; may use 0.9% saline in young or hypotensive patients
    c. The rate of fluid replacement varies with the age of the patient and the presence of severe heart or renal disease
      (1) The usual rate of infusion is 1L over the first hour, 300-500 ml/hr for the next 12 hours
      (2) Continue the infusion at a rate of 200-300 ml/hr until the serum glucose level is below 250-300 ml/hr, and then change the hydrating solution to D_5W to prevent hypoglycemia, replenish free water, and introduce additional glucose substrate (necessary to suppress lipolysis and ketogenesis)
2. Insulin administration
    a. The patient should be given an initial loading IV bolus of $0.15 - 0.2$ U/kg of regular insulin followed by a constant infusion at a rate of 0.1 U/kg/hr (e.g., 25 U of regular insulin in 250 ml of 0.9% saline at 70 ml/hr = 7 U/hr for 70 kg patient)
    b. Monitor serum glucose hourly for the first 2 hours then q2-4h
    c. The goal is to decrease serum glucose level by 50 mg/dl/hr (following an initial drop because of rehydration); if the serum glucose level is not decreasing at the expected rate, increase the rate of insulin infusion

Table 12-7 Initial potassium replacement in patients with DKA and normal renal function

Initial Serum Potassium Level (MEq/L)	Suggested Potassium Replacement* (mEq KCl/L)
>5.3	No KCl added to first liter of IV hydrating solution
5.0-5.3	10
4.5-5.0	20
4.0-4.5	30
3.5-4.0	40
<3.5	>40

*Per liter of hydrating solution.

    d. When the serum glucose level approaches 250-300 mg/dl, decrease the rate of insulin infusion to 2-3 U/hr and continue this rate until the patient has received adequate fluid replacement

    e. Approximately 30 minutes before stopping the IV insulin infusion, administer an IM dose of regular insulin (dose varies with patient's demonstrated insulin sensitivity); this IM dose of regular insulin is necessary because of the extremely short life of the insulin in the IV infusion[73]

3. Potassium replacement:

    a. Total body potassium loss in DKA is approximately 300-500 mEq; the rate of replacement varies with the patient's serum potassium level, degree of acidosis ($\downarrow$ pH = $\uparrow$ K level), and renal function (potassium replacement should be used with caution in patients with renal failure)

    b. Table 12-7 lists some guidelines for potassium replacement therapy in patients with normal renal function (as a rule of thumb, potassium administration may be started when there is no ECG evidence of hyperkalemia)

    c. Monitor serum potassium level hourly for the initial 2 hours, then q2-4h

    d. Monitor urine output hourly

4. Correct metabolic acidosis

    a. Vigorous hydration and correction of hyperglycemia usually restores normal pH

    b. Use bicarbonate judiciously (recent studies indicate that bicarbonate therapy in patients with severe DKA [arterial blood pH 6.9 to 7.15] will not shorten clinical recovery time or significantly improve biochemical variables[45]); restrict bicarbonate use only to severe metabolic acidosis (e.g., arterial pH <6.9)

5. Correct hypophosphatemia: obtain a serum phosphorus level on admission and after 24 hours of therapy

6. Use lab data flow sheet to closely monitor the patient (Table 12-8)

Complications

1. Cerebral edema should be suspected when the patient's sensorium remains impaired despite improvement of metabolic parameters

    a. Etiology is controversial; it may be secondary to an extremely rapid

Table 12-8 DKA flow sheet

Time (hr)	0	1	2	4	6	8	10	12	16	20	24
Serum glucose											
Serum potassium											
pH or HCO_3											
Insulin infusion (U/hr)											
IV fluids (ml/hr)											
Type of IV solution											
Urine output (ml/hr)											
Mental status											
Pulse											
Respiration											
Blood pressure											

decrease in the serum glucose level and to osmotic disequilibrium caused by rapid and early use of hypotonic fluids
  b. Diagnosis: a CT scan of the brain will demonstrate narrowing of the ventricular system compatible with cerebral edema
  c. Therapy
    (1) Mannitol and low–molecular weight dextran
    (2) Large doses of corticosteroids (controversial)
2. Cardiac dysrhythmias
  a. Caused by electrolyte abnormalities and acidosis
  b. Closely monitor potassium, magnesium, and calcium levels and correct any abnormalities
3. Shock: caused by severe hypovolemia, infection, or cardiac dysfunction
4. Hypoglycemia
5. MI
6. Acute pancreatitis

12.3 HYPEROSMOLAR COMA

Definition
Hyperosmolar coma is a state of extreme hyperglycemia, marked dehydration, serum hyperosmolarity, altered mental status, and absence of severe ketoacidosis. It occurs in non–insulin dependent diabetics.

Etiology
1. Infections (20%-25%), e.g., pneumonia, urinary tract infection, sepsis
2. New or previously unrecognized diabetes (30%-50%)
3. Reduction or omission of diabetic medication
4. Stress (MI, CVA)

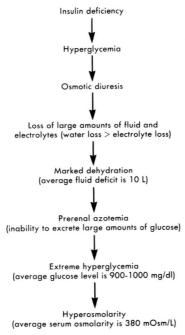

Figure 12-2
Pathophysiology of hyperosmolar state.

5. Drugs
   a. Phenytoin, diazoxide may lead to impaired insulin secretion
   b. Diuretics may result in excessive dehydration
   c. Hypertonic alimentation may cause dehydration secondary to osmotic diuresis

·   ·   ·

The patient is usually an elderly or bed-confined diabetic with impaired thirst (or inability to communicate thirst) usually presenting after an interval of 1-2 weeks of prolonged osmotic diuresis. Fig. 12-2 illustrates the pathophysiology of hyperosmolar coma.

Symptoms
1. Mental obtundation, seizures
2. Polyuria
3. Nausea and vomiting (not as severe as in patients with DKA)

Physical exam

1. Evidence of extreme dehydration (poor skin turgor, sunken eyeballs, dry mucous membranes)
2. Neurologic defects (reversible hemiplegia, focal seizures)
3. Orthostatic hypotension, tachycardia
4. Evidence of precipitating factors (pneumonia, infected skin ulcer)

Lab results[74]

1. Hyperglycemia: serum glucose usually >600 mg/dl
2. Hyperosmolarity: serum osmolarity usually >340 mOsm/L
3. Serum sodium: may be low, normal, or high; if normal or high the patient is severely dehydrated since normally an elevated blood sugar will draw fluid from intracellular space decreasing the serum sodium
4. Serum potassium: may be low, normal, or high; regardless of the initial serum level, the total body loss is approximately 5-15 mEq/kg
5. Serum bicarbonate: usually >12 mEq/L (average is 17 mEq/L)
6. Arterial pH: usually >7.2 (average 7.26); both serum bicarbonate and arterial pH may be lower if lactic acidosis is present
7. BUN: azotemia (prerenal) is usually present (BUN = 60-90 mg/dl)
8. Phosphorus: hypophosphatemia (average loss is 70-140 mM)
9. Calcium: hypocalcemia (average loss is 50-100 mEq)
10. Magnesium: hypomagnesemia (average loss is 50-100 mEq)

Therapy

1. Vigorous fluid replacement: Infuse 1000-1500 ml/hr for the initial 1-2 L, then decrease the rate of infusion to 500 ml/hr and monitor urine output, blood chemistries, and blood pressure; use normal saline (0.9% saline) if the patient is hypotensive, otherwise use 0.45% saline (slower infusion rate may be used initially in patients with compromised cardiac status and a history of CHF)[72]
2. Replace electrolytes and monitor serum levels frequently (Table 12-9)
   a. Monitor urine output hourly
   b. Monitor ECG continuously
3. Correct hyperglycemia
   a. Vigorous IV hydration will decrease the serum glucose level in most patients by 20 mg/dl/hr; a regular insulin IV bolus is often not necessary

Table 12-9   Suggested potassium replacement in diabetics with hyperosmolar state and normal renal function

Initial Serum Potassium Level (mEq/L)	Suggested Initial Potassium Replacement (mEq KCl/hr)*
>5.2	No initial potassium replacement necessary
4-5.2	10
3.2-4.0	20
<3.2	≥30

*If urine output is adequate.

b. Low dose insulin infusion at 1-2 U/hour (e.g., 25 U regular insulin in 250 ml 0.9% saline at 20 ml/hr) until the serum glucose level approaches 250-300 mg/dl, then the patient is started on regular insulin SC q6h with the dosage based on the serum glucose level:

<200 mg/dl: no insulin coverage
201-250 mg/dl: 2 U
251-300 mg/dl: 4 U
301-350 mg/dl: 6 U
351-400 mg/dl: 8 U
>400 mg/dl: notify physician

c. There is no need to give an IM dose of regular insulin when the infusion is stopped (unlike in DKA) since the majority of patients will not need any further insulin therapy for at least 6 hours

4. Rule out precipitating factors: obtain blood and urine cultures
5. Monitor all critical parameters (see Table 12-8)

12.4 HYPOGLYCEMIA
Iradj Nejad

Definition

Hypoglycemia can be arbitrarily defined as a plasma glucose level <50 mg/dl. To establish the diagnosis, the following three things are necessary:

1. Presence of symptoms
   a. Adrenergic: sweating, anxiety, tremors, tachycardia, palpitations
   b. Neuroglycopenic: seizures, fatigue, syncope, headache, behavior changes, visual disturbances
2. Low plasma glucose level in symptomatic patient
3. Relief of symptoms following ingestion of carbohydrates

Classification

1. Reactive hypoglycemia
   a. Hypoglycemia usually occurs 2-4 hours after a meal rich in carbohydrates
   b. These patients never have symptoms in the fasting state and rarely experience loss of consciousness secondary to their hypoglycemia
   c. Patients who have had subtotal gastrectomy will rapidly absorb carbohydrates causing an early and very high plasma glucose level followed by a late insulin surge that reaches its peak when most of the glucose has been absorbed and results in hypoglycemia
   d. Congenital deficiencies of enzymes necessary for carbohydrate metabolism and functional (idiopathic) hypoglycemia are additional causes of reactive hypoglycemia
2. Fasting hypoglycemia
   a. Symptoms usually appear in the absence of food intake (at night or during early morning)
   b. Etiology: factitious hypoglycemia, insulinoma, non–islet cell neoplasms, hormonal deficiency, liver disease, renal disease, and ethanol-induced hypoglycemia

Table 12-10   Lab differentiation of factitious hypoglycemia and insulinoma

Lab Test	Insulinoma	Exogenous Insulin	Sulfonylurea
Plasma insulin level	↑	↑ ↑	↑
Insulin anti-bodies	None*	Present	None*
Plasma/urine sulfonylurea levels	Absent	Absent	Present
C-peptide	↑	N/ ↓	↑

*May be present if the patient has had prior insulin injections.
KEY: ↑ , Increased; ↓ , decreased; N, normal.

Diagnosis

In a normal person, when the plasma glucose level is low (e.g., fasting state) the plasma insulin level is also low. Any patient presenting with fasting hypoglycemia of unexplained cause should have the following tests drawn during the hypoglycemic episode (see Table 12-10 for interpretation of results).

1. Plasma insulin level
2. Insulin antibodies
3. Plasma and urine sulfonylurea levels
4. C-peptide

Factitious hypoglycemia should be considered, especially if the patient has ready access to insulin or sulfonylureas (e.g., medical/paramedical personnel, family members who are diabetic or who are in the medical profession).

1. To diagnose factitious hypoglycemia secondary to sulfonylureas, screen serum and urine to determine the presence of sulfonylureas.
2. To diagnose factitious hypoglycemia secondary to insulin, measure:
   a. Plasma free insulin level, which is markedly increased following exogenous insulin injection.
   b. Insulin antibodies, which are usually present after an exogenous insulin injection, but may be absent if a more purified insulin preparation or if human insulin has been used (this test is not useful if the patient has a history of previous insulin use).
   c. C-peptide (connecting peptide): insulin is synthesized by the pancreas as a single chain polypeptide formed of A and B chains joined by the C-peptide. This single chain polypeptide (proinsulin) is broken down and secreted into the bloodstream as insulin and C-peptide in a 1:1 ratio. Exogenous insulin does not contain C-peptide, thus C-peptide levels are elevated in patients with insulinoma, but not following exogenous insulin injection.

Pancreatic islet cell neoplasms (insulinoma) are usually small (<3 cm in size), single, insulin-producing adenomas. Measurement of inappropriately elevated serum insulin levels despite an extremely low plasma glucose level after prolonged fasting (24-72 hours) is pathognomonic for these neoplasms.

The insulinoma can be located by CT scanning of pancreas and abdomen; if inconclusive, angiography or percutaneous transportal venous sampling (to measure a step up in insulin levels) can be attempted.

Other causes of hypoglycemia are as follows:

1. Non–islet cell neoplasms: tumors of mesodermal origin located in the peritoneal or retroperitoneal cavity. It is believed that they cause hypoglycemia or inhibit hepatic glucose production via a nonsuppressible insulin-like activity (NSILA).
2. Deficiency of counterregulatory hormones (e.g., glucagon catecholamines, cortisol, growth hormone) can also cause hypoglycemia.
3. Liver disease can deplete hepatic glycogen storage.
4. Chronic renal disease can result in increased insulin level and poor nutritional status.

12.5 HYPERLIPOPROTEINEMIAS

Definition

Hyperlipoproteinemias are characterized by an elevation of cholesterol or triglyceride level. As a rule of thumb, for a patient older than 20 the upper limit of normal serum cholesterol is 180 mg/dl plus the patient's age. A cholesterol/HDL ratio >4.5 is associated with increased risk of coronary artery disease.

Diagnosis

1. Measure fasting levels of plasma cholesterol, triglycerides, and high-density lipoprotein cholesterol (HDL)
2. If hyperlipoproteinemia is detected, perform serum lipoprotein electrophoresis to determine which class of lipoprotein is affected; Table 12-11 describes the electrophoretic mobility of the various lipoproteins
3. Calculations: if triglycerides are <400 mg/dl and lipoprotein electrophoresis does not detect chylomicrons and type III hyperlipoproteins (see Table 12-12), the very low–density lipoproteins (VLDL) and the low–density lipoprotein (LDL) cholesterol can be calculated using the following formulas:[24]

$$\text{VLDL cholesterol} = \frac{\text{triglyceride level}}{5}$$

$$\text{LDL cholesterol} = \text{total cholesterol} - (\text{VLDL cholesterol} + \text{HDL cholesterol})$$

Classification and therapy

Lipoprotein abnormalities are generally classified into six major categories based on the plasma lipoprotein pattern. Table 12-12 describes the major

Table 12-11 Lipoprotein electrophoresis: electrophoretic mobility

Chylomicrons	Origin
VLDL	Preβ
LDL	β
HDL	α

Table 12-12 Classification, clinical manifestations, and therapy of hyperlipoproteinemias[24,35,39,40,56]

Type	I	IIa	IIb	III	IV	V
Plasma lipoprotein pattern	↑ Chylomicrons	↑LDL	↑LDL, ↑VLDL	↑ Abnormal ILDL	↑ VLDL	↑ VLDL, ↑ chylomicrons
Cholesterol	N	↑	↑	↑	N	N/↑
Triglyceride	↑	N	↑	↑	↑	↑
Prevalence	Very rare	Common	Common	Uncommon	Common	Uncommon
Risk of atherogenesis	No increase	↑↑	↑↑	↑↑	No increase/mild ↑	No increase
Clinical signs and symptoms	Eruptive xanthomas Lipemia retinalis Pancreatitis Hepatosplenomegaly	Xanthelasma Tuberous xanthomas Tendinous xanthomas Arcus corneae	Xanthelasma Tuberous xanthomas Tendinous xanthomas Arcus corneae	Tuberous xanthomas Tendinous xanthomas Peripheral vascular disease ↑ Incidence of diabetes mellitus Hyperuricemia	↑ Incidence of diabetes mellitus Hyperuricemia Infrequent eruptive and tuberous xanthomas	Eruptive xanthomas Pancreatitis ↑ Incidence of diabetes mellitus Lipemia retinalis Arthritis Emotional lability
Recommended diet	Low fat diet (dietary fat <30% of total calories)	Low cholesterol diet (<300 mg/day) ↑ Polyunsaturates to maintain polyunsaturated/saturated fats ratio of approximately 1:1	Low cholesterol diet ↑ Polyunsaturates to maintain polyunsaturated/saturated fats ratio of approximately 1:1	Low cholesterol diet Low fat diet Avoid alcoholic beverages	Low cholesterol diet Low saturated fats Low calorie, restricted simple carbohydrates Avoid alcoholic substances	Dietary restriction of fat and cholesterol Avoid alcoholic beverages
Possibly beneficial medications	None	Cholestyramine Colestipol Nicotinic acid Probucol	Cholestyramine Colestipol Nicotinic acid Probucol Nicotinic acid Clofibrate Gemfibrozil	Nicotinic acid Clofibrate Gemfibrozil	Gemfibrozil (useful in diabetic patients) Nicotinic acid (useful in recurrent pancreatitis)	

KEY: ↑, Increased; N, normal; ILDL, intermediate low-density lipoproteins; LDL, low-density lipoproteins; VLDL, very low-density lipoproteins.

Table 12-13 Drug therapy of hyperlipoproteinemias[24,35,39,40,56]

Agent	Dosage	Effect	Indications
Cholestyramine (Questran)	8 mg PO bid-tid Maximum daily dosage is 32 g	↓ LDL cholesterol May ↑ triglyceride levels	Type II hyperlipoproteinemia
Clofibrate (Atromid-S)	1 mg PO bid	↓ VLDL cholesterol ↓ Triglycerides May ↑ HDL cholesterol	Type III, IV hyperlipoproteinemias Occasionally useful in type IIb hyperlipoproteinemias
Colestipol (Colestid)	5 mg PO tid Maximum daily dosage is 30 g	↓ LDL cholesterol	Type II hyperlipoproteinemias
Gemfibrozil (Lopid)	600 mg PO bid	↓ VLDL cholesterol ↓ LDL cholesterol ↑ HDL cholesterol	Type III, IV, V hyperlipoproteinemias
Nicotinic acid (Niacin)	Initial dosage is 100 mg PO tid with meals Average dosage is 1 g PO tid Maximum daily dosage is 9 g	↓ VLDL cholesterol ↓ LDL cholesterol ↓ Triglycerides ↑ HDL cholesterol	Type II, III, IV, V hyperlipoproteinemias
Probucol (Lorelco)	500 mg PO bid	↓ LDL cholesterol ↓ HDL cholesterol	Type II hyperlipoproteinemias

KEY: ↑, Increases; ↓, decreases.

laboratory and clinical characteristics of each category and the suggested therapeutic approach. Table 12-13 outlines drug therapy of hyperlipoproteinemias.

| 12.6 | ANTERIOR PITUITARY DISORDERS

HYPOPITUITARISM
Etiology and classification
1. Primary hypopituitarism
   a. Postpartum vascular insufficiency of anterior pituitary (Sheehan's syndrome)
      (1) Seen in postpartum patients with a history of hemorrhagic crisis at delivery or in the immediate postpartum period
      (2) Suspect in any postpartum patient who fails to resume menses or does not lactate
   b. Ischemic necrosis of pituitary secondary to sickle cell anemia, vasculitis, diabetes mellitus
   c. Neoplasms (primary or metastatic)
   d. Granulomatous diseases (sarcoidosis, Wegener's granulomatosis)
   e. Cavernous sinus thrombosis
   f. Infections (TB, mycoses, syphilis, meningitis)
   g. ''Empty sella syndrome''
      (1) Primary ''empty sella syndrome'': protrusion of the third ventricle (subarachnoid cistern) in the sella turcica; it is difficult to diagnose by conventional CT scan because the CSF fluid in the empty sella has the same density as fluid from a cystic pituitary tumor, but it can be readily diagnosed by magnetic resonance imaging (MRI)[32] or by injecting metrimazide (a water-soluble, iodine contrast agent) into the subarachnoid space via LP and outlining the parasellar contents
      (2) Secondary ''empty sella syndrome'': decrease in size of the pituitary caused by various etiologies (irradiation, surgery)
   h. Aneurysmal dilation of internal carotid artery
   i. Radiation therapy for neck and head tumors
   j. Other: surgical destruction, lymphocytic hypophysitis, hemochromatosis, chronic renal failure, familial
2. Secondary hypopituitarism
   a. Hypothalamic abnormalities: tumors, inflammation (sarcoidosis, TB), trauma, radiation, subarachnoid hemorrhage, infections (encephalitis, meningitis), lipid storage diseases
   b. Lesions of pituitary stalk: trauma, surgery, aneurysms, or tumor compression

Clinical presentation
1. Symptoms secondary to mass effect
   a. Visual disturbances
      (1) Bitemporal hemianopsia: most common defect; it is caused by compression of the optic chiasm
      (2) Superior bitemporal defect: earliest defect
      (3) Loss of central vision: caused by pressure on the posterior part of the chiasm (location of the papulomacular bundle of fibers)

    b. Headaches

    c. Seizures (rare)

2. Hormonal effects

    a. Growth hormone deficiency: initial hormonal deficiency; there are no clinical manifestations in adults

    b. Gonadal dysfunction: amenorrhea in menstruating women, impotence in men

    c. Hypothyroidism: often mistaken for depression

    d. ACTH deficiency: develops in later stages of hypopituitarism; can manifest with an Addisonian crisis during a period of stress, such as surgery, or infection

Diagnosis

1. Endocrine tests

    a. Demonstration of target gland deficiency (e.g., measurement of testosterone levels in an impotent man)

    b. Measurement of pituitary hormones (e.g., decreased plasma FSH and LH levels in an impotent man with low testosterone levels indicate hypogonadism caused by central defect [secondary hypogonadism])

    c. Tests of pituitary reserve: cortisol and GH levels fluctuate widely in response to stress or diurnal variation, but their deficiency can be demonstrated by using the following provocative testing methods:

       (1) Metyrapone test (Fig. 12-3)

          (a) Metyrapone competitively inhibits the adrenal enzyme 11-β hydroxylase necessary for the conversion of 11-deoxycortisol to cortisol; the resulting low cortisol level stimulates the normal pituitary (via feedback mechanism) to release ACTH, and

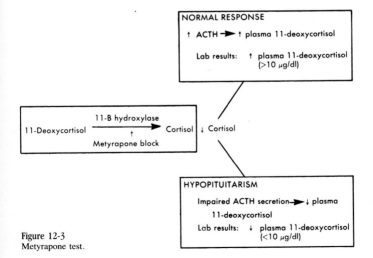

Figure 12-3
Metyrapone test.

thereby increases adrenal production of 11-deoxycortisol until the 11-deoxycortisol levels are sufficiently elevated to compete with all the metyrapone available (thus eliminating the block to cortisol formation)
- (b) An elevated plasma 11-deoxycortisol level following 3 g PO dose of metyrapone overnight is proof of adequate ACTH reserve
- (c) Caution: the metyrapone test produces adrenal insufficiency and can result in Addisonian crisis in patients with known primary or secondary insufficiency)
- (2) Insulin tolerance test (ITT)
  - (a) Obtain fasting plasma glucose, cortisol level, and GH level
  - (b) Start the patient on an insulin infusion at 0.1 U/kg/hr
  - (c) Measure plasma glucose, cortisol, and GH at 30, 45, 60, and 90 minutes
  - (d) Stop the insulin infusion when the blood sugar falls to half the control value or if the patient becomes symptomatic
  - (e) Interpretation: the induced hypoglycemia should result in a rise in cortisol (>7 μg/dl) and growth hormone (>9 ng/dl) in a patient with an intact hypothalamic-pituitary-adrenal axis
  - (f) Caution: this test must be performed only under close medical supervision; it is contraindicated in patients suspected of having adrenal insufficiency, seizure disorders, or cardiovascular disease
2. Additional tests
   - a. A lateral skull x-ray is useful in screening for large pituitary tumors; it can identify erosions or abnormalities in the shape of the sella and may also show lytic lesions in the skull, directing the diagnosis toward a primary breast or lung neoplasm, but its value is limited by many false-positive and false-negative results
   - b. CT of head: with coronal views and contrast enhancement

Therapy

Therapy is aimed at treating the cause of the pituitary failure and providing adequate hormone replacement.

ANTERIOR PITUITARY HYPERFUNCTION SECONDARY TO PITUITARY NEOPLASMS

The diagnosis and therapy of hormone-secreting pituitary adenomas varies with the type of hormone secreted. This section will discuss hypersecretion of growth hormone, ACTH, and prolactin.

Growth hormone

Excessive growth hormone (GH) secretion will result in *gigantism* (extreme height, wide hands and feet, prognathism) if it occurs before closure of the epiphyses or *acromegaly* if it occurs after epiphyseal closure.
1. History: obtain old photos for comparison and inquire about family history (acromegaly can present as a manifestation of multiple endocrine neoplasia [MEN])

2. Physical exam
   a. Excessive size of hands and feet with ''spade-like'' digits (because of increased width of distal bone tufts), sausage-shaped fingers
   b. Characteristic facies (broad jaw, protrusion of supraorbital ridges, gap teeth, prominent forehead)
   c. Oily skin, acanthosis nigricans, excessive sweating
   d. Enlargement of skeletal muscles, increase in size of visceral organs
   e. Deep voice, weakness
   f. Diastolic hypertension, decreased libido, galactorrhea
   g. Abnormalities secondary to pituitary enlargement (headaches, visual disturbances)
3. X-ray findings: degenerative arthritis
   a. Thickening of outer skull table, enlarged sella turcica
   b. Tufting of phalanges, narrowed carpal tunnels
4. Lab results
   a. Elevated fasting serum GH level (>10 ng/ml)
   b. Nonsuppression of GH secretion (failure to decrease GH concentration below 2 ng/ml) after an oral glucose tolerance test; if the glucose tolerance test is equivocal, thyrotropin-releasing hormone (TRH) injection will paradoxically stimulate GH secretion in acromegalic patients
   c. Glucose intolerance and hypercalciuria may also be present
   d. Increased plasma somatomedin C level (insulin-like growth factor I)
5. Therapy
   a. Surgery
      (1) Transfrontal surgery if there is suprasellar extension of the tumor
      (2) Transsphenoidal surgery if the tumor is confined to the sella turcica[68]
   b. Pituitary irradiation results in a higher incidence of hypopituitarism than surgery, therefore in patients in whom fertility is an important consideration (e.g., young patients) it should be regarded as a second choice
   c. Bromocriptine (dopamine agonist) will paradoxically reduce GH levels in some patients with acromegaly; however, shrinkage of tumor size is uncommon in these patients
   d. Combination of above treatments

ACTH

Glucocorticoid excess secondary to an ACTH-secreting pituitary adenoma will result in Cushing's disease. This is one of the many causes of Cushing's syndrome described in section 12.11. Therapy of ACTH-secreting pituitary adenomas:
1. Transsphenoidal microsurgery can result in selective removal of the adenoma, preservation of pituitary function, and minimal morbidity if performed by an experienced neurosurgeon[12]
2. Pituitary irradiation
   a. Heavy-particle irradiation produces high cure rates but also a greater incidence of hypopituitarism than conventional irradiation
   b. Conventional radiation therapy may be preferred to heavy-particle irradiation in children[30]

3. Neuropharmacotherapeutic drugs
   a. Cyproheptadine (serotonin antagonist) controls ACTH secretion in some patients with Cushing's disease
   b. Metyrapone inhibits adrenal cortisol biosynthesis and may be useful in debilitated patients who cannot tolerate surgery

Prolactin

Prolactin secretion, unlike other pituitary hormones, is regulated by tonic inhibition. Dopamine is the major prolactin inhibiting factor.
1. Etiology of hyperprolactinemia
   a. Pituitary tumors
   b. Drugs: phenothiazines, methyldopa, reserpine, MAO inhibitors, androgens, progesterone, cimetidine, tricyclic antidepressants, haloperidol, meprobamate, chlordiazepoxide, estrogens, narcotics
   c. Hepatic cirrhosis, renal failure, primary hypothyroidism
   d. Ectopic prolactin-secreting tumors (hypernephroma, bronchogenic carcinoma)
   e. Infiltrating diseases of the pituitary (sarcoidosis, histiocytosis)
   f. Head trauma
   g. Pregnancy
   h. Idiopathic hyperprolactinemia
2. Clinical manifestations
   a. Men: decreased libido, impotence, decreased facial and body hair, small testicles, delayed puberty (due to decreased testosterone secondary to inhibition of gonadotropin secretion)
   b. Women: amenorrhea and galactorrhea, oligomenorrhea, anovulation
   c. Both sexes: headache, visual field defects (caused by tumor expansion)
3. Diagnosis
   a. Lab results
      (1) Elevated serum prolactin level
         (a) Normal mean levels are 8 ng/ml (women) and 5 ng/ml (men)
         (b) Levels >300 ng/ml are virtually diagnostic of prolactinomas
      (2) TRH stimulation test: the normal response is an increase in serum prolactin levels by 100% within 1 hour of TRH infusion; failure to demonstrate an increase in prolactin level is suggestive of pituitary lesion
   b. Magnetic resonance imaging (MRI) is the procedure of choice in the radiographic evaluation of pituitary disease[32]; in absence of MRI, a radiographic diagnosis is best accomplished with a high-resolution CT scanner and special coronal cuts through the pituitary region; angiography should be considered to rule out aneurysm in patients with a large soft tissue mass in the sellar region and prolactin levels <100 ng/ml
4. Therapy
   a. Transsphenoidal resection: the success rate is dependent on the location of the tumor (entirely intrasellar), experience of the neurosurgeon, and size of the tumor (<10 mm in diameter)
   b. Medical therapy is preferred when fertility is an important consideration

(1) Bromocriptine (dopamine agonist): dosage is 2.5-10 mg/day; it decreases the size of the tumor and lowers the prolactin level into the normal range when the initial serum prolactin is <200 ng/ml, but initial values greater than 1000 ng/ml may be difficult to reduce[51]

(2) Pergolide mesylate: preliminary reports indicate that this drug effectively treats prolactinomas and is better tolerated than bromocriptine

c. Pituitary irradiation is useful as adjunctive therapy of macroadenomas (≥10 mm in diameter)

[12.7] **FLUID HEMOSTASIS DISORDERS**

DIABETES INSIPIDUS

Definition

Diabetes insipidus (DI) is a polyuric disorder resulting from insufficient production of antidiuretic hormone (ADH), pituitary (neurogenic) diabetes insipidus, or unresponsiveness of the renal tubules to ADH (nephrogenic diabetes insipidus).

Etiology

1. Neurogenic diabetes insipidus
   a. Idiopathic
   b. Neoplasms of brain or pituitary fossa (craniopharyngiomas, metastatic neoplasms from breast or lung)
   c. Posttherapeutic neurosurgical procedures (e.g., hypophysectomy)
   d. Head trauma (e.g., basal skull fracture)
   e. Granulomatous disorders (sarcoidosis or tuberculosis)
   f. Histiocytosis (Hand-Schüller-Christian disease, eosinophilic granuloma)
   g. Familial
   h. Other: interventricular hemorrhage, aneurysms, meningitis, postencephalitis)
2. Nephrogenic diabetes insipidus
   a. Drugs: lithium, amphotericin B, demeclocycline, methoxyflurane anesthesia
   b. Familial
   c. Metabolic hypercalcemia or hypokalemia

Clinical manifestations

1. Polyuria: urine volumes usually range 2.5-6 L/day
2. Polydipsia (predilection for cold or iced drinks)
3. Neurologic manifestations (seizures, headaches, visual field defects)
4. Evidence of volume contraction

Lab results

1. Decreased urine specific gravity (≤1.005)
2. Decreased urine osmolarity (usually <200 mOsm/kg H_2O)
3. Hypernatremia, increased plasma osmolarity, hypercalcemia, hypokalemia

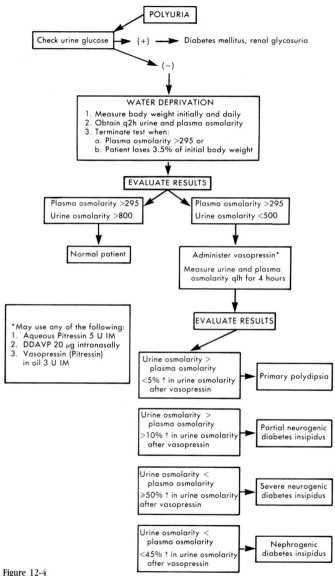

Figure 12-4
Diagnostic flowchart for diabetes insipidus.

Differential diagnosis

1. Diabetes insipidus
2. Primary polydipsia
3. Osmotic diuresis (glucose, mannitol, urea)

Diagnosis

Fig. 12-4 illustrates the diagnostic approach to a patient with suspected diabetes insipidus.

Therapy

1. Partial neurogenic diabetes insipidus
   a. Chlorpropamide (Diabinese) 250-375 mg PO qd; it potentiates the ADH effect on the kidney
   b. If chlorpropamide is inadequate to control the polyuria, the patient will require ADH replacement (see below)
2. Severe neurogenic diabetes insipidus: various ADH preparations are available
   a. Vasopressin tannate in oil: 2.5-5 U IM q24-72h; useful for long-term management because of its long life (the ampul must be shaken well before injection)
   b. DDAVP (1-deamino-8-D-arginine vasopressin): 2.5-20 μg administered intranasally q12-24h
   c. Aqueous vasopressin: 5-10 U SC/IM q4-6h; short acting, useful only for short-term therapy
3. Nephrogenic diabetes insipidus
   a. Adequate hydration
   b. Low sodium diet and chlorothiazide to induce mild sodium depletion
   c. Polyuria of DI secondary to lithium can be ameliorated by using amiloride (5 mg PO bid initially, increased to 10 mg PO bid after 2 weeks)[3]

SYNDROME OF INAPPROPRIATE ANTIDIURETIC HORMONE SECRETION

Definition

Syndrome of inappropriate antidiuretic hormone secretion (SIADH) is characterized by excessive secretion of ADH in absence of normal osmotic or physiologic stimuli (increased serum osmolarity, decreased plasma volume, hypotension).

Etiology

1. Neoplasms: lung, duodenum, pancreas, brain, thymus, bladder, prostate
2. Pulmonary disorders: pneumonia, TB, bronchiectasis, emphysema, status asthmaticus
3. Intracranial pathology: trauma, neoplasm, infections, hemorrhage, hydrocephalus
4. Postoperative period: surgical stress, ventilators with positive pressure, anesthetic agents
5. Drugs: chlorpropamide, thiazide diuretics, vasopressin, oxytocin, chemotherapeutic agents (vincristine, vinblastine, cyclophosphamide), car-

bamazepine, phenothiazines, MAO inhibitors, tricyclic antidepressants, narcotics, nicotine
6. Other: acute intermittent prophyria, Guillain-Barré syndrome

Clinical manifestations

1. The patient is generally normovolemic or slightly hypervolemic
2. Confusion, lethargy, and seizures may be present if the hyponatremia is severe or of rapid onset
3. Manifestations of the underlying disease may be evident (e.g., fever from an infectious process, or headaches and visual field defects from an intracranial mass)

Lab results

1. Hyponatremia
2. Urine osmolarity greater than serum osmolarity
3. Urinary sodium >30 mEq/L
4. Normal BUN, creatinine (indicate normal renal function and absence of dehydration)
5. Other criteria: normal thyroid, adrenal, and cardiac function; no recent use of diuretics

Therapy

1. Fluid restriction to 500-1000 ml/day
2. Demeclocycline (Declomycin) 300-600 mg PO bid may be useful in patients with chronic SIADH (e.g., secondary to a neoplasm), but use with caution in patients with hepatic disease; its side effects include nephrogenic DI and photosensitivity
3. In emergency situations (seizures, coma), SIADH can be treated with a combination of hypertonic saline and furosemide; this increases the serum sodium by causing diuresis of urine that is more dilute than plasma[28]

12.8 EATING DISORDERS

ANOREXIA NERVOSA
Definition

Anorexia nervosa is a prolonged illness that occurs mostly in female adolescents. It is characterized by severe self-induced weight loss, amenorrhea, and a specific psychopathology.[54]

Diagnosis[18]

1. An intense fear of becoming obese that does not diminish as weight loss progresses
2. Disturbance of body image (e.g., claiming to "feel fat" even when emaciated)
3. Weight loss of at least 25% of original body weight; if under 18 years of age, weight loss from original body weight plus weight gain expected from growth charts may be combined to make 25%
4. Refusal to maintain body weight over minimum normal weight for age and height

Symptoms

1. Amenorrhea
2. Sleep disturbances[17]
3. Cold intolerance
4. Early satiety, abdominal pain, and constipation or diarrhea

Physical exam

1. Severe malnutrition (cachexia), often masked by oversized clothes
2. Bradycardia, hypotension, hypothermia, bradypnea
3. Dry skin with excessive growth of lanugo
4. Peripheral edema may be present

Lab results

1. Endocrine abnormalities[23]
   a. Decreased FSH, LH, T_4, T_3, estrogens, urinary 17-OH steroids, estrone, and estradiol
   b. Normal free T_4, TSH
   c. Increased cortisol, GH, RT_3, T_3RU
   d. Absence of cyclic surge of LH
2. Leukopenia, thrombocytopenia, anemia
3. Increased plasma β-carotene levels, decreased fibrinogen

Treatment

1. Hyperalimentation of severely malnourished patients
2. Feed with assistance; patient should never eat alone and observation by the nursing staff or family is recommended
3. Psychiatric evaluation and therapy
4. Routine monitoring of patients with prolonged QT interval; sudden death in these patients is often caused by ventricular tachydysrhythmias related to QT interval prolongation[29]

BULIMIA

Definition

Bulemia is characterized by episodic, uncontrollable eating binges, self-induced vomiting, repeated attempts at weight loss by severe dieting aided by vomiting and laxatives, depressed mood and self-depreciation following binges[23]

Pathophysiology

According to some authors,[54] bulemia is a chronic phase of anorexia nervosa with the primary symptom being recurrent gorging on food and with the psychopathology consisting of an exaggerated fear of becoming fat. Others[21] consider it a distinct syndrome from anorexia nervosa.

Clinical features

In a recent series of 275 bulimic patients, Mitchel et al[44] noted the following features:

1. Eating binges: 100%
2. Self-induced vomiting: 88%
3. Laxative abuse: 60%

4. Diuretic abuse: 33%
5. Problems with alcohol or other drugs: 33%
6. Mean age of patients at the onset of bulimia is 17 years

Physical exam

1. Scars on the back of the hand from rubbing against the upper incisors when inducing vomiting
2. Patient is not usually emaciated and the physical exam may be entirely normal

Lab results

Abnormalities secondary to vomiting and laxative abuse may be evident (e.g., hypokalemia).

Therapy

1. Psychiatric evaluation and therapy
2. Management of medical complications

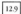 **THYROID DISORDERS**

INTERPRETATION OF THYROID FUNCTION STUDIES
(see Table 12-14)

1. Serum thyroxine (T_4)
   a. Thyroid function screening test; if results are within 75%-80% of the lab reference value, any further testing of asymptomatic patients is not likely to be productive[52]
   b. Test measures both circulating thyroxine bound to protein (represents >99% of circulating T_4) and unbound (free) thyroxine
   c. Values vary with protein binding; changes in the concentration of T_4, secondary to changes in thyroid binding globulin (TBG), can be caused by the following:

Increased TBG ($\uparrow T_4$)	Decreased TBG ($\downarrow T_4$)
Pregnancy	Androgens
Estrogens	Nephrotic syndrome
Acute infectious hepatitis	Acromegaly
Oral contraceptives	Hypoproteinemia
Familial	Dilantin, ASA, high-dose penicillin
	Chronic debilitating illness

   d. To eliminate the suspected influence of protein binding on thyroxine values, two additional tests are available: T_3 resin uptake, free thyroxine
2. T_3 resin uptake (T_3RU) measures the percentage of free T_4 (not bound to protein); it does not measure serum T_3 concentration
3. Free thyroxine directly measures unbound thyroxine by equilibrium dialysis, but it is expensive and difficult to quantitate; the free thyroxine index (FTI) can also be easily calculated by multiplying $T_4 \times T_3RU$ and dividing the result by 100:

Table 12-14   Use and interpretation of thyroid function tests

T_4	T_3RU	FTI	Comments
N	N	N	Normal; no additional thyroid studies necessary
N/↓	N/↓	N/↓	Order TSH; if normal, patient is euthyroid, but if ↑ patient is hypothyroid
N/↑	N/↑	N/↑	Order T_3; if ↑, early hyperthyroidism is present; if N or borderline ↑, order TRH
↑	↑	↑	Thyroid gland palpable (enlarged): hyperthyroidism
↑	↑	↑	Thyroid gland not palpable: order RAIU to rule out iatrogenic ingestion of thyroid hormone (↓ RAIU)
↑	↑	↑	Tender thyroid gland: order RAIU to rule out subacute thyroiditis (↓ RAIU)
↑	↑	↑	Patient appears clinically euthyroid: order TSH, if ↑, there is peripheral resistance to thyroid hormone
↓	↓	↓	Patient appears clinically euthyroid: liothyronine (Cytomel) ingestion is likely; T_3 is ↑
↓	↓	↓	Patient appears clinically hypothyroid: order TSH; if ↑, primary hypothyroidism is present, if N/↓, secondary hypothyroidism
↑	N/↓	N	↑ T_4 secondary to ↑ TBG, no additional thyroid studies necessary
N/↓	↑	N	↑ T_3RU secondary to ↓ TBG; no additional thyroid studies necessary

KEY. ↑, Increased; ↓, decreased; N, normal.

$$FTI = \frac{T_4 \times T_3RU}{100}$$

Normal values = 1-4

The FTI corrects for any abnormal T_4 values secondary to protein binding
4. Thyroid stimulating hormone (TSH) is measured by radioimmunoassay; used to diagnose primary hypothyroidism (the increased TSH level is the earliest thyroid abnormality to be detected)
5. Serum T_3
  a. Bound to TBG, therefore serum T_3 levels are subject to the same protein binding limitations as serum T_4
  b. Elevated in hyperthyroidism (usually earlier and to a greater extent than serum T_4)
  c. Useful in diagnosing:
    (1) T_3 hyperthyroidism (thyrotoxicosis): increased T_3, normal FTI

   (2) Toxic nodular goiter: increased T_3, normal or increased T_4
   (3) Iodine deficiency: normal T_3, possibly decreased T_4
   (4) Thyroid replacement therapy with liothyronine (Cytomel): normal T_4, increased T_3 if patient is symptomatically hyperthyroid
   d. Not ordered routinely, but it is indicated when hyperthyroidism is suspected and T_4, T_3RU, and FTI are inconclusive
6. Thyrotropin releasing hormone (TRH) stimulation is used to diagnose clinically suspected hyperthyroidism when the lab tests are inconclusive
   a. Method
      (1) Measure baseline TSH level
      (2) Inject 500 μg of TRH IV
      (3) Measure TSH levels at 30, 45, and 60 minutes
   b. Interpretation: Fig. 12-5 illustrates the TSH response to TRH stimulation in various endocrine disturbances
7. Radioactive iodine uptake (RAIU) measures the thyroid's ability to concentrate iodine
   a. Method
      (1) Give a PO dose of radioactive iodine (^{131}I)
      (2) Measure the amount of iodine taken up by the thyroid 24 hours later
   b. Interpretation
      (1) Normal 24-hour RAI uptake is 10%-30%

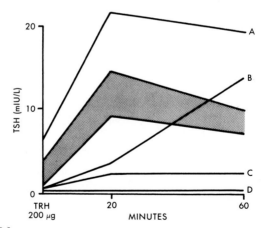

Figure 12-5
TSH response to TRH. The shaded area indicates normal response. *A*, Primary hypothyroidism; *B*, hypothalamic (tertiary) hypothyroidism; *C*, pituitary (secondary) hypothyroidism; *D*, hyperthyroidism with suppressed TSH. From Rock, R.C.: Interpreting thyroid tests in the elderly: updated guidelines, Geriatrics, **40**(12):67, 1985.

(2) An overactive thyroid shows an increased uptake whereas an underactive thyroid (hypothyroidism, subacute thyroiditis) shows a decreased uptake

c. Indications

(1) Iatrogenic ingestion of thyroid hormone by a clinically hyperthyroid patient will result in increased serum T_4, and serum T_3RU, but the RAIU is decreased instead of increased, as it would be in other causes of hyperthyroidism

(2) Subacute thyroiditis: the patient will have increased serum T_4 and serum T_3RU, but decreased RAIU because of the follicular cells' inability to concentrate iodine

(3) Pre-^{131}I-therapy for hyperthyroidism to calculate the ^{131}I dose to be administered

HYPERTHYROIDISM
Etiology

1. Graves' disease
2. Toxic multinodular goiter
3. Toxic adenoma
4. Iatrogenic and factitious
5. Transient hyperthyroidism
   a. Subacute thyroiditis
   b. Hashimoto's thyroiditis
6. Rare causes: hypersecretion of TSH (e.g., pituitary neoplasms), struma ovarii, ingestion of large amounts of iodine in a patient with preexisting thyroid hyperplasia or adenoma (Jod-Basedow phenomenon), hydatiform mole

Graves' disease

1. Definition: hypermetabolic state characterized by thyrotoxicosis, diffuse goiter, and infiltrative ophthalmopathy; infiltrative dermopathy is occasionally present
2. Pathogenesis: abnormalities are caused by thyroid-stimulating antibodies (TS Ab), which activate thyroid adenylate cyclase and compete with TSH for receptors on thyroid cell membranes.
3. Symptoms
   a. Tachycardia (resting rate >90 beats/minute), palpitations, atrial fibrillation
   b. Tremor, anxiety, irritability, emotional lability
   c. Proximal muscle weakness
   d. Heat intolerance, sweating
   e. Increased appetite, hyperdefecation
   f. Weight loss, weight gain from increased appetite (rare)
   g. Insomnia
   h. Menstrual dysfunction (oligomenorrhea, amenorrhea)
4. Physical exam
   a. General features
      (1) Tachycardia, tremor, hyperreflexia
      (2) Fine, smooth, or velvety skin, warm and moist hands
      (3) Onycholysis (brittle nails)
      (4) Diffuse goiter, bruit over thyroid

b. Features unique to Graves' disease
   (1) Infiltrative ophthalmopathy: exophthalmos, lid retraction, lid lag
   (2) Infiltrative dermopathy: pretibal myxedema (raised, hyperpigmented areas involving the pretibial region and the feet)
   (3) Thyroid acropachy: clubbing of fingers associated with periosteal new bone formation in other skeletal areas
   NOTE: Elderly hyperthyroid patients may have only subtle signs (weight loss, tachycardia, fine skin, brittle nails) this form is known as apathetic hyperthyroidism. Coexisting medical disorders (most commonly cardiac disease), may also mask the symptoms. These patients often have unexplained CHF, worsening of angina or new onset atrial fibrillation that is resistant to treatment.
5. Lab results
   a. Increased T_4, T_3RU, and FTI
   b. Increased T_3; see p. 177
   c. TRH stimulation test diagnostic of hyperthyroidism: use this test only when the serum T_4, T_3RU, FTI and T_3 are inconclusive
6. Medical therapy
   a. Antithyroid drugs (thionamides): propylthiouracil (PTU) and methimazole (Tapazole) inhibit thyroid hormone synthesis by blocking production of thyroid peroxidase (PTU and methimazole) or inhibit peripheral conversion of T_4 to T_3 (PTU)
      (1) Dosage
         (a) PTU: 100 mg PO q8h
         (b) Methimazole: 10 mg PO q8h
      (2) Side effects
         (a) Granulocytopenia occurs in 0.5% of patients (obtain baseline WBC before starting therapy); monitoring of WBC is generally not helpful because granulocytopenia is of sudden onset
         (b) Aplastic anemia
         (c) Skin rash (3%-5% of patients)
      (3) Comments
         (a) Both drugs cross the placenta and inhibit the fetal thyroid gland, therefore patient should be advised against pregnancy while taking thionamides; if patient is pregnant, use the smallest effective dose
         (b) PTU is preferred over methimazole during pregnancy because it crosses the placenta to a lesser degree[43]
         (c) Clinical response may be delayed up to 2 weeks after onset of therapy because of the stored supply of thyroid hormone
         (d) Prolonged therapy may cause hypothyroidism
      (4) Duration of therapy
         (a) Continue treatment for 6 weeks to 1 year after the patient becomes clinically euthyroid and the T_4 level returns to normal
         (b) After discontinuation, measure the T_4 level periodically to confirm the euthyroid state
         (c) If the T_4 level begins to rise (indicating early hyperthyroidism), restart the patient on antithyroid therapy or give radioactive iodine
         (d) If the patient becomes hypothyroid, start L-thyroxine (see therapy for hypothyroidism)

  b. Propranolol: alleviates the β-adrenergic symptoms of hyperthyroidism (tachycardia, tremor)
  - (1) Initial dosage: 20-40 mg PO q6h; dosage is gradually increased until symptoms are controlled
  - (2) Contraindications: bronchospasm, CHF
  c. Radioactive iodine therapy (^{131}I)
  - (1) Treatment of choice for men and for women over the age of 21
  - (2) High incidence of postradiotherapy hypothyroidism,[63] therefore these patients should be frequently evaluated for the onset of hypothyroidism
  - (3) Radioactive iodine therapy is contraindicated during pregnancy (can cause fetal hypothyroidism)
7. Surgical therapy: subtotal thyroidectomy
  a. Indications
  - (1) Pregnant patient who cannot be adequately managed with low doses of PTU, or who develops side effects with antithyroid medication
  - (2) Any patient who refuses radioactive iodine and cannot be adequately managed with thionamides
  b. Complications: hypothyroidism, hypoparathyroidism, and damage to recurrent laryngeal nerve

Toxic multinodular goiter

1. Incidence: usually seen in women over the age of 55 with a history of multinodular goiter for many years, whereas Graves' disease is typically seen in young women
2. Clinical presentation: onset is usually insidious and clinical phenomena (tachycardia, tremor, heat intolerance) may be masked by manifestations of coexisting diseases (e.g., a patient with ASHD may have CHF secondary to atrial fibrillation with a fast ventricular response)
3. Therapy: Radioactive iodine (^{131}I) after the patient has been made euthyroid with thionamides

Toxic adenoma

1. Diagnosis: thyroid scan demonstrates increased uptake (hot nodule)
2. Therapy
  a. Surgical removal of the adenoma is preferred in young hyperthyroid patients and patients with very large adenoma
  b. Medical: radioactive iodine (^{131}I) therapy is used mainly in elderly patients who would tolerate surgery poorly

THYROID STORM
Definition
Thyroid storm is characterized by an abrupt, severe exacerbation of thyrotoxicosis

Etiology
1. Major stress (infection, MI, surgery, DKA) in an undiagnosed hyperthyroid patient
2. Inadequate therapy in a hyperthyroid patient

Symptoms

1. Fever ($>100°$ F)
2. Marked anxiety and agitation, psychosis
3. Hyperhydrosis, heat intolerance
4. Marked weakness and muscle wasting
5. Tachydysrhythmias, palpitations
6. Hyperdefecation
7. Elderly patients may have a combination of tachycardia, CHF, and mental status changes

Physical exam

1. Goiter
2. Tremor, tachycardia, fever
3. Warm, moist skin
4. Lid lag, lid retraction, proptosis
5. Altered mental status (psychosis, coma, seizures)
6. Other: evidence of precipitating factors (infection or trauma)

Lab results

Increased T_4, T_3RU, T_3, and FTI

Therapy[37]

If the diagnosis is strongly suspected, start immediate therapy without waiting for lab confirmation.

1. Specific therapy
   a. To inhibit hormonal synthesis
      (1) Propylthiouracil (PTU) 400 mg initially (PO or via NG tube) then 400 mg PO q6h
      (2) If the patient has gastric or intestinal obstruction, methimazole (Tapazole) 80-100 mg can be administered PR, followed by 30 mg PR q8h
   b. To inhibit release of stored thyroid hormone
      (1) Iodide (sodium iodide) 250 mg IV q6h, potassium iodide (SSKI) 5 gtt PO q8h, or Lugol's solution 10 gtt q8h; administer a thionamide (PTU or methimazole) 1 hour *before* the iodide to prevent the oxidation of iodide to iodine and its incorporation in the synthesis of additional thyroid hormone
      (2) Corticosteroids: dexamethasone 2 mg IV q6h or hydrocortisone 100 mg IV q6h for approximately 48 hours
         (a) Inhibit thyroid hormone release
         (b) Impair peripheral generation of T_3 from T_4
         (c) Provide additional adrenal cortical hormone to correct deficiency (if present)
   c. To suppress peripheral effects of thyroid hormone
      (1) β-adrenergic blockers: propranolol 10-40 mg PO q4-6h; in acute situations propranolol may also be given IV 1 mg/minute for 2-10 minutes under continuous ECG and blood pressure monitoring
      (2) β-adrenergic blockers must be used with caution in patients with CHF or bronchospasm

(3) Cardioselective β-blockers (e.g., atenolol 100 mg PO qd) may be more appropriate for patients with bronchospasm, but these patients must be closely monitored for exacerbation of bronchospasm since these agents lose their cardioselectivity at high doses

2. Supportive therapy
   a. Control fever: use acetaminophen 300-600 mg q4h or cooling blanket if necessary, but do not use aspirin because it displaces thyroid hormone from its binding protein
   b. Digitalize patients with CHF: these patients may require higher than usual digitalis dosages, particularly to control atrial fibrillation
   c. Nutritional care: replace fluid deficit aggressively; use solutions containing glucose and add multivitamins to the hydrating solution
   d. Rule out and treat any precipitating factors: obtain blood and urine cultures; use IV antibiotics if infection is strongly suspected

HYPOTHYROIDISM

Etiology

1. Primary hypothyroidism (thyroid gland dysfunction) is the cause of >90% of the cases of hypothyroidism
   a. Hashimoto thyroiditis (chronic lymphocytic thyroiditis)
   b. Idiopathic myxedema (possibly a nongoitrous form of Hashimoto's thyroiditis)
   c. Previous treatment of hyperthyroidism (^{131}I therapy, subtotal thyroidectomy)
   d. Subacute thyroiditis
   e. Radiation therapy of the neck (usually for malignant disease)
   f. Iodine deficiency or excess
   g. Drugs (lithium, PAS, sulfonamides, phenylbutazone, thiourea)
   h. Congenital (approximately 1:4000 live births)
   i. Prolonged treatment with iodides
2. Secondary hypothroidism: pituitary dysfunction, postpartum necrosis, neoplasm, infiltrative disease causing deficiency of TSH
3. Tertiary hypothyroidism: hypothalmic disease (granuloma, neoplasm, or irradiation causing deficiency of TRH)
4. Tissue resistance to thyroid hormone (rare)

Symptoms

1. Fatigue, lethargy, weakness
2. Constipation, weight gain (usually <15 lbs)
3. Muscle weakness, muscle cramps, arthralgias
4. Cold intolerance
5. Slow speech with hoarse voice (caused by myxedematous changes in the vocal cords)
6. Slow cerebration with poor memory

Physical exam

1. Skin is dry, coarse, thick, cool and sallow (yellow color caused by carotenemia); nonpitting edema in the skin of the eyelids and hands (myxedema) secondary to infiltration of the subcutaneous tissues by a hydrophilic mucopolysaccharide substance

2. Hair is brittle and coarse; loss of outer one third of eyebrows
3. Facies: dulled expression, thickened tongue, and thick, slow moving lips
4. Thyroid gland may or may not be palpable (depending on the cause of the hypothyroidism)
5. Heart sounds are distant; pericardial effusion may be present
6. Pulse: bradycardia
7. Neurologic
   a. Delayed relaxation phase (return phase) of deep tendon reflexes
   b. Cerebellar ataxia
   c. Hearing impairment, poor memory
   d. Peripheral neuropathies with paresthesias, carpal tunnel syndrome

Lab results

1. Decreased T_4, T_3RU, and FTI
2. Increased TSH (TSH level may be normal if patient has secondary or tertiary hypothyroidism)
3. Increased serum cholesterol, triglycerides, LDH, SGOT, and MM band of CPK
4. Decreased Hb/Hct, hyponatremia
5. TRH stimulation test is useful to distinguish secondary from tertiary hypothyroidism (see Fig. 12-5)

Therapy

Start replacement therapy with L-thyroxine (Synthroid) 25-100 μg/day depending on the patient's age and the severity of the disease. May increase dose q2-4 weeks depending on the patient's clinical response. Elderly patients and patients with coronary artery disease should be started with ≤25 μg/day (higher doses may precipitate angina). The average maintenance dose of L-thyroxine is 2 μg/kg/day.

MYXEDEMA COMA
Definition

Myxedema coma is a life-threatening complication of hypothyroidism characterized by profound lethargy or coma and usually accompanied by hypothermia.

Contributing factors

1. Sepsis
2. Exposure to cold weather
3. CNS depressants (sedatives, narcotics, antidepressants)
4. Trauma, surgery
5. CVA, hypoglycemia, CO_2 narcosis

Symptoms

1. Elderly patients, profoundly lethargic or comatose
2. Hypothermia (rectal temperature <35° C (95° F); hypothermia is often missed by using ordinary thermometers graduated only to 34.5° C or if the mercury is not shaken below 36° C
3. Bradycardia, hypotension (secondary to circulatory collapse)
4. Delayed relaxation phase of DTR, areflexia

Lab results

1. Markedly increased TSH (if primary hypothyroidism)
2. Decreased T_4, T_3RU, and FTI
3. Other: CO_2 retention, hypoxia, acidosis, hyponatremia, macrocytic anemia, hypoglycemia
4. Draw cortisol level and blood cultures on admission to rule out adrenal insufficiency or sepsis

Therapy

If diagnosis is strongly suspected, initiate immediate treatment without waiting for confirmatory lab results (mortality in myxedema coma is 20%-50%).

1. L-thyroxine: 2 $\mu g/kg$ IV infused over 5-15 minutes, then 100 μg IV q24h
2. Hydrocortisone hemisuccinate: 100 mg IV bolus then 50 mg IV q12h or 25 mg q6h by continuous IV until plasma cortisol level is normal; glucocorticoids are given to treat possible associated adrenocortical insufficiency, but avoid large doses because they may impair conversion of T_4 to T_3
3. IV hydration: usually with D_5NS to correct hypotension and hypoglycemia (if present); avoid overhydration and possible water intoxication because clearance of free water is impaired in these patients
4. Prevent further heat loss, cover the patient but avoid external rewarming because it may produce vascular collapse
5. Support respiratory function: intubation and mechanical ventilation may be required
6. Rule out and treat precipitating factors, such as sepsis
7. Monitor patient in an intensive care unit

THYROIDITIS[26]

Thyroiditis is an inflammatory disease of the thyroid. It is clinically categorized as acute, subacute, and chronic thyroiditis.

Acute suppurative thyroiditis

1. Etiology: bacterial thyroid infection (usually seen in immunocompromised host) or following a penetrating injury to neck
2. Symptoms: fever, malaise, tenderness over thyroid
3. Lab results: increased WBC with ''shift to left,'' normal thyroid function studies, normal 24-hour RAI uptake
4. Therapy: IV antibiotics, drainage of abscess (if present)

Subacute thyroiditis (de Quervain's thyroiditis)

Subacute granulomatous thyroiditis

1. Etiology: possibly postviral; usually follows a respiratory illness
2. Symptoms: exquisitely tender, enlarged thyroid, fever, and generalized malaise
3. Lab results: markedly increased sedimentation rate, increased WBC with ''shift to left,'' low RAI uptake, increased serum thyroglobulin levels, and increased or normal T_4 level
4. Treatment
   a. The disease is self-limited, hyperthyroidism is transient and resolves spontaneously over a few weeks in >90% of patients; relapses may occur

b. Serial measurements of serum thyroglobulin (Tg) levels are useful in monitoring the course of subacute thyroiditis[41]

c. Pain can be treated with aspirin 650 mg qid; prednisone 20-40 mg qd may be used if aspirin is insufficient, but it should be gradually tapered off over several weeks

d. Symptoms of hyperthyroidism can be controlled with β-adrenergic blockers

e. Thionamides are not indicated in subacute thyroiditis

f. Some patients will develop transient hypothyroidism requiring thyroxine therapy for 3-6 months

Subacute lymphocytic thyroiditis (painless thyroiditis)

1. Etiology is unknown, but is probably autoimmune; usually seen postpartum

2. Symptoms
   a. Normal or slightly enlarged nontender thyroid gland
   b. Tachycardia, tremor, heat intolerance, insomnia, anxiety, and other signs of hyperthyroidism

3. Lab results
   a. Increased T_4, T_3RU, T_3, and FTI
   b. Decreased 24-hour RAI uptake
   c. Increased serum thyroglobulin (acute phase)
   d. Low or absent antimicrosomal antibody

4. Therapy: self-limited disease; symptoms of initial hyperthyroid phase can be controlled with β-adrenergic blockers; hypothyroid phase should be treated with thyroid hormone replacement therapy; recovery is generally seen in about 75% of patients

Chronic thyroiditis

Hashimoto's thyroiditis

1. Pathophysiology
   a. Autoimmune disease (patient may also have pernicious anemia or other autoimmune disorders)
   b. There is progressive destruction of thyroid gland by an inflammatory process
   c. Histologically there is marked lymphocytic infiltration of thyroid
   d. Antimicrosomal antibodies are detected in over 90% of patients

2. Symptoms
   a. Diffuse, firm enlargement of the thyroid gland; thyroid gland may also be of normal size (atrophic form with clinically manifested hypothyroidism)
   b. Patient may have signs of hyper- or hypothyroidism, depending on the stage of the disease

3. Therapy: if patient is hypothyroid, L-thyroxine therapy will correct hypothyroidism and suppress goiter

Riedel's thyroiditis is a rare condition characterized by fibrous infiltration of the thyroid with subsequent hypothyroidism; this condition may be mistaken with carcinoma of the thyroid

EVALUATION OF PATIENT WITH
THYROID NODULE
History and physical exam

1. History of prior head and neck irradiation (increased risk of thyroid cancer)
2. Family history of pheochromocytoma or carcinoma of the parathyroids (medullary carcinoma of the thyroid is a component of multiple endocrine neoplasia II)
3. Dysphagia/hoarseness (may indicate infiltrative malignant neoplasm)
4. Increased likelihood that nodule is malignant
   a. Nodule increasing in size
   b. Regional lymphadenopathy
   c. Fixation to adjacent tissues
   d. Age less than 40, male sex

Diagnostic tests

1. Fine-needle aspiration biopsy is the best initial diagnostic study; the accuracy can be as high as 97%,[53,71] but it is directly related to the level of experience of the physician and the cytopathologist interpreting the aspirate Evaluation of results:
   a. Normal cells: may repeat biopsy during present evaluation or reevaluate patient after 3-6 months of suppressive therapy (L-thyroxine, 150 mg PO qd)
      (1) Failure to suppress indicates increased likelihood of malignancy
      (2) Reliance on repeat needle biopsy is preferable to routine surgery for nodules not responding to thyroxine[27]
   b. Malignant cells: surgery
   c. Hypercellularity: thyroid scan
      (1) Hot nodule: ^{131}I therapy if the patient is hyperthyroid
      (2) Warm or cold nodule: surgery (follicular adenoma *vs* carcinoma)
2. Thyroid ultrasound to evaluate the size of the thyroid, and the number, composition (solid *vs* cystic), and dimensions of the thyroid nodule(s); solid thyroid nodules have a higher incidence of malignancy, but cystic nodules can also be malignant
3. Thyroid scan with (^{99m}Tc) pertechnetate
   a. Classifies nodules as hyperfunctioning (hot), normally functioning (warm), or nonfunctioning (cold); cold nodules have a higher incidence of malignancy
   b. Scan has difficulty evaluating nodules near the thyroid isthmus or at the periphery of the gland
   c. Normal tissue over a nonfunctioning nodule may mask the nodule as "warm" or normally functioning

•   •   •

Both thyroid scan and ultrasound provide information regarding the risk of malignant neoplasia based on the characteristics of the thyroid nodule, but their value in the initial evaluation of a thyroid nodule is limited because neither one provides a definite tissue diagnosis.

THYROID CARCINOMA

There are four major types of thyroid carcinomas: papillary, follicular, anaplastic, and medullary.

Papillary carcinoma

1. Characteristics
   a. Most common type (50%-60%)
   b. Most frequent in women during second or third decade
   c. Histologically "psammona bodies" (calcific bodies present in the papillary projections) are pathognomonic; they are found in 35%-45% of papillary thyroid carcinomas
   d. Majority are not pure papillary lesions, but are mixed papillary follicular carcinomas
   e. Spread is via lymphatics and by local invasion
2. Therapy
   a. Total thyroidectomy is indicated if the patient has:
      (1) Extrapyramidal extension of carcinoma
      (2) Papillary carcinoma limited to thyroid, but a positive history of irradiation to the head and neck
      (3) Lesion larger than 2 cm
   b. Lobectomy with isthmectomy (associated with careful exploration of the other lobe) may be considered in patients with intrathyroidal papillary carcinoma smaller than 2 cm and no history of neck and head irradiation; must follow surgery with supressive therapy of thyroid hormone because these tumors are TSH responsive
   c. Radiotherapy with ^{131}I (after total thyroidectomy), followed by thyroid suppression therapy with triiodothyronine can be used in metastatic papillary carcinoma

Follicular carcinoma

1. Characteristics
   a. More aggressive than papillary carcinoma
   b. Incidence increases with age
   c. Tends to metastasize hematogenously to bone, producing pathologic fractures
   d. Tends to concentrate iodine (useful for radiation therapy)
2. Therapy
   a. Total thyroidectomy
   b. Radiotherapy with ^{131}I followed by thyroid suppression therapy with triiodothyronine is useful in patients with metastases

Anaplastic carcinoma

1. Characteristics
   a. Very aggressive neoplasm
   b. Two major histologic types
      (1) Small cell: less aggressive (5-year survival approximately 20%)
      (2) Giant cell: death usually within 6 months of diagnosis
2. Therapy
   a. At diagnosis, this neoplasm is rarely operable; palliative surgery is indicated for extremely large tumor compressing the trachea
   b. Management is usually restricted to radiation therapy or chemotherapy with combination of doxorubicin, cisplatin, and other antineoplastic agents; these measures rarely provide significant palliation

Medullary carcinoma

1. Characteristics
   a. Unifocal lesion: found sporadically in elderly patients
   b. Bilateral lesions: associated with pheochromocytoma and hyperparathyroidism; this combination is known as multiple endocrine neoplasia II (MEN II) and is inherited as an autosomal dominant disorder (see section 12.14)
2. Diagnosis
   a. Increased plasma calcitonin assay (these tumors produce thyrocalcitonin)
   b. Screen family members; normal family members who are at risk can be identified by using provocative testing with IV pentagastrin or calcium infusion to stimulate thyrocalcitonin release from neoplastic cells
3. Treatment
   a. Thyroidectomy
   b. Patients and their families should be screened for pheochromocytoma and hyperparathyroidism

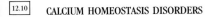 **CALCIUM HOMEOSTASIS DISORDERS**

PHYSIOLOGY

1. Serum calcium levels are controlled mainly by parathyroid hormone (PTH) and vitamin D (1,25 dihydroxy vitamin D), and to a lesser extent by calcitonin
   a. The three organs involved in calcium metabolism are bone, kidneys, and intestine
   b. The effect of calcium-regulating hormones on each are summarized in Table 12-15
2. Calcium is found in plasma in three major forms:
   a. Bound to plasma proteins, particularly albumin (35%-40%)
   b. Free (ionized) calcium (45%-50%)
   c. Bound to complexing ions: phosphate, citrate, carbonate (10%-15%)
3. The standard serum calcium level measures the total serum calcium level, but the only physiologically active form is the free (ionized) calcium; any factor that decreases the free (ionized) calcium (e.g., alkalosis) can produce hypocalcemic crises, whereas factors that affect only the protein-bound calcium will not provoke symptoms of hypocalcemia (Table 12-16)

HYPERCALCEMIA
Etiology

1. Malignancy: increased bone resorption via osteoclast-activating factors, secretion of PTH-like substances, prostaglandins E_2, direct erosion by tumor cells, transforming growth factors, colony-stimulating activity;[46] hypercalcemia is common in the following neoplasms:
   a. Solid tumors: breast, lung, pancreas, kidneys, ovary
   b. Hematologic cancers: myeloma, lymphosarcoma, adult T-cell lymphoma, Burkitt's lymphoma
2. Hyperparathyroidism: increased bone resorption, GI absorption, and renal absorption; etiology:

Table 12-15   Hormonal action in calcium homeostasis

Hormone	Action		Result	
	Bone	Kidneys	Intestine	Serum Ca	Serum PO$_4$
PTH	↑ Ca resorption ↑ PO$_4$ resorption	↑ Ca resorption ↑ Phosphate excretion ↑ Conversion of vita- min D to active form	↑ Ca absorption (via vitamin D)	↑	→
1,25 dihydroxy vitamin D	↑ Ca resorption	Undetermined	↑ Ca absorption ↑ PO$_4$ absorption	↑	←
Calcitonin	↑ Ca resorption	↑ Excretion of calcium phosphate	—	→	→

KEY: Ca, calcium; PO$_4$, phosphorus; ↑, increase; ↓, decrease.

Table 12-16 Effects of hypoalbuminemia and alkalosis on serum calcium

Condition	Effect	Result	Symptoms of Hypocalcemia
Decreased albumin	Decreased protein-bound Ca	Decreased total serum, but normal free (ionized) Ca	Absent
Alkalosis	Increased protein-bound Ca	Normal total serum Ca, but decreased free (ionized) Ca	May be present

    a. Parathyroid hyperplasia, adenoma
    b. Hyperparathyroidism of renal failure
3. Granulomatous disorders: increased GI absorption (e.g., sarcoidosis)
4. Paget's disease: increased bone resorption, seen only during periods of immobilization
5. Vitamin D intoxication, milk-alkali syndrome: increased GI absorption
6. Thiazides: increased renal absorption
7. Other causes: familial hypocalciuric hypercalcemia, thyrotoxicosis, adrenal insufficiency, prolonged immobilization, vitamin A intoxication, recovery from acute renal failure, lithium administration, pheochromocytoma

Symptoms

1. GI: constipation, anorexia, nausea, vomiting, pancreatitis, ulcers
2. CNS: confusion, obtundation, psychosis, lassitude, depression, coma
3. Genitourinary: nephrolithiasis, renal insufficiency, polyuria, decreased urine-concentrating ability, nocturia
4. Musculoskeletal: myopathy, weakness, osteoporosis, pseudogout
5. Other: hypertension, metastatic calcifications, band keratopathy

Diagnostic studies

1. History:
    a. Family history of hypercalcemia, such as MEN syndromes or familial hypocalciuric hypercalcemia (latter is a benign autosomal dominant condition of increased serum Ca, decreased fractional excretion of Ca, and a normal PTH level; parathyroidectomy is not indicated)
    b. Inquire about intake of milk and antacids (milk-alkali syndrome), intake of thiazides, lithium, large doses of vitamin A or D
    c. Inquire whether patient has any bone pain (multiple myeloma, metastatic disease), or abdominal pain (pancreatitis, PUD)
2. Physical exam
    a. Look for evidence of primary neoplasm (e.g., breast, lung)
    b. Check eyes for evidence of band keratopathy (found in medial and lateral margins of the cornea)

Table 12-17   Interpretation of initial lab studies

Lab Test	Hyperparathyroidism	Familial Hypocalciuric Hypercalcemia	Sarcoidosis
Serum Ca	↑	↑	↑
Serum PO$_4$	↓	↓	↑
24-hour urine Ca	N/↑	↓	↑ ↑
Alkaline phosphatase	N/↑	N	N

KEY: ↑, Increased; ↓, decreased; N, normal; Ca, calcium; PO$_4$, phosphorus.

Table 12-18   Use of iPTH and urinary cyclic AMP in the differential diagnosis of hypercalcemia

iPTH	Urinary Cyclic AMP	Diagnosis
↑ ↑	↑ ↑	Primary hyperparathyroidism
N/↓	N/↓	Probable occult malignancy

KEY: ↑, Increased; ↓, decreased; N, normal; iPTH, parathyroid hormone by radioimmunoassay.

3. Lab results
    a. Initial lab studies should include: serum calcium, albumin, PO$_4$, magnesium, alkaline phosphatase, electrolytes, BUN, creatinine and 24–hour urine calcium (see Table 12-17 for interpretation of results)
    b. If the history is suggestive of excessive intake of vitamin D (e.g., food faddists with intake of megadoses of fat-soluble vitamins), a serum vitamin D level (1,25 dihydroxy vitamin D) is indicated
    c. The iPTH distinguishes primary hyperparathyroidism from hypercalcemia caused by malignancy when the serum calcium level is >12 mg/dl; below this value there is considerable overlap and the differentiation between these two major causes of hypercalcemia is extremely difficult[31]
    d. A very high level of urinary cyclic AMP is strongly suggestive of primary hyperparathyroidism, although certain nonparathyroid malignancies have also been shown to produce elevated levels of urinary cyclic AMP[65]
    e. Table 12-18 describes the use of PTH and cyclic AMP in the differential diagnosis of hypercalcemia
4. Radiologic evaluation
    a. Bone survey may show evidence of subperiosteal bone resorption (suggesting PTH excess)
    b. Bone scan may show hot spots in association with lytic lesions
5. ECG: shortening of the QT interval

Therapy

1. Acute severe hypercalcemia (serum calcium >13 mg/dl or symptomatic patient)
   a. Vigorous IV hydration with normal saline followed by IV furosemide q4-6h
      (1) Normal saline infusion will increase urinary calcium excretion by inhibiting proximal tubular sodium and calcium reabsorption; the addition of a loop diuretic further inhibits calcium and sodium transport downstream from the proximal tubule
      (2) Use normal saline with caution in patients with cardiac or renal insufficiency to avoid fluid overload
      (3) Monitor serum electrolytes, and magnesium and calcium levels frequently; complications of the above regimen include decreased potassium, magnesium, and sodium
   b. Calcitonin: 4 U/kg q12h
      (1) The initial dose is given IV following initial skin testing for allergy; subsequent doses may be given SC
      (2) Particularly useful in hypercalcemia associated with hyperphosphatemia because it also increases urinary phosphate excretion; however, it is indicated only when saline hydration and furosemide are ineffective
   c. Mithramycin: 25 μg/kg by slow IV infusion (over 6 hours); this is the most potent of all antihypercalcemic agents
      (1) It lowers serum calcium within 12-24 hours by inhibiting bone resorption
      (2) Its use should be restricted to emergency treatment of severe hypercalcemia
      (3) May cause hepatotoxicity, nephrotoxocity, and thrombocytopenia (usually seen following repeated IV doses)
   d. Etidronate disodium (Didronel): 7.5 mg/kg/day in 250 ml of saline, infused over 2 hours on one to four consecutive days
      (1) Etidronate and other diphosphonates inhibit bone resorption by osteoclasts; recent studies[55] have found the use of etidronate safe and effective in lowering hypercalcemia in patients with malignant disease
      (2) The serum calcium level will be lowered to normal range within 2-5 days in approximately 75% of patients
2. Chronic hypercalcemia
   a. Identify and treat underlying disease (e.g., vitamin D intoxication, sarcoidosis)
   b. Discontinue potential hypercalcemic agents (e.g., thiazide diuretics)
   c. If the hypercalcemia is caused by a parathyroid adenoma, parathyroidectomy is the treatment of choice
   d. Unless contraindicated, these patients should maintain a high daily intake of fluids (3-5 L/day) and of sodium chloride (>400 mEq/day) to increase renal calcium excretion
   e. Medications
      (1) Glucocorticoids: hydrocortisone 3-5 mg/kg/day IV initially, then prednisone 30 mg PO bid
         (1) The calcium-lowering action of corticosteroids occurs via decreased intestinal calcium absorption; they are very effective

in hypercalcemia secondary to breast carcinoma, myeloma, sarcoidosis and vitamin D intoxication
- (b) Their use in acute hypercalcemia is limited because it takes 48-72 hours before the serum calcium shows a significant decline
- (2) Oral phosphates: 1-3 g/day in divided doses (e.g., Neutra-Phos 250-500 mg PO q6h)
  - (a) Phosphates lower serum calcium by decreasing GI calcium absorption and bone resorption
  - (b) Not useful in acute hypercalcemia because their calcium-lowering effect will not be apparent for 2-3 days
  - (c) Oral phosphates are contraindicated in renal insufficiency or any other medical conditions with elevated serum phosphate levels
- (3) Indomethacin: 75-150 mg/day
  - (a) Prostaglandin synthetase inhibitor
  - (b) It is only effective in prostaglandin-mediated hypercalcemia

HYPOCALCEMIA
Etiology
1. Renal insufficiency: hypocalcemia caused by
   a. Increased calcium deposits in bone and soft tissue secondary to increased serum PO_4 level
   b. Decreased production of 1,25 dihydroxy vitamin D
   c. Excessive loss of 25-OHD (nephrotic syndrome)
2. Hypoalbuminemia: each decrease in serum albumin of g/L will decrease calcium by 0.8 mg/dl
3. Vitamin D deficiency
   a. Malabsorption
   b. Inadequate intake
   c. Decreased production of 1,25 dihydroxy vitamin D (vitamin D–dependent rickets, renal failure)
   d. Decreased production of 25-OHD (parenchymal liver disease)
   e. Accelerated 25-OHD catabolism (phenytoin, phenobarbital)
   f. End-organ resistance to 1,25 dihydroxy vitamin D
4. Hypomagnesemia: hypocalcemia caused by
   a. Decreased PTH secretion
   b. Inhibition of PTH effect on bone
5. Pancreatitis, hyperphosphatemia, osteoblastic metastases: hypocalcemia is secondary to increased calcium deposits (bone, abdomen)
6. Pseudohypoparathyroidism: autosomal recessive disorder characterized by short stature, shortening of metacarpal bones, obesity, and mental retardation; the hypocalcemia is secondary to congenital end-organ resistance to PTH

Symptoms
1. Neuromuscular irritability
   a. Chvostek's sign: facial twitch following gentle tapping over the facial nerve
   b. Trousseau's sign: carpopedal spasm following inflation of blood pres-

Table 12-19 Differentiation of hypoparathyroidism from vitamin D deficiency

Disorder	Serum Calcium	Serum PO₄	Alkaline Phosphatase
Hypoparathyroidism	↓	↑	N
Vitamin D deficiency	↓	↓	↑

KEY: ↑, Increase; ↓, decrease; N, normal

sure cuff above the patients systolic blood pressure for a 2 to 3 minute duration

c. Tetany, paresthesias, myopathy, seizures, muscle spasm or weakness

2. Psychiatric disturbances: psychosis, depression, impaired cognitive function
3. Soft-tissue calcifications, ocular cataracts
4. Cardiovascular manifestations: dysrhythmias, CHF (caused by decreased myocardial contractility), increased QT interval, hypotension

Diagnostic tests

1. Serum albumin: to rule out hypoalbuminemia
2. BUN, creatinine: to rule out renal failure
3. Serum magnesium: to rule out severe hypomagnesemia
4. Serum PO₄, alkaline phosphatase: to differentiate hypoparathyroidism from vitamin D deficiency (see Table 12-19)
5. Serum PTH level by radioimmunoassay should be ordered only when above tests are inconclusive
   a. Markedly increased PTH: pseudohypoparathyroidism
   b. Increased PTH: vitamin D deficiency
   c. Decreased PTH: hypoparathyroidism

Therapy

1. Hypoalbuminemia
   a. Improve nutritional status
   b. Calcium replacement is not indicated since the free (ionized) calcium is normal
2. Hypomagnesemia: correct the magnesium deficiency
   a. Severe hypomagnesemia (serum magnesium level <0.8 mEq/L): give 1 g (8 mEq) of a 10% magnesium sulfate solution IV slowly (over 15 minutes)
   b. Moderate-to-severe hypomagnesemia (serum magnesium level 0.8-1.3 mEq/L): give one 2 ml ampul of a 50% magnesium solution IM; may repeat q4-6h
3. Acute, severe symptomatic hypocalcemia caused by hypoparathyroidism or vitamin D deficiency: give a slow IV bolus (over 15 minutes) of 10-30 ml of a 10% calcium gluconate solution
4. Chronic hypocalcemia caused by hypoparathyroidism or vitamin D deficiency

Table 12-20 Common vitamin D preparations

Vitamin	Trade Name	Preparations	Vitamin D Content	Dosage
Ergocalciferol (vitamin D_2)	Calciferol	Tab: 1.25 mg	50,000 U/ 1.25 mg	1.25-2.50 mg/day
Dihydro-tachysterol	DHT	Tab: 0.125 and 0.4 mg	50,000 U/ 0.25 mg	0.25-1.0 mg/day

    a. Calcium supplementation: 1-4 g/day of elemental calcium (e.g., calcium carbonate 650 mg PO qid will provide 1 g of elemental calcium/day)
    b. Vitamin D replacement (Table 12-20)
5. Chronic hypocalcemia caused by renal failure
    a. Reduction of hyperphosphatemia with phosphate binding antacids (Amphojel, Basojel, Alternajel)
    b. Vitamin D and oral calcium supplementation (as noted above)

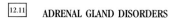 **ADRENAL GLAND DISORDERS**

CUSHING'S SYNDROME
Definition
Cushing's syndrome is characterized by glucocorticoid excess secondary to exaggerated adrenal cortisol production or chronic glucocorticoid therapy.

Etiology
1. Chronic glucocorticoid therapy
2. Pituitary ACTH excess (Cushing's disease)
3. Adrenal neoplasms
4. Ectopic ACTH production (neoplasm of lung, pancreas, kidney, thyroid, thymus)

Symptoms
1. Hypertension
2. Obesity
3. Hirsutism, menstrual irregularities, hypogonadism, infertility
4. Diabetes mellitus, osteoporosis (bone pain and fractures)
5. Psychosis, emotional lability
6. Skin fragility, hemorrhagic diathesis, poor wound healing

Physical exam
1. Ecchymoses, red-purple abdominal striae, acne, facial plethora, hyperpigmentation (when there is ACTH excess)
2. Central obesity with rounding of the facies (moon facies), thin extremities
3. Fat accumulation in dorsocervical spine (buffalo hump) and supraclavicular areas
4. Muscle wasting with proximal myopathy

NOTE: The above characteristics are not commonly present in Cushing's syndrome secondary to ectopic ACTH production. Many of these tumors secrete a biologically inactive ACTH that does not activate adrenal steroid synthesis.[27] These patients may only have weight loss and weakness.

Initial lab results

1. Hypokalemia, hypochloremia, metabolic alkalosis, hyperglycemia, hypercholesterolemia
2. Increased 24-hour urinary free cortisol (>100 μg/24 hours)

Diagnosis

1. The classic diagnostic approach is outlined in Fig. 12-6
2. Recently a new overnight, high-dose dexamethasone suppression test has been developed by Tyrrell et al. to diagnose Cushing's syndrome[70]
   a. Measure baseline plasma cortisol level (7 AM)
   b. Give patient 8 mg of dexamethasone PO at 11 PM
   c. Measure cortisol level at 7 AM the following morning
   d. Interpretation: suppression of plasma cortisol level to $>50\%$ of baseline indicates Cushing's disease
   e. This test has a sensitivity of 92%, a specificity of 100%, and diagnostic accuracy of 93%; these values equal or exceed those of the standard 2-day test whether based on suppression of plasma cortisol or urinary 17-hydroxysteroids

Therapy

1. Pituitary adenoma: transsphenoidal resection is the therapy of choice in adults
2. Adrenal neoplasm
   a. Surgical resection of the affected adrenal
   b. Glucocorticoid replacement therapy for approximately 9-12 months after the surgery to allow time for the contralateral adrenal to recover from its prolonged suppression
   c. Mitotane 6-12 g/day in divided doses can be used to control cortisol excess in patients with residual or nonresectable carcinoma[60]
   d. Metyrapone and aminoglutethimide can be used in patients who do not respond to or are unable to tolerate mitotane
3. Ectopic ACTH
   a. Surgical resection of the ACTH-secreting neoplasm
   b. Control of cortisol excess with metyrapone, aminoglutethimide, or ketoconazole[60]
   c. Control of the mineralocorticoid effects of cortisol and 11-deoxycorticosteroid with spironolactone[69]

PRIMARY ADRENOCORTICAL DEFICIENCY
Definition

Primary adrenocortical deficiency (Addison's disease) is characterized by inadequate secretion of corticosteroids caused by partial or complete destruction of the adrenal glands.

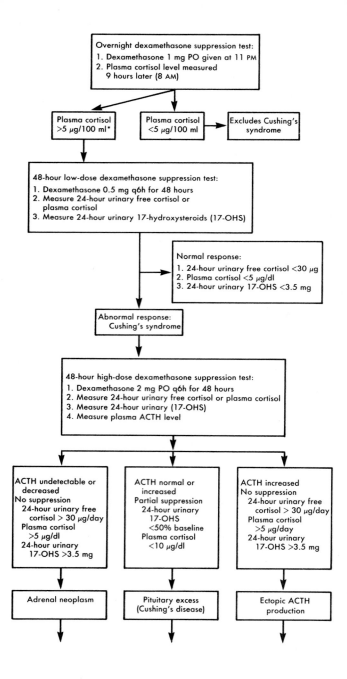

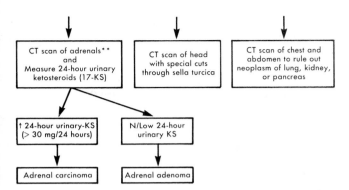

*Failure to suppress endogenous cortisol secretion can also be seen in patients with agitated depression, severe stress, alcoholism, anorexia nervosa, and in patients taking oral contraceptives. Corticotropin–releasing factor (CRF) is useful in evaluating Cushing's syndrome and in differentiating it from hypercortisolism of psychiatric origin.[59]

**A "routine" CT scan of the abdomen (with cuts >1 cm) is inappropriate to identify adrenal masses. The radiographer must be instructed to perform multiple small tomographic cuts through the adrenal area.[14]

Figure 12-6
Diagnostic approach to Cushing's syndrome.

Etiology

1. Autoimmune destruction of the adrenals
2. Tuberculosis
3. Carcinomatous destruction of the adrenals
4. Adrenal hemorrhage (anticoagulants, trauma, coagulopathies, pregnancy, sepsis)
5. Adrenal infarction (arteritis, thrombosis)
6. Other: sarcoidosis, amyloidosis, postoperative, fungal infection

Symptoms[5]

1. Weakness, anorexia, weight loss (100%)
2. Increased pigmentation (>90%)
3. Hypotension (85%-90%)
4. GI disturbances (abdominal pain, diarrhea, constipation) (>50%)
5. Other: hypoglycemic manifestations, salt craving, poor response to stress

Physical exam

1. Hyperpigmentation: more prominent in palmar creases, buccal mucosa, pressure points (elbows, knees, knuckles), perianal mucosa, and around areolas of nipples

2. Hypotension
3. Generalized weakness
4. Amenorrhea and loss of axillary hair in females

Lab results

1. Increased K^+, decreased Na^+ and Cl^-
2. Decreased glucose
3. Increased BUN and creatinine (prerenal azotemia)
4. Mild normocytic, normochromic anemia, neutropenia, lymphocytosis, eosinophilia (significant dehydration may mask the hyponatremia and anemia)
5. Decreased 24-hour urine cortisol, 17-OHCS, and 17-KS, and increased ACTH (if primary adrenocortical insufficiency)

Radiologic evaluation

1. Chest x-ray film: may reveal a small-sized heart
2. Abdominal x-ray film: adrenal calcifications may be noted if the adrenocortical insufficiency is secondary to TB or fungus
3. Abdominal CT scan: small adrenal glands generally indicate either idiopathic atrophy or long-standing TB, whereas enlarged glands are suggestive of early TB or potentially treatable diseases[75]

Diagnosis

1. A screening test can be performed for primary adrenal insufficiency
   a. Give 0.25 mg of cosyntropin (synthetic ACTH) IV/IM after measuring the basal cortisol level
   b. Measure the plasma cortisol levels again after 30 and 60 minutes
   c. A rise <10 mg/dl is suggestive of primary adrenal insufficiency if the patient's basal cortisol level is < 20 μg/dl
2. If the clinical picture is highly suggestive of adrenocortical insufficiency, the diagnosis can be made with the following test[22]
   a. On day before starting the test and on each day of the test collect 24-hour urine for 17-OHCS, and for creatinine (to evaluate adequacy of collection)
   b. Each day of the test (3 days) the patient is given dexamethasone 0.5 mg IV bid and fludrocortisone 0.1 mg PO qd, these are continued daily until the test results are known to avoid acute adrenal insufficiency
   c. ACTH 40 U mixed in 500 ml of D_5NS is infused over 8 hours each day of the test
3. The interpretation of the above test is summarized in Table 12-21
4. Secondary adrenocortical insufficiency can be distinguished from primary adrenal insufficiency by
   a. Absence of hyperpigmentation
   b. Decreased plasma ACTH level
   c. No significant impairment of aldostrone secretion (since aldosterone secretion is under control of the renin-angiotensin system)
   d. There may be additional evidence of hypopituitarism (e.g., hypogonadism, hypothyroidism)
   e. Absence of 11-deoxycortisol response to metyrapone

Table 12-21   Interpretation of 3-day test for adrenocortical insufficiency

Interpretation	Cortisol (Baseline)	ACTH (Baseline)	17-OHCS (Baseline)	17-OHCS (Day 1)	17-OHCS (Day 2)	17-OHCS (Day 3)
Normal response	N	N	N			
Primary adrenocortical insufficiency (Addison's disease)	↓	↑	N/↓	↓ No increase or small increase ↓	↓ No increase or small increase ↓	↓ No increase or small increase ↓
Secondary adrenocortical insufficiency (caused by pituitary dysfunction)	↓	↓	N/↓			

KEY: N, Normal; ↑, increase; ↓, decrease.

Therapy[4,47]

1. Chronic adrenocortical insufficiency
   a. Hydrocortisone 15-20 mg PO qAM and 5-10 mg in late afternoon, or prednisone 5 mg in AM and 2.5 mg at hs
   b. 9-α-fludrohydrocortisone 0.05-0.1 mg PO qAM; this mineralocorticoid replacement is necessary if the patient has primary adrenocortical insufficiency
   c. Periodic monitoring of serum electrolytes, vital signs, and body weight; liberal sodium intake
   d. Instruct patient to increase glucocorticoid replacement in times of stress and to receive parenteral glucocorticoids if diarrhea or vomiting occurs
2. Addisonian crisis: acute complication of adrenal insufficiency characterized by circulatory collapse, dehydration, nausea, vomiting, and hypoglycemia
   a. Draw plasma cortisol level; do not delay therapy until confirming lab results are obtained
   b. Administer hydrocortisone 100 mg IV q6h for 24 hours; if patient shows good clinical response, gradually taper dosage and change to oral maintenance dose (usually prenisone 7.5 mg/day)
   c. Provide adequate volume replacement with D_5NS until hypotension, dehydration, and hypoglycemia are completely corrected
   d. Identify and correct any precipitating factor (e.g., sepsis, hemorrhage)

DISORDERS OF MINERALOCORTICOID SECRETION
Physiology

1. Mineralocorticoids participate in the regulation of sodium and potassium balance by promoting
   a. Reabsorption of sodium in the cortical collecting tubules
   b. Secretion of potassium in the cortical collecting tubules
   c. Secretion of hydrogen ion in the collecting tubules
2. The principal sodium-retaining hormone, aldosterone, is regulated by several mechanisms[6]: renin-angiotension system, ACTH, and potassium
   a. The concentration of renin in the blood is the principal regulator
   b. Renin is secreted in response to several signals (renal perfusion pressure, β-adrenergic signals, fluid composition of the distal nephron at the macula densa)
   c. Renin stimulates aldosterone secretion by acting on angiotensinogen and splitting off a decapeptide, angiotensin I, which is then converted to angiotension II by an enzyme; angiotensin II stimulates adrenal production of aldosterone and also produces arterial vasoconstriction

Hypoaldosteronism

1. Etiology
   a. Hyporeninemic hypoaldosteronism: decreased aldosterone production secondary to decreased renin production; the typical patient has renal disease secondary to various factors (e.g., diabetes mellitus, interstitial nephritis, multiple myeloma)
   b. Aldosterone deficiency found in association with deficiency of adrenal glucocorticoid hormones (e.g., Addison's disease, bilateral adrenalectomy)

    c. Rarer causes: idiopathic hypoaldosteronism, unresponsiveness to aldosterone (pseudohypoaldosteronism)

2. Initial lab results[4]
   a. Increased potassium, normal or decreased sodium
   b. Hyperchloremic metabolic acidosis (caused by absence of hydrogen–secreting action of aldosterone)
   c. Increased BUN and creatinine (secondary to renal disease)
   d. Hyperglycemia (diabetes mellitus is common in these patients)
3. Treatment
   a. Treat primary condition
   b. Judicious use of 9-α-fluorocortisol (0.05-0.1 mg PO qAM) in patients with aldosterone deficiency associated with deficiency of adrenal glucocorticoid hormones

Hyperaldosteronism

1. Classification
   a. Primary aldosteronism (Conn's syndrome): aldosterone hypersecretion secondary to bilateral adrenal hyperplasia or aldosterone-secreting adenomas
   b. Secondary aldosteronism: excessive aldosterone secretion secondary to stimulation of the renin-angiotensin system; it is seen in association with chronic liver disease, chronic diuretic therapy, pregnancy, renal artery stenosis, renin-secreting neoplasms, Bartter's syndrome, hypovolemia, and sodium depletion
2. Diagnosis: see Fig. 12-7 for diagnostic evaluation of hypertensive patients with suspected aldosteronism, this is simplification of the various tests necessary for the diagnosis
3. Therapy[4]
   a. Aldosterone secreting adenoma: unilateral adrenalectomy after correction of blood pressure and hypokalemia with:
      (1) Spironolactone (aldosterone antagonist): 200-400 mg/day or
      (2) Amiloride (potassium-sparing diuretic): 20-40 mg/day
   b. Bilateral hyperplasia
      (1) Control hypokalemia with spironolactone or amiloride
      (2) Control hypertension with antihypertensive agents

12.12 PHEOCHROMOCYTOMA

Pathophysiology

Pheochromocytomas are catecholamine-producing tumors that originate from chromaffin cells of the adrenergic system. They generally secrete both norepinephrine and epinephrine, but norepinephrine is usually the predominant amine.

Characteristics[42]

1. "Rough rule of 10"
   a. 10% are extraadrenal
   b. 10% are malignant
   c. 10% are familial
   d. 10% occur in children
   e. 10% involve both adrenals
   f. 10% are multiple (other than bilateral adrenal)

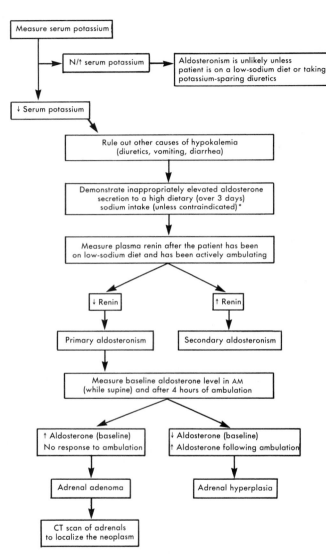

Figure 12-7
Diagnostic evaluation of hypertensive patient with suspected aldosteronism.

2. Clinical presentation: ''Five H's''
   a. Headache   d. Hypermetabolism
   b. Hypertension   e. Hyperglycemia
   c. Hyperhydrosis

Symptoms

1. Hypertension can be sustained (55%) or paroxysmal (45%)
2. Headache (80%): usually paroxysmal in nature and described as ''pounding'' and severe
3. Palpitations (70%): can be present with or without tachycardia
4. Hyperhydrosis (60%): most evident during paroxysmal attacks of hypertension

•   •   •

The above symptoms often arise in a dramatic and explosive fashion following sudden catecholemine release in response to a particular stimulus (e.g., sudden pressure in the area of the tumor, exercise, ingestion of certain foods, surgery). The paroxysms can last from less than 1 minute to several hours. Their frequency varies from once every few months to multiple daily episodes.

Diagnosis

1. Obtain family history: approximately 10% of pheochromocytomas are familial (see MEN)
2. Screening for pheochromocytoma should be considered in patients with[8,34]
   a. Malignant hypertension
   b. Poor response to antihypertensive therapy
   c. Paradoxical hypertensive responses
   d. Hypertension during induction of anesthesia, parturition, surgery, or thyrotropin–releasing hormone testing
   e. Hypertension associated with imipramine or desipramine
   f. Neurofibromatosis (increased incidence)
   g. von Hippel-Lindau disease (increased incidence)
3. Physical exam may be entirely normal if done in a symptom-free interval; during a paroxysm the patient may demonstrate marked increase in both systolic and diastolic pressure, profuse sweating, visual disturbances (caused by hypertensive retinopathy), dilated pupils (secondary to catecholamine excess), paresthesias in the lower extremities (caused by severe vasoconstriction), tremor, tachycardia
4. Lab results
   a. Increased 24-hour urine metanephrine level: this is the most accurate urine test for the diagnosis of phochromocytoma,[49] urinary vanillylmandelic acid or free catecholamines are less reliable
   b. Increased plasma catecholamines: according to some investigators[8] this test has the highest sensitivity for detecting pheochromocytoma
   c. Clonidine suppression test[9]: clonidine administration will cause a decrease in plasma catecholamine levels in patients with essential hypertension but have no effect in patients with pheochromocytoma

Locating the pheochromocytoma

1. Abdominal CT scan: useful in locating pheochromocytomas >0.5 inches in diameter[66]
2. Scintigraphy with ^{131}I-MIBG[61]: this norepinephrine analog localizes in adrenergic tissue; it is particularly useful in localizing extraadrenal pheochromocytomas
3. Selective vena cava sampling for norepinephrine levels: useful when CT scan and scintigraphy are unsuccessful; some investigators report a 97% success rate with this procedure[2]

Surgical therapy

1. Preoperative stabilization
   a. Volume expansion: done to prevent postoperative hypotension
   b. α Blockade to control hypertension: phenoxybenzamine (Dibenzyline) 10 mg PO bid-qid
   c. β Blockade: to be used only following α blockade
      (1) Useful to prevent catecholamine-induced dysrhythmias
      (2) Some investigators[9] do not recommend routine preoperative β blockade in absence of documented dysrhythmias; they advocate the use of IV propranolol (1-2 mg) intraoperatively if dysrhythmias develop during surgery
2. Hypertensive crises pre- and intraoperatively should be controlled with phentolamine (Regitine) 2-5 mg IV q5min; second drug of choice is nitroprusside used in combination with β-adrenergic blockers

12.13   CARCINOID SYNDROME

Definition

Carcinoid syndrome is characterized by paroxysmal vasomotor disturbances, diarrhea, and bronchospasm.

Pathophysiology

The symptoms are caused by the action of biologically active amines and peptides (serotonin, bradykinin, histamine) produced by tumors arising from enterochromaffin cells.

Organ distribution and characteristics

1. Carcinoids are principally found in the following organs:
   a. Appendix (40%)
   b. Small bowel (20%, 15% in ileum)
   c. Rectum (15%)
   d. Bronchi (12%)
   e. Esophagus, stomach, colon (10%)
   f. Ovary, biliary tract, pancreas (3%)
2. Carcinoid tumors do not usually produce the syndrome unless liver metastases are present or primary tumor does not involve the gastrointestinal tract
3. The appearance of the carcinoid syndrome often correlates directly with the tumor burden (increased tumor size = increased incidence of carcinoid syndrome) and with the presence of metastases

4. Carcinoids of the appendix and rectum have a low malignancy potential and they rarely produce the clinical syndrome; metastases are also uncommon if the size of the primary lesion is more than 2 cm in diameter

Clinical manifestations

1. Cutaneous flushing (90%)
   a. The patient usually has red-purple flushes involving face, neck, and upper trunk
   b. The flushing episodes last from a few minutes to hours (longer lasting flushes are usually associated with bronchial carcinoids)
   c. Flushing may be triggered by emotion or occur spontaneously
   d. Dizziness, tachycardia, and hypotension may be associated with the cutaneous flushing
2. Diarrhea (>70%): often associated with abdominal cramping and audible peristaltic rushes
3. Intermittent bronchospasm (25%): characterized by severe dyspnea and wheezing
4. Facial telangiectasia
5. Endocardial fibrosis: predominantly involves the endocardium, chordae, and valves of the right heart and can result in right-sided CHF

Lab results

1. Increased 24-hour urinary 5-hydroxy-indole-acetic acid (5-HIAA): a metabolite of serotonin (5 hydroxytryptamine)
2. False elevations can be seen with ingestion of certain foods (bananas, pineapples, eggplant, avocados, walnuts) and certain medications (acetaminophen, caffeine, guaifenesin, reserpine); therefore, these patients should be on a restricted diet when the test is ordered

Therapy

1. Surgical resection of tumor
   a. Can be palliative and result in prolonged asymptomatic periods
   b. Percutaneous embolization and ligation of the hepatic artery can decrease the bulk of the tumor in the liver and provide palliative treatment of the carcinoid syndrome
   c. Surgical manipulation of the tumor can cause severe vasomotor abnormalities and bronchospasm (carcinoid crisis): somatostatin is effective in reversing some of the symptoms[67]
2. Cytotoxic chemotherapy: combination chemotherapy with 5-fluorouracil and streptozotocin can be used in patients with unresectable or recurrent carcinoid tumors[10]
3. Control of clinical manifestations
   a. Diarrhea: usually responds to Lomotil (diphenoxylate with atropine)
   b. Flushing: can be controlled by the combined use of histamine H_1 and H_2 receptor antagonists (e.g., diphenhydramine 50 mg PO q6h and cimetidine 300 mg PO q6h)[50]
   c. Somatostatin analog is useful in severely symptomatic patients in need of clinical improvement before being treated with more aggressive measures[36]
4. Nutritional support: supplemental niacin therapy is used to prevent pellagra because these patients utilize dietary tryptophan for serotonin synthesis

MULTIPLE ENDOCRINE NEOPLASIA

Definition

Syndrome of multiple endocrine neoplasia (MEN) occurring familially in an autosomal dominant pattern. The endocrine neoplasms in these syndromes may be expressed as hyperplasia, adenoma, or carcinoma, and may develop synchronously or metachronously.[58]

Classification

1. MEN I (Wermer's syndrome)
   a. Tumors or hyperplasia of pituitary, pancreatic islet cells (insulinoma, gastrinoma, glucagonoma), or parathyroid
   b. Possible associated conditions
      (1) Adrenocortical adenoma or hyperplasia
      (2) Thyroid adenoma or hyperplasia
      (3) Renal cortical adenoma
      (4) Carcinoid tumors
      (5) Gastrointestinal polyps
      (6) Multiple lipomas
   c. Clinical manifestations[58]
      (1) Peptic ulcer and its complications
      (2) Hypoglycemia
      (3) Hypercalcemia and/or nephrocalcinosis
      (4) Headache, visual field defects, secondary amenorrhea
      (5) Multiple subcutaneous lipomas
      (6) Other: flushing, acromegaly, Cushing's syndrome, hyperthyroidism
2. MEN II (Sipple's syndrome, MEN IIa)
   a. Associated with[64] medullary thyroid carcinomas (MTC), pheochromocytoma, and hyperparathyroidism
   b. Clinical manifestations[13]
      (1) Neck mass (due to MTC)
      (2) Hypertension
      (3) Headache, palpitations, sweating
      (4) Hypercalcemia, nephrocalcinosis, osteitis fibrosa cystica
3. MEN III (multiple mucosal neuroma syndrome, MEN IIb)
   a. Associated with[34] medullary thyroid carcinoma (MTC), pheochromocytoma, and multiple mucosal neuromas
   b. Possible associated conditions: intestinal ganglioneuromatosis, marfanoid habitus
   c. Clinical manifestations[38]
      (1) Neck mass (due to MTC)
      (2) Headache, palpitations, sweating, hypertension
      (3) Mucosal neuromas (initially noted as whitish, yellow-pink nodules involving lips and anterior third of tongue[11])
      (4) Marfan-like habitus (with absence of cardiovascular abnormalities and lens subluxation)
      (5) Peripheral neuropathy (caused by neuromatous plaques overlying the posterior columns of the spinal cord, cauda equina, and sciatic nerve)[19]

References

1. AMA Division of Drugs and American Society for Clinical Pharmacology and Therapeutics: AMA drug evaluations, ed. 5, Philadelphia, 1983, W.B. Saunders Co.

2. Allison, D.J., Brown, M.J.: Role of venous sampling in locating a pheochromocytoma, Br. Med. J. **286:**1122, 1983.

3. Battle, D.C., Von Riotte, A.B., and Gaviria, M.: Amelioration of polyuria by amiloride in patients receiving long-term lithium therapy, N. Engl. J. Med. **312:**408, 1985.

4. Baxter, J.D.: Adrenocortical hypofunction. In Wyngaarden, J.B., and Smith, L.H., Jr., (editors): Cecil textbook of medicine, ed. 17, Philadelphia, 1985, W.B. Saunders Co.

5. Baxter, J.D., and Tyrrell, J.B.: The adrenal cortex. In Felig, P., Baxter, J.D., Broadus, A.H., Frohman, L.A. (editors): Endocrinology and metabolism, New York, 1900, McGraw-Hill Book Co.

6. Best, C.H.: Best and Taylor's physiological basis of medical practice, ed. 11, Baltimore, 1985, Williams and Wilkins, Co.

7. Biglieri, F.G., and Baxter, J.D.: The adrenal. In Felig, P., Baxter, J.D., Broadus, A.E., and Frohman, L.A., (editors): Endocrinology and metabolism, New York, 1981, McGraw-Hill Book Co.

8. Bravo, E.L., and Gifford, R.W., Jr.: Pheochromocytoma: diagnosis, localization and management, N. Engl. J. Med. **311:**1298, 1984.

9. Bravo, E.L., et al.: Clonidine-suppression test: a useful aid in the diagnosis of pheochromocytoma, N. Engl. J. Med. **305:**623, 1981.

10. Brennan, M., and MacDonald, J.: Carcinoid tumors. In De Vita, V. Jr., Hellman, S., and Rosenbery, S., (editors): Cancer, principles and practice of oncology, New York, 1985, J.B. Lippincott Co.

11. Brown, R.S., et al.: The syndrome of multiple mucosal neuromas and medullary thyroid carcinoma in childhood: importance of recognition of the phenotype for the early detection of malignancy, J. Pediatr. **86**(1):77, 1975.

12. Burch, W.M.: Cushing's disease: a review, Arch. Intern. Med. **145:**1106, 1985.

13. Cance, W.G., and Wells, S.A.: Multiple endocrine neoplasia type IIa, Curr. Probl. Surg., 1985.

14. Carpenter, P.C.: Cushing's syndrome: update of diagnosis and management, Mayo Clin. Proc. **61:**49, 1986.

15. Chava, N.R.: Use of the ECG in the clinical management of diabetic ketoacidosis, Pract. Cardiol. **12**(1):77, 1986.

16. Crapo, P.O., Reuven, G., Plefsky, J, and Alto, P.: Post-prandial plasma-glucose and insulin response to different complex carbohydrates, Diabetes, **26:**1178, 1977.

17. Crisp, A.H., et al.: Clinical features of anorexia nervosa: a study of a consecutive series of 102 female patients, J. Psychosom. Res. **24:**179, 1980.

18. Diagnostic and statistical manual of mental disorders III, Washington, D.C., American Psychiatric Association, 1980.

19. Dyck, P.J., et al.: Multiple endocrine neoplasia, type 2b: phenotype recognition, neurological features and their pathological basis, Ann. Neurol. **6:**302, 1979.

20. Expert committee on diabetes mellitus, World Health Organization, WHO Technical Report, 1980, p. 646.

21. Fairburn, C.G.: Bulimia nervosa, Br. J. Hosp. Med. **26:**537, 1983.

22. Federman, D.D.: The adrenal. In Rubenstein, E., and Federman, D.D., (editors): New York, 1985, Scientific American, Inc.

23. Federman, D.D.: Pituitary. In Rubenstein, E. and Federman, D.D., (editors): New York, 1986, Scientific American, Inc.

24. Flier, J.S., and Underhill, L.H.: Pathogenesis and management of lipoprotein disorders, N. Engl. J. Med. **312:**1300, 1985.

25. Hall, P.M., Cook, J., Sheldon, J., Rutheford, S., and Gould, B.J.: Proteins in the diagnosis of diabetes mellitus and impaired glucose tolerance, Diabetes Care, **7:**147, 1984.

26. Hamburger, J.I.: The various presentations of thyroiditis, Ann. Intern. Med. **104**:219, 1986.

27. Hamburger, J.: Consistency of sequential needle biopsy findings for thyroid nodules, Arch. Intern. Med. **147**:97, 1987.

28. HSU, T.H.: Disorders of the pituitary gland, In Harvey, A.M., Johns, R.J., McKusick, V.A., Owens, A.H., and Ross, R.S., (editors): The principles and practice of medicine, ed. 21, New York, 1984, Appleton-Century-Crofts.

29. Isner, J.M., et al.: Sudden death in anorexia nervosa, Ann. Intern. Med. **102**:49, 1985.

30. Jennings, A.S., Liddle, G.W., and Orth, D.N.: Results of treating childhood Cushing's disease with pituitary irradiation, N. Engl. J. Med. **297**:957, 1977.

31. KAOPC: Parathyroid hormone assay, Mayo Clin. Proc., **57**:596, 1982.

32. Kaufman, B.: Magnetic resonance imaging of the pituitary gland, Radiol. Clin. North Am. **22**:795, 1984.

33. Kem D., et al.: Saline suppression of plasma aldosterone in hypertension, Arch. Inter. Med. **128**:380, 1971.

34. Khairi, M.R., et al.: Mucosal neuroma, pheochromocytoma and medullary thyroid carcinoma: multiple endocrine neoplasia, type 3, Medicine, **54**:89, 1985.

35. Knoben, J.E., and Anderson, P.O.: Handbook of clinical drug data, ed. 5, 1983, Drug Intelligence Publications, Inc.

36. Kvols, L.K.: Metastatic carcinoid tumors and the carcinoid syndrome: a selective review of chemotherapy and hormonal therapy, Am. J. Med. **81**(68):49, 1986.

37. Larsen, P.R.: The thyroid. In Wyngaarden, J.B., and Smith, L.H., (editors): Cecil textbook of medicine, vol. 2, ed. 17, Philadelphia, 1985, W.B. Saunders Co.

38. Leshin, M.: Multiple endocrine neoplasia. In Wilson, J.D., and Foster, D.W., (editors): Williams textbook of endocrinology ed. 7, Philadelphia, 1985, W.B. Saunders Co.

39. Levy, R.I., Morganroth, J., and Rifkind, B.M.: Treatment of hyperlipidemias, N. Engl. J. Med. **290**:1295, 1974.

40. Levy, R.I., and Rifkind, B.M.: Lipid lowering drugs and hyperlipidemias, Drugs, **6**:12, 1973.

41. Maddedu, G., et al.: Serum thyroglobulin levels in the diagnosis and follow-up of subacute "painful" thyroiditis, Arch. Intern. Med. **145**:243, 1985.

42. Manger, W.M., Gifford, R.W., and Hoffman, B.B.: Pheochromocytoma: a clinical and experimental overview, Curr. Probl. Cancer, **9**(5):1985.

43. Marchant, B., et al.: The placental transfer of propylthiouracil, methimazole and carbimazole, J. Clin. End. Metab. **45**:1187, 1977.

44. Mitchell, J.E., et al.: Characteristics of 275 patients with bulimia, Am. J. Psychiatry, **142**:482, 1985.

45. Morris, L.R., et al.: Bicarbonate therapy in severe diabetic ketoacidosis, Ann. Intern. Med. **105**:836, 1986.

46. Mundy, G.R., et al: The hypercalcemia of cancer, N. Engl. J. Med., **310**:1718, 1984.

47. National Diabetes Data Group: Classification and diagnosis of diabetes mellitus and other categories of glucose intolerance, Diabetes **28**:1039, 1979.

48. Ney, R.L.: Disorders of the adrenal gland. In Harvey, A.M., Johns, R.J., McKusick, V.A., Owens, A.H., Ross, R.S., (editors): Principles and practice of medicine, ed. 21, New York, 1984, Appleton-Century-Crofts.

49. Plouin, P.F., et al.: Biochemical tests for diagnosis of pheochromocytoma: urinary versus plasma determinations, Br. Med. J. **282**:853, 1981.

50. Pyles, J.D., et al.: Histamine antagonists and carcinoid flush, N. Engl. J. Med. **302**:234, 1980.

51. Robbins, R.J.: Medical management of prolactinomas. In Robbins, R.J., and Olefsky, (editors): Prolactinomas, New York, 1986, Churchill Livingstone.

52. Rock, R.C.: Interpreting thyroid tests in the elderly: updated guidelines, Geriatrics, **40**(12):61, 1985.

53. Rojeski, M., and Gharib, H.: Nodular thyroid disease, evaluation and management, N. Engl. J. Med. **313**(7):428, 1985.

54. Russell, G.F.M.: Anorexia nervosa. In Wyngaarden, J.B., and Smith, L.A., Jr., (editors): Cecil textbook of medicine, ed. 17, Philadelphia, 1985, W.B. Saunders Co.

55. Ryzen, E., et al.: Intravenous etidronate in the management of malignant hypercalcemia, Arch. Intern. Med. **145**:449, 1985.

56. Samuel, P.: Drug treatment of hyperlipidemia, Am. Heart J. **100**:873, 1980.

57. Schimke, R.N.: Disorders affecting multiple endocrine systems. In Petersdorf, R.G., et al. (editors): Harrison's principles of internal medicine, ed. 10, New York, 1983, McGraw-Hill Book Co.

58. Schimke, R.N.: Genetic aspects of multiple endocrine neoplasia, Ann. Rev. Med. **35**:25, 1984.

59. Schuermeter, T.H.: Pharmacologic and pharmacokinetic properties of corticotropin-releasing factor in humans. In Chrousos, G.P. (moderator): Clinical applications of corticotropin-releasing factor, Ann. Int. Med. **102**:344, 1985.

60. Shepard, F.A., et al.: Ketoconazole, use in the treatment of ectopic adrenocorticotropic hormone production in Cushing's syndrome in small-cell lung cancer, Arch. Intern. Med. May, 1985.

61. Sisson, J.C., et al.: Locating pheochromocytomas by scintigraphy using ^{131}I-metaiodobenzylguanidine, CA **34**:86, 1984.

62. Skyler, J.S., Siegler, D.E., and Reeves, M.L.: A comparison of insulin regimens in insulin-dependent diabetes mellitus, Diabetes Care, **5**(1):11, 1982.

63. Sridama, V., et al.: Long term follow-up study of compensated low dose ^{131}I therapy for Graves' disease, N. Engl. J. Med. **311**:426, 1984.

64. Steiner, A.L., and Goodman, A.D.: Study of kindred with pheochromocytoma, medullary thyroid carcinoma, hyperparathyroidism and Cushing's disease: multiple endocrine neoplasia, type 2, Medicine, **47**:371, 1968.

65. Stewart, A.F., et al.: Biochemical evaluation of patients with malignancy associated hypercalcemia: evidence for humoral and non-humoral groups, N. Engl. J. Med., **303**:1377, 1980.

66. Stewart, B.H., et al.: Localization of pheochromocytoma by computerized tomography, N. Engl. J. Med. **299**:460, 1978.

67. Thulin, L., et al.: Efficacy of somatostatin in a patient with carcinoid syndrome, Lancet, **2**:43, 1978.

68. Tucker, H., et al.: The treatment of acromegaly by transsphenoidal surgery, Arch. Int. Med. **140**:795, 1980.

69. Tyrrell, J.B.: Cushing's syndrome, In Wyngaarden, J.B., and Smith, L.A., Jr., (editors): Cecil textbook of medicine, ed. 17, Philadelphia, 1985, W.B. Saunders Co.

70. Tyrrell, J.B., et al.: An overnight high: dose dexamethasone suppression test for rapid differential diagnosis of Cushing's syndrome, Ann. Intern. Med. **104**:180, 1986.

71. Van Herle, A.J., et al.: The thyroid nodule, Ann. Intern. Med. **96**:221, 1982.

72. Vignati, L., et al.: Coma in diabetics. In Marble, A., Krall, L., Bradley, R., Christlieb, A.R., Soeldner, J.S., (editors): Joslin's diabetes mellitus, ed. 12, Philadelphia, 1985, Lea and Febiger.

73. Vignati, L., et al.: Coma in diabetes. In Marble, A., Krall, L., Bradley, R., Christlieb, A.R., Soeldner, J.S. (editors): Joslin's diabetes mellitus, ed. 12, p. 537., Philadelphia, 1985, Lea and Febiger.

74. Vignati, L., et al.: Hyperosmolar coma. In Marble, A., Drall, L. Bradley, R., Christlieb, A.R., Soeldner, J.S., (editors): Joslin's diabetes mellitus, ed. 12, Philadelphia, 1985, Lea and Febiger.

75. Vita, J.A., et al.: Clinical clues to the cause of Addison's disease, Am. J. Med., **78**:461, 1985.

76. Williams, G.H., and Dluhy, R.G.: Diseases of the adrenal cortex. In Petersdorf, R.G., et al. (editors): Harrison's principles of internal medicine, ed. 10, New York, 1983, McGraw-Hill Book Co.
77. Zinman, B., Zuniga-Guajardo, S., and Kelly, D.: Comparison of the long-term effects of exercise in glucose control in Type I diabetes, Diabetes Care, 7:515, 1984.

Gastroenterology

13

ACUTE GASTROINTESTINAL BLEEDING
Saul Feldman

Patients with acute GI hemorrhage must be approached in a multidisciplinary manner. The evaluating team should include the family physician/internist, a gastroenterologist, a radiologist, and a gastrointestinal surgeon. The initial assessment is directed toward:

1. Evaluating the extent (severity) of the bleeding
2. Locating the site of the bleeding:
   a. Upper GI bleeding (above ligament of Treitz)
   b. Lower GI bleeding (below ligament of Treitz)

After a brief initial assessment, the physician should immediately stabilize the patient with volume expanders (Ringer's lactate or normal saline) until blood is available (after patient's blood is typed and cross-matched).

History and physical exam

Although the history and the physical exam may be somewhat limited by the patient's condition, they should be performed to evaluate the severity, duration, location, and cause of the bleeding (see p. 79-80 for the differential diagnosis of GI bleeding). The following are some salient points to note when taking the patient's history:

1. Drug history (aspirin, steroids, "blood thinners," nonsteroidal antiinflammatory drugs [NSAID])
2. Prior GI or vascular surgery
3. History of GI diagnosis or bleeding
4. History of smoking (increased risk of PUD)
5. Alcohol intake (gastritis, esophageal varices)
6. Symptoms of peptic ulcer
7. Associated diseases (ASHD, diabetes, hypertension, renal failure)
8. Protracted retching and vomiting (consider gastric or gastroesophageal tear [Mallory-Weiss])
9. Weight loss, anorexia (consider carcinoma)

Physical exam

1. Vital signs
   a. Document tachycardia, hypotension, and postural changes; a pulse increase of more than 20 beats/minute or a postural fall in systolic blood pressure greater than 10-15 mm Hg usually indicates blood loss greater than 1 L

b. Patients taking β-adrenergic blockers or vasodilators may not demonstrate significant variations of the vital signs

2. Cardiorespiratory exam: murmurs (increased incidence of angiodysplasia in patients with aortic stenosis), pulmonary rales, JVD (to determine rapidity of volume replacement)

3. Abdominal exam
   a. Observe for masses, tenderness, distention
   b. Auscultate for bowel sounds or abdominal bruits
   c. Look for evidence of liver disease (hepatomegaly, splenomegaly, abnormal vascular patterns, gynecomastia, spider angiomata, palmar erythema, testicular atrophy)

4. Digital rectal exam: check for masses, strictures, hemorrhoids; test stool for occult blood and inspect it for abnormalities (tarry, blood-streaked, bright red, mahogany color)

5. Skin: check for jaundice (liver disease), ecchymoses (coagulation abnormality), cutaneous telangiectasia (Rendu-Osler-Weber's disease), buccal pigmentation (Peutz-Jeghers' syndrome) and other mucocutaneous changes (Ehlers-Danlos' syndrome)

6. Look for evidence of metastatic disease (cachexia, firm nodular liver)

7. Insert NG tube to determine if the bleeding is emanating from the upper GI tract (presence of bright red blood clots or coffee ground guaiac-positive aspirate); however, a guaiac-negative aspirate does not rule out UGI bleeding since it could have subsided or the patient could be bleeding from the duodenal bulb without reflux into the stomach

Initial management

1. Stabilize patient: insert a large-bore (16 gauge) IV catheter and administer Ringer's lactate or normal saline; the rate of volume replacement is based on the estimated blood loss, clinical condition, and history of cardiovascular disease

2. Type and cross-match for 2-8 units of packed RBC (depending on estimated blood loss) and transfuse prn

3. Initial lab evaluation
   a. Hemoglobin/hematocrit
      (1) Initial value should be considered as erroneously high until blood volume is replaced
      (2) After bleeding ceases, the hemogram may continue to decrease for up to 6 hours and full equilibration may require 24 hours
      (3) The hematocrit generally falls by about 2-3 points for every 500 ml of blood lost
   b. BUN: in absence of renal disease, a BUN may help determine the severity of the bleeding; a simultaneous creatinine level may also be of value, as the disparity in the BUN/creatinine ratio will reveal the extent of the bleeding more accurately
   c. Prothrombin time (PT), partial thromboplastin time (PTT), and platelet count should be done to exclude bleeding disorders; they should also be assessed before endoscopy or other invasive procedures
   d. Other initial lab measurements to be drawn include liver function tests, serum electrolytes, glucose, and white blood cell count

Investigational tools (Fig. 13-1)

Endoscopic evaluation

1. Upper endoscopy is indicated when blood or guaiac-positive material is obtained from NG tube aspirate or if lower endoscopy is negative
2. Flexible signoidoscopy should be performed initially if lower GI bleeding is suspected; it helps to diagnose anal disease, colitis, and neoplasms in the lower colon
3. Colonoscopy should be performed if sigmoidoscopy is not diagnostic and bleeding appears to be colonic in origin; most useful in cases of AV malformations, colitis, neoplasms, and intussusception

Radiologic evaluation

1. Barium enema (BE)
    a. It should not be performed initially because it precludes other modes
    b. A double-contrast BE should be initiated after sigmoidoscopy, colonoscopy, arteriography, and nuclear scanning have been done
    c. The BE may be therapeutic in some cases of bleeding secondary to diverticular disease or intussusception
2. Upper GI series should be ordered only after utilizing endoscopy, arteriography, and nuclear scans; when ordering a GI series, the investigator must specify whether an esophagram or a small bowel series is desired
3. Radionuclide scans
    a. Technetium 99 pertechnetate scan (Meckel scan) selectively tags acid-secreting cells (gastric mucosa); it is used most often in unexplained bleeding in infants and young adults
    b. Technetium sulfur colloid scan is very sensitive in detecting low bleeding rates; its major drawbacks are:
        (1) Short half-life (difficulty in detecting intermittent bleeding)
        (2) Affinity of the colloid for liver and spleen (colonic bleeding may be missed if it originates in a region superimposed on areas of liver or spleen uptake)
    c. Technetium (^{99m}Tc)–labeled red blood cell scan: its major advantage over the sulfur colloid scan is its long duration; it is useful for intermittent bleeding because the patient can be monitored for GI bleeding for up to 24 hours
4. Selective angiography
    a. Occasionally first test ordered in actively bleeding patients
    b. May also be therapeutic since vasoconstrictors, autologous clots, or gelfoam emboli can be administered intraarterially at the time of angiography to occlude the bleeding vessel
    c. Major drawbacks are the high rate of bleeding (>0.5 ml/minute) necessary for diagnosis and the risk of allergic reaction to contrast dye

Therapy

The treatment of acute GI bleeding may require multiple modalities and will be mentioned only briefly.

1. Correct bleeding abnormalities by administering fresh frozen plasma or vitamin K if the patient has a coagulopathy
2. H_2-receptor antagonists, sucralfate, and antacids are indicated only in cases of probable peptic ulcer or gastritis; H_2-blockers can cause liver

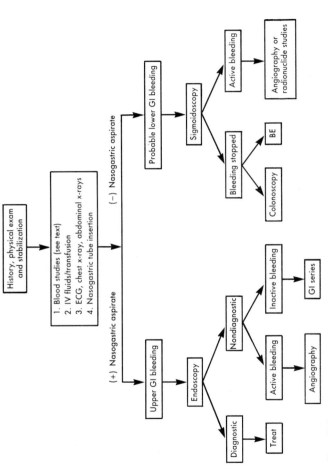

Figure 13-1
Management of acute GI bleeding.

toxicity and many serious drug interactions, so they should be used with caution

3. Vasopressin (Pitressin) infusion is used in the management of significant variceal bleeding
   a. Mix 20 U of vasopressin in 100 ml of D_5W (0.2 U/ml)
   b. The infusion rate initially is 0.2 U/minute (1 ml/minute via continuous infusion pump), but it can be increased by 0.2-0.3 U q30min prn to control esophageal bleeding; maximum dosage is 0.9 U/minute
   c. Relative contraindications are severe coronary artery disease and peripheral or cerebrovascular disease because of increased risk of angina, MI, tachycardia, TIA, CVA, and hypertension
   d. Concomitant administration of nitrates may be indicated in patients with ASHD
   e. Vasopressin is only a temporizing measure; many patients will experience rebleeding when vasopressin is stopped

4. Endoscopy
   a. Sclerotherapy for bleeding varices
   b. Laser therapy (directed through the endoscope) may be used in proven bleeding from ulcerations, AV malformations, or neoplasms
   c. Cauterization with bipolar electrode is a useful modality to stop bleeding from ulcerations

5. Balloon tamponade by inserting a Sengstaken-Blakemore (SB) tube or Minnesota quadruple tube (modification of SB tube with a port to suction above the esophageal balloon)
   a. Balloon tamponade is indicated for severe bleeding from esophageal varices
   b. It should be inserted only by experts since it can result in esophageal rupture and pulmonary aspiration

6. Radiologic modalities: localized infusion of vasopressin, autologous clots, or foreign coagulating substances (e.g., gelfoam) in the bleeding vessel during or following arteriography

7. Surgery is indicated at the onset of diagnosis of aortoduodenal fistula, but it is not suggested as the initial therapy in other causes of GI bleeding until a definitive diagnosis is made and other noninvasive modalities are attempted; exceptions to the conservative approach are:
   a. Rebleeding in a hospitalized patient
   b. Bleeding episode requiring transfusion of more than 6 units of blood
   c. Endoscopic visualization of a ''naked'' vessel in a peptic ulcer

13.2 PEPTIC ULCER DISEASE (PUD)

Etiology

Peptic ulcers result from an imbalance between mucosal defense mechanisms (protective factors) and various mucosal damaging mechanisms (Table 13-1).

Anatomic location

1. Duodenal ulcers: 90%-95% occur in the first portion of the duodenum
2. Gastric ulcers: occur most frequently in the lesser curvature, near the angularis

Table 13-1   Factors involved in the pathogenesis of peptic ulcers[41]

Protective Factors	Aggressive Factors
Mucosal barrier: pH-mucus gradient formed by a mixture of bicarbonate (secreted by gastric and duodenal epithelia) and gastric mucus	Acid secreted by parietal cells
	Pepsin secreted as pepsinogen by chief cells
	Bile acids play a significant role in the pathogenesis of gastric ulcer and esophagitis
Adequate blood supply to gastric mucosa and submucosa	Decreased blood flow to gastric mucosa
Competent sphincters (pyloric and LES) block reflux of bile salts into the stomach and esophagus	Incompetent pylorus or LES
Medications	Medications
Histamine H_2-receptor antagonists	Aspirin
	Nonsteroidal antiinflammatory drugs (NSAID)
Antacids	Glucocorticoids
Sucralfate	Cigarette smoking
Bismuth compounds	Gastrinoma
Anticholinergics	Stress (particularly following trauma)
Prostaglandins of A and E classes	Alcohol

Clinical manifestations

1. Duodenal ulcer: patient usually has epigastric pain occurring 3-4 hours after eating; the pain is described as a burning, aching, boring, gnawing " pressure on the abdomen" that awakens the patient from sleep and is usually relieved by ingesting antacids or food (however, many patients with active duodenal ulcers may be asymptomatic)
2. Gastric ulcer: the patient has epigastric pain similar to duodenal ulcer, but the pain is not usually relieved by food; food may actually precipitate the symptoms

Physical exam

The physical exam is often unremarkable. The patient may have epigastric tenderness, tachycardia, pallor, hypotension (from acute or chronic blood loss), nausea and vomiting (if the pyloric channel is obstructed), boardlike abdomen and rebound tenderness (if perforated), and hematemesis or melena (if bleeding ulcer).

Diagnostic modalities

1. Endoscopy
   a. Highest accuracy (approximately 90%-95%)
   b. Useful to identify superficial or very small ulcerations
   c. Essential to diagnose gastric ulcers (4% of gastric ulcers diagnosed as benign by UGI series are eventually diagnosed as gastric carcinoma)

    d. Additional advantages over UGI series include:
      (1) Possible biopsy of suspicious looking ulcers
      (2) Electrocautery of bleeding ulcers
      (3) Measurement of gastric pH in suspected gastrinoma (e.g., patient with multiple ulcers)
      (4) Diagnosis of esophagitis, gastritis, duodenitis
    e. Its major disadvantage is its higher cost
2. UGI series: conventional UGI barium studies identify approximately 70%-80% of PUD; accuracy can be increased to about 90% by using double contrast

Complications

1. GI bleeding (20%)
    a. Clinical manifestations: hematemesis, melena, hematochezia (if rapid transit time)
    b. Physical exam: pallor, hypotension, tachycardia, diaphoresis
    c. Diagnosis: endoscopy (after the patient has been stabilized)
    d. Therapy
      (1) IV hydration with NS, blood transfusion
      (2) Surgery if bleeding persists
2. Perforation (10%)
    a. Clinical manifestations: severe abdominal pain, epigastric pain with radiation to back or RUQ (if penetrating ulcer)
    b. Physical exam: boardlike abdomen, rebound tenderness, severe epigastric tenderness
    c. Diagnosis: x-ray studies of abdomen may reveal free air in the peritoneal cavity
    d. Therapy: surgery
3. Gastric outlet obstruction (5%)
    a. Clinical manifestations: nausea, vomiting of undigested food, epigastric pain unrelieved by food or antacids
    b. Physical exam: large amount of air and fluid in the stomach, "succussion splash" may be heard
4. Posterior penetrations: manifested by severe back pain, pancreatitis

Medical therapy

Medical treatment is aimed at neutralizing gastric acidity (antacids), reducing acid production (H_2-blockers), increasing mucosal protection (sucralfate), and decreasing risk factors (e.g., cigarette smoking).
1. Antacids[14]
    a. They decrease the hydrogen ion concentration; the duration of their effect is directly related to their potency (Table 13-2) and to the length of time the antacid remains in the stomach (duration is prolonged if given after meals)
    b. Dosage is 30 ml of antacid given 1 and 3 hours after meals and hs
    c. Duration of therapy is 6-8 weeks
2. Histamine H_2-receptor antagonists[23]
    a. They decrease gastric acid secretion by blocking histamine H_2-receptors on parietal cells

Table 13-2 Composition and acid neutralizing capacity of selected antacid preparations

Product	Dosage Forms*	Active Ingredients† AH	MH	CC	SI	Sodium Content mg	mEq	ANC‡
AlternaGel	Liq	600	—	—	—	2	0.09	16
Amphojel	Susp	320	—	—	—	6.9	0.30	7
	Tab	600	—	—	—	2.8	0.12	18
Camalox	Susp	225	200	250	—	2.5	0.11	18
	Tab	225	200	250	—	1.5	0.07	18
Delcid	Liq	600	665	—	—	12	0.53	42
Gelusil	Liq, tab	200	200	—	25	0.7	0.03	12
Maalox	Susp	225	200	—	—	1.4	0.06	13
	Tab	200	200	—	—	0.8	0.04	9
Maalox plus	Susp	225	200	—	25	1.3	0.06	13
	Tab	200	200	—	25	0.9	0.04	9
Maalox TC	Susp	600	300	—	—	0.8	0.3	28
Milk of magnesia	Susp	—	310	—	—	1.3	<0.01	14
	Tab	—	310	—	—	0.9	0.01	14
Mylanta	Liq, tab	200	200	—	20	0.7	0.03	12
Mylanta II	Liq, tab	400	400	—	30	1.3	0.06	24
Riopan	Susp, tab	480§	—	—	—	0.1	<0.01	14
Riopan plus	Susp, tab	480§	—	—	20	0.1	<0.01	14
Silain gel	Liq	280	285	—	25	4.8	0.21	15
Titralac	Liq	—	—	1000	—	11	0.48	20
	Tab	—	—	420	—	0.3	0.01	8
WinGel	Liq, tab	180	160	—	—	<2.5	0.10	12

From DiGregorio, G.J., Barbieri, E.J., and Piraino, A.J.: Handbook of commonly prescribed drugs, 1984, Medical Surveillance Inc.

*Liq, liquid; Susp, suspension; Tab, tablet.

†AH, aluminum hydroxide; MH, magnesium hydroxide; CC, calcium carbonate; SI, simethicone; in mg per 5 ml or per tablet.

‡Acid neutralizing capacity in mEq per 5 ml or per tablet.

§As magaldrate, a complex of aluminum and magnesium hydroxides.

   b. Dosage
     (1) Cimetidine (Tagamet)
       (a) PO: 300 mg q6h, 400 mg bid, or 800 mg qhs
       (b) IV: 300 mg q6h
     (2) Ranitidine (Zantac)
       (a) PO: 150 mg bid or 300 mg qhs
       (b) IV: 50 mg q8h
     (3) Famotidine (Pepcid): 20 mg PO bid or 40 mg PO qhs
   c. Duration of therapy is 8 weeks
3. Sucralfate (Carafate)[29]
   a. Sucralfate is a disaccharide with negatively charged radicals that adhere to positively charged proteins on the surface of the ulcer crater and form a protective coating that shields the ulcer from acid and pepsin
   b. The action of sucralfate requires an acidic environment, therefore simultaneous ingestion of H_2-blockers or antacids should be avoided
   c. Dosage is 1 g 30-60 minutes before meals and at hs
   d. Duration of therapy is 6-8 weeks
4. Experimental agents: prostaglandins of A and E classes[31]

Ancillary therapy

1. Stop cigarette smoking:[46] cigarette smoking increases the risk of PUD, decreases the healing rate, and increases the frequency of recurrence
2. Avoid salicylates and nonsteroidal antiinflammatory drugs (NSAID)
3. Prophylaxis of patients at risk for PUD:[43] patients on prolonged mechanical ventilation, ICU patients receiving steroids or admitted following severe trauma should receive a prophylactic regimen of antacids or H_2-blockers to prevent PUD
4. Special diets have been proved *unrelated* to ulcer development or healing; however, avoid foods that cause symptoms

•   •   •

   Medical and ancillary therapy will result in complete healing of approximately 80%-90% of peptic ulcers. Surgery should be performed when the patient has undergone an adequate course of medical therapy with an unsatisfactory response (inadequate healing, multiple recurrences).

Recurrence

The recurrence rate for untreated PUD is approximately 70%-80%. Treatment will decrease the recurrence rate approximately 20%-30%. Patients with recurrent ulcers should be retreated for an additional 8 weeks and then placed on prophylactic therapy with cimetidine 400 mg PO qhs, ranitidine 150 mg PO qhs, or famotidine 20 mg PO qhs.

Suggested follow-up

1. Duodenal ulcer: no further evaluation necessary if patient is asymptomatic after 8 weeks of therapy
2. Gastric ulcer: repeat endoscopy should be done after 4-6 weeks of therapy; further management will depend on the results of the endoscopy:

a. Completely healed ulcer requires no further follow-up
b. Partially healed ulcer:
   (1) >50% healing and exfoliative cytology negative for carcinoma requires continued medical therapy for 6 more weeks and then reevaluate patient
   (2) >50% healing but exfoliative cytology postive for carcinoma requires surgery
   (3) <50% healing requires surgery

13.3   INFLAMMATORY BOWEL DISEASE

Inflammatory bowel diseases (IBD) is a chronic inflammatory disorder of the GI tract of undetermined etiology. The incidence is increased in young adults and Jews, but decreased in blacks. IBD is subdivided into two major groups:
1. Crohn's disease
2. Ulcerative colitis/proctitis

Lab results
1. Decreased hemoglobin/hematocrit, decreased potassium, decreased magnesium, decreased calcium
2. Decreased albumin
3. Vitamin B_{12} deficiency, folate deficiency (more common in Crohn's disease)

Table 13-3   Comparison of inflammatory bowel diseases

Crohn's Disease	Ulcerative Colitis
Clinical Manifestations	
RLQ abdominal pain	Diarrhea often bloody and accompanied by tenesmus
Fever, dehydration, weight loss	Constipation may be present in some patients with significant rectal involvement
Anorexia, nausea, vomiting	Fever, dehydration, weight loss
Diarrhea	Abdominal pain, anorexia, nausea, vomiting
Physical Exam	
RLQ tenderness	Abdominal distention
Abdominal mass may be present (usually formed by adjacent loops of bowel)	Abdominal tenderness
	Extraintestinal manifestations may be present:
Anorectal disease (perirectal abscesses, fissures, fistulas)	Iritis, uveitis, episcleritis
	Arthritis
Extraintestinal manifestations same as in ulcerative colitis	Erythema nodosum
	Pyoderma gangrenosum
	Aphthous stomatitis

Differential diagnosis

1. Bacterial infections
   a. Acute: *Campylobacter, Yersinia, Salmonella, Shigella,* gonococcal proctitis, *Chlamidiae, E. coli* (toxigenic), *C. difficile* (pseudomembranous colitis)
   b. Chronic: Whipple's disease, TB enterocolitis
2. Irritable bowel syndrome
3. Protozoal and parasitic infections (amebiasis, giardiasis)
4. Abdominal lymphoma
5. Carcinoma of ileum or colon
6. Carcinoid tumors
7. Celiac sprue
8. Mesenteric adenitis
9. Diverticulitis
10. Appendicitis
11. Polyarteritis nodosa
12. Radiation enteritis
13. Collagenous colitis
14. Fungal infections *(Histoplasma, Actinomyces)*
15. α Chain disease
16. Endometriosis

Complications

1. Intestinal obstruction
2. Intestinal perforation
3. Malabsorption
4. Electrolyte abnormalities (secondary to diarrhea)
5. GI hemorrhage
6. Anemia (from chronic blood loss), hypoproteinemia, vitamin B_{12} and folate deficiencies
7. Carcinoma of colon or bile ducts, primary sclerosing cholangitis, and pericholangitis (in ulcerative colitis)
8. Fistulas (in Crohn's disease)
9. Toxic megacolon

Table 13-4   Endoscopic features of Crohn's disease and ulcerative colitis

Crohn's Disease	Ulcerative Colitis
Asymmetric and discontinuous disease	Very friable mucosa
Deep, longitudinal fissures	Diffuse, uniform erythema replacing the usual mucosal vascular pattern
Cobblestone appearance	Rectal involvement
Aphthous ulcers	
Mucosa friability not usually present	
Strictures	

Table 13-5   Radiographic differences between Crohn's disease and ulcerative colitis

Crohn's Disease	Ulcerative Colitis
Deep ulcerations (often longitudinal and transverse)	Fine, superficial ulcerations
Segmental lesions (skip lesions)	Continuous involvement (including rectum)
Strictures	Shortening of the bowel
Fistulas	Symmetric bowel contour
Cobblestone appearance of the mucosa (caused by submucosal inflammation)	Decreased mucosal pattern
"Thumbprinting" common	

Diagnosis

1. Sigmoidoscopy is done to establish the presence of mucosal inflammation; Table 13-4 describes the endoscopic differences between ulcerative colitis and Crohn's disease
2. Air-contrast barium enema: see Table 13-5 for interpretation of results
3. Pathologic differences: Crohn's disease can be further distinguished from ulcerative colitis by:
   a. Presence of transmural involvement
   b. Frequent presence of noncaseating granulomas and lymphoid aggregates

Therapy

Medical therapy

1. Control of inflammatory process
   a. Avoid oral feedings during acute exacerbation to decrease colonic activity; a low-roughage diet may be helpful in *early* relapse
   b. Sulfasalazine[4] is effective in ulcerative colitis and in Crohn's disease confined to the colon; dosage is 500 mg PO bid initially, increased qd or qod by 1 g until therapeutic dosages of 4-6 g/day are achieved
   c. Steroids: methylprednisolone[28] or prednisone (e.g., prednisone 40-60 mg/day); steroid retention enemas may be useful in patients with ulcerative colitis limited to the rectum and accompanied by severe tenesmus
   d. Immunosuppressants (azathioprine, 6-mercaptopurine[38]) have been used in severe IBD refractory to above measures; however, their role has been questioned
2. Correction of nutritional deficiencies
   a. Correct existing electrolyte disorders, anemia, and vitamin deficiencies
   b. IV alimentation in severe cases (peripheral or central)
3. Psychotherapy is very important because of the chronicity of the diseases and the relatively young age of the patients

4. Treatment of complications
   a. Fulminant colitis or toxic megacolon (midtransverse colon $\geq$6 cm in diameter)
      (1) IV corticosteroids
      (2) Broad spectrum IV antibiotics (e.g., cefoxitin plus gentamycin)
      (3) Vigorous IV hydration and correction of any electrolyte abnormalities
      (4) Nasogastric suction
      (5) Correct anemia, and metabolic and nutritional abnormalities
      (6) Surgical intervention if there is no marked improvement with the above measures
   b. Anal fistulas and other perineal diseases
      (1) IV metronidazole[9] (Flagyl) 20 mg/kg/day in divided doses
      (2) Surgical repair
      (3) Extensive bowel resection if the patient develops recurrent retrovaginal or rectovesicular fistulae
   c. Intestinal obstruction
      (1) Nasogastric suction
      (2) IV hydration
      (3) IV steroids
      (4) Surgical intervention if no improvement
   d. Abscess formation
      (1) IV antibiotics
      (2) IV steroids
      (3) IV hydration

Surgical therapy
Surgery is indicated in patients with ulcerative colitis who fail to respond to intensive medical therapy. Colectomy is usually curative in these patients and it also eliminates the high risk of developing adenocarcinoma of the colon (10%-20% of patients develop it after 10 years with the disease). In Crohn's disease, surgery is generally not curative (postoperative recurrence rate >50%) therefore, it is generally reserved for treatment of severe complications (e.g., intractable recurrent rectovaginal, rectovesicular fistulae or intractable obstruction).

 DIARRHEA

Definition
Diarrhea is defined as frequent passage of loose or watery stool.

Diagnostic approach to new-onset diarrhea
History
1. Travel history (traveler's diarrhea)
   a. Recent travel to areas or countries with poor sanitation: consider toxigenic *E. coli*, parasites *(Giardia, Entamoeba histolytica)*
   b. See Table 13-6 for causes of acute bacterial diarrheas and Table 13-7 for clues to common parasitic diarrheas
   c. Outdoor living in wilderness areas with ingestion of water from streams: consider *Giardia* (particularly in Rocky Mountains region)

Table 13-6 Acute bacterial diarrheas

	S. aureus	C. perfringens	Enterotoxigenic E. coli	V. cholerae	Salmonella (non-typhoid)	Shigella	Campylobacter fetus ssp. jejuni
Stool volume	Moderate to large	Moderate	Moderate to large	Large	Variable	Variable	Small to moderate
Blood	—	—	—	—	±	51%	71%
Fecal WBCs	—	—	—	—	85%	69%-91%	87%
Vomiting	++	±	±	—	—	—	29%
Fever	—	—	Low-grade	—	+	+	57%
Abdominal pain	—	+	+	—	+	+	86%
Rapid diagnosis*	—	—	—	—	—	—	Dark-field microscopy or fuchsin stain
Incubation period	2-4 hr	12-16 hr	1-2 weeks	6 hr-5 days	6-24 hr	24-48 hr	2-11 days
Duration of illness†	Few hours	Few hours	3-7 days	4-5 days	1-7 days	4 days-2 weeks	4-5 days
Duration of shedding†	—	—	—	—	Variable	Variable	Few days to 7 weeks

	Food	Meat, poultry	Food, water	Water	Food, animals, humans	Fecal-oral	Food, pets, humans
Mode of transmission							
Enterotoxin	+	+	+	+	±	—	Role in disease is unclear
Therapy*	Supportive	Supportive	Bismuth subsalicylate; tetracycline may be helpful	Supportive	Contraindicated except in life-threatening cases	Ampicillin or trimethoprim-sulfamethoxazole	Erythromycin
Comments		Generally mild illness	History of recent travel is suggestive	Very high stool volume; rare in children <1 yr old	Generally mild illness	Peripheral differential WBC count may show increased band: segmented ratio	Reactive arthritis may occur, especially associated with HLA-B27 antigen

From Appenheimer, A.T.: Emergency decisions, p. 21, Sept., 1985.
*Within first few hours of presentation.
†In untreated cases.

Table 13-7 Clues to common parasitic diarrheas

| | Organism | |
	Giardia	E. histolytica
Stool volume	Variable	Small to moderate
Stool consistency	Bulky, foul-smelling	Watery and mild to explosive and purulent
Blood	—	39%
Fecal WBCs	—	7%
Vomiting	—(nausea)	—
Fever	—	Low-grade
Abdominal symptoms	Distention, cramps, flatulence	Pain
Rapid diagnosis*	Stool exam†	Stool exam†
Incubation	Unknown	Unknown
Duration	Weeks	Weeks-years
Duration of shedding (if untreated)	Prolonged	Years
Transmission	Water, humans	Fecal-oral
Enterotoxin	—	—
Therapy	In adults, quinacrine or metronidazole, in children furazolidone	Metronidazole and diiodohydroxyquin
Comments	Malabsorption is common	Proctoscopy may be necessary for diagnosis

From Appenheimer, A.T: Emergency decisions, p. 21, Sept., 1985.
*Within first few hours of presentation.
†High incidence of false-negatives.

2. Temporal characteristics
   a. Duration of diarrhea: diarrhea of short duration (1-3 days) associated with mild symptoms is usually of viral etiology (Table 13-8); diarrhea lasting longer than 3 weeks is unlikely to be bacterial
   b. Time of day: nocturnal diarrhea is common with diabetic neuropathy
   c. Relationship to meals
      (1) Sudden onset within hours after a particular meal: consider diarrhea secondary to toxins *(Staphylococcus aureus,* toxigenic *E. coli, Clostridium perfringens, Bacillus cereus, Vibrio parahaemoliticus)*
      (2) Diarrhea secondary to *Salmonella, Shigella, Campylobacter* and *Yersinia* has a longer incubation period
   d. Related to stress: consider "functional" diarrhea

Table 13-8   Clues to two common viral diarrheas

	Organism	
	Rotavirus	Norwalk Agent
Population	Usually infants 6-24 mo	Older children, adults
Stool volume	Moderate to large	Moderate to large
Stool consistency	Watery	Watery
Blood	—	—
Fecal WBCs	3%	3%
Vomiting	Common	+
Fever	+	+
Abdominal pain	− (or minor)	+
Rapid diagnosis*	Immunologic	Not useful
Incubation	1-3 days	1-2 days
Duration	2-3 days (vomiting) 4-5 days (diarrhea)	1-2 days
Transmission	Fecal-oral	Fecal-oral
Therapy	Oral rehydration if possible; supportive medical therapy	Supportive medical therapy; bismuth subsalicylate
Comments	Severe dehydration not uncommon	Mild malabsorption

From Appenheimer, A.T.: Emergency decisions, p. 21, Sept. 1985.
*Within first few hours of presentation.

3. Diet
   a. Ingestion of foods containing sorbitol or mannitol may cause osmotic diarrhea
   b. Diarrhea following ingestion of dairy food products may be caused by lactose intolerance
   c. Shellfish ingestion: Norwalk agent
   d. Chinese food: *B. cereus*
4. Activities
   a. Long distance runners may experience bloody diarrhea secondary to bowel ischemia
   b. Institutionalized patients have a higher incidence of bacterial and parasitic infections
5. Medications
   a. Almost any drug can cause diarrhea; following is a list of commonly used drugs that may cause diarrhea:
      (1) Magnesium-containing antacids
      (2) Methylxanthines (caffeine, theophylline)
      (3) Laxatives

      (4) Lactulose

      (5) Colchicine

      (6) Quinidine and other antidysrhythmic agents

      (7) Nutritional supplements

   b. Antibiotic—induced pseudomembranous colitis should be suspected in any patient receiving antibiotics: a positive test for *C. difficile* toxin confirms the diagnosis

6. Sexual habits: male homosexuals have a high incidence of bacterial and parasitic intestinal infections (e.g., *Giardia lamblia, Entamoeba histolytica,*[27] *Cryptosporidium, Salmonella, Shigella, Campylobacter*)

7. Relevant medical history
   a. Surgical history (ileal resection, gastrectomy, cholecystectomy)
   b. Abdominal irradiation
   c. Diabetes mellitus
   d. Hyperthyroidism
   e. Watery diarrhea in elderly patient with chronic constipation may be caused by fecal impaction
   f. Immunocompromised host (*Cryptosporidium, Salmonella*)

8. Associated symptoms
   a. Tenderness, fever, weight loss (inflammatory bowel disease)
   b. Abdominal pain and significant weight loss (carcinoma of pancreas or other malignancies)
   c. Weight loss despite good appetite (malabsorption, hyperthyroidism)
   d. Diarrhea and PUD (Zollinger-Ellison's syndrome, gastrinoma)
   e. Flushing and bronchospasm (carcinoid syndrome)

9. Characteristics of the stool (from patient's history)
   a. Large, foul smelling (malabsorption)
   b. Increased mucus (irritable bowel syndrome)
   c. Watery stools (psychosomal disturbances, fecal impaction, IBD, pancreatic cholera [VIP])

Physical exam

1. Rectal fistulas, RLQ abdominal mass (Crohn's disease)
2. Arthritis, iritis, uveitis, erythema nodosum (IBD)
3. Abdominal masses (neoplasms of colon, pancreas, or liver, diverticular abscess [LLQ mass], IBD)
4. Flushing, bronchospasm (carcinoid syndrome)
5. Buccal pigmentation (Peutz-Jegher's syndrome)
6. Increased pigmentation (Addison's disease)
7. Ammoniacal or urinary breath odor (renal failure)
8. Ecchymosis (vitamin K deficiency secondary to malabsorption of fat soluble vitamins)
9. Fever (IBD, infectious diarrhea)
10. Goiter, tremor, tachycardia (hyperthyroidism)
11. Lymphadenopathy (neoplasm, lymphoma, TB)
12. Macroglossia (amyloidosis)

Initial evaluation

1. Lab tests
   a. CBC: markedly increased WBC with "shift to left" may indicate infectious process; decreased hemoglobin/hematocrit may indicate anemia from blood loss

b. Serum electrolytes: decreased potassium from diarrhea, increased sodium from dehydration

c. BUN, creatinine: indicated if physical exam shows evidence of significant dehydration

d. pH: hyperchloremic acidosis may be present

e. Stool sample
   (1) Occult blood (positive in IBD, bowel ischemia, some bacterial infections)
   (2) Löeffler's alkaline methylene blue stain for fecal leukocytes (positive in inflammatory diarrhea caused by *Salmonella, Campylobacter, Yersinia*)
   (3) Bacterial cultures and sensitivity *(Salmonella, Shigella, Campylobacter, Yersinia)*
   (4) Ova and parasites
   (5) *Clostridium difficile* titer to rule out pseudomembranous colitis in patients receiving antibiotics
   (6) Modified Ziehl-Nielsen stain or auramine stain in immunocompromised patients with suspected *Cryptosporidium* infection[13]

2. Procedures
   a. Sigmoidoscopy (without cleansing enema) is indicated in patients with:
      (1) Bloody diarrhea (sigmoidoscopy may reveal neoplasm, inflammatory changes caused by IBD, bacterial agents, or amebiasis)
      (2) Suspected antibiotic-induced pseudomembranous colitis (sigmoidoscopy will show raised, white-yellow exudative plaques adherent to the colonic mucosa)
   b. Abdominal x-rays (flat plate and upright) are indicated in patients with abdominal pain or evidence of obstruction

Initial treatment
1. NPO
2. IV hydration
3. Correct electrolyte abnormalities
4. Discontinue possible causative agents (e.g., antacids containing magnesium)
5. Antiperistaltic agents (loperamide, diphenoxylate) should be used with caution in patients suspected of having IBD or infectious diarrhea
6. If diarrhea persists and a bacterial or parasitic organism is identified, antibiotic therapy should be started:
   a. *Giardia* (quinacrine, metronidazole)
   b. *E. histolytica* (metronidazole, diodohydroxyquin)
   c. *Shigella* (ampicillin, trimethoprim sulfamethoxazole)
   d. *Campylobacter* (erythromycin)
   e. *Clostridium difficile* (vancomycin, metronidazole)[50]
   NOTE: Antibiotics are contraindicated in *Salmonella* infections unless caused by *S. typhosa* or if patient is septic

Evaluation of patient with chronic or recurrent diarrhea
Etiology of chronic diarrhea
1. Drug induced (including laxative abuse)
2. Irritable bowel syndrome
3. Inflammatory bowel disease

4. Lactose intolerance
5. Malabsorptive diseases (e.g., mucosal disease, pancreatic insufficiency, bacterial overgrowth)
6. Parasitic infections (giardiasis, amebiasis)
7. Functional diarrhea
8. Postsurgical (partial gastrectomy, ileal resection, cholecystectomy)
9. Endocrine disturbances
   a. Diabetes mellitus
   b. Hyperthyroidism
   c. Addison's disease
   d. Gastrinoma (Zollinger-Ellison's syndrome)
   e. Vipoma (pancreatic cholera)
   f. Carcinoid tumors (serotonin)
   g. Medullary carcinoma of thyroid (calcitonin)
10. Pelvic irradiation
11. Colonic carcinoma (e.g., villous adenoma)

Diagnosis
1. History, physical exam, and initial lab evaluation are the same as for new onset diarrhea

---

Lab Differentiation of Secretory and Osmotic Diarrhea

Obtain 24-hour stool collection and measure:
1. Volume (normal = <250 ml/day): if the volume is increased, make patient NPO and observe effect on diarrhea:
    a. Persistence of high volume diarrhea indicates secretory diarrhea
    b. Decreased diarrhea indicates osmotic diarrhea
2. pH >5.5 indicates carbohydrate malabsorption (osmotic diarrhea)
3. Osmolality (normal = <290 mOsm): >290 mOsm indicates osmotic diarrhea
4. Electrolytes (sodium, potassium): there are 2 methods to differentiate osmotic from secretory diarrhea based on the stool electrolyte values:
    a. Multiply sum of sodium + potassium by 2 and compare to stool osmolality

    $2 (Na + K)$ = measured stool osmolality indicates secretory diarrhea

    $2 (Na + K)$ < measured stool osmolality indicates osmotic diarrhea
    b. Calculate osmotic gap (OG): $O.G. = 290 - 2 (Na + K)$
       (1) >20 indicates osmotic diarrhea
       (2) <20 indicates secretory diarrhea

If all the above lab tests indicate malabsorption, additional work-up for malabsorption should proceed as indicated in section 13.5.

2. Additional lab evaluation
   a. Examine stool for presence of fat droplets (use Sudan III stain) and meat fibers, their presence indicates malabsorption
   b. If CBC shows macrocytic anemia, then obtain vitamin B_{12} and RBC folate levels to rule out megaloblastic anemia secondary to malabsorption
   c. Sodium hydroxide test for laxative derived phenolphtalein should be done in patients suspected of laxative abuse
   d. If Sudan stain is suggestive of malabsorption, additional lab exams indicative of malabsorption are: decreased serum albumin, serum carotene, serum cholesterol, serum calcium, and serum PO_4, and increased prothrombin time
   e. Define mechanism of diarrhea
      (1) Secretory diarrhea results from impaired absorption or excessive intestinal secretion of electrolytes (fecal fluid contains large amounts of electrolytes); following is a list of common causes of secretory diarrhea:
         (a) Enteric infections
         (b) Neoplasms of exocrine pancreas (VIP, GIP, secretin, glucagon)
         (c) Bile salt enteropathy
         (d) Villous adenoma
         (e) Inflammatory bowel disease
         (f) Carcinoid tumor
         (g) Celiac sprue
      (2) Osmotic diarrhea results from impaired water absorption secondary to osmotic effect of nonabsorbable intraluminal molecules; following is a list of common causes of osmotic diarrhea:
         (a) Lactose and other disaccharide deficiencies
         (b) Drug induced (lactulose, sorbitol, sodium sulfate, antacids)
         (c) Postsurgical (gastrojejunostomy, vagotomy and pyloroplasty, intestinal resection)

13.5 MALABSORPTION SYNDROME

Definition

Malabsorption syndrome is defined as impaired intestinal absorption manifested by steatorrhea and various nutritional deficiencies.

Etiology

1. Pancreatic exocrine insufficiency
   a. Chronic pancreatitis
   b. Pancreatic resection
   c. Pancreatic carcinoma
   d. Cystic fibrosis
2. Mucosal absorptive defect
   a. Gluten-induced enteropathy (celiac disease)
   b. Tropical spruce
   c. Whipple's disease
   d. Intestinal lymphangiectasia (lymphatic obstruction is also present)
   e. Lymphoma (lymphatic obstruction is also present)

    f. Amyloidosis
    g. Scleroderma
    h. Crohn's disease
    i. Intestinal resection (inadequate absorptive surface)
3. Bacterial proliferation in small bowel
    a. Afferent loop stasis (Billroth II subtotal gastrectomy)
    b. Blind loops, fistulas, strictures, multiple diverticula
    c. Diabetic neuropathy, hypothyroidism, vagotomy, and other causes of motor abnormalities
4. Other
    a. Endocrine and metabolic disorders (hyperthyroidism, carcinoid, vipoma, gastrinoma)
    b. Drugs (neomycin, cholestyramine)
    c. Liver disease, *Giardia* infection, disaccharide deficiency, abetalipoproteinemias

Signs and symptoms

1. Steatorrhea: foul-smelling, bulky, greasy stools
2. Diarrhea: often preceded by abdominal cramps
3. Malnutrition, weight loss
4. Excessive gas and bloating
5. Edema secondary to hypoalbuminemia
6. Generalized weakness, fatigue secondary to anemia (iron, folate, vitamin B_{12} deficiencies)
7. Neuropathy secondary to malabsorption of vitamin B group
8. Pathologic fractures secondary to decreased calcium and vitamin D
9. Purpura secondary to vitamin K deficiency

Lab results

1. Decreased serum albumin, serum carotene, and serum cholesterol
2. Decreased serum calcium and serum phosphorus
3. Increased prothrombin time
4. Decreased hemoglobin/hematocrit, increased MCV, decreased vitamin B_{12}, folate, and serum iron

Diagnostic studies

1. An x-ray of the small bowel is useful in the initial evaluation of malabsorption. The classic finding in malabsorption is a nonspecific segmentation of barium in the small bowel (moulage sign). A small bowel series can also detect intestinal fistulas, multiple diverticuli, motility problems, and other contributing factors to bacterial overgrowth.
2. Bentiromide test:[51] bentiromide is a synthetic peptide attached to PABA. Chemotrypsin separates benteromide from PABA and a by-product of the latter is excreted in the urine as arylamine. Decreased arylamine urinary excretion following ingestion of bentiromide is suggestive of pancreatic insufficiency (chemotrypsin deficiency).
3. Serum trypsin-like immunoreactivity test shows decreased immunoreactivity in pancreatic insufficiency.

The diagnosis of pancreatic insufficiency can be confirmed by adding pancreatic extract preparations (e.g., pancrease) to the patient's meals. A repeat

72-hour stool examination for fat (on an 80 g fat/day diet) will demonstrate increased fat absorption.

Treatment

The therapeutic approach varies with the etiology of the malabsorption.
1. Pancreatic insufficiency is treated by adding pancreatic extract and sodium bicarbonate to the patient's diet
2. Intestinal bacterial overgrowth is treated with broad-spectrum antibiotics (tetracycline, ampicillin) and surgical repair of strictures or other lesions causing stasis
3. In mucosal abnormalities, treat the specific disorder (e.g., antibiotic therapy for Whipple's disease; gluten-free diet [no wheat, barley, or oat grain] in patients with celiac disease)

Additional lab evaluation (Fig. 13-2)

1. Examine stool for fat droplets (use Sudan III stain) and meat fibers; their presence indicates malabsorption
2. Quantitate the degree of steatorrhea with a 72-hour fecal fat measurement on a diet of 80 g fat/day
   a. Normal excretion is 6 g fat/24 hours (>95% absorption)
   b. Excretion of more than 6 g fat/day indicates malabsorption
3. Perform a D-xylose absorption test to determine if the malabsorption is due to a mucosal lesion; a 5-hour urine xylose excretion less than 4.5 g following ingestion of 25 g of D-xylose indicates mucosal disease or bacterial overgrowth
4. Further define the mucosal lesion with a small bowel biopsy (PO)
   a. Following is a list of mucosal abnormalities identifiable with small bowel biopsy.
      (1) Celiac and tropical sprue
      (2) Whipple's disease
      (3) Lymphoma
      (4) Intestinal parasites
      (5) Amyloidosis
      (6) Eosinophilic gastroenteritis
      (7) Other: intestinal lymphangiectasia, abetalipoproteinemias, systemic mastocytosis, agammaglobulinemia, collagenous sprue
   b. A jejunal aspirate should be obtained at the time of biopsy and examined for the presence of intestinal parasites (*Giardia*)
5. Useful tests in suspected bacterial overgrowth are:
   a. 24-hour urine collection for Indican (by-product of the action of intestinal bacteria on tryptophan); increased 24-hour Indican excretion is suggestive of bacterial overgrowth
   b. Carbon-14 xylose breath test
   c. Shilling test demonstrating vitamin B_{12} malabsorption with subsequent correction after tetracycline or ampicillin administration
6. If the D-xylose absorption test is normal, pancreatic insufficiency should be suspected
7. Secretin test is useful to document pancreatic insufficiency
   a. Under fluoroscopic guidance, a tube is placed in the second part of the duodenum and pancreatic secretions are collected

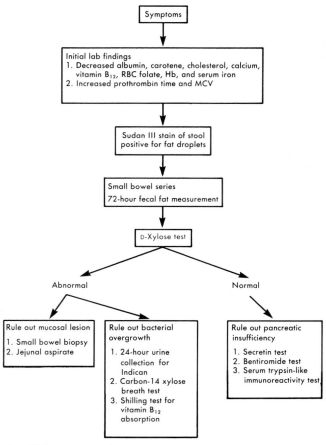

Figure 13-2
Diagnostic approach to malabsorption.

b. The patient is then given an IV dose of secretin (pancreatic secret-agogue) and pancreatic secretions are again measured

c. Pancreatic exocrine deficiency is proven by a decreased total pancreatic fluid output and decreased bicarbonate secretion

d. This test is very sensitive and specific for pancreatic insufficiency, but it is invasive and requires excellent patient cooperation

POLYPOSIS SYNDROMES

Definition

Polyposis is a hereditary syndrome characterized by multiple colonic adenomas and is further subdivided by the presence or absence of extracolonic signs.[26]

Clinical importance

The identification of colonic adenomatous polyps is extremely important because there is evidence that adenomatous tissue can transform into colorectal cancer.[24] The chance of a polyp becoming cancerous depends on:

1. The histologic type: villous adenoma carries the highest malignant potential; incidence of malignant degeneration can be found in up to 60% of villous adenomas at the time of diagnosis
2. Size of the polyp: 1-2 cm polyps have a 5%-10% incidence of malignancy; the malignant potential increases to 10%-40% for polyps larger than 2 cm

Characteristics and classification

Table 13-9 compares the characteristics of the various types of polyps. Table 13-10 describes the major inherited gastrointestinal polyposis syndromes. The risk of colon cancer varies with each polyposis syndrome. It is very high in patients with Gardner's syndrome and Turcot's syndrome, and in familial polyposis it approaches nearly 100% by the age of 40.

Identification and treatment

Patients with polyposis syndromes should be regularly examined for colon carcinoma, beginning in the second decade of life. The exams should consist of a biannual fecal occult blood test, an annual sigmoidoscopy, and colonoscopy every 1 to 3 years (depending on the age of the patient). Asymptomatic carriers of the familial polyposis genotype can be identified by the presence of increased levels of ornithine decarboxylase in biopsy specimens of colonic mucosa.[25] Surgical treatment varies from total colectomy and ileostomy to subtotal colectomy with regular rectal exams. The latter is preferred by the majority of patients because it enables them to have normal bowel movements. However, the rate of carcinoma recurring in the rectal stump is extremely high and many surgeons prefer total colectomy.

13.7   CARCINOMA OF THE COLON

Risk factors

1. Hereditary polyposis syndromes
   a. Familial polyposis (high risk)
   b. Gardner's syndrome (high risk)
   c. Turcot's syndrome (high risk)
   d. Peutz-Jeghers' syndrome (low-moderate risk)
2. Inflammatory bowel disease (predominantly ulcerative colitis)
3. Family history of "cancer family syndrome"
4. Heredofamilial breast cancer and colon carcinoma
5. History of previous colorectal carcinoma

Text continued on p. 241.

Table 13-9 Comparison of polyp types

	Juvenile	Peutz-Jeghers	Hyperplastic	Hyperplastic Adenomatous	Adenomatous
Size (cm)	0.1 to 3.0	0.1 to 3.0	Range from several microscopic crypts to 0.5	0.3 to 3.0+	Unicryptal to 100+
Sessile	±	±	+	+	+
Pedunculated	+	+	±*	+	+
Gland architecture	Disorganized	Disorganized	Organized	Organized	Tubular, villous, mixed
Smooth muscle	None	Present	None	None	May be splayed into polyp
Cell type	Mature colonic epithelial cells	Mature colonic epithelial cells	Immature cells at base of cysts, hypermature cells at surface	Tends to be uniform	Tends to be uniform at any level
Gland lumen	Tends to be straight; if regenerated, tends to be branched	Tends to be straight, tubular	Serrated, particularly in upper crypt	Serrated	Straight tubular
Pseudoinvasion	±	+	–	? Probably will be encountered in the future	+

Secretory activity	Present, inspissated, normal thickness, goblet cells	Present, normal thickness, goblet cells	Hypermature goblet with distended cytoplasm	Variable, tends to be decreased, no distended goblet	Variable, usually
Surface lumen collagen table	Normal	Normal	Thickened	Thinner than normal	Thinner than normal
Mitoses	Normal	Normal	−	±	+
Nuclei	Inconspicuous vesicular, basal	Inconspicuous vesicular, basal	Inconspicuous vesicular/basal base, hyperchromatic, crowded	Crowded, elongated hyperchromatic, often significant dysplasia	Crowded, elongated hyperchromatic, often dysplasia
Relation to cancer	±	±	−	+	+
Polyposis syndrome	+	+	−	?	+

From Fenoglio-Preiser, C.M., and Hutter, R.V.P.: CA 35(6):338, 1985.

KEY: +, Present; −, absent; ±, sometimes present.

*Pedunculated lesions have been described, but the figures suggest that they are mixed hyperplastic adenomatous polyps.

Table 13-10 Mutiple polyposis syndromes

Location	FP	GS	TS	JPC	CCS	GJP	PJS	CD
Esophagus	–	–	–	–	+	+	–	+
Small intestine	+	+	–	–	++	++	+++	+
Colon-rectum	+++	+++	+++	+	+++	+++	++	+
Nose	–	–	–	–	–	–	+	
Bronchi	–	–	–	–	–	–	+	
Urinary system	–	–	–	–	–	–	+	
Polyp type	A	A	A	J	J	J	H	H
Present at birth	±	±	±	+	+	+	+	+
Extraintestinal manifestations	None	Epidermoid cysts Fibromas Dental abnormalities Osteomas Lymphoid polyps Gastric manifestations Abdominal desmoids Retroperitoneal fibrosis Thyroid, adrenal carcinoma Duodenal carcinoma	Medulloblastoma Glioblastoma Ependymoma Cancer of thyroid				Gonadal stromal tumors Mucocutaneous pigmentation Endocervical lesions	Congenital anomalies Thyroid tumors Breast hypertrophy

From Fenoglio-Preiser, C.M., and Hutter, R.V.P.: CA 35(6):339, 1985.

KEY: FP, Familial polyposis; GS, Gardner's syndrome; TS, Turcot's syndrome; CD, Cowden's disease; JPC, juvenile polyposis coli; CCS, Cronkhite-Canada's syndrome; GJP, generalized juvenile polyposis; PJS, Peutz-Jeghers' syndrome; A, adenomatous polyp; J, juvenile polyp; H, hamartomatous polyp.

6. First-degree relatives with colorectal carcinoma
7. Age over 40
8. Possible dietary factors (high fat or meat diet, beer drinking, reduced vegetable consumption)

Distribution

1. 70%-75%
   a. Rectosigmoid and rectum (30%-33%)
   b. Descending colon (40%-42%)
2. 25%-30%
   a. Transverse colon (10%-13%)
   b. Cecum and ascending colon (25%-30%)
3. 50% of rectal cancers are within reach of the examiner's finger
4. 50% of colon cancers are within reach of the sigmoidoscope

Clinical presentation

Initially vague and nonspecific (weight loss, anorexia, malaise). It is useful to divide colon cancer symptoms into those commonly associated with the right colon and those commonly associated with the left colon since the clinical presentation varies with the location of the carcinoma.

1. Right colon
   a. Anemia (iron deficiency secondary to chronic blood loss)
   b. Dull, vague, uncharacteristic abdominal pain may be present or patient may be completely asymptomatic
   c. Rectal bleeding is often missed because blood is admixed with feces
   d. Obstruction is unusual because of large lumen
2. Left colon
   a. Change in bowel habits (constipation, diarrhea, tenesmus, pencil-thin stools)
   b. Rectal bleeding (bright red blood coating the surface of the stool)
   c. Intestinal obstruction is frequent because of small lumen

Physical exam

a. May be completely unremarkable
b. Digital rectal exam can detect approximately 50% of rectal cancers
c. Palpable abdominal masses indicate metastases or complications of colorectal carcinoma (abscess, intussusception, volvulus)
d. Abdominal distention and tenderness are suggestive of colonic obstruction
e. Hepatomegaly is indicative of hepatic metastases

Staging and prognosis (Table 13-11)

Diagnosis

Early identification of patients with surgically curable disease (Duke's A,B) is necessary since survival is directly related to the stage of the carcinoma at the time of diagnosis (see Table 13-11). The following are suggested screening intervals for colorectal cancer in the general population:

1. Yearly digital rectal exam starting at age 40-50
2. Fecal occult blood testing with guaiac-impregnated test cards
   a. Should be done yearly starting at age 40-50
   b. Test six specimens, two from each of three consecutive bowel movements

c. Patients should be instructed to avoid red meat, vitamin C, and high peroxidase foods (e.g., horseradish, turnips) during the testing period to avoid false positives
d. Women should not be tested during or immediately following a menstrual period (false positives)
e. Aspirin and nonsteroidal antiinflammatory drugs (NSAID) should be avoided during testing (occult blood from UGI bleed)
f. Refer to Fig. 13-3 for evaluation of patients with positive fecal occult blood

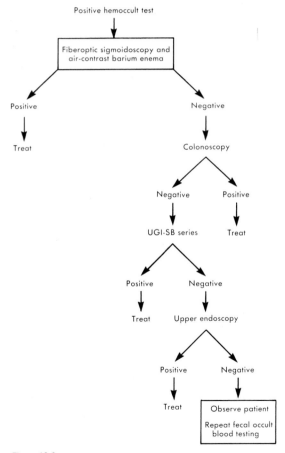

Figure 13-3
Evaluation of asymptomatic patients with positive fecal occult blood.

Table 13-11   Staging of colon cancer: Duke's classification (modified)

Stage	Tumor Involvement	Approximate 5-Year Survival
A	Confined to mucosa	80%
B_1	Confined to muscularis	66%
B_2	Penetrates the muscularis	50%-54%
C_1	Confined to bowel wall	30%-43%
C_2	Penetrates the bowel wall	15%-22%
D	Distant metastases	0-14%

3. Proctosigmoidoscopy: recommended in all individuals over the age of 40; if negative for 2 consecutive years, repeat every 3-5 years

Therapy

1. Surgical resection
2. Radiation therapy is a useful adjunct for rectal and anal carcinoma
3. Results of adjuvant chemotherapy (5-fluorouracil, hydroxyurea, methyl-CCNU) have generally been disappointing

Role of carcinoembryonic antigen (CEA)[16]

1. CEA should not be used as a screening test for colorectal cancer since it can be elevated in many other conditions (smoking, IBD, alcoholic liver disease)

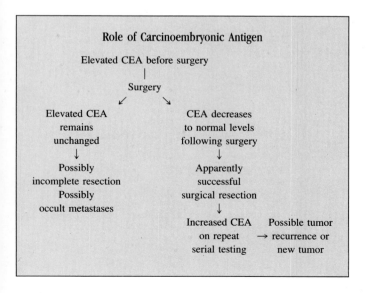

Role of Carcinoembryonic Antigen

Elevated CEA before surgery

Surgery

Elevated CEA remains unchanged → Possibly incomplete resection / Possibly occult metastases

CEA decreases to normal levels following surgery → Apparently successful surgical resection → Increased CEA on repeat serial testing → Possible tumor recurrence or new tumor

2. A normal CEA level does not exclude the diagnosis of colorectal cancer
3. A baseline CEA level is indicated in all patients with colorectal cancer since it can be used postoperatively as a measure of completeness of tumor resection or to monitor tumor recurrence (see the boxed material on p. 243)

13.8   DIVERTICULAR DISEASE

Definition
Colonic diverticula are herniations of mucosa and submucosa through the muscularis. They are generally found along the colon's mesenteric border at the site where the vasa recta penetrate the muscle wall (anatomic weak point).

Characteristics
1. More common in elderly patients (increased incidence with old age)
2. Found most commonly in sigmoid colon (area of highest intraluminal pressure)
3. Increased incidence in western nations is believed to be secondary to low intake of dietary fiber, which results in lessened fecal bulk, narrowing of colonic lumen, increased intraluminal pressure, and evagination of colonic mucosa and submucosa through anatomically weak areas

Clinical manifestations[2]
1. Diverticulosis: asymptomatic presence of multiple colonic diverticula
   a. Physical exam is generally normal
   b. Usually discovered as an incidental finding on barium enema
   c. No specific treatment
2. Painful diverticular disease: caused by distortion of the colonic lumen secondary to muscular hypertrophy
   a. Usual complaint is LLQ pain, often relieved by defecation
   b. Constipation is common; it often alternates with diarrhea
   c. Distinguished from diverticulitis by absence of fever, leukocytosis, or other evidence of peritoneal inflammation
   d. Barium enema will demonstrate multiple diverticula and muscle spasm ("saw-tooth" appearance of the lumen)
   e. Treatment consists of high-fiber diet; bulk laxatives (e.g., psyllium preparations) are helpful in most patients
3. Diverticulitis: inflammatory process or localized perforation of diverticulum
   a. Main clinical features are fever and LLQ pain
   b. Digital rectal exam reveals muscle spasm, guarding, rebound and significant tenderness
   c. Lab results reveal leukocytosis and left shift
   d. Diagnosis can be confirmed by barium enema (pericolonic mass, fistula, or stricture formation); barium enema can be hazardous and should not be performed in the acute stage because it may produce free perforation

   e. A CT scan can also be used to diagnose actue diverticulitis; typical findings are evidence of inflammation outside the bowel wall, fistulas, or abscess formation
   f. Treatment of diverticulitis consists of
      (1) IV antibiotics
         (a) Ampicillin (to cover enterococcus) in mild diverticulitis
         (b) In moderate to severe diverticulitis, gram-negative aerobes and bacteroides fragilis should be aggressively covered (possible antibiotic choices are cefoxitin, or an aminoglycoside plus clindamycin or metronidazole)
      (2) Liquid diet and stool softener for mild disease; bowel rest for moderate to severe disease
      (3) Surgical treatment consists of resection of involved area and reanastomosis (if feasible), otherwise a diverting colostomy is performed and reanastomosis performed when the infection has been controlled; surgery should be considered in patients with:
         (a) Repeated episodes of diverticulitis
         (b) Poor response to full medical therapy
         (c) Abscess or fistula formation
         (d) Obstruction
         (e) Peritonitis
         (f) Immunocompromised patients[37]
4. Hemorrhage: 70% of diverticular bleeding occurs in the right colon[1]
   a. Bleeding is painless and stops spontaneously in the majority of patients; it is usually caused by erosion of a blood vessel by a fecalith present within the diverticular sac
   b. Medical therapy consists of blood replacement and correction of volume and any clotting abnormalities
   c. The bleeding site can be identified by:
      (1) Arteriography if the bleeding is faster than 1 ml/minute; advantages of arteriography are the possible infusion of vasopression directly into the artery supplying the bleeding vessel[3] or selective arterial embolization[17]
      (2) Technetium-99m sulfur colloid
      (3) Technetium-99m labeled RBC
      (4) Emergent colonoscopy after rapid cleansing of the colon with a nonabsorbable solution ingested by the patient or instilled into the stomach via nasogastric tube
   d. Surgical resection is necessary if bleeding does not stop spontaneously after administration of four to five units of packed RBC or recurs with severity within few days[20]

| 13.9 | ACUTE PANCREATITIS

Etiology
1. In more than 90% of all cases:
   a. Biliary tract disease
   b. Alcohol
2. Drugs (thiazides, azathioprine, furosemide, sulfonamides, corticosteroids, tetracycline, estrogens, valproic acid)

3. Abdominal trauma
4. Surgery
5. ERCP
6. Infections (predominantly viral infections)
7. Peptic ulcer (penetrating duodenal ulcer)
8. Pancreas divisum
9. Idiopathic
10. Pregnancy
11. Vascular (vasculitis, ischemia)
12. Hyperlipoproteinemias (types I, IV, V)
13. Hypercalcemia
14. Pancreatic carcinoma (primary or metastatic)
15. Renal failure
16. Hereditary pancreatitis
17. Other: scorpion bite, obstruction at ampullar region (neoplasm, duodenal diverticula, Crohn's disease), hypotensive shock

Diagnosis

History
1. History of alcohol abuse or recent abdominal trauma
2. Patient taking drugs that may cause pancreatitis
3. Any associated illnesses
   a. Cholelithiasis: possible impacted stone or passage of stone
   b. PUD: possible posterior penetrating ulcer
   c. Hyperlipoproteinemias, renal failure, and hypercalcemia all have an increased incidence of pancreatitis
4. History of recurrent abdominal pains
   a. Pancreatitis usually manifests with boring abdominal pain located in the epigastrium
      (1) The pain may be localized or radiate to back and RUQ
      (2) Partial relief is at times obtained by sitting forward
   b. Patients with pancreas divisum often have recurrent abdominal pain following ingestion of small amounts of alcohol

Differential diagnosis
1. PUD
2. Acute cholecystitis, biliary colic
3. High intestinal obstruction
4. Early acute appendicitis
5. Mesenteric vascular obstruction
6. DKA
7. Pneumonia
8. MI
9. Renal colic
10. Ruptured aortic aneurysm

Physical exam
1. Epigastric tenderness and guarding
2. Hypoactive bowel sounds (secondary to ileus)
3. Tachycardia, shock (secondary to decreased intravascular volume)
4. Confusion (secondary to metabolic disturbances)
5. Fever
6. Tachycardia, decreased breath sounds (atelectasis, pleural effusions, ARDS)
7. Abdominal mass

8. Jaundice (secondary to obstruction or compression of biliary tract)
9. Ascites (secondary to tear in pancreatic duct, leaking pseudocyst)
10. Palpable abdominal mass (pseudocyst, phlegmon, abscess, carcinoma)
11. Evidence of hypocalcemia (Chvosteck's sign, Trousseau's sign)
12. Evidence of intraabdominal bleeding (hemorrhagic pancreatitis)
    a. Bluish discoloration around the umbilicus (Cullen's sign)
    b. Bluish discoloration involving the flanks (Grey-Turner's sign)
13. Tender subcutaneous nodules (caused by subcutaneous fat necrosis)

Lab results
1. Pancreatic enzymes
   a. Amylase
      (1) Increased serum amylase: usually elevated in the inital 3-5 days of acute pancreatitis; normal serum amylase levels may be found in acute pancreatitis in:
         (a) Patients presenting 3-5 days after onset of symptoms
         (b) Hyperlipemia (will mask elevated amylase)
         (c) Up to 31% of cases of acute alcoholic pancreatitis[47]
         Note: Serum amylase is not specific for pancreatitis and may be elevated in other illnesses (salivary gland dysfunction, mesenteric infarction, diabetic ketoacidosis)
      (2) Isoamylase determination:[22] separation of pancreatic and salivary isoenzyme components of amylase is helpful in excluding occasional cases of salivary hyperamylasemia
      (3) Urinary amylase determinations
         (a) To diagnose acute pancreatitis in patients with lipemic serum
         (b) To rule out elevated serum amylase secondary to macro-amylasemia
   b. Serum lipase levels are elevated in acute pancreatitis and the elevation is less transient than serum amylase; concomitant evaluation of serum amylase and lipase increases the diagnostic accuracy of acute pancreatitis[36]
   c. Elevated serum trypsin levels are diagnostic of pancreatitis (in absence of renal failure); measurement is made by radioimmunoassay (this test is not readily available in most labs)
2. Additional lab tests
   a. CBC
      (1) WBC: an increase may indicate sepsis or abscess
      (2) Hematocrit: initially increased secondary to hemoconcentration; decreased hematocrit may indicate hemorrhage or hemolysis (DIC)
   b. BUN: usually increased secondary to dehydration or renal impairment caused by pancreatitis
   c. Serum glucose: elevation in a previously normal patient correlates with the degree of pancreatic malfunction
   d. Liver profile
      (1) SGOT and LDH: increased secondary to tissue necrosis
      (2) Bilirubin and alkaline phosphatase: increased secondary to common bile duct obstruction

  e. Serum calcium: decreased secondary to saponification, precipitation, and decreased PTH response

  f. ABG
   (1) PaO_2: decreased secondary to ARDS, atelectasis, or pleural effusion
   (2) pH: decreased secondary to lactic acidosis, respiratory acidosis and renal insufficiency

  g. Serum electrolytes
   (1) Potassium is increased secondary to acidosis or renal insufficiency
   (2) Sodium is increased because of dehydration

Radiographic evaluation of suspected acute pancreatitis

1. Abdominal plain film may reveal
 a. Localized ileus (sentinel loop)
 b. Pancreatic calcifications
 c. Blurring of left psoas shadow
 d. Dilatation of transverse colon
 e. Calcified gallstones
2. Chest x-ray may reveal
 a. Elevation of one or both diaphragms
 b. Pleural effusion(s)
 c. Basilar infiltrates
 d. Plate-like atelectasis
3. Abdominal ultrasonography is useful in detecting gallstones and pancreatic pseudocysts; its major limitation is the presence of distended bowel loops overlying the pancreas
4. Computed tomography (CT) is superior to ultrasonography in identifying pancreatitis and defining its extent,[33,45] and it also plays a role in diagnosing pseudocysts (they appear as well-defined areas surrounded by a high-density capsule[32]); GI fistulation or infection of a pseudocyst can also be identified by the presence of gas within the pseudocyst[34]

Endoscopic retrograde cholangiopancreatography (ERCP)

Generally accepted indications for ERCP in pancreatitis are:[38]
1. Recurrent pancreatitis of unknown etiology
2. Preoperative planning in patients with chronic pancreatitis
3. Suspicion of pseudocyst not detected by sonography or CT scanning
NOTE: ERCP should not be performed during acute stage of disease

Determination of prognosis

When the illness is mild and self-limited with edema as the predominant inflammatory response, mortality is usually less than 5%.[6] Ranson et al.[39] have identified "early objective criteria" (see the boxed material on p. 249) that permit early identification of the risk of major complications or death from acute pancreatitis. The mortality varies with the numbers of risk factors present:
1. Less than three risk factors: mortality is approximately 1%
2. Three to four risk factors: 15% mortality
3. Five to six risk factors: 40% mortality
4. More than seven risk factors: mortality approaches 100%

Treatment

General measures

1. Maintain adequate intravascular volume with vigorous IV hydration
2. NPO until the patient is clinically improved, stable, and hungry
3. Nasogastric suction is useful in severe pancreatitis to decompress the abdomen and decrease vomiting
4. Control pain: all analgesics may effect the sphincter of Oddi; meperidine (Demerol) is preferred because it produces less constriction of the sphincter
5. Correct metabolic abnormalities: e.g., replace calcium and magnesium if necessary

Specific measures

1. Peritoneal lavage: there is continuing debate about the usefulness of peritoneal lavage in early alcohol-related acute pancreatitis with ascites; early studies showed a definite benefit,[48] but a recent study[30] demonstrated that peritoneal lavage did not significantly alter mortality or morbidity
2. IV antibiotics: should not be used prophylactically; their use is justified if the patient has evidence of septicemia, pancreatic abscess, or pancreatitis secondary to biliary calculi
   Appropriate antibiotic therapy should cover:
   a. *Bacteroides fragilis* and other anaerobes (cefoxitin, metronidazole, or clindamycin, plus aminoglycoside)
   b. Enterococcus (ampicillin)
3. Surgical therapy has a limited role in acute pancreatitis
   a. Gallstone-induced pancreatitis: cholecystectomy is indicated as soon as the acute pancreatitis subsides[40]
   b. Perforated peptic ulcer
   c. Excision or drainage of necrotic or infected foci

Prognostic Signs in Acute Pancreatitis

At Admission or Diagnosis

Age >55 years (70 for gallstones)
White blood cell count >16,000/cu mm
Blood glucose >200 mg/dL
Serum lactic dehydrogenase >350 IU/L
Serum glutamic-oxaloacetic transaminase >250 IU

During Initial 48 Hours

Hematocrit fall >10%
Blood urea nitrogen rise > 5 mg/dL
Serum calcium level <8 mg/dL
Arterial oxygen pressure <60 mmHg
Base deficit >4 mEq/L
Estimated fluid sequestration >6,000 mL

From Ranson, J.H.C.: Am. J. Gastroenterol. 77:633, 1982.

4. Identification and treatment of complications
   a. Pseudocyst[7]
      (1) Definition: round or spheroid collection of fluid, tissue, pancreatic enzymes, and blood; it is distinct from adjacent structures
      (2) Diagnosis: CT scan or sonography
      (3) Therapy: CT scan or ultrasound-guided percutaneous drainage, (with a pigtail catheter left in place for continuous drainage) has been used by some,[21] but the recurrence rate is high; the conservative approach is to reevaluate the pseudocyst (with CT scan or sonography) after 6-7 weeks and surgically drain it if the pseudocyst has not decreased in size (pseudocysts ≥ 5 cm in diameter have an increased incidence of perforation, hemorrhage, or infection)
   b. Phlegmon
      (1) It represents pancreatic edema
      (2) Diagnosis: CT scan or sonography
      (3) Treatment: general supportive measures; it usually resolves spontaneously
   c. Pancreatic abscess
      (1) Diagnosis: CT scan demonstrates presence of air bubbles in the retroperitoneum[15]; cultures of fluid obtained from percutaneous aspiration usually identify the bacterial organism
      (2) Therapy: surgical drainage and IV antibiotics
   d. Pancreatic ascites
      (1) Etiology: usually caused by leaking pseudocyst or tear in pancreatic duct; increased incidence is seen in pancreatitis secondary to trauma or alcohol
      (2) Diagnosis: paracentesis reveals very high amylase and lipase levels in the pancreatic fluid; ERCP may demonstrate the lesion (e.g., ductal rupture)
      (3) Treatment: surgical correction
   e. GI bleeding: caused by alcoholic gastritis, bleeding varices (secondary to cirrhosis or portal vein thrombosis following inflammation of tail of the pancreas), stress ulceration, or disseminated intravascular coagulation (DIC)
   f. Renal failure: caused by hypovolemia resulting in oliguria or anuria, cortical or tubular necrosis (shock, DIC), or thrombosis of renal artery or vein
   g. Hypoxemia: caused by ARDS, pleural effusion(s), or atelectasis

---

| 13.10 | **ACUTE VIRAL HEPATITIS**

Etiology

Acute viral hepatitis may be caused by any of the following (Table 13-12):
1. Hepatitis A virus (HAV)
2. Hepatitis B virus (HBV)
3. Hepatitis non-A, non-B viruses (NANB)
4. Delta agent (needs HBV for replication)

Table 13-12 Selected features of four causes of viral hepatitis

	Type A Hepatitis	Type B Hepatitis	Non-A, Non-B Hepatitis	Delta Hepatitis
Virus	27 nm, RNA	42 nm, DNA	No specific confirmable virus	35 nm, RNA core:delta Ag surface:HgsAg
Antigens	HA Ag	HBsAg, HBcAg, HBeAg	Not identifiable by assay	Delta Ag
Antibodies	Anti-HAV	Anti-HBs, anti-HBc, anti-HBe	Not identifiable by assay	Anti-delta
Spread	Fecal-oral	Parenteral	Parenteral	Parenteral
Mean incubation (range)	30 days (15 to 45)	75 days (40 to 180)	50 days (15 to 150)	40 days (30 to 50)
Onset	Abrupt	Insidious	Insidious	Often abrupt
Severity of acute bout	Usually mild	Often severe	Often mild	Often severe
Jaundice	50%	33%	20%	Unknown
Chronicity	None	5% to 10%	20% to 40%	Unknown
Recovery	99%	85% to 90%	Variable	Unknown
Mortality	0.1%	1% to 3%	1% to 2%	Unknown
Treatment	Supportive	Supportive	Supportive	Supportive
Prophylaxis	ISG	HBIG, hepatitis B vaccine	?ISG	Unknown

From Sass, M. A., and Cianflocco, A. J.: Resident & Staff Physician, **PC**: 19, 1985.

Table 13-13   Hepatitis nomenclature

Abbreviation	Term	Comments
Hepatitis A		
HAV	Hepatitis A virus	Etiologic agent of "infectious" hepatitis; a picornavirus; single serotype
Anti-HAV	Antibody to HAV	Detectable at onset of symptoms; lifetime persistence
IgM anti-HAV	IgM class antibody to HAV	Indicates recent infection with hepatitis A; positive up to 4-6 months after infection
Hepatitis B		
HBV	Hepatitis B virus	Etiologic agent of "serum" or "long-incubation" hepatitis; also known as Dane particle
HBsAg	Hepatitis B surface antigen	Surface antigen(s) of HBV detectable in large quantity in serum; several subtypes identified
HBeAg	Hepatitis B e antigen	Soluble antigen; correlates with HBV replication, high titer HBV in serum, and infectivity of serum
HBcAg	Hepatitis B core antigen	No commercial test available
Anti-HBs	Antibody to HBsAg	Indicates past infection with and immunity to HBV, passive antibody from HBIG, or immune response from HBV vaccine
Anti-HBe	Antibody to HBeAg	Presence in serum of HBsAg carrier suggests lower titer of HBV
Anti-HBc	Antibody to HBcAg	Indicates past infection with HBV at some undefined time
IgM anti-HBc	IgM class antibody to HBcAg	Indicates recent infection with HBV; positive for 4-6 months after infection

Delta Hepatitis

δ virus	Delta virus	Etiologic agent of delta hepatitis; may only cause infection in presence of HBV
δ-Ag	Delta antigen	Detectable in early acute delta infection
Anti-δ	Antibody to delta antigen	Indicates past or present infection with delta virus

Non-A Non-B Hepatitis

NANB	Non-A, non-B hepatitis	Diagnosis of exclusion
		At least two candidate viruses; epidemiology parallels that of hepatitis B

Epidemic Non-A, Non-B Hepatitis

Epidemic NANB	Epidemic non-A, non-B hepatitis	Causes large epidemics in Asia, North Africa; fecal-oral or waterborne

Immune Globulins

IG	Immune globulin (previously ISG, immune serum globulin, or gamma globulin)	Contains antibodies to HAV, low titer antibodies to HBV
HBIG	Hepatitis B immune globulin	Contains high titer antibodies to HBV

Reproduced from the Immunization Practices Advisory Committee, Centers for Disease Control; Atlanta, Ga., Ann. Intern. Med. **103**:391, 1985.

Table 13-14 Interpretation of hepatitis profiles

IgM Anti-HAV	HBsAg	IgM Anti-HBc	Anti-HBs	HBeAg	Anti-HBe	Interpretation
-	-	-	-	-	-	Clinical acute hepatitis may be caused by non-A, non-B hepatitis, other viral infection, or liver toxin
+	-	-	-	-	-	Acute type A hepatitis
-	+	-	-	+	-	Late incubation period or early acute type B hepatitis
-	+	+	-	+	-	Acute type B hepatitis with persistent viral replication (HBsAg+) and high degree of infectivity (HBeAg+)
-	+	+	-	-	+	Acute type B hepatitis with favorable prognosis for resolution (seroconversion of HBeAg to anti-HBe)
-	-	+	-	-	-/+	Acute infection nearly resolved (core window)
-	-	+/-	+	-	-/+	Convalescent phase of type B hepatitis with recovery and immunity
-	-	-	+	-	-	Past type B hepatitis long before with recovery and immunity, passive transfer of antibody (HBIG), or hepatitis-B vaccine

From Sass, M.A., and Cianflocco, A.J.: Resident & Staff Physician, **PC**:33, 1985.

Diagnostic criteria

1. History
   a. Blood transfusions: non-A, non-B hepatitis; hepatitis B (now rare since testing of blood for HBV)
   b. IV drug abuse: hepatitis B; non-A, non-B hepatitis
   c. Travel history to underdeveloped countries: hepatitis A
   d. Ingestion of raw shellfish: hepatitis A
   e. Contact with children attending a day care center: hepatitis A
   f. Exposure to others with hepatitis: hepatitis A
   g. History of hepatitis B: delta hepatitis
   h. Homosexuals: all types of hepatitis
2. Clinical manifestations
   a. Anorexia, nausea, vomiting
   b. Generalized malaise, fever, myalgias
   c. Loss of taste for cigarettes and food
   d. Diarrhea, abdominal pain
   e. Dark urine, light colored stool
   f. Pruritus
   g. Patient may be asymptomatic
3. Physical exam
   a. Jaundice
   b. Tender hepatomegaly
   c. Splenomegaly in 20% of cases
   d. Posterior cervical adenopathy (rare)
   e. Rash (rare)
   f. Arthritis (rare)
   g. Physical exam may be normal
4. Lab results
   a. Liver profile
      (1) Greatly increased ALT (SGPT), and AST (SGOT)
      (2) Increased bilirubin (both direct and indirect)
      (3) Normal or minimally elevated alkaline phosphatase
   b. Prothrombin time (PT), glucose are usually normal; increased PT or decreased glucose indicate severe liver damage
   c. Serologic tests: the nomenclature of the various serologic tests for infectious hepatitis is described in Table 13-13; Table 13-14 summarizes the interpretation of these serologic tests

Diagnoses[42]

1. Acute hepatitis A is diagnosed by
   a. Detection of HAAg (IgM) in patient's serum
   b. Fourfold rise in total serum anti-HAAg (IgM and IgG) in samples drawn 2-4 weeks apart (controversial)
2. Acute hepatitis B is diagnosed by
   a. Detection of HBs Ag or
   b. Anti-HBc
      (1) Anti-HBc (IgM): acute infection
      (2) Anti-HBc (IgG): acute infection is present only if there is a fourfold rise in this titer

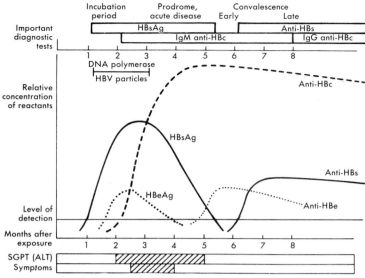

Figure 13-4
Serologic and clinical patterns observed during acute HBV infection. *SGPT,* Serum glutamic pyruvic transaminase; *ALT,* alanine aminotransferase. Patients who do not resolve the hepatitis B infection (chronic carrier state) will demonstrate persistance of HBsAg and will not have an elevation of anti-HBs. Reproduced from Hollinger, F.B., and Dienstag, J.L.: Lennette, E.H., Balows, A., Hausler, W.J., Jr., and Shadomy, H.J., (editors): Manual of clinical microbiology, ed. 4, Washington, D.C., 1985, American Society for Microbiology.

     (3) Anti-HBc is particularly useful as a serologic marker of acute hepatitis during the ''core antibody window'' period when both HBsAg and anti-HBs may be negative (Fig. 13-4)
  3. Non-A, non-B hepatitis: there is no specific serologic test available; diagnosis is made by excluding HAV, HBV, drugs, and other infectious agents (Epstein-Barr virus, CMV)
  4. Delta hepatitis: is diagnosed by the presence of delta antigen or antibody to delta antigen in the patient's serum

Treatment

1. General measures
  a. Avoid strenuous activity and ingestion of excessive amounts of hepatotoxic agents (e.g., alcohol)

Table 13-15 Recommendation for hepatitis B prophylaxis after percutaneous exposure

| | Exposed Person | |
Source	Unvaccinated	Vaccinated
HBsAg positive	One dose of HBIG* immediately Initiate hepatitis B vaccine series†	Test exposed person for anti-HBs If inadequate antibody (<10 sample ratio units by RIA or negative by EIA), give one dose of HBIG* immediately plus hepatitis B vaccine booster dose
Known source High risk of being HBsAg positive	Initiate hepatitis B vaccine series† Test source for HBsAg; if positive, give one dose of HBIG* immediately	Test source for HBsAg only if exposed person is vaccine nonresponder; if source is HBsAg positive, give one dose of HBIG* immediately plus hepatitis B vaccine booster dose
Low risk of being HBsAg positive	Initiate hepatitis B vaccine series	Nothing required
Unknown source	Initiate hepatitis B vaccine series	Nothing required

Reproduced from Immunization Practices Advisory Committee, Centers for Disease Control, Atlanta, Ga., Ann. Intern. Med. **103**:391, 1985.

*One dose of hepatitis B immune globulin (HBIG) is 0.06 ml/kg body weight IM. HBsAg, hepatitis B surface antigen; RIA, radioimmunoassay; EIA, enzyme immunoassay; anti-HBsAg.

†Hepatitis B vaccine series is 20 µg IM for adults, 10 µg IM for infants or children under 10 years of age. The first dose is given within 1 week of exposure, and the second and third doses, 1 and 6 months later, respectively.

  b. Correct any metabolic abnormalities (hypoglycemia, elevated PT)
  c. Protein and salt restriction is indicated only if hepatic failure is present
  d. Hospitalization is rarely indicated
2. Postexposure prophylaxis
  a. Hepatitis A: single IM dose of 0.02 ml/kg of immune globulin (IG) as soon as possible
  b. Hepatitis B: refer to Table 13-15 for recommendations after percutaneous exposure
  c. Prophylaxis after sexual exposure to a HBsAg positive partner is essentially the same as after percutaneous exposure

LIVER FAILURE

Etiology

1. Alcohol abuse
2. Primary or metastatic neoplasm
3. Obstruction of common bile duct (stone, stricture, pancreatitis, neoplasm)
4. Drugs (e.g., acetaminophen, isoniazid, methyldopa)
5. Hepatotoxins (e.g., carbon tetrachloride, phosphorus, halothane, beryllium, vinyl chloride)
6. Hepatic congestion (e.g., CHF, constrictive pericarditis, tricuspid insufficiency, thrombosis of hepatic veins, obstruction to inferior vena cava)
7. Primary biliary cirrhosis
8. Hemochromatosis
9. Chronic active hepatitis
10. Acute fulminant viral hepatitis
11. Reye's syndrome
12. Wilson's disease
13. Primary sclerosing cholangitis
14. α-1-antitrypsin deficiency
15. Infiltrative diseases (amyloidosis, glycogen-storage diseases, hemochromatosis)
16. Hepatic cysts or abcesses
17. Shock and sepsis
18. Other: parasitic infections (amebiasis, shistosomiasis, toxoplasmosis, leptospirosis), brucellosis and other bacterial infections, idiopathic portal hypertension, congenital hepatic fibrosis, heat stroke, systemic mastocytosis

Diagnosis

History

1. Alcohol abuse: alcoholic liver disease
2. Onset of symptoms following drug ingestion (drug-induced liver failure)
   a. Cholestasis: oral contraceptives, anabolic steroids, and chlorpromazine
   b. Hepatic necrosis: INH, acetaminophen, and methyldopa
   c. Hepatic granulomas: allopurinol, quinidine, and sulfonamides
   d. Fatty metamorphosis: methotrexate and tetracycline
3. Onset of symptoms following exposure to toxins (toxin-induced liver failure)
4. Hypoglycemia and increased PT in patient with acute viral hepatitis (fulminant hepatitis)
5. History of hepatitis B (chronic active hepatitis, primary hepatic neoplasm)
6. Anorexia, severe weight loss, weakness (metastic neoplasm)
7. History of inflammatory bowel disease (primary sclerosing cholangitis)
8. History of pruritus, hyperlipoproteinemia, and xanthomas in middle-aged or elderly female (primary biliary cirrhosis)
9. History of Raynaud's phenomenon, sclerodactyly and telangiectasia—CRST syndrome
10. Impotence, diabetes, hyperpigmentation (hemochromatosis)

11. Liver failure and neurologic disturbances (Wilson's disease—hepatolenticular degeneration)
12. Family history of ''liver disease'' (hemochromatosis—positive family history in 25% of patients; α-1-antitrypsin deficiency)
13. Postoperative jaundice (consider halothane toxicity)
14. History of recurrent episodes of RUQ pain (biliary tract disease)

Physical exam: Possible findings in patients with liver failure
1. Skin: jaundice, palmar erythema (alcohol abuse), spider angiomata, ecchymosis (thrombocytopenia or prothrombin deficiency), dilated superficial periumbilical veins (caput medusae), increased pigmentation (hemochromatosis), xanthomas (primary biliary cirrhosis), needle tracks (viral hepatitis)
2. Lymph nodes: lymphadenopathy (neoplasm, infectious process)
3. Eyes: Kayser-Fleischer rings (corneal copper deposition seen in Wilson's disease), scleral icterus
4. Breath: fetor hepaticus (musty odor of breath and urine found in severe hepatic failure)
5. Chest: gynecomastia in men indicates chronic liver disease
6. Abdomen
    a. Tender hepatomegaly (acute viral hepatitis, congestive hepatomegaly)
    b. Rock-hard liver (neoplasm—primary or metastatic)
    c. Small nodular liver (cirrhosis)
    d. Palpable, nontender gallbladder—Courvoisier's sign (neoplastic extrahepatic biliary obstruction)
    e. Tender gallbladder and positive Murphy's sign (cholecystitis)
    f. Palpable spleen (hepatitis, cirrhosis)
    g. Venous hum auscultated over periumbilical veins (portal hypertension)
    h. Hepatic bruit and friction rub (hepatoma)
    i. Ascites (portal hypertension, hypoalbuminemia)
7. Rectal exam
    a. Hemorrhoids (portal hypertension)
    b. Guaiac-positive stool (alcoholic gastritis, bleeding esophageal varices, PUD)
8. Genitalia: testicular atrophy in males (chronic liver disease)
9. Extremities
    a. Pedal edema (hypoalbuminemia, right-sided heart failure)
    b. Finger clubbing
10. Neurologic
    a. Flapping tremor—asterixis (hepatic encephalopathy)
    b. Choreoathetosis, dysarthria (Wilson's disease)

Lab results
1. Routine admission lab results
    a. Decreased hemoglobin/hematocrit (consider GI bleeding)
    b. Increased MCV (caused by RBC membrane abnormalities)
    c. Increased BUN, creatinine (prerenal azotemia, hepatorenal syndrome); the BUN can also be ''normal'' or low if the patient has severely diminished liver function
    d. Decreased sodium (dilutional hyponatremia)

    e. Decreased potassium (caused by secondary aldosteronism or urinary losses)

    f. Decreased glucose in a patient with liver disease indicates severe liver damage

2. Liver function studies[11]

    a. Serum transaminases

        (1) Alcoholic hepatitis and cirrhosis: mild elevations of ALT (SGPT) and AST (SGOT), usually to <500 IU; AST > ALT (ratio >2:1)

        (2) Extrahepatic obstruction: moderate elevations of ALT and AST to levels <500 IU

        (3) Viral, toxic, or ischemic hepatitis: extreme elevations (>500 IU) of ALT and AST

        (4) Transaminases may be normal despite significant liver disease in patients with jejuno-ileal bypass operations, hemochromatosis, or following methotrexate injection

    b. Alkaline phosphatase is present in liver, bone, placenta, and intestine

        (1) Significant elevations of hepatic alkaline phosphastase occur in extrahepatic obstruction (calculi, strictures, neoplasm, pancreatitis), primary biliary cirrhosis, and primary sclerosing cholangitis

        (2) Measure serum 5'-nucleotidase to determine if the elevated alkaline phosphatase is of hepatic origin; elevation of 5'-nucleotidase implies a hepatobiliary source

        (3) A more reliable method to identify hepatic alkaline phosphatase is to fractionate the elevated alkaline phosphatase with polyarylamide gel electrophoresis

    c. Serum lactate dehydrogenase (LDH) of hepatic origin (LDH$_5$ by isoenzyme determination) is significantly elevated in metastatic disease to the liver; lesser elevations are seen with hepatitis, cirrhosis, extrahepatic obstruction, and congestive hepatomegaly

    d. Serum γ glutamyl transpeptidase (GTT) is elevated in alcoholic liver disease

    e. Serum bilirubin: refer to p. 83 for a listing of the major causes of conjugated and unconjugated hyperbilirubinemia

    f. Urine bilirubin: present in hepatitis, hepatocellular jaundice, and biliary obstruction

    g. Serum albumin: significant liver disease results in hypoalbuminemia; refer to Chapter 20 for a listing of the various causes of low serum albumin

    h. Prothrombin time (PT): an elevated PT in patients with liver disease indicates severe liver damage and poor prognosis

3. Additional tests

    a. Presence of hepatitis B surface antigen (HBsAg) implies acute or chronic active hepatitis B

    b. Presence of antimitochondrial antibody is suggestive of primary biliary cirrhosis or chronic active hepatitis

    c. Elevated serum copper, decreased serum ceruloplasmin is diagnostic of Wilson's disease

    d. Protein immunoelectrophoresis

        (1) Decreased α-1-globulins (α-1 antitrypsin deficiency)

        (2) Increased IgA (alcoholic cirrhosis)

        (3) Increased IgM (primary biliary cirrhosis)

        (4) Increased IgG (chronic active hepatitis)

e. Coagulation factors
  (1) Advanced liver disease will result in deficiency of vitamin K–dependent factors (II, VII, IX, X) and factor V
  (2) Factor VIII is not affected by liver disease, and so it can be used to distinguish DIC from coagulopathy of liver disease
f. An elevated level of serum ferritin is suggestive of hemochromatosis
g. An elevated blood ammonia level is suggestive of hepatocellular dysfunction; serial values can be useful in following patients with hepatic encephalopathy, however, there is poor correlation between blood ammonia level and the degree of hepatic encephalopathy[12]
h. Serum cholesterol is elevated in cholestatic disorders

Radiographic evaluation
1. Ultrasonography is the procedure of choice for detection of gallstones
2. CT scanning is useful for
  a. Detecting hepatic mass lesions
  b. Assessing hepatic fat content[10]
  c. Identifying idiopathic hemochromatosis[18]
  d. Early diagnosis of Budd-Chiari's syndrome[5]
3. Technetium-99m sulfur colloid scanning is useful for
  a. Diagnosing hepatic cirrhosis: there is a shift of colloid uptake to the spleen and vertebral bone marrow
  b. Identifying hepatic adenoma: "cold" defect is noted
  c. Diagnosing of Budd-Chiari's syndrome[49]: there is increased uptake by caudate lobe
4. Endoscopic retrograde cholangiopancreatography (ERCP) is the procedure of choice for diagnosing periampullary carcinoma and common duct stones[44]; it is also used for diagnosing primary sclerosing cholangitis
5. Percutaneous transhepatic cholangiography (PTC) is useful when evaluating patients with cholestatic jaundice and dilated intrahepatic ducts by ultrasonography[35]
6. Percutaneous liver biopsy is useful in
  a. Evaluating hepatic filling defects
  b. Undiagnosed hepatocellar disease/hepatomegaly
  c. Persistently abnormal liver function tests
  d. Diagnosing: hemochromatosis, primary biliary cirrhosis, Wilson disease, glycogen storage diseases, chronic hepatitis, type I Crigler-Najjar's syndrome, infiltrative diseases (sarcoidosis, tuberculosis), and primary or secondary carcinoma

Therapy
Eliminate cause of liver failure
1. Correct any mechanical obstruction to bile flow (e.g., calculi, strictures)
2. Avoid any hepatotoxins (e.g., ethanol)
3. Therapy of underlying cardiovascular disorders in patients with cardiac cirrhosis
4. Remove excess body iron with phlebotomy and desferroxamine in patients with hemochromatosis
5. Remove copper deposits with D-penicillamine in patients with Wilson's disease

Treatment of complications
1. Ascites
   a. Bed rest
   b. Fluid (1000-1500 ml/day) and salt restriction (250-500 mg/day)
   c. Spironolactone (aldosterone antagonist)
   d. Furosemide may be added if ascites is refractory to above measures
   e. Therapeutic paracentesis may be necessary if there is respiratory embarassment caused by massive ascites
   f. Peritoneovenous shunt (Le Veen shunt) may be indicated in some patients with intractable ascites
2. Esophagogastric varices: Bleeding is the major cause of death in patients with cirrhosis and hypertension; the following is a step-wise approach to the management of bleeding esophageal varices:
   a. Resuscitation (IV fluids and blood transfusion) and correction of any coagulation abnormalities
   b. IV vasopressin *or*
   c. Emergency endoscopic sclerotherapy
   d. Balloon tamponade
   e. Emergency portacaval or splenorenal shunt if above measures fail to stop the bleeding
   NOTE: Endoscopic sclerotherapy should be undertaken even if bleeding is controlled with vasopressin or balloon tamponade because of the high recurrence rates of variceal hemorrhage when these measures are stopped
3. Hepatic encephalopathy: abnormal mental status occurring in patients with severe impairment of liver function and consequent accumulation of toxic products not metabolized by the liver; management consists of the following:
   a. Identifying and treating precipitating causes (UGI bleeding, hypokalemia, sepsis, alkalosis, increased dietary protein, and acute infections)
   b. Reducing toxic protein metabolites
      (1) Restricting protein intake (30-40 g/day)
      (2) Reducing colonic ammonia production
         (a) Lactulose is a nonabsorbable synthetic disaccharide that acidifies the intestinal lumen; the increase in hydrogen ions facilitates the conversion of ammonia (NH_3) to ammonium (NH_4^+), which is then excreted in the stool; refer to Chapter 21 for dosage of lactulose
         (b) Neomycin is an antibiotic used to lower the concentration of urease-containing bacteria in the intestinal flora, thereby decreasing ammonia production; dosage is 1 g PO q4-6h or given as a 1% retention enema solution (1 g in 100 ml of isotonic saline)
         (c) A combination of lactulose and neomycin can be used when either agent is ineffective alone
   c. Provide adequate calories to prevent protein catabolism
4. Hepatorenal syndrome is usually a lethal complication of severe liver disease. It may occur following vigorous reduction of effective blood volume (e.g., paracentesis, GI bleeding, diuretics) or in the absence of any precipitating events. Diagnosis is suspected when oliguria with concentrated

urine and low urine sodium develop in a patient with severe liver disease. The hepatorenal syndrome must be differentiated from prerenal azotemia since the renal function studies are similar in both conditions (urine sodium <10 mEq/L, U/P osm >1, U/P creatinine >30/1, usually normal renal sediment). Acute tubular necrosis must also be considered as a cause of the renal failure. Urinary sodium excretion will be high and urinary osmolarity will be approximately 300 mOsmol/kg.

References

1 Almy, T.P., and Naitove, A.: Diverticular disease of the colon. In Sleisenger, M.H., and Fordtran, J.S., (editors): Gastrointestinal disease, ed. 3, Philadelphia, 1983, W.B. Saunders Co.

2. Almy, T.P., and Howell, D.A.: Diverticular disease of the colon, N. Eng. J. Med. **302**:324, 1980.

3. Athanosoulis, C.A., et al.: Mesenteric arterial infusions of vasopressin for hemorrhage from colonic diverticulosis, Am. J. Surg. **129**(2):212, 1975.

4. Azad Khan, A.K., et al.: Optimum dose of sulfasalazine for maintenance treatment in ulcerative colitis, Gut, **12**:232, 1980.

5. Baert, A.L., et al.: Early diagnosis of Budd-Chiari syndrome by computed tomography and ultrasonography: report of five cases, Gastroenterol. **84**:587, 1983.

6. Banks, P.A.: Clinical manifestations and treatment of pancreatitis. In Geokas, M.C., (moderator): Acute pancreatitis, Ann. Intern. Med. **103**:86, 1985.

7. Bradley, E.L., III: Pancreatic pseudocysts. In Bradley, E.L. III (editor): Complications of pancreatitis: medical and surgical management, Philadelphia, 1982, W.B. Saunders Co.

8. Brady, P.G.: Endoscopic retrograde cholangiopancreatography, its role in diagnosis and therapy of pancreatitis, Post Grad. Med. **79**:253, 1986.

9. Brandt, L.S., et al.: Metronidazole therapy for perineal Crohn's disease: a follow-up study, Gastroenterol. **83**:383, 1982.

10. Bydder, G., et al.: Accuracy of computed tomography in diagnosis of fatty liver, Br. Med. J. **281**:1042, 1981.

11. Chopra, S., and Griffin, P.H.: Laboratory tests and diagnostic procedures in evaluation of liver disease, Am. J. Med. **79**:221, 1985.

12. Conn, H.O., and Lieberthal, M.M.: Blood ammonia determination. In Conn, H.O., and Lieberthal, M.M., (editors): The hepatic coma syndromes and lactulose, Baltimore 1978, Williams and Wilkins, Co.

13. Current, W.L., et al.: Human cryptosporidiosis in immunocompetent and immunodeficient persons: studies of an outbreak and experimental transmission, N. Engl. J. Med. **308**:1251, 1983.

14. Englert, E., Jr., et al.: Cimetidine, antacid, and hospitalization in the treatment of benign gastric ulcer: a multicenter double blind study, Gastroenterol. **74**:416, 1978.

15. Federle, M.P., and Jeffrey, R.B.: Computed tomography of pancreatic abscesses, A.J.R., **136**:879, 1981.

16. Go, V.L., and Zacheck, N.: The role of tumor markers in the management of cancer, Cancer **50**(suppl):2618, 1982.

17. Goldberger, L.E., and Bookstein, J.J.: Transcatheter embolization for treatment of diverticular hemorrhage, Radiol. **122**(3):613, 1977.

18. Howard, J.M., et al.: Diagnostic efficacy of hepatic computed tomography in the detection of body iron overload, Gastroenterol. **84**:209, 1983.

19. Immunization Practices Advisory Committee, Centers for Disease Control, Atlanta, Ga. Ann Intern. Med. **103**:391, 1985.

20. Johnson, H.C.L., Jr., and Block, M.A.: Diverticular disease, current trends in therapy, Post Grad. Med. **78**(3): 75, 1985.

21. Karlson, K.B., et al.: Percutaneous drainage of pancreatic pseudocysts and abscesses, Radiol **142**:619, 1982.

22. Kolars, J.C., Ellis, C.J., and Levitt, M.D.: Comparison of serum amylase pancreatic isoamylase and lipase in patients with hyperamylasemia, Dig. Dis. Sci. **29**(4): 289, 1984.

23. Korman, M.G., et al.: Ranitidine in duodenal ulcer: incidence of healing and effect of smoking, Dig. Dis. Sci. **27**:712, 1982.

24. Lane, N., et al.: Defining the precursor tissue of ordinary large bowel cancer: implications for cancer prevention. In Lipkin, M., and Good, R.A., (editors): Gastrointestinal tract cancer, New York, 1978. Plenum Press.

25. Luk, G.D., and Baylin, S.B.: Ornithine decarboxylase as a biologic marker in familial colonic polyposis, N. Engl. J. Med. **311**:80, 1984.

26. Lynch, H.T., Rozen, P., and Schuelke, G.S.: Hereditary colon cancer: polyposis and nonpolyposis variants, CA **35**(2): 95;, 1985.

27. McMillan, A., et al.: Amoebiasis in homosexual men, Gut, **25**:356, 1984.

28. Malchow, H., et al.: European cooperative Crohn's disease study: results of drug treatment, Gastroenterol. **86**:249, 1984.

29. Martin, F., et al.: Comparison of the healing capacities of sucralfate and cimetidine in the short-term treatment of duodenal ulcer: a double-blind randomized trial, Gastroenterol. **82**:401, 1982.

30. Mayer, A.D., et al.: Controlled clinical trial of peritoneal lavage for the treatment of severe acute pancreatitis, N. Eng. J. Med. **312**(7):399, 1985.

31. Miller, T.A.: Protective effects of prostaglandins against gastric mucosal damage: current knowledge and proposed mechanism, Am. J. Physiol. **245**:G601, 1983.

32. Moossa, A.R.: Diagnostic tests and procedures in acute pancreatitis, N. Engl. J. Med. **310**:639, 1984.

33. Moossa, A.R.: The impact of computed tomography and ultrasonography on surgical practice, Bull. Am. Coll. Surg. **67**(11):10, 1982.

34. Moossa, A.R.: Pancreatic pseudocysts in children, J.R. Coll. Surg. Edinb. **19**:149, 1974.

35. Mueller, P.R., Van Sonnenberg, E., and Simeone, J.F.: Fine needle transphepatic cholangiography: indications and usefulness, Ann. Intern. Med. **95**:567-572, 1982.

36. Orda, R., et al.: Lipase turbidimetric assay and acute pancreatitis Dig. Dis. Sci. **29**(4):294, 1984.

37. Perkins, J.D., et al.: Acute diverticulitis: comparison of treatment in immunocompromised patients, Am. J. Surg. **148**(6):745, 1984.

38. Present, D.H., et al.: Treatment of Crohn's disease with 6-mercaptopurine: a long-term, randomized, double-blind study, N. Engl. J. Med. **302**:981, 1980.

39. Ranson, J.H.C.: Etiological and prognostic factors in human pancreatitis, Am. J. Gastroenterol. **77**(9):633, 1982.

40. Ranson, J.H.: The timing of biliary surgery in acute pancreatitis, Ann. Surg. **189**(5):654, 1979.

41. Richardson, C.T.: Pathogenetic factors in peptic ulcer and disease, AM. J. Med. **79**(supp 2C): 1, 1985.

42. Sarver, D.K.: Hepatitis in clinical practice, Post Grad. Med. **79**(4):194, 1986.

43. Schuster, D.P., et al.: Prospective evaluation of risk of upper gastrointestinal bleeding after admission to medical intensive care unit, Am. J. Med. **76**:623, 1984.

44. Siegal, J.H., and Yatto, R.P.: Approach to cholestasis: an update, Arch. Intern. Med. **142**:1897, 1982.

45. Silverstein, W., et al.: Diagnostic imaging of acute pancreatitis: prospective study using CT and sonography, Am. J. Roentgenol. **137**:497, 1981.

46. Sontag, S., et al.: Cimetidine, cigarette smoking, and recurrence of duodenal ulcer, N. Engl. J. Med. **311**:690, 1984.

47. Spechler, S.J., et al.: Prevalence of normal serum amylase levels in patients with acute alcoholic pancreatitis, Dig. Dis. Sci. **28**(10):865, 1983.

48. Stone, H.H., and Fabian T.C.: Peritoneal dialysis in the treatment of acute alcoholic pancreatitis, Surg. Gynecol. Obstet. **150**:878, 1980.

49. Tavill, A.S., and Wood, E.J.: The Budd-Chiari syndrome: correlation between hepatic scintigraphy and the clinical, radiological and pathological findings in nineteen cases of hepatic venous outflow obstruction, Gastroenterol. **68**:509, 1975.
50. Teasley, D.G., et al.: Prospective randomised trial of metronidazole versus vancomycin for *Clostridium difficile* associated diarrhea and colitis, Lancet, **2**:1043, 1983.
51. Toskes, P.P.: Bentiromide as a test of exocrine pancreatic function in adult patients with pancreatic exocrine insufficiency: determination of appropriate dose and urinary collection interval, Gastroenterol. **85**:565, 1983.

14 Hematology/Oncology

APPROACH TO THE PATIENT WITH ANEMIA
Robert Burd

Definition

Anemia can be defined as a reduction below normal limits in the amount of hemoglobin or in the volume of red blood cells (hematocrit) in a sample of peripheral venous blood.

Etiology

1. Decreased red blood cell production
   a. Deficiency of hematinic agents
   b. Bone marrow failure
2. Increased red cell destruction or loss
   a. Hemolysis
   b. Hemorrhage

Diagnosis

1. History
   a. Family and ethnic history: inquire about thalassemia, sickle cell anemia, splenectomy, cholelithiasis at an early age
   b. Drug and toxic exposures: e.g., chloramphenicol, methyldopa, quinidine, benzene, alkylating agents
   c. Obstetric and menstrual history: "excessive" menstrual bleeding is a frequent cause of iron deficiency anemia in menstruating women
   d. External blood loss: GI, GU (inquire about melena, hematochezia, hematuria)
   e. Dietary habits: poor dietary habits and alcohol intake may result in folic acid deficiency
   f. Rapidity of onset: gradual onset is suggestive of bone marrow failure or chronic blood loss whereas sudden onset of symptoms suggests hemolysis or acute hemorrhage
2. Physical exam
   a. General appearance: evaluate nutritional status
   b. Vital signs: hypotension, tachycardia (acute blood loss)
   c. Skin: pallor, jaundice (hemolysis), petechiae, purpura (thrombocytopenia)
   d. Mouth: glossitis (pernicious anemia, iron deficiency anemia)

e. Heart: listen for flow murmurs, prosthetic valves (increased RBC destruction)

f. Abdomen: splenomegaly (hemolysis, neoplasms, infiltrative disorders)

g. Rectum: examine stool for occult (or gross) blood

h. Lymph nodes: infiltrative lesions, infections

3. Lab results

  a. Hemoglobin and hematocrit: provide a guide to diagnosis and severity of anemia; refer to Chapter 20 for normal values

  b. Reticulocyte count

    (1) Should be performed before any therapeutic maneuvers

    (2) Reticulocyte counts below 1% indicate inadequate marrow production, counts above 4% indicate RBC destruction or acute blood loss

    (3) However, the reticulocyte count should be considered in light of the degree of anemia and the shift of reticulocytes to the peripheral blood

    (4) Further laboratory studies should be determined by the result of the reticulocyte count

  c. Mean corpuscular volume (MCV): classifies anemia as normocytic, microcytic, or macrocytic

    (1) Normocytic anemia: the reticulocyte count is used to distinguish excess destruction or blood loss (high reticulocyte count) from decreased production (low reticulocyte count); a bone marrow examination is of value in distinguishing the following causes of normocytic anemia and reticulocytopenia

      (a) Marrow hypoplasia (toxic drugs, radiation)

      (b) RBC aplasia

      (c) Marrow infiltration (myeloma, lymphoma, leukemia)

      (d) Myelofibrosis

      (e) Renal insufficiency

    (2) Microcytic anemia

      (a) Iron deficiency is the most common cause

      (b) Thalassemia, anemia of chronic disease, and sex-linked sideroblastic anemia are other causes

      (c) The peripheral smear and RBC count may help distinguish iron deficiency from thalassemia minor (relatively high RBC count and basophilic stippling in the latter)

      (d) Assess iron stores by determining the serum ferritin (or marrow iron stain if ferritin unavailable); if ferritin is low, iron deficiency is proven, but if normal or elevated appropriate work-up for thalassemia (hemoglobin A_2), sideroblastic anemia, and anemia of chronic disease (low serum iron, low TIBC, increased ferritin, decreased reticulocytes) should be obtained

    (3) Macrocytic anemia

      (1) Because reticulocytes have a large diameter, an elevated reticulocyte count will read out as an elevated MCV; if the reticulocyte count is elevated, hemolytic studies (haptoglobin, LDH, indirect bilirubin) are indicated

(b) If hemolysis is confirmed, determine the cause with Coombs' test; other studies (as suggested by RBC morphology) may be indicated

(c) If the reticulocyte count is normal and RBCs are macrocytic, vitamin B_{12} or folate deficiency is possible, therefore RBC folate, serum vitamin B_{12}, and serum folate level should be obtained

(d) The presence of a megaloblastic bone marrow would enhance the diagnosis of vitamin B_{12} or folate deficiency; if the bone marrow exhibits dyserythropoiesis or WBC abnormalities, a myelodysplastic anemia is the cause of the macrocytic anemia

(e) A systematic and logical search, with avoidance of a ''shotgun'' diagnostic or therapeutic approach will yield the correct diagnosis

d. Review peripheral blood smear: red blood cell morphology should be evaluated for:

(1) Size
   (a) normal RBC have a diameter equal to that of the nucleus of a mature lymphocyte
   (b) Macrocytosis indicates megaloblastic anemia, liver disease, or refractory anemia
   (c) Microcytosis is seen with iron deficiency, hemoglobinopathies, and sideroblastic anemia

(2) Shape
   (a) Spherocytes (hereditary spherocytosis, immune, or other hemolytic states)
   (b) Tear drop cells (myeloproliferative diseases, pernicious anemia, thalassemia)
   (c) Helmet cells (microangiopathic hemolysis, severe iron deficiency)
   (d) Sickle cell (Hb SS)

(3) Color
   (a) Hypochromasia (iron deficiency, sideroblastic anemias)
   (b) Hyperchromasia (megaloblastic anemia, spherocytosis)

e. Morphology of WBC and platelets should be noted and any abnormal cells identified; additional abnormalities of diagnostic value that may be present on peripheral smears are the following:

(1) Basophilic stippling: lead poisoning, thalassemia, hemolytic states

(2) Heinz bodies (denatured Hb): unstable hemoglobinopathies, some hemolytic anemias; identification of Heinz bodies requires supravital stain

(3) Howell-Jolly bodies (nuclear fragments): hemolytic and megaloblastic anemias, splenectomy

(4) Cabot ring (nuclear remnants): megaloblastic anemias

(5) Pappenheimer bodies: postsplenectomy, hemolytic, sideroblastic, and megaloblastic anemias

(6) Rouleaux formation: multiple myeloma, Waldenstrom's macroglobulinemia

(7) Presence of parasites: e.g., plasmodium in malaria
(8) Nucleated RBCs: extramedullary hematopoiesis, hypoxia, hemo-lysis
(9) Target cells: hemoglobinopathies, iron deficiency, liver disease

14.2 MICROCYTIC ANEMIA

Etiology

1. Iron deficiency
2. Chronic disease
3. Sideroblastic anemia (sex-linked)
4. Thalassemia

Peripheral blood smear

1. Iron deficiency: microcytic, hypochromic RBCs with a wide area of central pallor
2. Chronic disease: normocytic or microcytic RBCs
3. Sideroblastic anemia: dimorphic population of cells (hypochromic cells and normochromic, normocytic cells); basophilic stippling may also be present
4. Thalassemia: basophilic stippling, target cells, high RBC count

Lab results

1. Serum ferritin: reflects the quantity of stored iron
   a. A low level is diagnostic of iron deficiency
   b. A normal or elevated level does not rule out iron deficiency because ferritin is an acute phase reactant and can be increased in the presence of infection, inflammation, or liver disease
2. A low serum iron and an elevated total iron-binding capacity indicate iron deficiency anemia (Table 14-1)
3. Reticulocyte count: should be viewed in relation to the degree of anemia; a frequently used correction method is the determination of the reticulocyte production index (RPI)[39]

$$RPI = \frac{\dfrac{(\text{Measured Hct/Normal Hct})}{} \times \text{Reticulocyte count}}{\text{Maturation factor}}$$

The maturation factor (MF) equals 1 if the patient's hematocrit is 45. Each 10 point decrease in the patient's hematocrit will increase the maturation factor by 0.5 (e.g., if the patient's hematocrit is 35, the MF is 1.5)
   a. The RPI subdivides anemias into two major classes:
      (1) RPI >3: proliferative anemia (hemolysis, hemorrhage, response to hematinic agents)
      (2) RPI <3: hypoproliferative anemia (marrow failure, iron deficiency, renal failure, endocrinopathies)

Table 14-1 differentiates the causes of microcytic anemias based on the initial lab evaluation.

Table 14-1   Lab differentiation of microcytic anemias

Abnormality	Ferritin	Serum Iron	TIBC
Iron deficiency	↓	↓	↑
Chronic disease	N/ ↑	↓	↓
Sideroblastic anemia	N/ ↑	↑	N
Thalassemia	N/ ↑	↑	N

KEY: N, Normal; ↑ , increased; ↓ , decreased.

Bone marrow exam (if indicated)

1. Iron deficiency
   a. Absent iron stores
   b. Absent sideroblasts
2. Chronic disease
   a. Normal or increased iron stores
   b. Absent or decreased sideroblasts
3. Sideroblastic anemia
   a. Normal or increased iron stores
   b. "Ringed" sideroblasts present
4. Thalassemia
   a. Normal or increased iron stores
   b. Normal or increased sideroblasts

Major causes of microcytic anemia

1. Iron deficiency anemia
   a. Lab results vary with the stage of deficiency
      (1) Absent iron marrow stores and decreased serum ferritin level are the initial abnormalities
      (2) Decreased serum iron and increased TIBC are the next abnormalities
      (3) Hypochromic microcytic anemia is present with significant iron deficiency
   b. Anemia is usually secondary to excessive blood loss (GI, GU); additional causes are iron malabsorption (postgastrectomy) and increased requirements (pregnancy)
   c. If the diagnosis of iron deficiency is made, it is mandatory to try to locate the site of iron loss (see Chapter 13, p. 243)
   d. Treatment consists of ferrous sulfate 325 mg PO tid for at least 6 months
2. Chronic disease states
   a. Anemia is often seen with chronic infection (e.g., TB, endocarditis), chronic inflammation (e.g., rheumatoid arthritis), or neoplasms
   b. It is caused by several mechanisms (e.g., decreased erythrocyte survival, slow iron release from macrophage iron storage pool)[26]
   c. Treatment is aimed at identification and therapy of underlying disease
3. Sideroblastic anemia
   a. It is characterized by ineffective erythropoiesis as a result of enzymatic defects in the mitochondria of RBCs[6]

b. Sideroblastic anemias can be hereditary or acquired (e.g., alcohol induced, idiopathic, drug-induced [INH]); they are also associated with various malignant disorders (e.g., Di Gugliermo's disease) and hemochromatosis[12]

c. Management consists of treatment of underlying disorder; the pyridoxine-responsive benign forms of sideroblastic anemia can be treated with pyridoxine 200 mg/day

2. Thalassemia

a. Hereditary disorders characterized by defective hemoglobin synthesis, broadly classified into α- or β-thalassemias according to the affected globin chain

b. The homozygous state of β-thalassemia (thalassemia major) is characterized by severe anemia and hepatosplenomegaly; patients with heterozygous β-thalassemia (thalassemia trait) have only mild anemia and microcytic indices without any significant clinical manifestations

c. The diagnosis of thalassemia trait is established by hemoglobin electrophoresis (elevation of HbA_2 from normal value of 2.5% to approximately 5% in β-thalassemia, or elevation of HbH in α-thalassemia)

d. The major points in the management of homozygous β-thalassemia are:

   (1) Periodic transfusions to maintain Hb approximately 10 g/dl
   (2) Chelation therapy with deferoxamine mesylate to achieve negative iron balance
   (3) Splenectomy between age 5-10
   (4) Ancillary measures (folic acid, vitamin C)

| 14.3 | NORMOCYTIC ANEMIA

Etiology

1. Hemolysis
2. Aplastic anemia
3. Acute hemorrhage (GI, GU), see Chapter 13, pp. 213-217
4. Renal failure, see Chapter 16
5. Myelophthisis (marrow replacement by fibrosis, tumor, or granulomatous substance)
6. Combined microcytic and macrocytic anemia (e.g, iron and folate deficiency)
7. Endocrine disorders (hypothyroidism, gonadal dysfunction, adrenal insufficiency)
8. Chronic inflammation (connective tissue disorders, infection, cancer)

Peripheral blood smear

1. Hemolysis: the findings vary with the cause of the hemolysis:

   a. Helmet cells, schistocytes: microangiopathic hemolysis
   b. Sickle cells, Howell-Jolly bodies: sickle cell anemia
   c. RBC fragments in a patient with a mechanical heart valve: traumatic hemolysis
   d. Spherocytes: hereditary spherocytosis, autoimmune hemolytic anemias
   e. Spur cells (very irregular borders with thorny projections): hepatic cirrhosis

2. Aplastic anemia: neutropenia, thrombocytopenia (unless pure red cell aplasia is present)
3. Myelophthisis: the peripheral smear shows a leukoerythroblastic picture (normoblasts, granulocyte precursors) caused by premature release from bone marrow

Lab results

1. Reticulocyte count: elevated with RBC destruction (hemolysis), decreased with RBC underproduction (e.g., aplastic anemia, myelophthisis)
2. Coombs' test
   a. Direct: detects the presence of antibody or complement on the surface of RBCs
   b. Indirect: detects the presence of anti-RBC antibodies freely circulating in the patient's serum
3. Lactic dehydrogenase (LDH): frequently elevated in patient with intravascular or extravascular hemolysis
4. Haptoglobin is a serum protein that binds hemoglobin, the hemoglobin-haptoglobin complex is then cleared by the liver; a low or absent haptoglobin indicates intravascular hemolysis
5. Indirect bilirubin: increased in both intravascular and extravascular hemolysis
6. Urine hemosiderin and urine hemoglobin: detected in moderate to severe intravascular hemolysis
7. Chromium-51 red cell survival: expensive and difficult test; it should not be done as part of the initial evaluation of hemolytic anemias
8. Additional studies depend on clinical presentation: BUN, creatinine (to rule out renal failure), and thyroid screening

Bone marrow exam

1. Aplastic anemia: scarcity or absence of erythropoietic and myelopoietic precursor cells; patients with pure red cell aplasia demonstrate only absence of RBC precursors in the marrow
2. Myelophthisis: replacement of normal marrow with fibrosis, granulomata or tumor cells (lymphoma, leukemia, metastatic carcinoma)

Selected causes of normocytic anemia

1. Hemolytic anemia
   a. Classification: see the list on p. 273
   b. Additional evaluation of selected patients with hemolytic anemia includes ANA (to rule out connective tissue diseases) and CT scan of chest and abdomen (to rule out lymphoma)
   c. Patients with suspected PNH (history of voiding brown or red urine upon arising in AM) should be screened with sucrose lysis test (sugar water test) and acidified serum test (Ham test)
   d. Treatment of hemolytic anemias varies with the cause
      (1) Drug induced
         (a) Discontinue drug
         (b) Immunosuppressive treatment with steroids (prednisone 60 mg/day) is indicated in symptomatic patients
         (c) Replace folic acid (folic acid 1 mg PO qd)

(2) Hemolysis secondary to hereditary spherocytosis: splenectomy
(3) Sickle cell anemia
  (a) Improve oxygenation (nasal O_2 to correct hypoxemia)
  (b) Treat any infections
  (c) Maintain adequate hydration (PO or IV)

Classification and Characteristics of Hemolytic Anemias

Acquired
1. Environmental factors
   a. Autoimmune: isohemagglutinins (e.g., transfusion reaction) or autoantibodies (e.g., warm [IgG] or cold [IgM])
      (1) Idiopathic
      (2) Drugs (three major mechanisms)
         (a) Antibody directed against Rh complex (e.g., methyldopa)
         (b) Antibody directed against RBC-drug complex (hapten-induced e.g., penicillin)
         (c) Antibody directed against complex formed by drug and plasma proteins; the drug–plasma protein–Ab complex causes destruction of RBC (innocent bystander [e.g., quinidine])
      (3) Underlying diseases
         (a) Connective tissue diseases (e.g., SLE)
         (b) Non-Hodgkin's lymphoma, CLL
         (c) Infections (e.g., mycoplasma)
   b. Nonimmune mediated
      (1) Microangiopathic (DIC, TTP, hemolytic-uremic syndrome, malignant hypertension)
      (2) Hypersplenism
      (3) Cardiac valve prosthesis
      (4) Giant cavernous hemangiomas
      (5) March hemoglobinuria
      (6) Physical agents (e.g., thermal injury)
      (7) Infections (e.g., malaria, *Clostridium welchii*)
      (8) Drugs (e.g., nitrofurantoin, sulfonamides)
      (9) Chemicals (e.g., heavy metals)
2. Membrane defects
   a. Paroxysmal nocturnal hemoglobinuria (PNH)
   b. Spur-cell anemia (caused by lipid alterations secondary to liver disease)
   c. Wilson's disease

Congenital
1. Defects of cell interior
   a. Hemoglobinopathies (SS disease, thalassemia, Hb SC, CC)
   b. Enzymopathies (e.g., G-6PD deficiency)
2. Membrane defects: hereditary spherocytosis, elliptocytosis

        (d) Pain relief during acute crisis
        (e) Replace folic acid, consider subcutaneous heparin
        (f) Avoid unnecessary transfusions
    (4) Transfusion reaction
        (a) Stop transfusion immediately
        (b) Maintain urine flow greater than 100 ml/hr with adequate hydration plus mannitol and diuretics
        (c) Save suspected unit for analysis
2. Aplastic anemia
    a. Etiology
        (1) Toxins (e.g., benzene)
        (2) Drugs (e.g., alkylating agents, antimetabolites, chloramphenicol, gold compounds)
        (3) Irradiation
        (4) Infections (e.g., non-A, non-B hepatitis)
        (5) Idiopathic
        (6) Inherited (Fanconi's anemia)
        (7) Associated with other disorders (e.g., leukemia, PNH)
    b. Treatment
        (1) Discontinue any offending drugs
        (2) Aggressive treatment and prevention of infections
        (3) Platelet and RBC transfusion prn
        (4) Two methods of immunosuppressive therapy are available
            (a) Antithymocyte globulin (ATG)[14]
            (b) 6-Methylprednisolone[43,29]
            The response to immunosuppressive therapy can be predicted using flow microflurometry[45]
        (5) The use of anabolic androgenic steroids is questionable[15] and is not recommended
        (6) In patients with severe aplastic anemia who have HLA-matched donors, transplanation of allogeneic marrow is the treatment of choice; patients with severe aplastic anemia who have marrow transplants before the onset of transfusion-induced sensitization have an excellent probability of long-term survival and normal life[5]

| 14.4 | MACROCYTIC ANEMIA

Etiology

1. Folate deficiency
2. Vitamin B_{12} deficiency
3. Chronic liver disease (the elevated MCV is multifactorial: ineffective erythropoiesis, hemolysis, acute blood loss)
4. Alcoholism (RBC membrane abnormalities)
5. Hypothyroidism (can also cause a normocytic anemia)
6. Elevated reticulocyte count (each increase in the reticulocyte count by 1% will increase the MCV by approximately 2 fL)
7. Some patients with aplastic or hypoplastic anemia may have macrocytic indices

Peripheral blood smear

Hypersegmented neutrophils (>6 lobes) are present in vitamin B_{12} deficiency.

Lab results[37]

1. Serum vitamin B_{12} level: a low level indicates vitamin B_{12} deficiency; exceptions are falsely low levels seen in patients with severe folate deficiency or falsely high or normal levels when vitamin B_{12} deficiency coincides with severe liver disease or CLL
2. Serum folate, RBC folate: both tests should be ordered because serum folate alone is very labile and does not accurately reflect tissue folate levels, whereas RBC folate is a good indicator of tissue stores but may be reduced in severe cobalamin deficiency
3. Reticulocyte count
4. Thyroid and liver function studies

Bone marrow exam

Examination of the bone marrow will demonstrate megaloblastic erythroid hyperplasia.

Selected causes of macrocytic anemia

1. Folate deficiency
   a. Decreased intake (alcoholism, poor diet)
   b. Increased requirements (hemolysis, pregnancy, dialysis)
   c. Impaired absorption (e.g., sprue, IBD)
   d. Drugs (e.g., phenytoin, methotrexate, ethanol, trimethoprim, antituberculous agents)
   e. Treatment: folic acid 1 mg PO qd
2. Vitamin B_{12} deficiency
   a. Etiology
      (1) Pernicious anemia
      (2) Malabsorption (small bowel disease, pancreatic insufficiency, gastric abnormalities)
      (3) Inadequate dietary intake (rare, usually seen in strict vegetarians)
      (4) Interference with vitamin B_{12} absorption (fish tapeworm, drugs)
   b. Clinical presentation: patients with severe deficiency can present with significant neurologic findings (paresthesias, ataxia, loss of position and vibration senses, memory impairment, depression, dementia)
   c. Diagnostic approach: Shilling test and work-up of malabsorption (see Chapter 13)
   d. Therapy: 1000 μg of vitamin B_{12} (cyanocobalamin) IM every week for 6 weeks followed by 500-1000 μg/month indefinately

| 14.5 |

ACUTE LEUKEMIAS[47]

Definition

Acute leukemia is a disorder characterized by uncontrolled proliferation of abnormal immature white blood cell progenitors. Proliferation of abnormal immature lymphocytes and their progenitors is known as *acute lymphoblastic leukemia (ALL)*. Proliferation of primitive myeloid cells (blasts) is called *acute nonlymphocytic leukemia (ANLL)*. The distinction between the two types has therapeutic and prognostic significance.

Etiology

1. Previous use of antineoplastic agents (e.g., chemotherapy of lymphoma, Hodgkin's disease, ovarian cancer, myeloma)
2. Chromosomal abnormalities (e.g., Down's syndrome [twenty-fold increase in the risk of acute leukemia], C-group trisomy, neurofibromatosis, Klinefelter's syndrome [increased risk of ANLL])
3. Environmental factors (e.g., ionizing radiation)
4. Toxins (e.g., benzene)
5. Drugs (e.g., choramphenicol, phenylbutazone)
6. Others: CML, PNH, polycythemia vera, myelodysplastic syndromes

Classification

The distinction between ALL and ANLL and the classification of the various subtypes is based on the following factors:
1. Cell morphology
   a. Lymphoblasts: very high nucleus/cytoplasm ratio, usually cytoplasmic granules are not present
   b. Myeloblasts: abundant cytoplasm, cytoplasmic granules often present (Auer rods)
2. Histochemical stains
   a. Peroxidase and Sudan black stains: negative in ALL; useful to distinguish nonlymphoid from lymphoid cells
   b. Chloracetate esterase: a pink cytoplasmic reaction identifies granulocytes; useful to distinguish granulocytes from monocytes in patients with ANLL
3. The French-American-British (FAB) cooperative study group has classified ALL into three groups (L-1 to L-3) based on cell size, cytoplasmic appearance, nuclear shape, and chromatin pattern; ANLL is subdivided into six categories (M-1 to M-6) based on the type and percentage of immature cells[22]

Characteristics and clinical presentation

1. ALL is primarily a disease of children (peak incidence between ages 2-10) whereas ANLL usually affects adults (most patients are 30-60 years old)
2. The patients generally come to medical attention because of the effects of the cytopenias:
   a. Anemia manifests with weakness and fatigue
   b. Thrombocytopenia can manifest with bleeding, petechiae, and ecchymoses
   c. Neutropenia can result in fever and infections
3. The peripheral WBC varies from $5000/mm^3$ to $>100,000/mm^3$
4. Occasionally patients may present with neurologic manifestations secondary to meningeal leukemia (usually ALL) or cerebral leukostasis (in ANLL) secondary to very elevated WBC counts ($>150,000/mm^3$)
5. Additional systemic manifestations of acute leukemia are pneumonia (secondary to granulocytopenia), dysphagia (secondary to oropharyngeal candidiasis), GI bleeding (secondary to thrombocytopenia), and acute prostatism (secondary to significant leukemic infiltration of the prostate)

6. Additional lab findings may include: elevated LDH and uric acid levels, decreased fibrinogen, and increased FDP secondary to DIC (more frequent in ANLL)
7. Physical exam may reveal petechiae and purpura (secondary to thrombocytopenia), evidence of infections (e.g., oropharyngeal candidiasis), lymphadenopathy, infiltration (e.g., gingival hypertrophy in patients with acute monocytic leukemia), and hepatosplenomegaly

Treatment[13,24]

1. Emergency treatment is indicated in patients with intracerebral leukostasis; it consists of one or more of the following:
   a. Cranial irradiation
   b. Leukapheresis
   c. Oral hydroxyurea (requires 48-72 hours to significantly lower the circulating blast count)
2. Urate nephropathy can be prevented by lowering uric acid level with allopurinol and urine alkalinization with acetazolamide
3. Infections must be aggressively treated with broad-spectrum antibiotics
   a. Any febrile neutropenic patient must have cultures taken and be promptly treated with IV antibiotics (e.g., mezlocillin or ticarcillin plus an aminoglycoside to provide adequate coverage against gram-negative bacteria)
   b. If evidence of infection persists despite adequate treatment with antibiotics, amphotericin B may be added to provide coverage against fungal infections (*Candida, Aspergillus*)
4. Correct significant thrombocytopenia (platelet counts <20,000/mm^3) with platelet transfusions
5. Bleeding secondary to DIC is treated with heparin
   a. Thrombocytopenia is not a contraindication to heparin therapy in these patients since bleeding from DIC is life-threatening
   b. Concomitant use of heparin and platelet transfusions is indicated in severely thrombocytopenic patients with DIC
6. Induction chemotherapy
   a. Intensive chemotherapy to destroy a significant number of leukemic cells and achieve remission; it usually consists of the following:
      (1) ANLL: cytarabine (Cytosar) and daunorubicin (Cerubidine), with or without 6-thioguanine
      (2) ALL: combination of vincristine (Oncovin), prednisone, L-asparaginase (Elspar), and daunorubicin (Cerubidine)
   b. It usually takes 28-32 days from the start of therapy to achieve remission
   c. The duration of remission is variable; the median duration of remission in an adult with ANLL is 1 year, but up to 50% of patients with ALL remain in remission for 2 or more years
7. Consolidation therapy
   a. It consists of aggressive courses of chemotherapy with or without radiotherapy shortly after complete remission has been obtained; it's purpose is to prolong the remission period or cure
   b. Complications of consolidation therapy are usually secondary to severe bone marrow suppression (anemia, thrombocytopenia, granulocytopenia)

     c. The risk of nonhematopoietic toxicity is also increased (e.g., GI tract ulceration and cardiac toxicity with use of daunorubicin)

  8. Meningeal prophylactic therapy is indicated in patients with ALL
     a. Intrathecal methotrexate is used with or without cranial irradiation
     b. Meningeal prophylaxis in adults with ANLL is controversial because meningeal leukemia is uncommon in these patients

  9. Maintenance therapy
     a. Its goal is to maintain a state of remission
     b. The drugs used and the duration of therapy vary with the type of acute leukemia
        (1) ALL: intermittent therapy for at least 3 years with combination of prednisone, vincristine, methotrexate, and mercaptopurine
        (2) ANLL: therapy is continued for at least 1 year; cytarabine and 6-thioguanine are commonly used

 10. Bone marrow transplantation
     a. Allogeneic
        (1) The marrow from an HLA-matched sibling is transplanted into the patient after complete remission is achieved with chemotherapy
        (2) Because of a higher incidence of graft-versus-host disease with advancing age, allogeneic marrow transplants are usually performed only in patients less than 40 years old
     b. Autologous
        (1) The patient's marrow is harvested after remission is achieved with chemotherapy
        (2) The patient is then irradiated and given high doses of cyclophosphamide to kill any residual leukemic cells
        (3) The previously harvested bone marrow is then returned to the patient; current research is directed at immunologic or chemotherapeutic manipulation of the marrow to destroy any residual leukemic cells before reimplantation

Complications of chemotherapy

The major complication is profound marrow depression with pancytopenia lasting 3-4 weeks. Treatment is aimed at RBC and platelet replacement and aggressive monitoring and treatment of suspected infections. Some investigators have recommended prophylaxis with antifungal and antibacterial agents in patients with acute leukemia who are receiving remission induction treatment.[18] Prophylactic administration of norfloxacin (400 mg PO q12h) in patients with acute leukemia and granulocytopenia may decrease the overall morbidity and frequency of gram-negative infections.[25]

| 14.6 | CHRONIC LEUKEMIA

CHRONIC LYMPHOCYTIC LEUKEMIA[10,21,33]
Definition
Chronic lymphocytic leukemia (CLL) is a lymphoproliferative disorder characterized by proliferation and accumulation of mature-appearing neoplastic lymphocytes.

Lab results

1. Peripheral lymphocytosis (generally $\geq 15,000/dl$) of well-differentiated lymphocytes
2. Monotonous replacement of the bone marrow by small lymphocytes (marrow contains $\geq 30\%$ well-differentiated lymphocytes)
3. Hypogammaglobulinemia and elevated LDH may be present at time of diagnosis
4. Anemia or thrombocytopenia, if present, indicate poor prognosis

Characteristics and clinical manifestations

1. CLL generally occurs in middle-aged and elderly patients (median age is 60 years); male to female ratio is $2:1$
2. The abnormal lymphocytes are B-cells 90% of the time (B-cell monoclonal disorder)
3. Clinical presentation varies with the stage of the disease; many patients are diagnosed on the basis of a CBC obtained following routine physical exam, other patients may come to medical attention because of weakness or fatigue (secondary to anemia) or lymphadenopathy
4. Physical exam reveals lymphadenopathy, splenomegaly, and hepatomegaly in the majority of patients

Staging

Rai and coworkers'[34] have divided CLL into five clinical stages
1. Stage 0 is characterized by lymphocytosis only
2. The coexistence of lymphocytosis and other factors increases the clinical stage
   a. Lymphadenopathy (I)
   b. Splenomegaly/hepatomegaly (II)
   c. Anemia (III)
   d. Thrombocytopenia (IV)

Prognosis

Prognosis is directly related to the clinical stage. For example, the average survival for patients in stage 0 (lymphocytosis alone) is 150 months, whereas for stage IV (lymphocytosis and thrombocytopenia), the average survival is only 19 months.

Treatment

The therapeutic approach varies with the clinical stage and presence or absence of symptoms:

Stage 0:	treatment is not indicated for asymptomatic patients
Stages I and II:	symptomatic patients are treated with chlorambucil; local irradiation therapy can be used for isolated symptomatic lymphadenopathy and for lymph nodes that interfere with vital organ function
Stages III and IV:	treatment consists of chlorambucil chemotherapy with or without prednisone

   a. Cyclophosphamide is used in patients who respond poorly to chlorambucil
   b. Splenic irradiation is useful in selected patients with advanced disease[4]

CHRONIC GRANULOCYTIC LEUKEMIA[10,41]

Definition

Chronic granulocytic leukemia (CGL) is a myeloproliferative disorder characterized by abnormal proliferation and accumulation of immature granulocytes.

Lab results

1. Elevated total leukocyte count (generally $>100,000/mm^3$) with wide spectrum of granulocytic forms
2. Bone marrow demonstrates hypercellularity with granulocytic hyperplasia
3. Philadelphia chromosome (shortening of long arms of chromosome G22, generally secondary to translocation of chromosomal material to the long arms of chromosome C9) is present in over 90% of patients with CGL; its presence is a major prognostic factor because the survival rate of patients with the Philadelphia chromosome is about eight times that of those without it
4. Leukocyte alkaline phosphatase (LAP) is markedly decreased (used to distinguish CGL from other myeloproliferative disorders)
5. Anemia and thrombocytosis are often present
6. Additional lab results are elevated vitamin B_{12} levels (caused by increased transcobalamin I from granulocytes) and elevated blood histamine levels (because of increased basophils)

Characteristics and clinical manifestations

1. CGL usually affects middle-aged patients
2. Common complaints at the time of diagnosis are weakness or discomfort secondary to an enlarged spleen (abdominal discomfort or pain)
3. CGL is characterized by a *chronic phase* lasting months to years, followed by an *accelerated myeloproliferative phase* manifested by poor response to therapy, worsening anemia, or decreased platelet count; this second phase then evolves into a terminal phase *(acute transformation)* characterized by elevated number of blast cells and numerous complications (e.g., sepsis, bleeding)
4. The median survival time from diagnosis of CGL is approximately 45 months; the median duration of the terminal phase is approximately 3 months
5. Physical exam in the chronic phase usually reveals splenomegaly; hepatomegaly is not infrequent, but lymphadenopathy is very unusual and generally indicates the accelerated myeloproliferative phase of the disease

Treatment

The therapeutic approach varies with the clinical phase and the degree of hyperleukocytosis.

1. Symptomatic hyperleukocytosis (e.g., CNS symptoms are treated with leukapheresis and hydroxyurea); allopurinol should also be started to prevent urate nephropathy following rapid lysis of the leukemic cells
2. Cytotoxic chemotherapy usually includes either hydroxyurea or busulfan; the major complications associated with busulfan are its long-term toxic effect (aplasia) and pulmonary fibrosis
3. Severe persistant thrombocytosis may require treatment with thiotepa or melphalan

4. Allogeneic marrow transplantation (following intense chemotherapy and radiotherapy to destroy residual leukemic cells) is the only curative treatment for CGL
   a. It should be considered in young patients (increased survival in patients younger than 30) with compatible siblings
   b. Early transplantation is also very important for patient survival; a recent study demonstrated that the probability of long-term survival for allogeneic graft recipients was 49%-58% for patients in the chronic phase, 15% in the accelerated phase and 14% for patients in the blastic phase[42]

14.7 HODGKIN'S DISEASE[16,32]

Definition
Hodgkin's disease is a malignant disorder of lymphoreticular origin, characterized histologically by the presence of multinucleated giant cells (Reed-Sternberg cells).

Characteristics and clinical manifestations
1. There is a bimodal age distribution (15-34 and over age 50)
2. The patient usually has painless lymphadenopathy, generally involving the cervical region; at times the disease is detected by the presence of mediastinal adenopathy on a routine chest x-ray exam
3. Symptomatic patients usually have the following manifestations:
   a. Fever and night sweats: when the fever has a cyclical pattern (days or weeks of fever alternating with afebrile periods), it is known as Pel-Ebstein fever
   b. Weight loss, generalized malaise
   c. Persistent, dry, nonproductive cough
   d. Pain associated with alcohol ingestion, often secondary to heavy eosinophil infiltration of the tumor sites
   e. Pruritus
   f. Others: superior vena cava syndrome and spinal cord compression are rare presentations
4. Initial lab evaluation generally reveals normochromic, normocytic/microcytic anemia, elevated sedimentation rate, and cutaneous anergy to common skin tests; elevated serum alkaline phosphatase, eosinophilia, lymphocytopenia, mild leukocytosis, and thrombocytosis may also be present

Histopathology
There are four main histologic subtypes, based on the number of lymphocytes and Reed-Sternberg cells and the presence of fibrous tissue: lymphocyte predominance, mixed cellularity, nodular sclerosis, and lymphocyte depletion. Nodular sclerosis is the most common type. Prognosis is generally best for lymphocyte predominance and worst for lymphocyte depletion. However, survival is more directly related to the pathologic and clinical stage rather than the histologic subtype.

Staging

1. The Ann Arbor staging classification[11] (Table 14-2) is commonly used; because of different therapeutic and prognostic implications, stage III has been subdivided into III_1 (involvement of upper abdomen, spleen, splenic and hilar nodes) and III_2 (involvement of lower abdominal nodes)
2. Proper staging requires the following:
   a. Detailed history and physical exam
   b. Surgical biopsy
   c. Lab evaluation (CBC, sedimentation rate, BUN, creatinine, alkaline phosphatase, liver function studies)
   d. Chest x-ray (PA and lateral)
   e. Bilateral bone marrow biopsy
   f. Bipedal lymphangiography
   g. Computed tomography
      (1) Chest: indicated when abnormal findings are noted on chest x-ray
      (2) Abdomen and pelvis: to supplement lymphangiographic findings
   h. Exploratory laparatomy and splenectomy
      (1) Decision to perform staging laparotomy depends on the therapeutic plan
      (2) It is generally recommended for patients with clinical stage I-IIA and I-IIB
      (3) It is valuable in identifying patients who can be treated with radiation alone

Treatment

1. The main therapeutic modalities are radiotherapy and chemotherapy; the indications for each varies with the pathologic stage and other factors
   a. Stages I and II: radiation therapy alone, unless large mediastinal mass is present (mediastinal to thoracic ratio ≥ 1.3); in the latter case, a combination of chemotherapy and radiation therapy is indicated
   b. Stage IIIA: treatment is controversial and varies with the anatomic substage
      (1) III_1A and minimum splenic involvement: radiation therapy alone may be adequate
      (2) III_2 or III_1A with extensive splenic involvement: there is disagreement whether chemotherapy alone or a combination of chemotherapy and radiotherapy is the preferred treatment modality

Table 14-2   Ann Arbor staging classification for Hodgkin's disease

Stage	Definition
I	Limited to one area
II	Involves two or more areas on the same side of the diaphragm
III	Involves two or more areas on both sides of the diaphragm
IV	Disseminated extralymphatic disease

NOTE: A, Asymptomatic; B, symptomatic (fever, sweats, weight loss >10% of body weight); S, splenic involvement; E, extralymphatic site.
From Carbone, P.P., et al.: Cancer Res. 31:1860, 1971.

  c. Stages IIIB and IV: the treatment of choice is chemotherapy with or
   without adjuvant radiotherapy
2. Various regimens can be used for combination chemotherapy; some commonly used regimens are:
  a. MOPP: nitrogen mustard, vincristine, procarbazine, and prednisone
  b. ABVD: doxorubicin (Adriamycin), bleomycin, vinblastine, and DTIC
  c. BCVPP: BCNU, cyclophosphamide, velban, procarbazine, and prednisone
3. Cure rates as high as 75%-80% are now possible with appropriate initial
 therapy

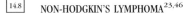

14.8   NON-HODGKIN'S LYMPHOMA[23,46]

Definition

Non-Hodgkin's lymphoma (NHL) is a heterogeneous group of malignancies
of the lymphoreticular system.

Characteristics and clinical manifestations

1. The median age at time of diagnosis is 50
2. Patients often have asymptomatic lymphadenopathy
  a. Involvement of extranodal sites can result in unusual presentations
   (e.g., GI tract involvement can simulate peptic ulcer disease)
  b. Pruritus is rare
  c. Fever, night sweats, and weight loss are less common than in Hodgkin's disease and their prognostic significance is less well defined
3. Initial lab evaluation may reveal only mild anemia

Histopathology and classification

Table 14-3 compares commonly used pathologic classifications of non-Hodgkin's lymphoma.

Staging

1. The Ann Arbor classification is also used to stage NHL (see Table 14-2)
2. Histopathology has greater therapeutic implications in NHL than in Hodgkin's disease
3. Proper staging usually requires the following:
  a. A thorough history and physical exam and an adequate biopsy
  b. Routine lab evaluation (CBC, sedimentation rate, urinalysis, BUN,
   creatinine, serum calcium, uric acid, liver function tests, serum protein
   electrophoresis)
  c. Chest x-ray (PA and lateral)
  d. Bone marrow evaluation (aspirate and four bone core biopsies)
  e. CT scan of abdomen and pelvis; CT scan of chest if chest x-ray film
   is abnormal
  f. Bone scan (particularly in patients with histiocytic lymphoma)
  g. Depending on the histopathology, the results of the above studies, and
   the planned therapy, some other tests may be performed: gallium scan
   (e.g., in patients with high-grade lymphomas), liver-spleen scan, lym-
   phangiogram, lumbar puncture, and staging laparotomy

Table 14-3 Comparison of pathologic classifications of non-Hodgkin's lymphoma

Working Formulation of Non-Hodgkin's Lymphomas for Clinical Usage[30]	Rappaport Classification[35]	Lukes and Collins[27]
Low grade		
ML,* small lymphocytic	Diffuse lymphocytic, well differentiated	Small lymphocytic and plasmacytoid lymphocytic
ML, follicular, predominantly small cleaved cell	Nodular, poorly differentiated lymphocytic	Small cleaved FCC,† follicular only or follicular and diffuse
ML, follicular, mixed small cleaved and large cell	Nodular, mixed lymphocytic-histiocytic	Small cleaved FCC, follicular; large cleaved FCC, follicular
Intermediate grade		
ML, follicular, predominantly large cell	Nodular histiocytic	Large cleaved or noncleaved FCC, follicular
ML, diffuse small cleaved cell	Diffuse lymphocytic, poorly differentiated	Small cleaved FCC, diffuse
ML, diffuse, mixed small and large cell	Diffuse mixed lymphocytic-histiocytic	Small cleaved, large cleaved and/or large noncleaved FCC, diffuse
ML, diffuse large cell	Diffuse histiocytic	Large cleaved or noncleaved FCC, diffuse
High grade		
ML, large cell immunoblastic	Diffuse histiocytic	Immunoblastic sarcoma, T-cell or B-cell type
ML, lymphoblastic	Lymphoblastic convoluted/nonconvoluted	Convoluted T-cell
ML, small noncleaved cell	Undifferentiated, Burkitt and non-Burkitt	Small noncleaved FCC
Miscellaneous		
Composite		
Mycosis fungoides		
Histiocytic		
Extramedullary plasmacytoma		
Unclassifiable		

*ML, malignant lymphoma.
†FCC, follicular center cell.
Modified from the National Cancer Institute—sponsored study of the classifications of non-Hodgkin's lymphomas. From Ultmann, J.E., Jacobs, R.H.: CA 35(2):66, 1985. Reproduced with permission of the American Cancer Society.

Treatment

The therapeutic regimen varies with the histologic type and the pathologic stage. The following are commonly used therapeutic modalities:

1. Low-grade NHL (e.g., nodular, poorly-differentiated lymphoma)
   a. Local radiotherapy for symptomatic obstructive adenopathy
   b. Deferment of therapy and careful observation in asymptomatic patients
   c. Single-agent chemotherapy with cyclophosphamide or chlorambucil
   d. Combination chemotherapy, alone or with radiotherapy
      (1) CVP: cyclophosphamide, vincristine, prednisone
      (2) CHOP: cyclophosphamide, doxorubicin, vincristine, (oncovin), prednisone
      (3) CHOP-Bleo: addition of bleomycin to CHOP
      (4) COPP: cyclophosphamide, vincristine, procarbazine, prednisone
      (5) BACOP: bleomycin, doxorubicin (Adriamycin), cyclophosphamide, vincristine, prednisone
2. Intermediate and high-grade lymphomas (e.g., diffuse histiocytic lymphoma)
   a. Combination chemotherapy, alone or with radiotherapy
      (1) Pro-MACE-MOPP:[20] prednisone, methotrexate, leucovorin, doxorubicin, cyclophosphamide, epipodophyllotoxin VP-16, mechlorethamine, vincristine, procarbazine, prednisone
      (2) COMLA: cyclophosphamide, vincristine, methotrexate, leucovorin, cystosine arabinoside (Ara-C)
      (3) M-BACOD: methotrexate, leucovorin, bleomycin, doxorubicin, cyclophosphamide, vincristine, dexamethasone
      (4) CHOP: cyclophosphamide, doxorubicin, vincristine, prednisone

Prognosis

Patients with low-grade lymphomas, despite their long-term survival, are rarely cured and the great majority (if not all) patients eventually die of the lymphoma, whereas patients with high-grade lymphomas may achieve a cure with aggressive chemotherapy.

14.9 MULTIPLE MYELOMA[3,31,40]

Definition

Multiple myeloma is a malignancy of plasma cells characterized by overproduction of intact monoclonal immunoglobulin or free monoclonal kappa or lambda chains.

Characteristics and clinical manifestations

1. The median age at diagnosis is 60 years; there is an increased incidence in blacks
2. The median survival is approximately 30 months with standard therapy
3. The patient usually comes to medical attention because of one or more of the following:
   a. Bone pain (back, thorax) or pathologic fractures caused by osteolytic lesions or osteoporosis
   b. Fatigue or weakness because of anemia secondary to bone marrow infiltration with plasma cells

   c. Recurrent infections as a result of multiple factors (deficiency of normal immunoglobulins, impaired neutrophil function, prolonged physical immobilization); common infecting organisms are *S. pneumoniae, S. aureus, H. influenzae, Pseudomonas, E. coli,* and *Klebsiella*

   d. Nausea and vomiting caused by uremia (renal failure secondary to myeloma kidney, hypercalcemia, amyloidosis, hyperuricemia)

   e. Confusion as a result of hypercalcemia from bone resorption secondary to osteoclast-activating factor (OAF) secreted by myeloma cells

   f. Neurologic complications, such as spinal cord or nerve root compression, carpal tunnel syndrome secondary to amyloid infiltration, blurred vision or blindness from hyperviscosity

Lab results

1. Normochromic, normocytic anemia; Rouleaux formation may be seen on peripheral smear
2. Hypercalcemia
3. Elevated BUN and creatinine
4. Proteinuria secondary to overproduction and secretion of free monoclonal kappa or lambda chains (Bence-Jones protein)
5. Tall, homogeneous monoclonal spike (M spike) is present on protein electrophoresis in approximately 75% of patients
   a. The increased immunoglobulins are IgG, IgA, IgE, and rarely IgM
   b. Some patients have no increase in immunoglobulins but increased light chains in the urine
   c. A very small percentage of patients have nonsecreting myeloma (no increase in immunoglobulins and no light chains in the urine), but have other evidence of the disease
6. Reduced anion gap secondary to the positive charge of the M proteins and to the frequent presence of hyponatremia in myeloma patients[9]
7. Bone marrow exam usually demonstrates nests or sheets of plasma cells

Radiologic evaluation

X-ray films of painful areas usually demonstrate punched out lytic lesions or osteoporosis. Bone scans are not useful since lesions are not blastic.

Diagnostic criteria

1. Presence of $\geq 10\%$ immature plasma cells in the marrow
2. Presence of serum or urinary monoclonal protein
3. Osteolytic bone lesions

Staging

Durie and Salmon[17] developed a clinical staging system correlated with tumor mass, response to treatment, and survival. It has recently been refined by Smith and Alexanian[40] and includes the degree of marrow plasmacytosis, the level of serum β_2 microglobulin,[7] and the level of normal immunoglobulins (see the boxed material on p. 287).

Treatment

1. Supportive measures
   a. Pain control with analgesics; radiation therapy and surgical stabilization may also be indicated

Tumor Mass Staging of Multiple Myeloma*

1. High tumor mass
   a. Characterized by one of the following:
      (1) Hemoglobin <8.5 gm/100 ml without renal failure or hypoferremia
      (2) Calcium >11.5 mg/100 ml† without bedridden status
   b. Supporting features often present:
      (1) Marrow plasmacytosis >40% on flow cytometry or suspension smears in most patients
      (2) IgM <20 mg/100 ml or IgA <40 mg/100 ml or IgG <400 mg/100 ml in about half the patients
      (3) Serum β_2 microglobulin >8.0 mg/liter without creatinine >1.8 mg/100 ml in about half the patients
2. Low tumor mass
   a. Characterized by all of the following:
      (1) Hemoglobin >10.5 gm/100 ml, unless other factors are causing anemia
      (2) + Calcium <11.0 mg/100 ml†
      (3) + IgG or IgA peak <5.0 gm/100 ml
      (4) + Serum β_2 microglobulin <4.5 mg/liter
   b. Supporting features often present:
      (1) Marrow plasmacytosis <20 percent on flow cytometry or suspension smears in most patients
      (2) IgM >50 mg/100 ml and IgA >100 mg/100 ml and IgG >750 mg/100 ml in about half the patients
3. Intermediate tumor mass: all other patients

*IgM, IgG, and IgA are normal immunoglobulins.
†Corrected calcium (mg/100 ml) = serum calcium (mg/100 ml) − serum albumin (gm/100 ml) + 4.0
From Smith L., Alexanian, R.: CA **35**(4):214, 1985. Used with permission.

   b. Control hypercalcemia (see Chapter 12, p. 193)
   c. Prompt diagnosis and treatment of any infection (see Chapter 15, pp. 313-315)
   d. Prevent renal failure by:
      (1) Adequate hydration
      (2) Control of hypercalcemia
      (3) Control of hyperuricemia (allopurinol and urine alkalinization)
      (4) Avoid nephrotoxic agents
      (5) Avoid dye contrast studies (e.g., IVP and CT scans with contrast)
   e. Preserve ambulation and mobility
2. Chemotherapy: commonly used regimens are:
   a. Melphalan and prednisone
   b. Vincristine, doxorubicin, and dexamethasone
   c. Vincristine, cyclophosphamide, doxorubicin, and prednisone

14.10 POLYCYTHEMIA VERA[1,8]

Definition

Polycythemia vera is a chronic myeloproliferative disorder characterized mainly by erythrocytosis (increase in RBC mass).

Differential diagnosis

1. Smoking
   a. Polycythemia is secondary to increased carboxyhemoglobin resulting in left shift in the hemoglobin dissociation curve
   b. Lab evaluation shows increased hematocrit, RBC mass, erythropoietin level, and carboxyhemoglobin
   c. Splenomegaly is not present on physical exam
2. Hypoxemia (secondary polycythemia): e.g., living for prolonged periods at high altitudes, pulmonary fibrosis
   a. Lab evaluation shows decreased arterial oxygen saturation and elevated erythropoietin level
   b. Splenomegaly is not present on physical exam
3. Erythropoietin-producing tumors: e.g., renal cell carcinoma
   a. The erythropoietin level is elevated in these patients, the arterial oxygen saturation is normal
   b. Splenomegaly may be present with metastatic neoplasms
4. Stress polycythemia (Gaisböck's syndrome, relative polycythemia)
   a. Lab evaluation demonstrates normal RBC mass, arterial oxygen saturation, and erythropoietin level; plasma volume is decreased
   b. Splenomegaly is not present on physical exam
5. Hemoglobinopathies associated with high O_2 affinity: a high P_{50} O_2 is present

Characteristics and clinical manifestations

1. Polycythemia vera is slightly more common in men and in patients of Jewish descent
2. Average age at onset is 60 years
3. The patient generally comes to medical attention because of symptoms associated with increased blood volume and viscosity or impaired platelet function
   a. Impaired cerebral circulation resulting in headache, vertigo, blurred vision, dizziness, TIA, CVA
   b. Fatigue, poor exercise tolerance
   c. Pruritus, particularly following bathing
   d. Bleeding: epistaxis, UGI bleeding (increased incidence of PUD)
   e. Abdominal discomfort secondary to splenomegaly
4. Physical exam generally reveals facial plethora, enlargement and tortuosity of retinal veins, and splenomegaly

Lab results

1. Elevated RBC count (>6 million/mm³), elevated hemoglobin (>18 g/dl in men, >16 g/dl in women), elevated hematocrit (>54% in men, >49% in women)
2. Increased WBC (often with basophilia), thrombocytosis is present in the majority of patients

3. Elevated leukocyte alkaline phosphatase, serum B_{12} level, and uric acid level are common

Diagnostic criteria

Diagnosis requires all three major criteria or the first two major criteria plus two minor criteria.

1. Major critera
   a. Increased RBC mass (≥36 ml/kg in men, ≥32 ml/kg in women)
   b. Normal arterial oxygen saturation ($\geq92\%$)
   c. Splenomegaly
2. Minor criteria
   a. Thrombocytosis ($>400,000/mm^3$)
   b. Leukocytosis ($>12,000/mm^3$)
   c. Elevated leukocyte alkaline phosphatase (>100)
   d. Elevated serum vitamin B_{12} (>900 pg/ml) or vitamin B_{12} binding protein (>2200 pg/ml)

Diagnostic step-wise approach

1. Measure RBC mass by isotope dilution using ^{51}Cr-labeled autologous RBCs; a high value eliminates stress polycythemia
2. Measure arterial saturation; a normal value eliminates polycythemia secondary to hypoxia
3. Measure carboxyhemoglobin; a normal value eliminates polycythemia secondary to smoking
4. Measure erythropoietin level; if elevated, obtain IVP and abdominal CT scan to rule out renal cell carcinoma
5. The diagnosis of hemoglobinopathy with high O_2 affinity is ruled out by a normal oxyhemoglobin dissociation curve

Treatment

1. Phlebotomy; the median survival time with phlebotomy is approximately 12 years
2. Radiophosphorus (^{32}P) produces hematologic remission in most patients, but it may result in an increased incidence of acute leukemia, therefore it should be reserved for older patients
3. Hydroxyurea can be used in conjuction with phlebotomy and appears to be free of leukemogenic effect

14.11 PLATELET DISORDERS

Thrombocytopenia

1. Definition: platelet count $<100,000/mm^3$
2. Clinical manifestations: ecchymoses, petichiae, purpura, menorrhagia, GI bleeding, epistaxes
3. Etiology
   a. Increased destruction
      (1) Immunologic
         (a) Drugs: quinine, quinidine, digitalis, procainamide, thiazide diuretics, sulfonamides, phenytoin, aspirin, penicillin, heparin
         (b) ITP: see p. 290

- (c) Transfusion reaction: transfusion of platelets with PLA-antigen in recipients without PLA-1 antigen
- (d) Fetal/maternal incompatibility
- (c) Vasculitis (e.g., SLE)
- (f) Autoimmune hemolytic anemia
- (g) Lymphoreticular disorders (e.g., CLL)
  - (2) Nonimmunologic
    - (a) Prosthetic heart valves
    - (b) TTP: see p. 291
    - (c) Sepsis
    - (d) DIC: see p. 291
    - (e) Hemolytic-uremic syndrome
- b. Decreased production
  - (1) Abnormal marrow
    - (a) Marrow infiltration (e.g., leukemia, lymphoma, fibrosis)
    - (b) Marrow suppression (e.g., chemotherapy, alcohol, radiation)
  - (2) Hereditary disorders
    - (a) Wiskott-Aldrich's syndrome: X-linked disorder characterized by thrombocytopenia, eczema, and repeated infections
    - (b) May-Hegglin's anomaly: increased megakaryocytes but ineffective thrombopoiesis
  - (3) Vitamin deficiencies (e.g., vitamin B_{12}, folic acid)
- c. Platelet sequestration and pooling
  - (1) Splenomegaly
  - (2) Cavernous hemangioma
- d. Dilutional, secondary to massive transfusion
4. Diagnostic approach to undetermined thrombocytopenia
- a. Thorough history (particularly drug history)
- b. Physical exam: evaluate for presence of spenomegaly (hypersplenism, leukemia, lymphoma)
- c. Examine peripheral blood smear, note platelet size and other abnormalities (e.g., fragmented RBC may indicate TTP)
- d. Check PT, PTT, bleeding time, Coomb's test
- e. Bone marrow exam

Idiopathic thrombocytopenic purpura (ITP)[28]

1. Definition: probable autoimmune disorder characterized by thrombocytopenia
2. Pathogenesis: The platelets contain an unidentified antigen with which antibodies react, thereby increasing the susceptibility of these platelets to phagocytosis by macrophages
3. Characteristics and clinical manifestations
- a. ITP can be subdivided into acute and chronic forms: the acute form is generally seen in children following a viral infection; the chronic form occurs more frequently in young women (age 20-40)
- b. The clinical presentation is characterized by various manifestations of thrombocytopenia (petechiae, purpura, epistaxes, GI bleeding, menorrhagia); splenomegaly is generally not present on physical exam
4. Lab results
- a. Thrombocytopenia
- b. Anemia may be present in patients with significant hemorrhage

   c. Peripheral blood smear reveals a decreased amount of platelets, and normal or increased platelet size

   d. Bone marrow reveals increased number of megakaryocytes

   e. Increased platelet-associated IgG

5. Treatment

   a. Prednisone 1-2 mg/kg qd, continued until the platelet count is normalized, then slowly tapered off

   b. Platelet transfusion only in case of life-threatening hemorrhage

   c. Have patient restrict physical activity and avoid any physical trauma

   d. Splenectomy is indicated in patients not responding to steroids

   e. Immunosuppression with vincristine or cyclophosphamide may be necessary if significant thrombocytopenia persists despite steroids and splenectomy

   f. Encouraging results have been reported with the use of IV gammaglobulins[19] and danazol[2]

6. Prognosis is excellent in children with the acute form (>90% recover within few months)

Thrombotic thrombocytopenic purpura[44]

1. Definition: rare disorder characterized by thrombocytopenia and microangiopathic hemolytic anemia

2. Characteristics and clinical manifestations

   a. Purpura (secondary to thrombocytopenia)

   b. Jaundice, pallor (secondary to hemolysis)

   c. Mucosal bleeding

   d. Fever

   e. Neurologic symptoms and signs (e.g., fluctuating levels of consciousness)

   f. Renal failure (secondary to renal cortical infarction)

3. Lab results

   a. Severe anemia and thrombocytopenia

   b. Elevated BUN and creatinine

   c. Hematuria and proteinuria

   d. Peripheral blood smear shows severely fragmented RBCs (schistocytes)

   e. No lab evidence of DIC (normal FDP, fibrinogen)

4. Treatment[38]

   a. Plasmapheresis with fresh frozen plasma replacement

   b. Vincristine[36]

14.12 DISSEMINATED INTRAVASCULAR COAGULATION

Definition

Disseminated intravascular coagulation (DIC) is characterized by generalized activation of the clotting mechanism

Etiology

1. Infections (e.g., gram-negative sepsis, viral infection)

2. Obstetric complications (e.g, dead fetus, amniotic fluid embolism, abruptio placentae)

3. Tissue trauma (e.g., burns)
4. Neoplasms (e.g., adenocarcinomas, acute promyelocytic leukemia)

Clinical manifestations

DIC manifests with profuse bleeding in association with any of the above clinical settings.

Lab results

1. Peripheral blood smear generally shows red blood cell fragments and low platelet count
2. Additional findings vary depending on whether the DIC is acute or chronic; Table 14-4 describes lab findings indicative of DIC
3. Coagulopathy secondary to DIC can be differentiated from that secondary to liver disease or vitamin K deficiency by measuring factors V, VIII, and X
   a. Decreased factors V and VIII are consistent with DIC
   b. Decreased factor V and normal factor VIII are seen in liver disease
   c. Normal factors V and VIII, but decreased factor X are associated with vitamin K deficiency

Therapy

1. Correct underlying cause (e.g., antimicrobial therapy for infection)
2. Replacement therapy with fresh-frozen plasma and platelets in patients with significant hemorrhage
3. Heparin therapy in selected cases (e.g., DIC associated with acute promyelocytic leukemia)

Table 14-4   Findings indicative of DIC

Test Parameter	Acute DIC	Chronic DIC
Fibrinogen (clottable)	↓ ↓ or ↓ ↓ ↓	N or ↑
Fibrinolytic activity	N rarely ↑	N rarely ↑
Fibrin breakdown products present	+ +	+
Soluble fibrin monomer complexes (protamine sulfate or ethanol gelation)	+ +	+
Platelet count	↓ ↓ to ↓ ↓ ↓	N to ↑
APTT (activated partial thromboplastin time)	↑ to ↑ ↑ to ↑ ↑ ↑	N
PT (prothrombin time)	↑	N
Thrombin time	↑ ↑	↑
RBC microangiopathy	—	↑

Reproduced from Jacobs, D.S., Kasten, B.L., Jr., Dermott, W.R., and Wolffson, W.L.: Laboratory test handbook with DRG index, St. Louis, 1984, Mosby/Lexi-Comp.

References

1. Adamson, J.W.: Polycythemia vera. In Petersdorf, R.G., et al., (editors): Harrison's principles of internal medicine, ed. 10, New York, 1983, McGraw Hill Book Co.

2. Ahm, Y.S., et al.: Danazol for the treatment of idiopathic thrombocytopenic purpura, N. Engl. J. Med. **308**:1396, 1983.

3. Alexanian, R., and Dreicer, R.: Chemotherapy for multiple myeloma, Cancer, **53**:583, 1984.

4. Al-Mondhiry, H., Stryker, J., and Kempin, S.: Splenic irradiation (SI) in chronic lymphocytic leukemia (CLL) [abstract], Proc. Am. Soc. Clin. Oncol. **3**:192, 1984.

5. Anasetti, C., et al.: Marrow transplantation for severe aplastic anemia, long-term outcome in fifty "untransfused" patients, Ann. Intern. Med. **104**:461, 1986.

6. Aoki, Y.: Multiple enzymatic defects in mitochondria in hematological cells of patients with primary sideroblastic anemia, J. Clin. Invest. **66**:43, 1980.

7. Bataille, R., Grenier, J., and Sany J.: Beta-2-microglobulin in myeloma: optimal use for staging, prognosis, and treatment—a prospective study of 160 patients, Blood, **63**:468, 1984.

8. Berlin N.I.: Diagnosis and classification of the polycythemias, Semin. Hematol. **12**:339, 1975.

9. Bloth, B., Christensson, T., and Mellstedt, H.: Extreme hyponatremia in patients with myelomatosis: an effect of cationic paraproteins, Acta Med. Scand. **203**:273, 1978.

10. Canellos, G.P.: Chronic leukemias. In DeVita, V.T., Hellman, S., and Rosenberg, S.A., (editors): Cancer: principles and practice of oncology, Philadelphia, 1985, J.B. Lippincott Co.

11. Carbone, P.P., et al.: Report of the committee on Hodgkin's disease staging, Cancer Res. **31**:1860, 1971.

12. Cartwright, G.E., et al.: Association of HLA-linked hemochromatosis with idiopathic refractory sideroblastic anemia, J. Clin. Invest. **65**:989, 1980.

13. Cassileth, P.A.: Adult acute nonlymphocytic leukemia, Med. Clin. North Am. **68**:675, 1984.

14. Champlin, R., Ho, W., and Gale, R.P.: Antithymocyte globulin treatment in patients with aplastic anemia: a prospective randomized trial, N. Engl. J. Med. **308**:113, 1983.

15. Champlin, R.E., et al.: Do androgens enchance the response to antithymocyte globulin in patients with aplastic anemia? A prospective randomized trial, Blood, **66**:184, 1985.

16. DeVita, V.T., Jr., Jaffe, E.S., and Hellman, S.: Hodgkin's disease and the non-Hodgkin's lymphomas. In DeVita, V.T., Hellman, S., and Rosenberg, S.A., (editors): Cancer: principles and practice of oncology, Philadelphia, 1985, J.B. Lippincott Co.

17. Durie, B.G.M., and Salmon, S.E.: A clinical staging system for multiple myeloma: correlation of measured myeloma cell mass with presenting clinical features, response to treatment, and survival, Cancer, **36**:842, 1975.

18. Estey, E., et al.: Infection prophylaxis in acute leukemia: comparative effectiveness of sulfamethoxazole and trimethoprim, ketoconazole, and a combination of the two, Arch. Intern. Med. **144**:1562, 1984.

19. Fehr, J., Hofmann, V., and Kappeler, U.: Transient reversal of thrombocytopenia in idiopathic thrombocytopenic purpura by high dose intravenous gamma globulin, N. Engl. J. Med. **306**:1254, 1982.

20. Fisher, R.I., et al.: Diffuse aggressive lymphomas: increased survival after alternating flexible sequences of ProMACE and MOPP chemotherapy, Ann. Intern. Med. **93**:304, 1983.

21. Gale, R.P., Foon, K.A.: Chronic lymphocytic leukemia: recent advances in biology and treatment, Ann. Intern. Med. **103**:101, 1985.

22. Gralnick, H.R., et al.: Classification of acute leukemia, Ann. Intern. Med. **87**:740, 1977.

23. Haller, D.G.: Non-Hodgkin's lymphomas, Med. Clin. North Am. **68**:741, 1984.
24. Jacobs, A.D., and Gale, R.P.: Recent advances in the biology and treatment of acute lymphoblastic leukemia in adults, N. Engl. J. Med. **311**:1219, 1984.
25. Karp, J.E., et al.: Oral norfloxacin for prevention of gram-negative bacterial infections in patients with acute leukemia and granulocytopenia, Ann. Intern. Med. **106**:1, 1987.
26. Lee, G.R.: The anemia of chronic disease, Semin. Hematol. **20**:61, 1983.
27. Lukes, R.J., and Collins, R.D.: Immunologic characterization of human malignant lymphomas, Cancer, **34**:1488, 1974.
28. McMillan, R.: Chronic idiopathic thrombocytopenic purpura, N. Engl. J. Med. **304**:1135, 1981.
29. Marmont, A.M., et al.: Treatment of severe aplastic anemia with sequential immunosuppression, Exp. Hematol. **11**:856, 1983.
30. National Cancer Institute—sponsored study of classification on non-Hodgkin's lymphoma: Summary and description of a working formulation for clinical usage. The non-Hodgkin's lymphoma pathological classification project, Cancer, **49**:2112, 1982.
31. Oken, M.M.: Multiple myeloma, Med. Clin. North Am. **68**:757, 1984.
32. Portlock, C.S.: Hodgkin's disease, Med. Clin. North Am. **68**:729, 1984.
33. Rai, K.R., et al.: Chronic lymphocytic leukemia, Med. Clin. North Am. **68**:697, 1984.
34. Rai, K.R., et al.: Clinical staging of chronic lymphocytic leukemia, Blood **46**:219, 1975.
35. Rappoport, H.: Tumors of the hematopoietic system. In Atlas of tumor pathology, Section 3, Fascicle 8. Washington, D.C.: Armed Forces Institute of Pathology, 1966.
36. Schreeder, M.T., and Prchal, J.T.: Successful treatment of thrombotic thrombocytopenic purpura by vincristine, Am. J. Hematol. **14**:75, 1983.
37. Schrier, S.L.: Anemia: production defects, Sci. Am. Med. **9**(5):10, 1985.
38. Sennett, M.L., and Conrad, M.E.: Treatment of thrombotic thrombocytopenic purpura: plasmapheresis, plasma transfusion, and vincristine, Arch. Intern. Med. **146**:266, 1986.
39. Skihne, B.S.: A practical approach to the initial diagnosis of anemia, Medical times, **114**:63, 1986.
40. Smith, L., Alexanian, R.: Treatment strategies for plasma cell myeloma, **35**:214, 1985.
41. Spiers, A.S.D.: Chronic granulocytic leukemia, Med. Clin. North Am. **68**:713, 1984.
42. Thomas, E.D., and Clift, R.A.: Marrow transplantation for the treatment of chronic myelogenous leukemia, Ann. Intern. Med. **104**:155-163, 1986.
43. Thomas, E.D., and Storb, R.: Acquired severe aplastic anemia: progress and perplexity, Blood, **64**:325, 1984.
44. Thompson, H.N., McCarthy, L.J.: Thrombotic thrombocytopenic purpura, Arch. Intern. Med. **143**:2117, 1983.
45. Torok-Storb, B., et al.: Subsets of patients with aplastic anemia identified by flow microfluorometry, N. Engl. J. Med. **312**:1015, 1985.
46. Ultmann, J.E., and Jacobs, R.H.: The non-Hodgkin's lymphomas, CA **35**:66, 1985.
47. Wiernik, P.H.: Acute leukemias of adults. In DeVita, V.T., Hellman, S., and Rosenberg, S.A., (editors): Cancer: principles and practice of oncology, Philadelphia, 1985, J.B. Lippincott Co.

Infectious Diseases

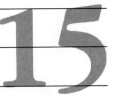

15.1   NOSOCOMIAL INFECTIONS
Joseph Herbin

Definition

A nosocomial infection is one that was not present nor incubating when the patient entered the hospital. It also includes any infection acquired during hospitalization and manifested clinically after hospital discharge (e.g., hepatitis B).

Predisposing factors

1. Surgery or other invasive procedures
2. Urinary or intravenous catheters
3. Immunocompromised host because of underlying disease (e.g., leukemia) or treatments (e.g., immunosuppressive agents)

Clinical manifestations

1. Fever; its absence does not rule out infection (particularly in elderly patients)
2. Change in mental status, delirium
3. Unexplained hypotension, tachycardia, tachypnea

Lab results

1. Alterations of WBC ranging from neutropenia to marked leukocytosis with shift to left
2. Metabolic acidosis
3. Hypernatremia, elevated BUN, creatinine (secondary to dehydration)

Common sites of infections

1. Urinary tract
2. Surgical wounds
3. Intravascular devices
4. Respiratory tract

Control of nosocomial infection

General principles

1. Handwashing is the single most important procedure for prevention of nosocomial infections[19]

a. In the absence of a true emergency, personnel should *always* wash their hands:
   (1) Before performing invasive procedures
   (2) Before taking care of particularly susceptible patients (e.g., immunocompromised patients, newborns)
   (3) Before and after touching any wounds
   (4) After situations likely to contaminate hands (e.g., contact with mucous membranes, blood or bloody fluids, secretions or excretions)
   (5) After touching inanimate sources that are likely to be contaminated with virulent or epidemiologically important microorganisms (e.g., urine measuring devices or secretion collection apparatus)
   (6) After caring for an infected patient or one likely to be colonized with microorganisms of special clinical or epidemiologic significance (e.g., bacteria resistant to multiple antibiotics)
   (7) Between contacts with different patients in high-risk units
b. Most routine, brief patient care activities other than those above (e.g., measuring blood pressure) do not require handwashing
c. Most routine hospital activities involving indirect patient contact (e.g., handling medication, food, or other objects) do not require handwashing

Selected nosocomial infections

1. Urinary tract infections (UTI) are the most common nosocomial infections
   a. Manifestations: most patients are asymptomatic, but 1% may develop bacteremia (chills, fever) and localized symptoms (dysuria, frequency, urgency, CVA tenderness)
   b. Contributing factors: Foley catheters, cystoscopy or surgery, obstruction with ureteral reflux
   c. Common organisms: gram-negative bacilli, *Escherichia, Pseudomonas aeruginosa, Proteus*/Providencia, group D streptococci, *Staphylococcus aureus,* and *Candida*
   d. Prevention
      (1) Insert Foley catheter only if absolutely necessary
      (2) Insert with aseptic technique
      (3) Keep system closed
      (4) Remove catheter as soon as possible
      (5) Treat "positive" cultures only if the patient is symptomatic
   e. Management of suspected UTI
      (1) Patient without Foley catheter:
         (a) Insert Foley catheter and record residual urine volume; if volume is >250 ml, leave catheter in
         (b) Obtain urinalysis and culture
         (c) Perform Gram stain of urine sediment
         (d) Treat symptomatic patients on the basis of Gram stain results
            • Gram-positive cocci: treat for enterococci and *S. aureus*
            • Gram-negative bacilli: treat for *Pseudomonas*

      (2) Patient with Foley catheter
- (a) Rule out other sources of infection
- (b) If no other sources are found and urine culture is positive, treat symptomatic patient based on culture results
- (c) If urine culture is negative, perform Gram stain of urine sediment and treat as described above

2. Surgical wound infection: a wound is considered infected if purulent material drains from it, even if cultures reveal no growth; most infections are confined to the incisional wound, the deep tissues are rarely involved

  a. Contributing factors: impaired host resistance (e.g., malnourished patient), poor surgical technique, surgery involving contaminated or potentially contaminated areas (e.g., traumatic lacerations), virulence, and number of organisms that contaminate the wound

  b. Common organisms: *S. aureus* is the most common pathogen isolated; other frequent pathogens include streptococci, gram-negative bacilli, and anaerobes

  c. Prevention: good surgical technique is the most important measure in the prevention of a wound infection; additional recommendations are:[20]

    (1) In elective surgery, the preoperative hospital stay should be as short as possible

    (2) If the patient is malnourished and surgery is not urgent, the patient should receive enteric or parenteral hyperalimentation before surgery

    (3) In elective surgery, all bacterial infections, except that for which the operation is performed, should be treated before surgery

    (4) When indicated (e.g., endocarditis prophylaxis), prophylactic antibiotics should be given just before surgery and discontinued promptly afterwards

    (5) If hair removal is necessary, clipping is preferable to shaving

    (6) The common accepted preoperative, intraoperative, and postoperative procedures should be strictly followed

    (7) Personnel should wash their hands before and after taking care of a surgical wound

    (8) Fresh or open wounds should be touched only with sterile gloves

    (9) Dressings should be removed or changed if wet or if the patient has signs suggestive of infection; wound drainage should be Gram stained and cultured

   (10) Patients with infected wounds should be placed on isolation precautions according to the hospital's infection control guidelines

  d. Management of infected surgical wounds

    (1) Inspect the wound thoroughly

    (2) If the wound is sutured or closed but shows signs of infection (erythema, foul smell, drainage), surgical evaluation is indicated with possible removal of sutures and exploration of the wound for presence of pus

    (3) If purulence is present, Gram stain and aerobic and anaerobic cultures should be obtained

    (4) Consider necrotizing cellulitis or fasciitis if symptoms are severe or if local findings are extensive; urgent surgical evaluation is indicated

     (5) If deep infection is suspected, obtain ultrasound or CT scan to rule out abscess formation

     (6) The choice of antibiotics depends on the Gram stain results; if no organisms are seen, treat for *S. aureus*

3. Intravascular device infection can result in septicemia, endocarditis, suppurative thrombophlebitis, tract infection, and local site infection

   a. Common organisms: *S. aureus* and *Staphylococcus epidermidis* are the most frequent infecting organisms; other organisms include gram-negative bacilli, *Candida,* enterococci, and diphtheroids

   b. Prevention

     (1) All major intravascular devices (e.g., CVP lines, A-lines) should be inserted using sterile technique and should be sutured to the skin to prevent movement

     (2) Whenever possible, use peripheral rather than central lines, percutaneous rather than cut-down insertion, and upper rather than lower extremities

     (3) When a device is inserted using unsterile technique (i.e., in an emergency situation) consider removal within 24 hours and replacement, using sterile technique

     (4) Remove all intravascular devices as soon as possible (increased risk of infection after 72 hours); culture catheter tip

   c. Management

     (1) If there is evidence of infection, immediately remove the intravascular device and obtain Gram stain and cultures

     (2) Antibiotic choice depends upon the Gram stain results; if no organism is seen, treat for *S. aureus*

4. Respiratory tract infection: pneumonia is the leading cause of death of all nosocomial infections

   a. Manifestations

     (1) Fever, dyspnea, cough, increased sputum production

     (2) Decreased arterial Po_2, leukocytosis

     (3) New or worsening infiltrate on chest x-ray film

     (4) Purulent sputum

   b. Risk factors

     (1) Severity of underlying disease (e.g., COPD, cancer, leukemia)

     (2) Surgery (thoracic or thoracoabdominal surgery)

     (3) Intubation or tracheostomy

     (4) Hospitalization in an intensive care unit (ICU)

     (5) Atelectasis

     (6) Excessive sedation

     (7) Immunosuppressive medication (e.g., steroids)

     (8) Antibiotic therapy

     (9) Advanced age

   c. Common organisms: *S. aureus* and gram-negative bacilli are the most common infecting organisms; less common are *haemophilus influenzae, Streptococcus pneumoniae,* anaerobes, *Legionella,* viruses, and fungi *(Candida, Aspergillus)*

   d. Prevention is difficult; measures include the following:

     (1) Prevention of atelectasis in postoperative patients by encouraging deep breathing and coughing in addition to incentive spirometry

  (2) Minimize excessive sedation to prevent aspiration
  (3) Avoid (if possible) the use of steroid immunosuppressive therapy
  (4) Minimize continuous ventilatory support
 e. Diagnosis of suspected respiratory tract infection
  (1) Chest x-ray: look for new or changing pulmonary infiltrates
  (2) Obtain a sputum specimen for Gram stain and culture; consider transtracheal aspiration if necessary to obtain an adequate sputum specimen
  (3) Obtain two or three blood cultures from different sites (not through an intravascular device)
  (4) Check arterial blood gases and WBC
 f. Management: the choice of antibiotics depends on the clinical setting, the sputum Gram stain, and the chest x-ray film
  (1) Gram-positive cocci: treat for *S. aureus*
  (2) Gram-negative bacilli: treat for *Pseudomonas aeruginosa*
  (3) Inconclusive Gram stain and
     (a) Localized infiltrate: consider gram-negative bacilli or *S. aureus;* treat with cephalosporin plus aminoglycoside
     (b) Diffuse infiltrates: consider *Legionella* (treat with erythromycin) or *Pneumocystis carinii* in immunocompromised host (treat with IV trimethoprim-sulfamethoxazole); aerobic gram-negative bacilli, gram-positive bacteria, anaerobes, and fungal pneumonia should also be considered in patients with diffuse infiltrates
  (4) If there is no significant clinical response to the initial antibiotics, fiberoptic bronchoscopy should be strongly considered

15.2 PRINCIPLES OF ANTIBIOTIC USE

Characteristics of commonly used antimicrobial agents

Cephalosporins
Cephalosporins are subdivided into three generations based on their gram-negative enteric bacillary activity
1. First generation
   a. Cefadroxil (Duricef, Ultracef), cefazolin (Ancef, Kefzol), cephalexin (Keflex), cephalothin (Keflin, Seffin), cephapirin (Cefadyl), and cephradine (Anspor, Velosef)
   b. Comments: excellent broad-spectrum activity against gram-positive cocci *(Staphylococcus aureus, Streptococcus pneumoniae);* limited activity against gram-negative bacilli, and poor coverage of enterococcus
2. Second generation
   a. Cefaclor (Ceclor), cefamandole (Mandol), cefonicid (Monocid), ceforanide (Precef), cefoxitin (Mefoxin), cefuroxime (Zinacef)
   b. Comments: more effective against gram-negative bacilli than first generation cephalosporins
      (1) Cefoxitin has excellent activity against *Bacteroides fragilis* and *Serratia* sp.
      (2) Cefuroxime crosses the blood-brain barrier (useful in the treatment of some forms of bacterial meningitis)

3. Third generation
   a. Cefoperazone (Cefobid), cefotaxime (Claforan), ceftazidime (Fortaz), ceftizoxime (Cefizox), ceftriaxone (Rocephin), and moxalactam (Moxam)
   b. Comments: broader activity against most enteric gram-negative bacilli
      (1) Cefotaxime, ceftriaxone, and moxalactam demonstrate good CSF penetration and are useful in the treatment of gram-negative meningitis
      (2) Moxalactam can significantly prolong bleeding time

Aminoglycosides

1. Common preparations: gentamicin, tobramycin, amikacin, kanamycin, neomycin, netilmicin, streptomycin
2. Comments
   a. Aminoglycosides have excellent activity against aerobic gram-negative rods, however they are ineffective against anaerobic organisms and streptococci
   b. Amikacin has the broadest spectrum of activity; it is useful in the treatment of gentamicin- or tobramycin-resistant bacteria
   c. Netilmicin is a new aminoglycoside similar to gentamicin but less nephrotoxic and ototoxic
   d. Kanamycin is infrequently used because of a high degree of bacterial resistance
   e. Neomycin is used orally to reduce intestinal bacteria in patients with hepatic encephalopathy

Penicillins

Can be subdivided into four generations based on an increasing spectrum of activity

1. First generation
   a. Penicillin G (aqueous, procaine, benzathine), phenoxymethyl penicillin (penicillin V), methicillin, oxacillin, dicloxacillin, nafcillin
   b. Comments
      (1) Penicillins G and V are useful against streptococci, most anaerobes found in the oral cavity, *Treponema pallidum, Clostridium,* nonpenicillinase–producing staphylococci, most *Neisseria* and *Bacteroides* sp. (except *B. fragilis*)
      (2) Methicillin, nafcillin, oxacillin, and dicloxacillin are effective against penicillinase-producing strains of *S. aureus*
2. Second generation
   a. Ampicillin and amoxicillin
   b. Comments
      (1) Broader spectrum against gram-negative organisms
      (2) Ineffective against penicillinase-producing bacteria, *Klebsiella,* and *Pseudomonas* strains
3. Third generation
   a. Carbenicillin and ticarcillin
   b. Comments
      (1) Increased activity against *P. aeruginosa, Enterobacter* sp., *Morganella morgagni,* and *Proteus* sp.
      (2) Ineffective against penicillinase-producing bacteria

(3) Less active against enterococci than ampicillin
(4) Often used in combination with an aminoglycoside to treat *P. aeruginosa* infections

4. Fourth generation
   a. Azlocillin, mezlocillin, and piperacillin
   b. Comments
      (1) Broader spectrum of activity than third generation penicillins
      (2) More active against enterococci
      (3) Greater activity against *P. aeruginosa* and *Klebsiella* strains
      (4) Inactive against penicillinase-producing staphylococci or ampicillin–resistant *Haemophilus influenzae*

Erythromycin

1. Active against most gram-negative cocci
2. Effective against *Mycoplasma pneumoniae, Legionella* sp., pneumococci, group A streptococci, *Chlamydiae,* and *Campylobacter jejuni*
3. Inactive against most gram-negative bacilli

Metronidazole

1. Effective against anaerobes (*B. fragilis, Clostridium, Fusobacterium*, anaerobic cocci); useful for intraabdominal and pelvic infections
2. Good CSF penetration; useful in the treatment of meningitis or brain abscess secondary to *B. fragilis*
3. Effective in the treatment of pseudomembranous colitis secondary to *Clostridium difficile*
4. Antiprotozoal useful for therapy of *Trichomonas* and *Entamoeba histolytica*

Trimethoprim-sulfamethoxazole

1. Indicated for *Pneumocystis carinii* pneumonia
2. Useful for treatment of outpatient UTI
3. Effective in otitis media (in penicillin-allergic patients) and in exacerbation in COPD

Vancomycin

1. Excellent activity against gram-positive bacteria (including methicillin-resistant staphylococci)
2. Useful in enterococcal infections in patients allergic to penicillin
3. Effective orally for pseudomembranous colitis secondary to *C. difficile*
4. Used in combination with gentamicin and rifampin for prosthetic valve endocarditis caused by methicillin-resistant *Staphylococcus*

Clindamycin

1. Effective against anaerobes (*B. fragilis*) and gram-positive cocci
2. Useful for intraabdominal infections and for infections secondary to gram-positive cocci in patients allergic to penicillin

Imipenem

1. New class of broad-spectrum antibiotics (Carbapenem); administered in combination with cilastin (Primaxin) to prevent rapid renal metabolism
2. Comments
   a. Effective against most bacterial pathogens, including anaerobes, *Listeria,* and *Nocardia*
   b. Ineffective against *Streptococcus faecalis* and some *Pseudomonas* sp.

Table 15-1   Antibiotic dosage reduction in patients with renal impairment

Extent of Reduction in Dosage	Agent	Serum Half-Life (hours)		Initial Dose	Subsequent Dose	Interval Between Subsequent Doses
		Normal	Anuric			
Major	Amikacin	2	44 (minimum function) 86 (anephric)	7.5 mg/kg	0.75 mg/kg	12 hr (avoid levels >35 µg/ml)
	Gentamicin	2	48-72	1.7 mg/kg (IM or IV)	0.17 mg/kg	8 hr (avoid levels >12 µg/ml)
	Kanamycin	3	30-80	7.5 mg/kg	0.75 mg/kg	12 hr
	Streptomycin	2-3	100-110	0.5 gm (IM)	0.25 g	16 hr
	Tobramycin	2-3	56-72	2.0 mg/kg (IM or IV)	0.17 mg/kg	8 hr (avoid levels >12 µg/ml)
	Vancomycin	6	240	7.0 mg/kg	1.5 mg/kg	24 hr (avoid levels >50 µg/ml)
Moderate	Acyclovir	2-2.5	20	6.2 mg/kg	6.2 mg/kg	24 hr
	Azlocillin	1.0	5.0	45 mg/kg (IV)	45 mg/kg	12 hr
	Carbenicillin	0.5-1.0	12.5	75 mg/kg (IV)	28 mg/kg	8 hr
	Cefamandole	1.0	11	25 mg/kg (IV)	15 mg/kg	12 hr
	Cefazolin	1.9	32	15 mg/kg (IM)	4 mg/kg	12 hr
	Cefonicid	4.4	50-65	30 mg/kg	7.5 mg/kg	72 hr
	Ceforanide	3.0	20-40	15 mg/kg	7.5 mg/kg	24 hr
	Cefoxitin	0.7-1.0	22	15 mg/kg (IV)	15 mg/kg	24 hr
	Ceftazidime	1.8	16-25	30 mg/kg	7.5 mg/kg	24 hr

	Ceftizoxime	1.7	25-36	30 mg/kg	7.5 mg/kg	24 hr
	Cefuroxime	1.4-1.8	20	15 mg/kg (IV)	15 mg/kg	24 hr
	Cephalexin	1.0	5-30	15 mg/kg	2 mg/kg	12 hr
	Cephalothin	0.5	3-18	30 mg/kg (IV)	7.5 mg/kg	12 hr
	Cephapirin	0.9	2.4	15 mg/kg	15 mg/kg	12 hr
	Cephradine	0.7	8-15	15 mg/kg	7.5 mg/kg	12 hr
	Imipenem	0.8-1.0	3.5	15 mg/kg (IV)	7.5 mg/kg	12 hr
	Moxalactam	2.2	19	25 mg/kg	7.5 mg/kg	12 hr
	Penicillin G	0.5	7-10	30,000 U/kg (IV)	10,000 U/kg	8 hr
	Ticarcillin	1-1.5	13	45 mg/kg IV	28 mg/kg	12 hr
	Trimethoprim	11	25	2 tabs (400 mg SMZ, 80 mg TMP/tab) (PO)	1 tab	12 hr
	Sulfamethoxazole	9	27			
None or minor	Amoxicillin	1.0	16	30 mg/kg (IM or IV)	15 mg/kg	12 hr
	Amphotericin B	$\frac{24}{15\ days}$	40	0.5 mg/kg IV	0.5 mg/kg IV	1-2 days
	Ampicillin	0.5-1.0	8-20	30 mg/kg (IM or IV)	15 mg/kg	12 hr
	Cefoperazone	1.6-2.4	4.2	30 mg/kg	20 mg/kg	12 hr
	Cefotaxime	1.5	2.7	30 mg/kg	30 mg/kg	12 hr
	Ceftriaxone	8	12-15	15 mg/kg	15 mg/kg	24 hr

Modified from Sanford, J.P.: Guide to antimicrobial therapy, 1985.

Clavulanate
1. β-Lactamase inhibitor; administered in combination with amoxicillin (Augmentin) or ticarcillin (Timentin)
2. Comments
   a. Augmentin has a spectrum similar to second generation cephalosporins and is active against enterococci
   b. Timentin has a spectrum similar to third generation cephalosporins

Quinolones
1. Norfloxacin and nalidixic acid are useful agents in urinary tract infections
2. Norfloxacin is effective against *P. aeruginosa* and most gram-negative bacilli

Antibiotic susceptibility testing[10]

1. MIC (minimum inhibitory concentration): lowest antibiotic concentration that inhibits visible growth of a standardized inoculum after overnight incubation
2. MBC (minimum bactericidal concentration): lowest concentration of an antibiotic necessary to kill 99.9% of bacterial cells when a mixture of bacteria and antibiotic have been incubated together
3. SBT (serum bactericidal titer): determined by inoculating dilutions of the patient's serum with the infecting bacterial isolate; diluted with no growth after 24 hours are then cultured without antibiotic (the SBT is the highest titer with a 99.9% kill)

Antibiotics in renal failure

Table 15-1 describes antibiotic dosage reduction necessary in patients with impaired renal function.

15.3   FEVER OF UNKNOWN ORIGIN

Definition[33]

A fever is considered to be of unknown origin (FUO) when it has been present for at least 3 weeks, with temperature elevations of 101° F (38.3° C), and of undetermined etiology after 1 week of investigation in a hospital.

Etiology

1. Neoplasm*
   a. Lymphomas, Hodgkin's disease
   b. Leukemias
   c. Hepatic neoplasms (primary or metastatic)
   d. Hypernephroma
   e. Carcinoma of lung
   f. Other: carcinoma of colon, prostate, thyroid
2. Infectious diseases
   a. Tuberculosis
   b. Bacterial endocarditis
   c. Intraabdominal infections (liver, subphrenic, renal, or perinephric abscess)
   d. Other: cholangitis, hepatitis, infectious mononucleosis, fungal infections, malaria, brucellosis

---

*Neoplasms have replaced infections as the commonest cause of FUO.[28]

3. Collagen-vascular diseases
   a. Allergic vasculitis
   b. Polymyalgia rheumatica
   c. SLE
   d. Rheumatoid arthritis
   e. Other: polyarteritis nodosa, juvenile rheumatoid arthritis, Wegener's granulomatosis, polymyositis
4. Drugs
   a. Barbiturates
   b. Antibiotics (sulfonamides, penicillins, nitrofurantoin, amphotericin B, INH, cephalosporins, rifampin, PAS, vancomycin, tetracyclines)
   c. Antihypertensives (methyldopa, hydralazine)
   d. Antidysrhythmics (procainamide, quinidine)
   e. Phenytoin
   f. Other: antihistamines, salicylates, cimetidine, bleomycin
5. Miscellaneous
   a. Factitious fever
   b. Pulmonary emboli
   c. Periodic fever
   d. Inflammatory bowel disease
   e. Other: subacute thyroiditis, familial Mediterranean fever (FMF), retroperitoneal hematoma

Diagnostic approach

When attempting to diagnose a FUO, think of unusual presentations of common diseases rather than rare diseases

History

1. Occupational history
   a. Rule out idiosyncratic reaction to fumes, dusts, chemicals (e.g., zinc or nickel)
   b. Consider diseases of animals (e.g., brucellosis, leptospirosis) in veterinarians, butchers, trappers, and workers in meat packing plants
2. Travel history: inquire about travel to areas endemic with malaria or enteric diseases
3. Duration of fever and associated symptoms
   a. Prolonged fever and significant weight loss: consider neoplasm
   b. History of myalgias, arthralgias: collagen-vascular diseases
   c. Dyspnea, cough: tuberculosis, multiple pulmonary emboli, sarcoidosis, lung neoplasm
   d. Abdominal pain: intraabdominal abscess, neoplasm
4. Family history of episodic or periodic fever: consider FMF, periodic fever
5. Current or recent drug use: rule out drug fever
6. IV drug addict: consider SBE, AIDS, ARC
7. Recent abdominal surgery: possible intraabdominal abscess
8. History of multiple hospitalizations and numerous diagnostic tests without elucidation of cause of fever: consider factitious fever
9. Homosexual patient: consider ARC and AIDS

Physical exam
1. Temperature: measure temperature rectally; if elevated and factitious fever is suspected, remeasure temperature immediately without leaving the room
2. Pulse: each increase in temperature of $1°$ F generally increases the pulse by 10 beats/minute
   a. Exceptions are typhoid fever (relative bradycardia), some viral infections, and use of β-adrenergic blockers
   b. A significant discrepancy between pulse and temperature indicates possible factitious fever
3. Skin
   a. Look for evidence of internal malignancy (e.g., acanthosis nigricans)
   b. Skin lesions (DLE, vasculitis, chronic meningococcemia, Lyme disease, erythema nodosum, Kaposi's sarcoma, rheumatic fever)
   c. Jaundice indicates hepatitis or neoplastic hepatic involvement
   d. Cool skin in a patient with "high temperature" is suggestive of factitious fever
   e. Examine skin for evidence of infection and insect or animal bites
4. Lymph nodes: generalized lymphadenopathy is suggestive of lymphoma, Hodgkin's disease, ARC, or AIDS
5. Head: tenderness and nodularity over the temporal artery is suggestive of temporal arteritis
6. Eyes: perform careful fundoscopic exam to rule out presence of choroid tubercles (indicative of tuberculosis)
7. Neck: rule out presence of thyroid nodules (suggestive of carcinoma)
8. Heart: the presence of new murmurs or variation of an existing cardiac murmur is suggestive of bacterial endocarditis
9. Abdomen: rule out presence of any palpable masses (neoplasm, abscess), hepatosplenomegaly (hepatitis, miliary TB, neoplasms)
10. Rectum
    a. Enlarged hard, nodular prostate is suggestive of carcinoma
    b. Guaiac-positive stool is suggestive of colon carcinoma, IBD
11. Joints: evidence of arthritis
12. Neurologic: presence of focal neurologic deficits is suggestive of cerebral neoplasm (primary or metastatic) or cerebral abscess

Lab results
1. CBC, examine peripheral smear for presence of parasites
2. Urinalysis, urine culture and sensitivity
3. Obtain three sets of paired blood cultures from different sites
4. Sedimentation rate (nonspecific, generally not helpful)
5. PPD, anergy panel, histoplasmin, coccidioidin
6. Obtain sputum for cytology and AFB stain
7. Liver function studies
8. ANA, rheumatoid factor
9. Mononucleosis test, CMV and other viral titers, ASLO and streptozyme titers
10. Serum calcium
11. CK

Radiographic evaluation
1. Chest x-ray films: look for evidence of TB, mediastinal adenopathy (sarcoidosis, neoplasm), cardiomegaly, failure (decompensation secondary to valvular lesions)
2. Abdominal x-ray films: indicated in patients with history of abdominal pain; look for evidence of calcifications (calculi, TB), obstruction (neoplasms), abdominal abscess

Additional diagnostic tests are indicated if the initial tests are nondiagnostic or if the history and physical exam suggest a particular diagnosis
1. Focal neurologic deficits: CT scan of head to rule out cerebral abscess, neoplasm
2. Lethargy, confusion: lumbar puncture to rule out meningitis, encephalitis, meningeal carcinomatosis
3. Lymphadenopathy: lymph node biopsy to rule out lymphoma or neoplasm, HIV titer
4. Cough, dyspnea: bronchoscopy to rule out TB or neoplasm if chest x-ray film shows abnormalities; consider gastric aspirate for acid-fast culture to rule out TBC; consider ventilation/perfusion scan to rule out pulmonary embolism
5. Hepatosplenomegaly or abdominal pain: CT scan of abdomen
6. Cardiac murmur: echocardiogram may show valve vegetation in SBE
7. Headache, tenderness over temporal area: temporal artery biopsy to rule out temporal arteritis
8. Bone pain: bone scan, metastatic bone series, protein electrophoresis
9. Guaiac-positive stool: colonoscopy or barium enema plus sigmoidoscopy
10. Hematuria: renal ultrasound, IVP, cystoscopy
11. Liver biopsy: useful in patients with hepatic dysfunction to rule out granulomatous liver disease
12. Bone marrow exam: useful in suspected lymphoma, myeloma, or miliary TBC
13. Gallium scan: used to detect occult infection or neoplasm, but it is rarely helpful
14. Exploratory laparotomy: indicated only when other tests (CT scan of abdomen, liver-spleen scan, or ultrasound) are nondiagnostic and an abdominal source of fever is suspected

| 15.4 | ACQUIRED IMMUNODEFICIENCY SYNDROME

Definitions
1. AIDS-related complex (ARC) is a syndrome characterized by the presence of lab abnormalities (e.g., inversion of T4/T8 ratio, detection of human immunodeficiency virus [HIV, formerly HTLV III or LAV]), anergy, and clinical abnormalities (e.g., weight loss, lymphadenopathy, fevers), but no discoverable opportunistic infections or secondary cancers[37]
2. AIDS: development of selected opportunistic diseases in a patient with lab evidence of HIV infection

Classification

The Centers For Disease Control (CDC) has classified patients with HIV infection into four major groups based on clinical characteristics*

Group I: acute infection
Mononucleosis-like syndrome associated with seroconversion

Group II: asymptomatic infection
Positive HIV antibody or viral culture; may be subclassified on basis of laboratory evaluation (CBC, platelet count, T-cell subset studies)

Group III: persistent generalized lymphadenopathy
Palpable lymphadenopathy ($>$ 1 cm) at two or more extrainguinal sites for more than 3 months in the absence of a concurrent illness or infection to explain the findings; may be subclassified on the basis of laboratory evaluation (see above)

Group IV: other HIV disease
1. Subgroup A (constitutional disease): one or more of the following: fever or diarrhea persisting more than 1 month or involuntary weight loss greater than 10% of baseline; and absence of a concurrent illness or infection to explain the findings
2. Subgroup B (neurologic disease): one or more of the following: dementia, myelopathy, or peripheral neuropathy; and absence of a concurrent illness or condition
3. Subgroup C (secondary infectious diseases): infectious disease associated with HIV infection and/or at least moderately indicative of a defect in cell-mediated immunity
   a. Category C-1: symptomatic or invasive disease due to one of 12 specified diseases listed in the surveillance definition of AIDS: *Pneumocystis carinii* pneumonia, chronic cryptosporidiosis, toxoplasmosis, extraintestinal strongyloidiasis, isosporiasis, candidiasis (esophageal, bronchial, or pulmonary), cryptococcosis, histoplasmosis, mycobacterial infection *(Mycobacterium avium* complex or *M. kansasii),* cytomegalovirus infection, chronic mucocutaneous or disseminated herpes simplex virus infection, and progressive multifocal leukoencephalopathy
   b. Category C-2: symptomatic or invasive disease due to one of six other specified diseases: oral hairy leukoplakia, multidermatomal herpes zoster, recurrent *Salmonella* bacteremia, nocardiosis, tuberculosis, and oral candidiasis (thrush)
4. Subgroup D (secondary cancers): diagnosis of one or more cancers known to be associated with HIV infection as listed in the surveillance definition of AIDS and at least moderately indicative of a defect in cell-mediated immunity: Kaposi's sarcoma, non-Hodgkin's lymphoma (small, noncleaved lymphoma or immunoblastic sarcoma), or primary lymphoma of the brain
5. Subgroup E (other conditions in HIV infection): clinical findings or diseases, not classifiable above, that may be attributable to HIV infection and are indicative of a defect in cell-mediated immunity; symptoms attri-

---

*From Centers For Disease Control: Classification system for human T-lymphotropic virus type III/ lymphadenopathy-associated virus infections, MMWR 35:334, 1986

butable to either HIV infection or a coexisting disease not classified else-
where; or clinical illnessess that may be complicated or altered by HIV
infection. These include chronic lymphoid interstitial pneumonitis and
constitutional symptoms, secondary infectious diseases, and neoplasms
not listed above

Serologic testing

HIV antibodies are initially detected by enzyme-linked immunosorbent assay
(ELISA). This assay is a highly sensitive and specific marker for HIV infection, particularly for screening and epidemiologic research.[56] To rule out
false positives, the standard confirmation assay used is the Western blot. This
technique uses electrophoretically banded proteins to identify viral core antigens or envelope antigens.[41] It is highly specific for the AIDS virus, but it
is not as sensitive as the ELISA test because more antibody is required to
result in a positive test.[47]

Pathophysiology

The causative agent of AIDS is a retrovirus that attacks the immune system,
resulting in numerous immunologic abnormalities[7] (quantitative and functional abnormalities of T lymphocytes, functional abnormalities of B lymphocytes and monocyte/macrophages, and serologic abnormalities). Because
of an impaired immune response, the individual is overwhelmed by "opportunistic infections" as well as certain forms of malignant tumors[14] (Kaposi's
sarcoma, angiosarcomas, B cell lymphomas, Burkitt's lymphoma, Hodgkin's
disease, T cell leukemias, squamous cell carcinomas, hairy cell leukemia).

Opportunistic infections in patients with AIDS

The major opportunistic infections in patients with AIDS are summarized in
Table 15-2. Therapeutic measures are only partially effective. Current research indicates that 3'-azido-3'-deoxythymidine (AZT), a thymidine analog
with potent antiviral activity against HIV in vitro, can prolong survival in
AIDS patients (particularly post-*Pneumocystis carinii* pneumonia) and may
be effective in slowing or reversing some AIDS-virus associated clinical abnormalities.[61] Table 15-3 summarizes the diagnostic and therapeutic approach to opportunistic infections in AIDS patients.

Kaposi's sarcoma (KS) in AIDS patients

KS is common in young homosexual men with AIDS. The Kaposi's sarcoma
identified in AIDS patients differs from the "classic" type usually found in
elderly Mediterranean men. Table 15-4 describes the major differences. Single-agent IV vinblastine (4-8 mg/week) is reported to be effective in controlling the malignancy in approximately 30% of patients and in temporarily
arresting tumor progression in 50% of patients.[54]

Prevention

1. Although the AIDS virus has been isolated from blood, semen, saliva,
   and other body fluids, the main modes of transmission are the following:
   a. Intimate sexual contact (particularly in homosexuals, although bi-di-
      rectional heterosexual transmission is increasing in frequency)[35]
   b. Use of or sharing of infected needles (IV drug abusers)

Table 15-2 Microorganisms causing opportunistic infections in AIDS patients

	Syndromes	Comment
Viruses		
Cytomegalovirus	Encephalitis, chorioretinitis, pneumonia, hepatitis, colitis, adrenalitis, disseminated infection	Found in almost all patients; liver, lungs, and colon are frequent sites of severe disease and biopsy usually needed to document. Responsible for clinical adrenal insufficiency. Characteristic chorioretinitis.
Herpes simplex virus	Persistent, recurrent, or disseminated skin ulcers	Herpes simplex virus type-2 perineal lesions are frequently an early occurrence; respond to antiviral therapy but recur.
Varicella-zoster	Local, severe, or disseminated infection	Tends to recur.
Epstein-Barr virus	Lymphoma	Aggressive B cell lymphomas seen, including central nervous system lesions.
Papovavirus-JC	Central nervous system infection	Progressive multifocal leukoencephalopathy is one of the major central nervous system diseases.
Adenoviruses	Colonization Disseminated infection	Regularly isolated, rarely cause symptomatic disease; high serotypes similar to those of bone-marrow transplant recipients.
Bacteria		
Commonly taking advantage of T cell defects		
Mycobacterium avium-intracellulare	Disseminated infection, severe gastrointestinal disease, massive intraabdominal lymphadenopathy	Usually serovar 4, remarkably heavy infection. Isolated regularly from blood and seen on acid-fast stain of stool. Portal of entry appears to be gastrointestinal tract. Poor response to therapy.
Mycobacterium tuberculosis	Adenitis, pulmonary infection, meningitis	Variable presentation. Responds to therapy. Some strains may be resistant.
Mycobacterium sp.	Disseminated infection	Usually accompanies other life-threatening infection.
Nocardia asteroides	Pulmonary-pericardial infection, brain abscess	Accompanies other opportunistic infection.
Salmonella sp.	Typhoidal syndrome, severe gastroenteritis with bacteremia	Recurs.

Listeria monocytogenes	Bacteremia	Responds promptly to therapy.
Legionella sp.	Pneumonias, cellulitis	Especially severe.
Commonly taking advantage of B cell defects		
Streptococcus pneumoniae	Pneumonia, bacteremia	Respond promptly to therapy.
Haemophilus influenzae	Pneumonia, bacteremia	May cause diffuse infiltrates resembling pneumocytosis.
Reasons uncertain		
Staphylococcus aureus	Bacteremia, skin infections, pneumonia	Pneumonias complicate pneumocystosis in patients with Kaposi's sarcoma
Clostridium perfringens	Bacteremia	Mild abdominal complaints. Transient. Secondary to Kaposi's sarcoma lesions of bowel?
Shigella sp.	Diarrhea, bacteremia	Persistent and recurrent.
Parasites		
Pneumocystis carinii	Pneumonia	Often large numbers of organisms seen, toluidine blue on bronchoalveolar lavage fluid an effective stain in our experience; prolonged therapy advisable ($\geq$3 weeks).
Toxoplasma gondii	Encephalitis, brain abscess	Brain abscess and encephalitis common; antibody response may be poor, especially IgM; prolonged therapy necessary.
Cryptosporidium sp.	Gastroenteritis	Illness varies from mild, self-limited diarrhea to cholera-like syndrome, unresponsive to any therapy; organisms seen by acid-fast stain or sucrose flotation.
Fungi		
Candida sp.	Oropharyngitis, esophagitis, vaginitis	Most disease is of the mucous membranes and esophagus; most isolates are *C. albicans*, but *C. tropicalis* has been identified.
Cryptococcus neoformans	Meningitis, disseminated infection, pneumonia	Pneumonias as well as meningitis seen; should look for antigen in serum as well as cerebrospinal fluid.
Histoplasma capsulatum	Disseminated infection	Seen in nonendemic areas in persons with residence to endemic areas in the past; should stain and culture marrow and peripheral blood buffy coat.
Aspergillus sp.	Pneumonia	Reported, but apparently very uncommon.

From Armstrong, D., et al.: Ann. Intern. Med. **103:**738, 1985.

Table 15-3 *Diagnosis and therapy for selected opportunistic infections in AIDS patients*

Opportunistic Infection	Diagnosis	Therapy
Pneumocystis carinii	Bronchoalveolar lavage Transbronchial biopsy	Trimethoprim-sulfamethoxazole, pentamidine
Cytomegalovirus (CMV)	Tissue biopsy and culture	DHPG is useful in suppressing virus replication, but it is not curative
Cryptosporidium	Colonoscopy with bowel biopsy, stool sample Auramine stain or modified acid-fast stain will detect organism	Spiramycin, furazolidone, DFMO
Candida albicans	Smear of throat swab	Nystatin oral suspension Clotrimazole troches Oral ketoconazole
Cryptococcus neoformans	India ink and Gram stain of CSF	Amphotericin B and flucytosine
Herpes simplex	Culture of material obtained by swab or biopsy of lesion	Topical acyclovir or IV acyclovir for 5 days
Mycobacterium avium-intracellulare	Blood cultures for *Mycobacteria*. Stool, bronchial washings, and urine smears and cultures for acid-fast bacilli[25]	Combination therapy with ansamycin, ethionamide, clofazimine Antituberculous drugs (INH, rifampin, ethambutol) may be partially effective in selected patients
Varicella-zoster virus	Swab or biopsy of lesion	Vidarabine or acyclovir
Toxoplasma gondii	CNS involvement is suggested by CT scan of head demonstrating ring-enhancing lesions Biopsy confirms diagnosis	Sulfonamide, pyrimethamine

From Armstrong, D., et al.: Ann. Intern. Med. **103**:738, 1985.

Table 15-4 Kaposi's sarcoma: classic versus AIDS-associated

Characteristic	AIDS-Associated KS	Classic KS
Initial clinical manifestations	Small pink or red macules widely distributed over the trunk; these macules eventually develop into the classic dark blue plaques	Large violet–dark blue macules present over the lower extremities
Visceral lesions	Common	Rare
Mean age of patients	<40 years old	>60 years old
Lymphadenopathy	Frequent	Rare
Course	Very aggressive	Indolent

2. Infection with AIDS virus by transfusion of blood or certain blood products (e.g., factor VIII) derived from infected donors is no longer a problem since donors are routinely screened for the presence of the HIV virus
3. The risk of HIV infection among health care workers appears to be low and related to needle-stick exposure.[57] The following are suggested practices for caring for AIDS patients:[34]
   a. Blood and body fluid (discharge precautions)
   b. Gloves should be worn when handling blood specimens, blood-soiled items, body fluids, excretions, and secretions
   c. Hands should be washed after removing gloves and before leaving the rooms of AIDS patients; halogenated soap and most common disinfectants (e.g., hydrogen peroxide, alcohol, creosol solution [Lysol]) destroy the virus
   d. Masks are recommended only for direct, sustained contact with a patient who is coughing extensively or a patient who is intubated and being suctioned
   e. Instruments that come in contact with blood secretions, excretion, or tissues (e.g., laryngoscopes, endotracheal tubes) should be sterilized before re-use
   f. Special care should be taken when handling sharp items (e.g., needles, scalpel blades)

15.5 INFECTIONS IN THE IMMUNOCOMPROMISED HOST

Definition

An immunocompromised host is one whose resistance to infection is impaired by an underlying disease or by immunosuppressive therapy.

Diagnostic considerations

1. The list of potential pathogens in the immunocompromised host is quite extensive and includes:

      a. Pathogens commonly affecting normal hosts
      b. Pathogens predominantly affecting compromised hosts
2. Specific immune deficits predispose to infection with specific microorganisms, thus the type of infection present in the immunocompromised host can often be predicted by the immune defect present
3. The clinical manifestations may be greatly modified or masked by the underlying illness:
      a. The patient may not be able to mount a fever response or a leukocytosis
      b. Pulmonary infiltrates in pulmonary infections may be absent or slow to develop because of leukopenia
      c. The clinical findings may be minimal (e.g., mild headache without meningismus in patients with cryptococcal meningitis, deep-seated abscesses without evidence of inflammation)
4. The infectious process may involve multiple organs and multiple agents (e.g., disseminated CMV, candidiasis, and *Pneumocystis pneumonia* in patients with AIDS)
5. Rapid diagnosis and initiation of therapy is crucial for patient survival

General approach to neutropenic patients with suspected infection

1. History
      a. Inquire about recent use of antibiotics, steroids, chemotherapeutic agents, and radiotherapy
      b. History of recurrent infections, recent travel, and exposure to contagious diseases
2. Physical exam
      a. Presence of skin lesions
         (1) Ecthyma gangrenosum: embolic skin manifestations of gram-negative bacilli; usually begins as a red macule (0.5-3 cm in diameter) then becomes more papular with central necrosis or vesicle formation surrounded by erythema
         (2) Mucormycosis: usually seen in diabetics; manifested as a black eschar on the palate and paranasal sinuses
      b. Evidence of fungal colonization (oropharynx, rectum, vagina)
      c. Evaluate mental status, look for evidence of meningismus or focal deficits
      d. Auscultate heart for presence of new murmurs or accentuation of an existing murmur (suggestive of bacterial endocarditis) particularly in IV drug addicts and patients with central lines
      e. Evidence of respiratory infection (decreased breath sounds, rales, rhonchi); the lungs are the most frequent site of infection in immunocompromised patients
3. Initial lab results
      a. CBC with differential count
      b. Urinalysis, urine culture, sensitivity, and Gram stain
      c. Blood cultures
      d. Sputum Gram stain, acid-fast stain, and cultures
      e. Culture, sensitivity, and Gram stain of any skin lesions
      g. Lumbar puncture, if indicated
4. Chest x-ray: look for infiltrates, lobar consolidation, cavitary lesions

Therapy of neutropenic patient (<500 PMNs) with FUO

1. Consider gram-negative organisms *(Pseudomonas, Klebsiella, E. coli)* and initiate IV antibiotic therapy with combination of
   a. Aminoglycoside (amikacin, tobramycin, gentamicin) plus
   b. β Lactam (azlocillin, mezlocillin) or selected cephalosporins with antipseudomonal activity (e.g., ceftazidime)
   Combination antimicrobial therapy is associated with increased patient survival when compared with single-drug therapy of *Pseudomonas* infections even if synergy cannot be demonstrated in vivo[2]
2. If fever persists and there is no clinical improvement in a patient with suspected pulmonary infection, add erythromycin to provide coverage against *Legionella*[11]
3. If there is no improvement after 5-7 days and all cultures are negative, consider adding amphotericin B for therapy of possible fungal infections
4. If progressive pulmonary involvement occurs, consider open lung biopsy

15.6 BACTEREMIA AND SEPSIS

Definitions[36]

1. Bacteremia: presence of viable bacteria in the blood as evidenced by a positive blood culture; bacteremia can be:
   a. Transient (e.g., dental extractions)
   b. Continuous or sustained (e.g., bacterial endocarditis)
   c. Intermittent (e.g., intermittent biliary tract obstruction)
2. Septicemia: bacteremia with clinical manifestations (fever, chills)
3. Septic shock: Life-threatening manifestation of bacteremia caused by the effects of bacteria cell wall substances (activation of the complement, coagulation, and kallikrein-kinin systems, ACTH/endorphin release)[32]

Septicemic septic shock

1. Etiology
   a. Gram-negative bacilli *(Escherichia coli, Pseudomonas, Proteus, Klebsiella, Enterobacter, Serratia)*
   b. Gram-positive organisms (*Staphylococcus aureus*, pneumococci, streptococci)
   c. Fungal infections
2. Sites of infection
   a. GU tract (most common site of sepsis in the elderly)
   b. GI tract
   c. Respiratory tract
   d. Wounds, infected IV lines
   e. Meninges
3. Predisposing factors: malnutrition, instrumentation or other invasive procedures, advanced age, immunosuppressive therapy, neoplastic diseases
4. Clinical manifestations
   a. Early phase
      (1) Hypotension
      (2) Hyperventilation (respiratory alkalosis)
      (3) Skin warm, dry

    (4) Fever (may not be present in elderly or chronically ill patients; some of these patients may actually manifest hypothermia)

    (5) Chills generally occur approximately 1 hour after the acute episode of bacteremia[4] at a time when the host has generally cleared the bloodstream of bacteria; the highest yield for blood cultures is before the onset of chills

    (6) Lab results: leukocytosis with shift to left or neutropenia

    (7) Hemodynamic monitoring: decreased PCWP and SVR, and increased CO

  b. Late phase

    (1) Significant hypotension

    (2) Skin cool and clammy

    (3) Oliguria

    (4) Metabolic acidosis (secondary to lactic acidosis)

    (5) Hemodynamic monitoring: decreased PCWP and CO, and increased SVR

5. Management

  a. Treat hypotension with saline infusion

    (1) Colloid plus crystalloid solutions may be necessary in selected patients

    (2) Vasopressors are indicated only when previous measures fail to correct the hypotension

  b. IV antibiotic therapy: early treatment is crucial for patient survival, (do not wait until all blood cultures have been obtained if necessary); use broad antibiotic coverage with combination of:

    (1) Aminoglycoside (amikacin, gentamicin, tobramycin)

    (2) Additional agents depending on suspected site of infection and predisposing factors:

      (a) Neutropenic patient: add a β lactam (ticarcillin, mezlocillin) to provide additional coverage of *Pseudomonas*

      (b) Suspected skin infection: add anti-staphylococcal agent (nafcillin, oxacillin)

      (c) Suspected intraabdominal focus: add cefoxitin, clindamycin, or metronidazole to cover anaerobic organisms, plus ampicillin to cover enterococci

      (d) Suspected pulmonary infection: add a cephalosporin (e.g., cefazolin)

      (e) Suspected UTI: add ampicillin to cover enterococci

  c. Monitor with a pulmonary artery catheter

  d. Low-dose dopamine is useful to maintain renal perfusion

  e. Drain any septic foci

  f. High-dose IV corticosteroids are controversial and studies have shown that they do not improve the overall survival of patients with severe late septic shock[44]; but if used, they should be administered within the first 4 hours of shock as a single dose (e.g., methylprednisolone sodium succinate, 30 mg/kg IV)

  g. Antibody to endotoxin helps to prevent gram-negative shock and improve survival in surgical patients[51] however, additional studies are necessary to clearly document its indications

CELLULITIS

Definition
Cellulitis is a superficial inflammatory condition of the skin. It is characterized by erythema, warmth, and tenderness of the area involved.

General approach
1. Lab tests
   a. Gram stain and culture (aerobic and anerobic) of:
      (1) Aspirated material from
         (a) Advancing edge of cellulitis
         (b) Any vesicles
      (2) Swab of any drainage material
      (3) Punch biopsy (in selected patients)
   b. Blood cultures
   c. ASO titer (in suspected streptococcal disease)
2. Despite the above measures, the cause of cellulitis remains unidentified in most patients[23]; in these patients initial antimicrobial therapy should cover both staphylococcal and streptococcal cellulitis (e.g., first-generation cephalosporin or penicillinase-resistant penicillin)

Identification and therapy[30]
1. Erysipelas
   a. Superficial spreading, warm, erythematous lesion distinguished by its indurated, elevated margin; lymphatic involvement and vesicle formation are common
   b. Generally secondary to group A β-hemolytic streptococci
   c. Commonly involves face and legs
   d. Gram stain reveals small gram-positive cocci in chains
   e. Therapy
      (1) PO: penicillin V, 250-500 mg qid
      (2) IM: penicillin G (procaine), 600,000 U bid
      (3) IV: penicillin G (aqueous), 4-6 million U/day
      NOTE: Use erythromycin, cephalosporins, clindamycin, or vancomycin in patients allergic to penicillin
2. Staphylococcal cellulitis
   a. Area involved is erythematous, hot, and swollen; differentiated from erysipelas by nonelevated, poorly demarcated margins
   b. Local tenderness and regional adenopathy are common
   c. Gram stain shows clusters of large gram-positive cocci
   d. Therapy
      (1) PO: dicloxacillin 250-500 mg qid
      (2) IV: oxacillin or nafcillin 1-2 g q4-6h
      (3) Use vancomycin in patients allergic to penicillin
      (4) Cephalosporins (cephalotin, cephalexin, cephradine) also provide adequate antistaphylococcal coverage
3. *Haemophilus influenzae* cellulitis
   a. Area involved has a blue red–purple red color
   b. Occurs mainly in children; it generally involves the face in children and the neck or upper chest in adults

c. Gram stain shows pleomorphic gram-negative rods; blood cultures are frequently positive
d. Therapy
   (1) PO: amoxicillin or cefaclor (Ceclor) 500 mg tid
   (2) IV: cefuroxime or amoxicillin; trimethoprim-sulfamethoxazole, or chloramphenicol may be used in patients allergic to penicillin
   (3) Amoxicillin is ineffective in ampicillin-resistant strains; IV cefuroxime is indicated in severely ill patients

15.8 URINARY TRACT INFECTIONS (UTI)

Definitions

1. Pyuria: presence of >10 leukocytes/ml of uncentrifuged urine
2. Bacteriuria
   a. "Significant" bacteriuria has been generally defined as the presence of >100,000 bacteria/ml of urine (in urine cultures)
   b. Counts between 10,000-100,000/ml can also be indicative of infection, especially in the presence of pyuria; it has been shown[45] that up to 50% of acutely dysuric women with gram-negative coliform infection of the urinary tract have <100,000 bacteria/ml of urine
   c. The presence of bacteria on urinalysis generally implies bacteria counts >30,000/ml

Diagnostic methods[51]

1. Urinalysis (clean-catch urine specimen)
2. Gram stain of urine
3. Urine culture
4. Test urine with dipstick containing leukocyte esterase assay to detect presence of neutrophils in the urine; the specificity of this test in predicting pyuria is >90%, sensitivity is >70%[9,16]
5. Blood cultures: indicated only in suspected pyelonephritis
6. IVP/cystoscopy/ultrasound: indicated in men with UTI and women with recurrent UTI; done to rule out obstruction, calculi, and papillary necrosis

Major risk factors

1. Indwelling Foley catheters
2. Obstruction to urine flow (strictures, calculi, neurogenic bladder)
3. Pregnancy
4. Female sex
5. Immunocompromised host

Common infecting organisms

1. *Escherichia coli*
2. *Proteus*
3. *Klebsiella*
4. Enterococci
5. *Pseudomonas*
6. *Staphylococcus*

Classification of dysuria

Dysuria (pain or discomfort on voiding) effects approximately 25% of all women yearly. Recognizing that dysuria can be caused by several disease entities, Komaroff[26,27] has categorized "acute dysuria" into the following seven entities, based on clinical and lab findings:

1. Acute pyelonephritis
2. Subclinical pyelonephritis
3. Chlamydial urethritis
4. Urethritis secondary to gonococci (also *Candida albicans, Trichomonas vaginilis,* herpes simplex)
5. Vaginitis
6. Lower urinary tract bacterial infection
7. No apparent infectious pathogen

Diagnosis and therapy[26,27]

The diagnostic and therapeutic approach to acute dysuria varies with the suspected cause; the salient points to each cause are described below:

1. Acute pyelonephritis
   a. Symptoms
      (1) Fever, frequency, dysuria, urgency
      (2) Flank pain or tenderness
      (3) Malaise, myalgias, anorexia
   b. Lab results
      (1) Urinalysis shows pyuria, bacteriuria
      (2) Gram stain of urine shows presence of bacteria and leukocytes
      (3) Urine culture counts generally >100,000 bacteria/ml of urine
      (4) Gram-negative rods are most commonly seen
      (5) Blood cultures are indicated in patients suspected of acute pyelonephritis
   c. Treatment: IV antibiotic therapy based on Gram stain of urine
      (1) If gram-negative rods or gram-positive cocci are present, the patient should be started on an aminoglycoside (gentamicin, tobramycin, netilmicin) plus ampicillin
      (2) In case of penicillin allergy and gram-positive cocci, use vancomycin plus an aminoglycoside; vigorous hydration is also indicated
2. Subclinical pyelonephritis
   a. Diagnosis
      (1) Clinical presentation undistinguishable from "lower tract" UTI (dysuria, frequency, urgency)
      (2) Increased incidence in diabetics and patients with recurrent UTI or history of childhood UTIs
      (3) Urinalysis shows pyuria, bacteriuria
      (4) Urine culture colony counts generally >100,000/ml
   b. Therapy
      (1) Preferred initial treatment is single dose amoxicillin 3 g, PO
         (a) Therapy with single-dose amoxicillin is also useful to differentiate bladder infection from subclinical pyelonephritis, since persistent infection or relapse within a few weeks of treatment indicates subclinical pyelonephritis which would dictate a 2 week course of therapy

        (b) Male patients, pregnant females, and any patient with underlying obstruction should be treated initially with 7-14 days of therapy

     (2) A follow-up urine culture (posttreatment) may be indicated following single-dose amoxicillin therapy[42]

3. Chlamydial urethritis
   a. Diagnosis
     (1) Dysuria present in a young, sexually active patient
     (2) Urinalysis shows pyuria without bacteriuria
     (3) Cervical discharge and edema
     (4) Diagnosis can be easily made with use of commercially available monoclonal antibodies[50]
   b. Treatment
     (1) Tetracycline 500 mg PO qid for 10 days
     (2) In pregnant women, use erythromycin 250 mg PO qid for 7 days
     (3) Both patient and sexual partner should be treated

4. Gonococcal urethritis
   a. Diagnosis
     (1) Dysuria and urethral discharge in a sexually active patient
     (2) Urinalysis shows pyuria without bacteriuria
     (3) Gram stain of urethral discharge shows polymorphonuclear leukocytes with intracellular gram-negative diplococci
   b. Treatment: see section 15.9

5. Vaginitis must be considered in any young woman presenting with symptoms of "dysuria"
   a. Diagnosis is made by vaginal exam
   b. Coexistence of vaginitis and urethritis (e.g., *Trichomonas vaginalis* can cause both) should be ruled out with exam and appropriate cultures

6. "Lower tract" UTI (cystitis, acute urethral syndrome)
   a. Diagnosis
     (1) Dysuria, frequency, urgency, suprapubic pain or fullness
     (2) Pyuria and bacteriuria seen on urinalysis
     (3) Urine culture is not cost effective[8] and should not be routinely obtained in suspected lower tract UTI
   b. Treatment: single-dose trimethoprim-sulfamethoxazole (TMP/SMX)[46] 320 mg/1600 mg (e.g., bactrim DS—two tablets) or amoxicillin 3 g PO; male patients, pregnant females, or any patient with underlying obstruction require 7-14 days of therapy (e.g., TMP/SMX 160 mg/800 mg PO bid or ampicillin 250-500 mg qid)

7. No apparent infectious pathogen
   a. These patients have dysuria but not pyuria
   b. The dysuria may be secondary to urethral trauma, interstitial cystitis, chemical agents, or estrogen deficiency (postmenopausal women)
   c. Antibiotic treatment is not indicated

Management of asymptomatic bacteriuria

The management of asymptomatic bacteriuria varies with the age of the patient and with the presence of associated conditions (pregnancy, immunosuppression).

1. Elderly patients
   a. Bacteriuria is common in the elderly
   b. It appears related to functional status and is generally transient
   c. Antibiotic treatment is generally not indicated[6]
2. Non-pregnant adults
   a. Antimicrobial therapy is controversial
   b. Single-dose treatment with TMP/SMX (320/1,600 mg) is generally indicated in diabetics, patients undergoing urologic manipulation, and immunocompromised patients
3. Pregnant women
   a. Treat pregnant patients; if untreated, they have a higher incidence of acute pyelonephritis and low–birth weight infants
   b. The choice of antibiotic depends on the results of urine culture and sensitivity; however, avoid antibiotics contraindicated in pregnancy

Management of recurrent UTI

1. Determine reason for recurrence:
   a. Superinfection: common in patients with indwelling catheters
   b. Reinfection: generally associated with sexual intercourse
   c. Resistant organism
2. Repeated infections with the same pathogen is an indication for cystoscopy and IVP to rule out underlying urinary tract disease
3. Prophylactic therapy with TMP-SMX (e.g., ½ tab at hs for 6 months) may be effective in some patients
4. Patients with recurring UTI following intercourse may benefit from post-coital prophylaxis (e.g., ½ tab TMP/SMX after coitus)

15.9 TREATMENT GUIDELINES FOR SELECTED SEXUALLY TRANSMITTED DISEASES*

Reducing risk of acquiring sexually transmitted diseases

The only effective way to *prevent* acquiring sexually transmitted diseases (STDs) is to *abstain* from all forms of sexual contact. To *reduce risk* of STD, those who are sexually active should:
1. Avoid multiple partners, anonymous partners, prostitutes, and other persons with multiple sex partners
2. Avoid sexual contact with persons who have a genital discharge, genital warts, genital herpes lesions or other suspicious genital lesions, or those with lab evidence of HIV infection or hepatitis B surface antigen
3. Avoid oral-anal sex to prevent enteric infections
4. Avoid genital contact with oral "cold sores"
5. Use condoms and diaphragms in combination with spermicides
6. Have a periodic exam for sexually transmitted agents and syndromes if at high risk for STD
7. Avoid oral-genital and anal intercourse to protect against HIV infection, gonococcal pharyngitis, and proctitis; the use of condoms will decrease the risk of transmitting or contracting these infections

*From Morbidity and Mortality Weekly Report, Oct. 18, **34**(4) 1985.

CHLAMYDIA TRACHOMATIS INFECTION

Chlamydia trachomatis is the most prevalent sexually transmitted bacterial pathogen in the United States today. Although lab tests for detection of *C. trachomatis* are becoming widely available, diagnosis and treatment are frequently based on the clinical syndrome. The following guidelines are for lab-documented infections caused by non-lymphogranuloma venereum strains of *C. trachomatis*. (See discussions under Gonococcal infections.)

Treatment of uncomplicated urethral, endocervical, or rectal infection

1. Tetracycline hydrochloride (HCI) 500 mg PO qid for 7 days, *or*
2. Doxycycline 100 mg PO bid for 7 days

GONOCOCCAL INFECTIONS

Treatment of uncomplicated urethral, endocervical, or rectal infection

An important concern in treatment for gonorrhea is coexisting chlamydial infection, documented in up to 45% of gonorrhea cases when adequate chlamydial cultures are performed. Concern also exists about the problem of patient compliance with multiple-day tetracycline/doxycycline regimens for gonococcal infections and for the potential selection of tetracycline-resistant isolates when incomplete doses are taken. To address these concerns, a single-dose regimen for gonorrhea should be administered just before a tetracycline or doxycycline regimen.

1. Amoxicillin 3 g or ampicillin 3.5 g PO *or* aqueous procaine penicillin G (APPG) 4.8 million U IM *or* ceftriaxone 250 mg IM
   a. Amoxicillin, ampicillin, and penicillin (but not ceftriaxone) are accompanied by probenecid 1.0 g PO
   b. *Comment:* APPG may be less desirable because of associated pain and toxicity
2. Tetracycline HCI 500 mg PO qid for 7 days *or* doxycycline 100 mg PO bid for 7 days
3. For patients in whom tetracyclines are contraindicated or not tolerated, the single-dose regimen may be followed by erythromycin base or stearate 500 mg PO qid for 7 days *or* erythromycin ethylsuccinate 800 mg PO qid for 7 days

Disseminated gonococcal infection

Hospitalization is recommended, especially for those who cannot reliably comply with treatment, have uncertain diagnoses, or have purulent synovial effusions or other complications. Attempts should be made to exclude endocarditis or meningitis. Several acceptable treatment schedules exist for the gonococcal arthritis/dermatitis syndrome, including the following:

1. Aqueous crystalline penicillin G 10 million U/day IV for at least 3 days followed by amoxicillin or ampicillin 500 mg PO qid for at least 7 days
2. Amoxicillin 3.0 g or ampicillin 3.5 g each with probenecid 10 g PO followed by amoxicillin or ampicillin 500 mg PO qid for at least 7 days
3. Cefoxitin 1.0 g IV qid for at least 7 days
4. Cefotaxime 500 mg IV qid for at least 7 days
5. Ceftriaxone 1.0 g IV once daily for 7 days

Penicillin-resistant *Neisseria gonorrhoeae*

Penicillinase-producing *Neisseria gonorrhoeae* (PPNG): Patients with proven PPNG infection or who are likely to have acquired gonorrhea in areas of high PPNG prevalence and their sex partners should receive spectinomycin 2.0 g IM or ceftriaxone 250 mg IM both followed by tetracycline, doxycycline, or erythromycin as outlined above; to treat pharyngeal gonococcal infection caused by PPNG, administer ceftriaxone 250 mg IM or nine tablets of trimethoprim/sulfamethoxazole (120 mg 3600 mg) per day in one daily dose for 5 days

GENITAL HERPES SIMPLEX VIRUS INFECTION

Genital herpes infection is a viral disease that may be chronic and recurring and for which no known cure exists. Acyclovir regimens provide partial control of the signs and symptoms of herpetic eruptions, but do not affect the subsequent risk, frequency, or severity of recurrences after the drug is discontinued.

First clinical episode

A careful history should be obtained to establish that this is the patient's first episode of genital herpes.

1. *To reduce symptoms:* acyclovir 200 mg PO 5 times daily for 7-10 days, initiated within 6 days of onset of lesions will shorten the median duration of first episode eruptions by 3 to 5 days and may reduce systemic symptoms in primary episodes
2. For patients who have severe symptoms or complications that necessitate hospitalization, an alternative regimen is acyclovir 5 mg/kg of body weight IVq8h for 5-7 days
   a. This treatment shortens the median course of first episodes by approximately 7 days
   b. Topical acyclovir ointment has marginal benefit in decreasing virus shedding, but has no significant effect on symptoms or healing time
   c. The above regimens are also useful for herpes simplex proctitis

Recurrent genital herpes

Since benefit to the patient may be minimal, treatment for recurrent episodes should be limited to those patients who typically have severe symptoms and who are able to begin therapy at the beginning of the prodrome or within 2 days of onset of lesions. Acyclovir 200 mg PO 5 times daily for 5 days initiated within 2 days of onset will shorten the mean clinical course by about 1 day. IV and topical acyclovir are not indicated for recurrences.

Sexually transmitted epididymo-orchitis

Sexually transmitted epididymo-orchitis occurs in young adults and is associated with presence of urethritis, absence of underlying genitourinary pathology, and absence of gram-negative rods on Gram stain of urine.

1. Amoxicillin 3 g PO, ampicillin 3.5 g PO, or aqueous procaine penicillin G 4.8 million U IM at 2 sites (each along with probenecid 1.0 g PO) or spectinomycin 2.0 g IM or ceftriaxone 250 mg IM *followed by*
2. Tetracycline HCl 500 mg PO qid for 10 days, *or*
3. Doxycycline 100 mg PO bid for 10 days, *or*

4. When tetracyclines are contraindicated or not tolerated: erythromycin base or stearate 500 mg PO qid for 7 days or erythromycin ethylsuccinate 800 mg PO qid for 7 days

SYPHILIS

Early syphilis

Early syphilis (primary, secondary, or latent syphilis of less than 1 year's duration) should be treated with benzathine penicillin G 2.4 million U total IM in a single dose. Patients who are allergic to penicillin should be treated with tetracycline HCl 500 mg PO qid for 15 days.

Syphilis of more than 1 year's duration

Syphilis of more than 1 year's duration (latent syphilis of indeterminate or more than 1 year's duration, cardiovascular, or late benign syphilis) except neurosyphilis, should be treated with benzathine penicillin G 2.4 million U IM once a week for 3 successive weeks (7.2 million U total). There are no published clinical data that adequately document the efficacy of drugs other than penicillin for syphilis of more than 1 year's duration. Cerebrospinal fluid (CSF) exams should be performed before therapy with these regimens. Patients who are allergic to penicillin should be treated with tetracycline HCl 500 mg PO qid for 30 days. Patient compliance with this regimen may be difficult, so care should be taken to encourage optimal compliance.

Neurosyphilis

Published studies show that a total dose of 6-9 million U of penicillin G over a 3- to 4-week period results in a satisfactory clinical response in approximately 90% of patients with neurosyphilis. Regimens employing benzathine penicillin in standard doses or procaine penicillin in doses under 2.4 million U/day do not consistently provide treponemicidal levels of penicillin in CSF, and several case reports document the failure of such regimens to cure neurosyphilis. Potentially effective regimens, none of which has been adequately studied, include:

1. Aqueous crystalline penicillin G 12-24 million U IV/day (2-4 million U q4h) for 10 days, followed by benzathine penicillin G 2.4 million U IM weekly for three doses
2. Aqueous procaine penicillin G 2.4 million U IM daily and probenecid 500 mg PO qid, both for 10 days, followed by benzathine penicillin G 2.4 million U IM weekly for three doses
3. Benzathine penicillin G 2.4 million U IM weekly for three doses

ACUTE PELVIC INFLAMMATORY DISEASE (PID): ENDOMETRITIS, SALPINGITIS, PARAMETRITIS, OR PERITONITIS

1. Regimen A
   a. Doxycycline 100 mg IV bid plus cefoxitin 2 g IV qid
   b. Continue IV drugs for at least 4 days and at least 48 hours after the patient improves; then continue doxycycline 100 mg PO bid to complete 10-14 days total therapy

2. Regimen B
   a. Clindamycin 600 mg IV qid plus Gentamicin 2 mg/kg IV followed by 1.5mg/kg tid in patients with normal renal function
   b. Continue IV drugs for at least 4 days and at least 48 hours after patient improves; then continue clindamycin 450 mg PO qid to complete 10-14 days total therapy

Ambulatory treatment

When the patient is not hospitalized, the following regimen is recommended:
1. Cefoxitin 2 g IM, amoxicillin 3 g PO, ampicillin 3.5 g PO, aqueous procaine penicillin G 4.8 million U IM at two sites, or ceftriaxone 250 mg IM; each of these regimens except ceftriaxone is accompanied by probenecid 1 g PO followed by doxycycline 100 mg PO bid for 10-14 days
2. Tetracycline HCI 500 mg qid maybe substituted for doxycycline, but it is less active against certain anaerobes and requires more frequent dosing; these are potentially important drawbacks in the treatment of PID

LYMPHOGRANULOMA VENEREUM: GENITAL, INGUINAL, OR ANORECTAL

Infection with a lymphogranuloma venereum (LGV) serotype of *C. trachomatis* should be treated with tetracycline HCI 500 mg PO qid for at least 2 weeks. The following alternative drugs are active against LGV serotypes in vitro, but have not been evaluated extensively in culture-confirmed cases.
1. Doxycycline 100 mg PO bid for at least 2 weeks
2. Erythromycin 500 mg PO qid for at least 2 weeks
3. Sulfamethoxazole 1 g PO bid for at least 2 weeks; other sulfonamides can be used in equivalent dosage

CHANCROID (*HAEMOPHILUS DUCREYI* INFECTION)

Chancroid may be a more common cause of genital ulcers than is presently recognized. The diagnosis is best made by isolation of *Haemophilus ducreyi* from ulcers or lymph nodes. The susceptibility of *H. ducreyi* to antimicrobial agents differs among geographic regions, and this should be taken into account when selecting therapy.
1. Erythromycin 500 mg PO qid for 7 days
2. Ceftriaxone 250 mg IM in a single dose
NOTE: Not evaluated in the United States, but probably effective

NONGONOCOCCAL URETHRITIS (NGU)

Urethritis not associated with *N. gonorrhoeae* is usually caused by *C. trachomatis* or *Ureaplasma urealyticum*. NGU requires prompt antimicrobial treatment of the patient and evaluation and treatment of sex partners.
1. Tetracycline HCI 500 mg PO qid for 7 days
2. Doxycycline 100 mg PO bid for 7 days

External genital/perianal warts

1. Cryotherapy (e.g., liquid nitrogen or carbon dioxide [dry ice])
2. Podophyllin 10 in compound tincture of benzoin

a. Apply carefully to each wart, avoiding normal tissue
b. Wash off thoroughly in 1-4 hours; some consultants use a longer period, but this must be individualized after patient tolerance and compliance have been established
c. Repeat once or twice weekly
d. If warts do not regress after four applications of podophyllin, alternative treatments are indicated
e. Podophyllin should not be used during pregnancy

TRICHOMONIASIS

1. Recommended regimen
   a. Metronidazole 2.0 g PO in a single dose
   b. Metronidazole may be administered in a dose of 250 mg PO tid for 7 days
2. Asymptomatic women with trichomoniasis should be treated the same as symptomatic women
3. Treatment failures
   a. Resistance of *Trichomonas vaginalis* to metronidazole has been observed, but it is rare
   b. Patients who fail treatment should be retreated with the same regimen
   c. Persistent failures should be managed in consultation with an expert
   d. Metronidazole 2 g PO qid for 3 days has been successful in patients infected with *T. vaginalis* strains mildly resistant to metronidazole, but experience with this regimen is limited

| 15.10 |

INFECTIOUS ARTHRITIS

Etiology

The type of infecting organism varies with the age of the patient and predisposing factors:

1. *Neisseria gonorrhoeae* is the most common organism in the 15-40 year old age group
2. *Staphylococcus aureus* is the most common cause of nongonococcal bacterial arthritis in adults; very common in patients with underlying rheumatoid arthritis
3. Streptococci (group A, nongroup A) is common in all age groups; they represent approximately 25% of cases of nongonococcal bacterial arthritis
4. Gram-negative bacilli are common in compromised hosts (e.g., malignancy, immunosuppression, chronic debilitating diseases) and IV drug addicts
5. *Haemophilus influenzae* is common in pediatric patients
6. *Staphylococcus epidermidis* is common in prosthetic joint infections
7. Lyme disease is caused by a spirochete *(Borrelia burgdorferi)* transmitted via the bite of a tick (Ixodes dammini and related species)[24,48]
8. Viral arthritis is associated with viral hepatitis, rubella infection or immunization, mumps
9. Others: *Mycobacterium tuberculosis,* atypical mycobacteria, fungal infections *(Candida,* coccidioidomycosis, sporotrichosis)

Predisposing factors

1. Septicemia
2. Immunosuppression (neoplasm, steroids)
3. Rheumatoid arthritis
4. IV drug abuse
5. Joint prosthesis
6. Penetrating wounds
7. Prior site of inflammation or damage
8. Other: deficiency of C_7, C_8, (increased risk of gonococcal arthritis), hypogammaglobulinemia, inherited disorders of chemotaxis

Diagnostic approach

1. History and physical exam
   a. Classic presentation consists of fever, erythema, pain, swelling, and limited motion of involved joint; however, these signs and symptoms may be absent or minimal, particularly in patients with rheumatoid arthritis or immunosuppression
   b. Nongonococcal arthritis is generally monoarticular; the knee is the joint most commonly involved
   c. Gonococcal arthritis usually presents with a migratory polyarthralgia and is often accompanied by tenosynovitis (inflammation of the tendon sheath) and a skin rash that usually involves the distal extremities; the typical patient with gonococcal arthritis is an otherwise healthy adult with a history of recent sexual contact
   d. Lyme disease often begins with a characteristic expanding annular skin lesion (erythema chronicum migrans), followed by intermittent attacks of joint swelling and pain in large joints; neurologic complications (aseptic meningitis, encephalitis, cranial neuritis) and cardiac abnormalities (AV block, myocarditis) may also be present
   e. *Pseudomonas aeruginosa* septic arthritis is usually associated with IV drug abuse and often involves the sternoclavicular joint
   f. Tuberculous arthritis is generally monoarticular and usually involves large joints
2. Arthrocentesis with analysis of joint fluid: refer to pp. 67-71 for procedure and interpretation of results
3. X-ray films of involved joints: indicated initially (and often following therapy), to rule out osteomyelitis; in septic arthritis, x-ray films early in the course generally reveal only the presence of joint effusion
4. Lab results
   a. WBC: peripheral leukocytosis is usually present
   b. Blood cultures (aerobic and anaerobic): indicated in all patients
   c. Skin cultures: should be done on any skin lesions
   d. Genitourinary cultures: indicated in suspected gonococcal arthritis
   e. Sedimentation rate: generally not helpful; if initially elevated, it may be useful in following response to therapy (progressive decrease of sedimentation rate with successful treatment)
   f. Serologic testing: antibody titers against *B. burgdorferi* are useful in suspected Lyme arthritis

Therapy[17, 38]

1. IV antibiotic therapy: based on results of Gram stain of synovial fluid
   a. Gram-negative cocci
      (1) In an adult patient consider *N. gonorrhoeae*
         (a) Treatment consists of penicillin G 10 million U/day for 3-5 days (depending on clinical response), followed by PO ampicillin 500 mg q6h or tetracycline
         (b) Erythromycin is generally not used because of its poor penetration in the synovial fluid
         (c) Penicillinase-producing strains of *N. gonorrhoeae* can be treated with spectinomycin
      (2) In a young child consider *H. influenzae* and treat with ampicillin IV 200 mg/kg/day in divided doses q6h; if allergic to penicillin, consider chloramphenicol or cefuroxime
   b. Gram-positive cocci: consider *S. aureus* and treat with oxacillin or nafcillin IV 9-12 g/day for at least 3 weeks; in patients allergic to penicillin, use vancomycin or cefazolin (Ancef)
   c. Gram-negative bacilli: consider *Pseudomonas* or *Escherichia coli*
      (1) Initial IV treatment consists of an aminoglycoside plus carbenicillin (or mezlocillin, azlocillin)
      (2) Suggested duration of treatment is 6-8 weeks, followed by 2-4 weeks of PO therapy in some cases
   d. Inconclusive Gram stain: treat according to presumed organism (based on age and risk factors)
      (1) In a compromised host use an aminoglycoside plus mezlocillin to cover for *P. aeruginosa*
      (2) In a young, otherwise healthy adult use penicillin G to cover for *N. gonorrhoeae*
      (3) In patients with suspected Lyme disease use benzathine penicillin 2-4 million U/week for 3 weeks, or IV penicillin G 20 million U/day for 10 days[49], or tetracycline
2. Drainage of infected joint: generally accomplished with needle aspiration; open drainage is generally reserved for prosthetic joint infections, inaccessible joints (e.g., hip), or inadequate drainage with needle aspiration
3. Joint immobilization: indicated in symptomatic patients; weight bearing by the infected joint should also be limited

15.11   **OSTEOMYELITIS**

Definition

Osteomyelitis is an infection involving bone and bone marrow.

Etiology

1. *Staphylococcus aureus* is the most common causative agent
2. Gram-negative bacilli: *Salmonella, Escherichia coli, Pseudomonas, Klebsiella*

   a. *Salmonella* is often seen in patients with sickle cell disease

   b. *Pseudomonas* is more frequent in IV drug addicts

   c. There is an increased incidence of gram-negative osteomyelitis in immunocompromised or chronically debilitated patients

3. *Haemophilus influenzae:* generally seen in infants and children

4. *Staphylococcus epidermidis:* often associated with prosthetic joints

5. Anaerobes often involve sacrum (associated with infected decubitus ulcers), skull, and hands (following human bites)

6. Others: streptococci, *Mycobacterium tuberculosis* (generally involves spine and results in compression fractures), fungi (*Candida albicans,* histoplasmosis)

Major predisposing factors

1. Sickle cell disease (bone infarcts, marrow thrombosis)
2. Compound fractures, open reduction of fractures
3. IV drug abuse
4. Peripheral vascular disease (atherosclerosis, diabetes mellitus)
5. Contiguous focus of infection (septic arthritis, otitis media, infected decubitus ulcer)
6. Trauma (particularly in children)

Diagnostic approach

1. History and physical exam
   a. Classic presentation consists of bone pain, fever, chills, and generalized malaise
     (1) There is significant tenderness over the bone and limitation of movement of the involved extremity
     (2) Osteomyelitis can also present with minimal, vague symptoms (e.g., vertebral osteomyelitis)
   b. History and physical exam often reveals one or more preexisting factors (see above)

2. Lab results
   a. Blood cultures
   b. WBC: peripheral leukocytosis is usually present
   c. Sedimentation rate: a normal value does not rule out osteomyelitis; an initially elevated sedimentation rate may be useful in following the course of the disease
   d. Aspirate and culture any joint effusions: refer to pp. 67-71 for arthrocentesis and interpretation of results

3. Radiographic evaluation
   a. Initial x-ray films may be normal because radiologic changes lag behind the clinical manifestations
   b. Initial changes consist of subperiosteal elevation and soft tissue swelling; these are then followed by lytic changes generally 3-4 weeks after the onset of disease
   c. Radionuclide scanning (technetium and gallium scans) can detect osteomyelitis early in its course; however, neoplasms, trauma, and other inflammatory processes may also produce positive radionuclide scans

Treatment

1. IV antibiotics
   a. The choice of antibiotic depends on the suspected likely pathogen (e.g., adult with suspected *S. aureus* osteomyelitis should be initially treated with IV oxacillin or nafcillin)
   b. Antibiotics are generally continued for 8-12 weeks following resolution of tenderness and local signs of swelling
2. Drainage of any infected joints
3. Immobilization of affected bone (plaster, traction)
4. Radiographic surveillance during and after treatment

| 15.12 | SPONTANEOUS BACTERIAL PERITONITIS |

Definition

Spontaneous bacterial peritonitis (SBP) is defined as the onset of bacterial peritonitis without an evident source of infection.

Pathogenesis

SBP usually occurs as a complication of hepatic ascites. The following mechanisms may account for bacterial seeding of the ascitic fluid:

1. Hematogenous transmission
2. Direct transmural passage following mucosal damage (ischemia, edema)
3. Bowel perforation following paracentesis (uncommon)[22]

Infecting organisms

1. *Escherichia coli*
2. Pneumococci
3. Others: enterobacter, streptococci, *Pseudomonas, Klebsiella*

Clinical manifestations

1. Fever
2. Abdominal pain and tenderness
3. Jaundice and encephalopathy
4. Hypoactive bowel sounds
5. Diarrhea
6. Sudden deterioration of mental status or renal function

Ascitic fluid analysis (see pp. 65, 68)[15,22,40]

1. Polymorphonuclear (PMN) cell count $>250/mm^3$ in ascitic fluid; this is the most sensitive and specific test for SBP if PMN cell count is $>500/mm^3$
2. Presence of bacteria on initial Gram stain of ascitic fluid
3. Lactic acid (lactate) >32 mg/dl[21]
4. pH <7.31 or arterial-ascetic fluid pH >0.1
5. Protein <1 g/dl
6. Glucose >50 mg/dl
7. Lactate dehydrogenase <225 mU/ml

Major distinguishing factors between SBP and secondary peritonitis (perforation of bowel wall)[40]

1. Presence of free air on abdominal x-ray films in secondary peritonitis
2. Common presence of multiple organisms and anaerobes in ascitic fluid in secondary peritonitis
3. Analysis of ascitic fluid in secondary peritonitis generally reveals: leukocyte count >10,000/mm^3, LDH >225 mU/ml, protein >1 g/dl and glucose <50 mg/dl

Therapy of SBP[13]

Cefotaxime (Claforan) 2 g IV q4h (in patients with normal renal function) or combination of an aminoglycoside and ampicillin

15.13	BACTERIAL MENINGITIS

Etiology

The type of infecting organism varies with the age of the patient and predisposing factors:

1. *Streptococcus pneumoniae* is common in adults and elderly patients; predisposing factors include blunt head trauma, otitis media, pneumonia, and CSF leaks
2. *Neisseria meningitidis* is common in young adults and children
3. *Haemophilus influenzae* is usually seen in preschool age children
4. *Listeria monocytogenes* is common in immunosuppressed patients (lymphoma, organ transplant recipients)
5. *Gram-negative bacilli* are usually seen in neonates (acquired in passage through birth canal) and in elderly patients
6. *Staphylococcus aureus* is seen in diabetics, patients with *S. aureus* pneumonia, or cancer

Diagnostic approach

1. History and physical exam
   a. The classic presentation consists of fever, headache, lethargy, confusion, and nuchal rigidity; these manifestations are not always present, particularly in infants, elderly, and immunocompromised patients
   b. Physical exam
      (1) Kernig's sign: resistance to knee extension following flexion of the patient's hips and knees by the examiner
      (2) Brudzinski's sign: rapid flexion of the neck elicits involuntary flexing of the knees in a supine patient
      (3) Altered mental status (confusion, lethargy)
      (4) Bulging fontanelle in infants
      (5) Petechial or purpuric rash generally involving the trunk or extremities; the rash is suggestive of meningococcal meningitis but can also be present in viral meningitis, other bacterial meningitis, bacterial endocarditis, and bacteremia secondary to staphylococci and other organisms
      (6) Papilledema is unusual and should raise the suspicion of brain abscess or mass lesion

2. Lab results
   a. WBC usually reveals leukocytosis with shift to the left, however leukopenia can also be present; peripheral lymphocytosis is usually suggestive of a viral etiology (aseptic meningitis)
   b. Blood cultures are appropriate; however, antibiotic therapy should not be delayed until all cultures are obtained if patient is very ill
3. Lumbar puncture: refer to pp. 59-62 for procedure, diagnostic studies, and interpretation of results; in bacterial meningitis, the classic findings on CSF examination are: elevated WBC (predominantly PMNs), decreased glucose, elevated protein, and positive Gram stain

Treatment

IV antibiotic therapy should be based on the results of the Gram stain and consideration of predisposing factors for specific organisms (e.g., age, head trauma, immunosuppression). Table 15-5 describes suggested initial treatment of bacterial meningitis in adults.

Table 15-5   Initial treatment of acute bacterial meningitis in adults[5,53]

Suspected Organism	Antibiotic of Choice	Second Choice
S. pneumoniae N. meningitidis	Penicillin G, 50,000 U/ kg IV q4h (18-24 million U/day)	Chloramphenicol 75-100 mg/kg/day IV in divided doses q6h
H. influenzae	Ampicillin 50 mg/kg IV q4h (12 g/day) plus chloramphenicol 75-100 mg/kg/day IV in divided doses q6h until susceptibility of the organism to ampicillin is determined	Cefuroxime or third-generation cephalosporin
L. monocytogenes	Ampicillin 50 mg/kg IV q4h (12 g/day)	Vancomycin 1 g IV q12h, or Trimethoprim-sulfamethoxazole (TMP-10 mg/kg/day and SMX-50 mg/kg/day)
S. aureus	Nafcillin 200 mg/kg/day IV in 6 doses (12-18 g/day) plus rifampin 750 mg PO qd[18]	Vancomycin 1 g q12h
Gram-negative bacilli	Third-generation cephalosporin* plus an aminoglycoside	Trimethoprim-sulfamethoxazole[29]

*e.g., Ceftazidime (Fortaz) 2 g IV q8h; cefotaxime (Claforan) 200 mg/kg/day IV in six equally divided doses.

Table 15-6   Suggested duration of therapy in bacterial meningitis[5,18,29,53]

Infecting Organism	Suggested Duration of Therapy
N. meningitidis	7-10 days
S. pneumoniae	12-14 days
H. influenzae, type B	14 days
Gram-negative bacilli	10-14 days after negative repeat CSF culture
L. monocytogenes	4-6 weeks
S. aureus	4-6 weeks

Suggested duration of therapy in bacterial meningitis

The duration of treatment varies with the infecting organism and the patient's clinical course. Guidelines are listed in Table 15-6.

Prophylaxis of bacterial meningitis[43]

1. Indications
   a. Meningococcal meningitis and *H. influenzae* meningitis (type B)
      (1) Members of the same household
      (2) Individuals who have had close contact with the index case (e.g., babysitter)
      (3) Hospital personnel who performed mouth-to-mouth resuscitation on the patient
      (4) Contacts at day care, school, or chronic care facilities should be considered on an individual basis
2. Prophylaxis
   a. Meningococcal meningitis
      (1) Adults: rifampin 600 mg PO bid for 2 days
      (2) Children: rifampin 10 mg/kg PO bid for 2 days
   b. *H. influenzae* meningitis
      (1) Adults: rifampin 600 mg PO qd for 4 days
      (2) Children: rifampin 20 mg/kg (maximum 600 mg) PO qd for 4 days

| 15.14 |

INFECTIVE ENDOCARDITIS

Etiology

1. Streptococci
   a. *S. viridans* is the single most common organism except for right-sided endocarditis and prosthetic valve endocarditis
   b. Enterococci (group D streptococci)
   c. Other streptococci
2. Staphylococci
   a. *Staphylococcus aureus* is the most common organism in right-sided endocarditis
   b. *Staphylococcus epidermidis* is the most common organism in prosthetic valve endocarditis
3. Others: fungi, gram-negative bacilli, gonococci, pneumococci

Risk factors

1. Rheumatic valvulitis
2. IV drug abuse
3. Congenital heart disease
4. Mechanical heart valves
5. Mitral insufficiency
6. Coarctation of aorta, VSD, PDA
7. Mitral valve prolapse
8. Marfan syndrome
9. Myxomas associated with calcification of the valves
10. Previous endocarditis
11. Mitral stenosis
12. Male gender
13. Black race

Diagnosis

1. History and physical exam
   a. Presence of any risk factors (see above)
   b. Physical exam may reveal
      (1) Heart murmur is usually present in subacute bacterial endocarditis (SBE), but may be absent in acute bacterial endocarditis and right-sided endocarditis
      (2) Fever is generally present; may be absent in elderly or immuno-compromised patients
      (3) Flame-shaped retinal hemorrhages with pale centers (Roth spots)
      (4) Painless erythematous papules and macules on the palms of the hands and soles of the feet (Janeway lesions)
      (5) Painful erythematous subcutaneous papules (Osler nodes)
      (6) Petechiae
      (7) Subungal splinter hemorrhages
      (8) Splenomegaly
      (9) Other: headaches, backache, arthralgias, confusion
2. Lab results
   a. Blood cultures: positive in 85%-95% of patients; negative cultures are usually secondary to:[52]
      (1) Prior antibiotic therapy (in preceding 2 weeks)
      (2) Fastidious organisms with special growth requirements (anaerobes, *Brucella, Neisseria, Corynebacterium*)
      (3) Slow-growing organisms *(Haemophilus, Actinobacillus)*
      (4) Fungi *(Candida, Aspergillus, Histoplasma, Cryptococcus)*
      (5) Improper collection of blood and cultures
   b. Decreased hemoglobin/hematocrit: usually secondary to decreased RBC production caused by inflammatory state
   c. Normal, elevated, or decreased WBC, usually with shift to left
   d. Assay of Teichoic acid antibody: can aid in the diagnosis of *S. aureus* endocarditis (e.g., IV drug addicts); an assay should be obtained on admission and repeated in 1-2 weeks in patients with suspected *S. aureus* endocarditis
   e. Urinalysis: may show hematuria with associated RBC casts

    f. Rheumatoid factor: positive in approximately 50% of cases after 6 weeks; its significance is unclear

    g. Sedimentation rate: generally elevated, not helpful

3. Echocardiography

    a. Useful to demonstrate valvular vegetations and to evaluate valvular damage and left ventricular function; however, a normal echocardiogram does not rule out endocarditis

    b. Two-dimensional echocardiography is preferred over M-mode echocardiography because of increased sensitivity (can detect 80%-85% of vegetations)[31]

    c. The incidence of complications (e.g., heart failure) is directly related to the size of the vegetation[60]

    d. Echocardiographically documented vegetations ≥1 cm in patients with right-sided infective endocarditis are associated with a lower response rate to appropriate medical therapy[39]

Special diagnostic considerations

1. Right-sided endocarditis

    a. Usually seen in IV drug addicts

    b. Physical exam usually reveals a murmur of tricuspid regurgitation (holosystolic, heard at left lower sternal border, increased by inspiration, decreased by expiration and Valsalva maneuver); evidence of right-sided heart failure may also be present (neck vein distention, congestive hepatomegaly)

    c. Blood cultures reveal *S. aureus* in the majority of cases

    d. Chest x-ray film may demonstrate peripheral wedge-shaped infiltrates with cavitation (septic pulmonary emboli)

2. Prosthetic valve endocarditis[58]

    a. Overall frequency is approximately 2%

    b. Overall mortality is 59%

    c. The microbiologic agent involved and the mortality are related to the time of onset of endocarditis after cardiac valve implantation

        (1) Early onset prosthetic valve endocarditis (within 2 months of implantation)

            (a) Frequency of endocarditis (0.78%)

            (b) Usually resulting from surgical infection

            (c) Staphylococci are the most common organisms (*S. epidermidis* the predominant organism)

            (d) Mortality (77%)

        (2) Late-onset prosthetic valve endocarditis (occurring more than 2 months postoperatively)

            (a) Frequency of endocarditis (1.1%)

            (b) Usually community-acquired infection

            (c) Streptococci are the predominant organisms

            (d) Overall mortality (46%)

Major complications of infective endocarditis

1. CHF caused by valvular destruction or associated myocarditis
2. Embolism

Text continued on p. 342.

Table 15-7 Antibiotic treatment* in infective endocarditis in adults

Infecting Organism	Recommended Treatment	Duration (Weeks)	Alternative Treatment	Duration (Weeks)
Streptococcus viridans and Streptococcus bovis (MIC ≤0.2 μg/ml)	†Aqueous penicillin G, 10-20 million U/day in equally divided doses q4h IV alone or plus	4	Vancomycin, 10 mg/kg body weight (not to exceed 500 mg) IV q6h, or Cephalothin, 2 g IV	4
	Streptomycin, 10 mg/kg body weight (not to exceed 500 mg) IM q12h, or	2		
	Procaine penicillin G,‡ 1.2 million U q6h IM, plus	2		
	Streptomycin, 10 mg/kg body weight (not to exceed 500 mg) IM q12h	2		
Streptococcus viridans and Streptococcus bovis (MIC >0.2 μg/ml)	Aqueous penicillin G, 20 million U/day IV in equally divided doses q4h, plus	4	Vancomycin, 10 mg/kg body weight (not to exceed 500 mg) IV q6h, plus Streptomycin, 10 mg/kg weight (not to exceed 500 mg) IM q12 h	4
	Streptomycin, 10 mg/kg body weight (not to exceed 500 mg) IM q12h	4		
Enterococci	Aqueous penicillin G, 20 million U/day IV in equally divided doses q4h, plus	4-6	Vancomycin, 10 mg/kg body weight (not to exceed 500 mg) IV q6h, plus	4-6

Organism		Weeks		Weeks
	Streptomycin, 0.5 g IM q12h, or ||Gentamicin, 1 mg/kg IM or IV q8h	4-6	||Streptomycin, 10 mg/kg body weight (not to exceed 500 mg) IM q12h, or Gentamicin, 1 mg/kg IM or IV q8h	4-6
Pneumococci, or group A streptococci	Aqueous penicillin, 10-20 million U/day IV in equally divided doses q4h	4	Vancomycin, 10 mg/kg body weight (not to exceed 500 mg) IV q6h, or §Cephalothin, 2 g IV q4h	4
Gonococci	Aqueous penicillin, 10-20 million U/day IV in equally divided doses q4h	4	Erythromycin, 500 mg IV q6h, or §Cefoxitin, 1-2 g IV q6h	4
Staphylococci: S. aureus or epidermidis (penicillin-sensitive)	Aqueous penicillin 12-20 million U/day IV either continuously or in equally divided doses q4h	4-6	Vancomycin, 10 mg/kg body weight (not to exceed 500 mg) IV q6h or §Cephalothin, 2 g IV q4h	4-6

From Reid, C.L., Chandraratna, P.A.N., and Rahimtoola, S.H.: Curr. Probl. Cardiol. 10(1), 1985. Reproduced with permission.

*Antibiotic dosages are given for patients with normal renal and hepatic function.

†Aqueous penicillin G used alone is recommended for most patients more than 65 years of age and those with impairment of eighth nerve function or impaired renal function, although the dosage of penicillin may need to be reduced depending on the degree of renal impairment.

‡Two-week therapy regimen should not be used in patients with shock, mycotic aneurysms, prosthetic valve endocarditis, or infections caused by nutritionally deficient variants.

§Other cephalosporin antibiotics in equivalent doses also may be effective; in vitro sensitivity testing is necessary. Potential cross-allergenicity between penicillins and cephalosporins may exist.

||Gentamicin is used when the enterococcus is resistant to 2,000 μg/ml of streptomycin.

Continued.

Table 15-7 Antibiotic treatment in infective endocarditis in adults—cont'd

Infecting Organism	Recommended Treatment	Duration (Weeks)	Alternative Treatment	Duration (Weeks)
S. aureus or epidermidis (penicillin-resistant)	β-Lactamase-resistant penicillin: Nafcillin, 12 g/day IV Oxacillin, 12 g/day IV Methicillin, 16 g/day IV	4-6	Vancomycin, 2 g/day IV or §Cephalothin, 2 g IV q4h	4-6 4-6
	Addition of gentamicin, 1 mg/kg IV q8h, may speed sterilization of blood	2-4	Addition of gentamicin, 1 mg/kg IV q8h, may speed sterilization of blood	2-4
	¶Addition of rifampin, 300 mg/day, may be of benefit in myocardial abscesses	Several weeks		
S. aureus or epidermidis (methicillin-resistant)	Vancomycin, 10 mg/kg body weight (not to exceed 500 mg) IV q6h	4-6		
	Addition of gentamicin, 1 mg/kg IV q8h, may speed sterilization of blood	4-6		
Gram-negative Pseudomonas aeruginosa	Carbenicillin, 30-40 g/day IV in equally divided doses q2-4h, or	4-6		

| | Piperacillin, 12-18 g/day IV in equally divided doses q4h, plus Gentamicin, 3-5 mg/kg/day IV in equally divided doses q8h, or Amikacin, 15 mg/kg/day IV in equally divided doses q8h; may require concomitant colistin or polymyxin B | |
| *Serratia marcescens* | Gentamicin, 3-5 mg/kg/day IV in equally divided doses q8h, or Amikacin, 15 mg/kg/day IV in equally divided doses q8h, plus Mezlocillin, 12-18 g/day IV in equally divided doses q8h, or Carbenicillin, 30-40 g/day IV in equally divided doses q2-4h (if strain is sensitive) | 4-6 |

¶This use of this agent is not listed in the manufacturer's directive.

Continued.

Table 15-7 Antibiotic treatment in infective endocarditis in adults—cont'd

Infecting Organism	Recommended Treatment	Duration (Weeks)	Alternative Treatment	Duration (Weeks)
Hemophilus parainfluenza	Ampicillin, 12-18 g/day IV in equally divided doses q6h, plus Gentamicin, 3-5 mg/kg/day IV in equally divided doses q8h; may also require Chloramphenicol, 3-6 g/day IV in equally divided doses q4-6h	4-6		
Enterobacteriaceae	Ampicillin 12-18 g/day in equally divided doses q6h, or Mezlocillin, 12-18 g/day IV in equally divided doses q4h, or Carbenicillin, 12-18 g/day IV in equally divided doses q2-4 hr, plus	4-6		

	Gentamicin, 3-5 mg/kg day IV in equally divided doses q8h, or Amikacin, 15 mg/kg day IV in equally divided doses q8h		Vancomycin, 10 mg/kg body weight (not to exceed 500 mg) IV q6h	4-6
Corynebacterium	Aqueous penicillin G, 10-20 million U/day in equally divided doses q4h IV, plus Gentamicin, 3-5 mg/kg/day IV in equally divided doses q8h	4-6	
Fungal (*Candida* sp.)	Amphotericin B, 1.5-3.0 g as a total dose IV (daily dose, 1.0-1.25 mg/kg) 5-Fluorocytosin, 150 mg/kg/day IV in equally divided doses q6h, plus Surgery		
(*Aspergillus* sp.)	Amphotericin B, 1.5-3.0 g as total IV dose (daily dose, 1.0-1.25 mg/kg), plus Surgery		

a. CNS: hemiplegia, sensory loss, aphasia, meningeal irritation, mycotic aneurysm, brain abscesses, seizures, headaches
b. Kidneys: hematuria secondary to focal glomerulonephritis, renal failure secondary to diffuse proliferative glomerulonephritis, renal emboli, and infarction
c. Coronary arteries: heart failure, angina, MI
d. Spleen: splenic infarct
3. Dysrhythmias
4. Pericarditis, myocardial abscess, myocarditis

Indications for Cardiac Surgery in Patients with Active Infective Endocarditis

Indications for Urgent Cardiac Surgery in Patients with Active Infective Endocarditis

1. Hemodynamic compromise
   a. Severe heart failure
   b. Valvular obstruction
2. Uncontrolled infection
   a. Fungal endocarditis
   b. Persistent bacteremia
   c. No effective antimicrobial agent available
3. Unstable prosthesis

Relative Indications for Cardiac Surgery in Active Native Valve Endocarditis

1. Etiologic bacteria other than "susceptible" streptococci
2. Relapse
3. Evidence for intracardiac extension of the infection
   a. Ruptured chordae tendineae or papillary muscle
   b. Rupture of sinus of Valsalva or ventricular septum
   c. Heart block
   d. Abscess demonstrated by echocardiography or catheterization
4. Two or more emboli
5. Vegetations demonstrated by echocardiography
6. Mitral valve preclosure by echocardiography

Relative Indications for Cardiac Surgery in Active Prosthetic Valve Endocarditis

1. Early prosthetic valve endocarditis
2. Nonstreptococcal late prosthetic valve endocarditis
3. Periprosthetic leak
4. Two or more emboli
5. Relapse
6. Evidence for intracardiac extension of infection

From Alsip, S.G., Blackstone, M.D., Kirklin, M.D., and Cobbs, C.G.: Am. J. Med. 78(suppl 6B):138, 1985. Reproduced with permission.

Indications for Endocarditis Prophylaxis

Procedures
1. Oral cavity and respiratory tract
   a. All dental procedures likely to induce gingival bleeding (not simple adjustment of orthodontic appliances or shedding of deciduous teeth)
   b. Tonsillectomy or adenoidectomy
   c. Surgical procedures or biopsy involving respiratory mucosa
   d. Bronchoscopy, especially with a rigid bronchoscope*
   e. Incision and drainage of infected tissue
2. Genitourinary and gastrointestinal tracts
   a. Cystoscopy
   b. Prostatic surgery
   c. Urethral catheterization (especially in the presence of infection)
   d. Urinary tract surgery
   e. Vaginal hysterectomy
   f. Gallbladder surgery
   g. Colonic surgery
   h. Esophageal dilatation
   i. Sclerotherapy for esophageal varices
   j. Colonoscopy
   k. Upper gastrointestinal tract endoscopy with biopsy
   l. Proctosigmoidoscopic therapy

Cardiac Conditions
1. Endocarditis prophylaxis recommended
   a. Prosthetic cardiac valves (including biosynthetic valves)
   b. Most congenital cardiac malformations
   c. Surgically constructed systemic-pulmonary shunts
   d. Rheumatic and other acquired valvular dysfunction
   e. Idiopathic hypertrophic subaortic stenosis
   f. Previous history of bacterial endocarditis
   g. Mitral valve prolapse with insufficiency†
2. Endocarditis prophylaxis not recommended
   a. Isolated secundum atrial septal defect
   b. Secundum atrial septal defect repaired without a patch 6 or more months earlier
   c. Patent ductus arteriosus ligated and divided 6 or more months earlier
   d. Postoperatively after coronary artery bypass graft surgery

Adapted from Shulman, S.T., et al.: Circulation, **70**:1123A, 1984. Used with permission.
*The risk with flexible bronchoscopy is low, but the necessity for prophylaxis is not yet defined.
†Definitive data to provide guidance in management of patients with mitral valve prolapse are particularly limited. In general, such patients are clearly at low risk of development of endocarditis, but the risk-benefit ratio of prophylaxis in mitral valve prolapse is uncertain.

Management

1. Medical
   a. Table 15-7 describes antibiotic treatment in adults, based on positive blood culture results
      (1) Antibiotic therapy (upon identification of the organism) should be guided by susceptibility testing (MIC, MBC)[59]
      (2) Peak serum bactericidal titers $\geq 1:64$ and trough bactericidal titers $\geq 1:32$ are recommended[55]
   b. Initial IV antibiotic therapy (before culture results) is aimed at the most likely organism; it should consist of vancomycin plus gentamicin in patients with prosthetic valves or patients with native valves but allergic to penicillin
      (1) In IV drug addicts, initial therpay consists of a penicillinase-resistant synthetic penicillin (oxacillin, nafcillin) plus gentamicin
      (2) In native valve endocarditis, initial therapy consists of combination of penicillin and gentamicin; a penicillinase-resistant penicil-

Table 15-8   Recommendations for prophylaxis of endocarditis

Standard Regimen	
For dental procedures and oral or upper respiratory tract surgery	Penicillin V 2 g PO 1 hr before, then 1.0 g 6 hr later
Special Regimens	
Parenteral regimen for high-risk patients; also for GI or GU tract procedures	Ampicillin 2 g IM or IV plus gentamicin 1.5 mg/kg IM or IV, 30 min before†
Parenteral regimen for patients allergic to penicillin	Vancomycin 1 g IV slowly over 1 hr, starting 1 hr before; add gentamicin 1.5 mg/kg IM or IV if GI or GU tract involved†
Oral regimen for patients allergic to penicillin (oral and respiratory tract only)	Erythromycin 1 g PO 1 hr before, then 0.5 g 6 hr later†
Oral regimen for minor GI or GU tract procedures	Amoxicillin 3 g PO 1 hr before, then 1.5 g 6 hr later†
Cardiac surgery, including implantation of prosthetic valves	Cefazolin 2 g IV at induction of anesthesia, repeated 8 and 16 hr later

From Durack, D.T.: Am. J. Med. 78(suppl 6B):155, 1985.

*These regimens are empiric suggestions; no regimen has been proved to be effective for prevention of endocarditis and prevention failures may occur with any regimen. These regimens are not intended to cover all clinical situations; the practitioner should evaluate safety and cost-benefit issues in each individual case. One or two additional doses may be given if the period of risk for bacteremia is prolonged.

†Pediatric dosages: ampicillin 50 mg/kg; erythromycin 20 mg/kg for first dose, then 10 mg/kg; gentamicin 2 mg/kg; penicillin V and amoxicillin, for children who weight more 60 pounds, use same as for adults, and children less than 60 pounds, use half the adult dose; vancomycin 20 mg/kg.

lin should be added in acute bacterial endocarditis or if *S. aureus* in suspected as one of the possible causative organisms
2. Surgery: indications for cardiac surgery in patients with active infective endocarditis are listed in the boxed material on p. 342

Prophylaxis for infective endocarditis

Cardiac conditions and procedures for which endocarditis prophylaxis is recommended are described in the boxed material on p. 343. Suggested antibiotic regimens for prophylaxis of bacterial endocarditis are listed in Table 15-8.[12]

References

1. Armstrong, D., et al.: Treatment of infections in patients with the acquired immunodeficiency syndrome, Ann. Intern Med. **103**:738, 1985.
2. Baltch, A.L., and Smith, R.P.: Combinations of antibiotics against *Pseudomonas aeruginosa,* Am. J. Med. **79**(suppl 1A):8, 1985.
3. Baumgartner, J.D., et al.: Prevention of gram-negative shock and death in surgical patients by antibody to endotoxin core glycolipid, Lancet **2**:59, 1985.
4. Bennett, I.V., Jr., and Beeson, P.B.: Bacteremia: a consideration of some experimental and clinical aspects, Yale J. Bio. Med. **26**:241, 1954.
5. Bolan, G., and Barza, M.: Acute bacterial meningitis in children and adults, Med. Clin. North Am. **69**:236, 1985.
6. Boscia, J.A., et al.: Epidemiology of bacteriuria in an elderly ambulatory population, Am. J. Med. **80**:208, 1986.
7. Bowen, D.L., Lane, H.C., and Fauci, A.S.: Immunopathogenesis of the acquired immunodeficiency syndrome, Ann. Intern. Med. **103**:704, 1985.
8. Carlson, K.J., and Mulley, A.G.: Management of acute dysuria: a decision-analysis model of alternative strategies, Ann. Intern. Med. **102**:244, 1985.
9. Chernow B., et al.: Measurement of urinary leukocyte esterase activity: a screening test for urinary tract infections, Am. Emerg. Med. **13**:150, 1984.
10. Cohen, S.H., and Jordan, G.W.: Clinical use of antimicrobial susceptibility data, Hosp. Physician, **88**:11-16, 1986.
11. Cordonnier, C., et al.: Legionnaire's disease and hairy-cell leukemia: An unfortuitous association? Arch. Intern. Med. **144**:2373, 1984.
12. Durack, D.T.: Current issues of prevention of infective endocarditis, Am. J. Med. **78**(suppl 6B):155, 1985.
13. Felisart, J., et al.: Cefotaxime is more effective than ampicillin-tobramycin in cirrhotics with severe infections, Hepatology **5**:457, 1985.
14. Fischinger, P.J.: Acquired immune deficiency syndrome: the causative agent and the evolving peropective, Curr. Probl. Cancer, **9**(1):4, 1985.
15. Garcia-Tsao, G., Conn, H.O., and Lerner, R.: The diagnosis of bacterial peritonitis: comparison of pH, lactate concentration, and leukocyte count, Hepatology **5**:91, 1985.
16. Gelbart, S.M., Chen, W.T., and Reid, R.: Clinical trial of leukocyte strips in routine use, Clin. Chem. **29**:997, 1983.
17. Goldenberg, D.L., and Reed, J.I.: Bacterial arthritis, N. Engl. J. Med. **312**(12):764, 1985.
18. Gordon, J.J., Harter, D.H., and Phair, J.P.: Meningitis due to *Staphylococcus aureus,* Am. J. Med. **78**:965, 1985.
19. Guidelines for Handwashing and Hospital Environmental Control, 1985, Center for Disease Control, 8.
20. Guidelines for Prevention of Surgical Wound Infections, 1985. Center for Disease Control, 7-9.
21. Guyton, B.J., and Achord, J.L.: The rapid determination of ascitic fluid L-lactate for the diagnosis of spontaneous bacterial peritonitis, Am. J. Gastroenterol. **78**:231, 1983.

22. Hoefs, J.C., and Runyon, B.A.: Spontaneous bacterial peritonitis, DM **31**:1, 1985.

23. Hook, E.W., and Hooton, T.M.: Microbiologic evaluation of cutaneous cellulitis in adults, Arch. Intern. Med. **146**:295, 1986.

24. Johnston, Y.E., et al.: Lyme arthritis: spirochetes found in synovial microangiopathic lesions, Am. J. Pathol. **118**:26, 1985.

25. Kiehn, T.E., et al.: Infections caused by *Mycobacterium avium* complex in immunocompromised patients: diagnosis by blood culture and fecal examination, antimicrobial susceptibility tests, and morphological and seroagglutination characteristics, J. Clin. Microb. **21**:168, 1985.

26. Komaroff, A.L.: Acute dysuria in women, N. Engl. J. Med. **310**:368, 1984.

27. Komaroff, A.L.: Urinalysis and urine culture in women with dysuria, Ann. Intern. Med. **104**:212, 1986.

28. Larson, E.B., and Featherstone, H.J.: Fever of unknown origin: diagnosis and follow-up of 105 cases, 1970-1980, Medicine, **61**:269, 1982.

29. Levitz, R., and Quintiliani, R.: Trimethoprim-sulfamethoxazole for bacterial meningitis, Ann. Intern. Med. **100**:881, 1984.

30. Magnussen, C.R.: Skin and soft tissue infections. In Reese, R.E., and Douglas, R.G., (editors): A practical approach to infectious diseases, Boston, 1983, Little, Brown, and Co.

31. Martin, R.P., et al.: Clinical utility of two-dimensional echocardiography in infective endocarditis, Am. J. Cardiol. **46**:379, 1980.

32. Parker, M.M., et al.: Profound but reversible myocardial depression in patients with septic shock, Ann. Intern.Med. **100**:483, 1984.

33. Petersdorf, R.G., and Wallace, J.F.: Fever of unknown origin, in Barondess, J.A., (editor): Diagnostic approaches to presenting syndromes, Baltimore, 1971, Williams and Wilkins Co.

34. Recommendations for preventing transmission of infection with human T-lymphotropic virus type III/Lymphadenopathy-associated virus in the workplace, MMWR, **34**(45):1985.

35. Redfield, R.R., Markham, P.D., and Solahuddin, S.Z.: Heterosexually acquired HTLV-III/LAV disease (AIDS-related complex with AIDS), JAMA, **254**:2094, 1985.

36. Reese, R.E.: Bacteremias and sepsis. In Reese, R.E., and Douglas, R.G., Jr., (editors): A practical approach to infectious diseases, Boston, 1983, Little, Brown, and Co.

37. Revision of the case definition of acquired immunodeficiency syndrome for national reporting: United States, MMWR, **34**:373, 1985.

38. Roberts, N.J., Jr.: Joint infections. In Reese, R.E., Douglas, R.G., Jr., (editors): A practical approach to infectious diseases, Boston, 1983, Little, Brown, and Co.

39. Robbins, M.J., et a..: Influence of vegetation size on clinical outcome of right-sided infective endocarditis, Am. J. Med. **80**:165, 1986.

40. Runyon, B.A., and Hoefs, J.C.: Ascitic fluid analysis in the differentiation of spontaneous bacterial peritonitis from gastrointestinal tract perforation into ascitic fluid, Hepatology, **4**:447, 1984.

41. Sangadharan, M.G., et al.: Antibodies reactive with human T-lymphotropic retrovirus (HTLV III) in the serum of patients with AIDS, Science, **224**:506, 1984.

42. Savard-Fenton, M., et al.: Single-dose amoxicillin therapy with follow-up urine culture, Am. J. Med. **73**:808, 1982.

43. Shapiro, E.: Prophylaxis for bacterial meningitis, Med. Clin. North Am. **69**(2):269, 1985.

44. Sprung, C.L., et al.: The effects of high-dose corticosteroids in patients with septic shock: a prospective controlled study, N. Engl. J. Med. **311**:1137, 1984.

45. Stamm, W.E., et al.: Diagnosis of coliform infection in acutely dysuric women, N. Engl. J. Med. **307**:463, 1982.

46. Stamm, W.E.: Management of recurrent urinary tract infections with patient administered single dose therapy, Ann. Intern. Med. **102**:302, 1985.

47. Status report on the acquired immunodeficiency syndrome, JAMA, **254**:1342, 1985.

48. Steere, A.C., et al.: The spirochetal etiology of Lyme disease, N. Engl. J. Med. **308**:733, 1983.

49. Steere, A.C.: Successful parenteral penicillin therapy in established Lyme arthritis, N. Engl. J. Med. **312**:873, 1985.

50. Tam, M.R., et al.: Culture-independent diagnosis of *Chlamydia trachomatis* using monoclonal antibioties, N. Engl. J. Med. **310**:1146, 1984.

51. Valenti, W.M.: Genitourinary infections. In Reese, R.E., and Douglas, R.G., Jr., (editors): A practical approach to infectious diseases, Boston, 1983, Little, Brown, and Co.

52. Van Scoy, R.E.: Culture negative endocarditis, Mayo Clin. Proc. **57**:149, 1982.

53. Van Voris, L.P., and Roberts, N.J., Jr.: Central nervous system infections. In Reese, R.E., and Douglas,R.G., Jr., (editors): A practical approach to infectious diseases, 1983, Little, Brown, and Co.

54. Volberding, P.A., et al.: Vinblastine therapy for Kaposi sarcoma in the acquired immunodeficiency syndrome, Ann. Intern. Med. **103**:335, 1985.

55. Weinstein, M.P., and Stratton, C.W.: Multicenter collaborative evaluation of a standardized serum bactericidal test as a prognostic indicator in infective endocarditis, Am. J. Med. **78**:262, 1985.

56. Weiss, S.H., et al.: Screening test for HTLV III (AIDS agent) antibody: specificity, sensitivity and applications, JAMA **253**:221, 1985.

57. Weiss, S.H., Saxinger, W.C., and Richtman, D.: HTLV-III infection among health care workers, JAMA, **254**:2089, 1985.

58. Wilson, W.R., Danielson, G.K., Giuliani, E.R., and Ceraci, J.E.: Prosthetic valve endocarditis, Mayo Clin. Proc. **57**:155, 1982.

59. Wilson, W.R., Giuliani, E.R., and Geraci, J.E.: General considerations in the diagnosis and treatment of infective endocarditis, Mayo Clin. Proc. **57**:81, 1982.

60. Wong, D.H., et al.: Clinical implications of large vegetations in infectious endocarditis, Arch. Intern. Med. **143**:1874, 1983.

61. Yarchoan, R., et al.: Response of human immunodeficiency virus associated neurologic disease to 3'-azido-3'-deoxythymidine, Lancet, **I**:132, 1987.

16 Nephrology

Nephrology

RENAL FAILURE
James Grant

Classification

1. Prerenal: secondary to decreased renal perfusion, volume contraction, CHF, and altered renal hemodynamics
2. Renal: associated with acute or chronic intrinsic renal disease (e.g., ATN, glomerulonephritis, vasculitis, interstitial disease)
3. Postrenal: obstructive uropathy (e.g., prostatic hypertrophy, bilateral ureteral obstruction, neurogenic bladder)

Prerenal failure

Etiology

1. Volume deficits: including extrarenal losses (e.g., hemorrhage, GI bleeding, inadequate fluid intake), third-spacing, and urinary losses secondary to diuretics or osmotically obligatory urine volumes
2. Low output states: including CHF, dysrhythmias, and pericardial disease
3. Decreased systemic vascular resistance as seen in sepsis, pancreatitis, pharmacologic resistence circuit unloaders, and cirrhosis
4. Decreased oncotic vascular volume support: nephrosis, severe catabolic states
5. Reversible prerenal insufficiency secondary to decreased renal blood flow can be seen with use of prostaglandin inhibitors (NSAID)
   NOTE: Renal dysfunction secondary to NSAID is also characterized by the following features[12]:
   a. Hyporeninemic hypoaldosteronism with resultant hyperkalemia (often associated with hyperchloremic metabolic alkalosis)
   b. Acute interstitial nephritis, often associated with proteinuria in the nephrotic range
6. Inhibition of intrinsic renal vascular modulation by ACE inhibitors
   NOTE: ACE inhibitors (Captopril, Enapril) can also lead to "non-prerenal" acute renal failure in patients with renal artery stenosis
7. Hepatorenal syndrome: labeled "prerenal" because when the involved kidney is transplanted to a normal host, it functions normally; it is associated with severe oliguria, a falling GFR with rising creatinine, but a persistently low urinary sodium level

Characteristics of prerenal failure
1. Decreased renal perfusion results in increased sodium and water reabsorption at the proximal tubule (in an attempt to reexpand circulating blood volume)
   a. Oliguria
   b. Decreased urine sodium (<20 mEq/L)
2. Serum sodium that reflects relative sodium-water losses and/or gains
3. Decreased distal tubular flow results in increased urea absorption and K^+ secretion
   a. Increased BUN
   b. Increased BUN/creatinine ratio
4. Increased renal ''threshold'' for plasma ions
   a. Increased HCO_3 absorption: contraction alkalosis
   b. Increased uric acid absorption: hyperuricemia
5. Increased ADH secretion: increased water absorption; urine osmolarity greater than serum osmolarity
6. Hyponatremia with free water loading until volume is restored

Treatment
1. Appropriate volume challenge in contracted patients
2. Maximize cardiac function
3. Discontinue offending drugs

Intrinsic renal failure

Etiology
1. Acute tubular necrosis(vasomotor nephropathy)
2. Acute allergic interstitial nephritis
3. Acute glomerular syndromes
4. Chronic intrinsic renal disease
5. Vascular disorders
6. Toxic nephropathies
7. Myeloma kidney
8. Tubular disorders

Characteristics of specific causes of intrinsic renal failure
1. Acute tubular necrosis (ATN) is the most common form of acute renal failure in the hospital setting
   a. Precipitating factors
      (1) Severe and protracted decrease in renal perfusion: prolonged prerenal failure, shock, hypovolemia, sepsis and low-output states, CABG surgery, aortic aneurysm repair
      (2) Pigment toxicity: transfusion reactions, rhabdomyolysis (seizures, crush injury), surgery in hyperbilirubinemic states
      (3) Aminoglycoside antibiotics
      (4) Radiographic dyes (arteriography, CT scan, pyelography)[2]
   b. Diagnostic features
      (1) Serial increases in creatinine and BUN vary with catabolic rate and protein intake
      (2) Oliguria or nonoliguria, but relatively fixed outputs
      (3) Variable response to high dose furosemide, may convert oliguria to nonoliguria

    (4) Pulmonary vascular congestion and hyperkalemia represent the most important parameters to follow; PA catheter may be necessary to monitor fluid status

    (5) Urine sodium is high, generally >30

    (6) Urine osmolarity is less than 350 mOsm/kg and generally fixed (300 mOsm/kg +/−)

    (7) Urine creatinine is low in relation to urine volume, leading to a U/P creatinine less than 20

    (8) Fractional excretion of sodium[13] (FE_{Na}) is greater than 1 (see Table 16-1)

    (9) Urine sediment contains "muddy-brown," renal tubular casts

    (10) Myoglobinuria and serum CPK elevations in rhabdomyolysis

    (11) Polyuric phase often heralds healing

2. Acute allergic interstitial nephritis

    a. Drug induced: methicillin, oxacillin, β lactams, trimethoprim-sulfamethoxazole, NSAIDs, cimetidine, rifampin, azathioprine, diuretics, or sulfa drugs

    b. Differentiated from ATN by: presence of a putative drug, rash, absence of polyuric phase, eosinophiles on stained urine sediment preparations, pyuria, lymphocyturia; positive Gallium scan may be helpful

    c. Biopsy may be necessary for diagnosis

    d. Course of the disease may be shortened by steroids

3. Acute glomerular syndromes

    a. Acute glomerulonephritis

        (1) Etiology

            (a) Prototypically poststreptococcal glomerulonephritis (PSGN)

                • Occurs 3-4 weeks after a streptococcal infection; pharyngitis or impetigo common

                • Manifested by hypertension, gross or microscopic hematuria, periorbital edema

                • Positive throat culture

                • Lab results: 1-3 g/24 hours protein excretion, low C_3, elevated antibodies to streptococcal antigens (ASO, antihyaluronidase, ANADase), low urinary sodium, active urinary sediment including RBC casts

                • Progressive resolution is usually the case, with normalization of C_3 and clearing of urinary findings

            (b) Other glomerular and systemic diseases may present as acute, nonprogressive, or slowly progressive glomerulonephritis although they can present with a rapidly progressive course; three important examples are:

                • Mesangiocapillary GN (hypocomplementemic GN): predominant in young females, insidious onset, and persistently low complement (C_3)

                • Lupus nephritis with focal involvement: positive ANA, anti-DNA, and anti-Sm, together with elements of the total clinical complex

                • IgA nephropathy (Berger's disease): usually presenting with recurrent hematuria following URIs; diagnosis requires renal biopsy with immunofluorescence to identify IgA deposits

    (2) Diagnosis: PSGN possible on clinical grounds

        (a) Alternative diagnoses require renal biopsy

        (b) Biopsy is mandatory if immunotherapy is considered

    (3) Treatment

        (a) If self-limited (e.g., PSGN), treatment consists of blood pressure control and symptomatic measures

        (b) With biopsy-proven diagnosis of a potentially progressive disease, immunosuppressive therapeutic measures are of value:

          • Alternate day steroids in mesangiocapillary GN

          • Pulse cyclophosphamide (Cytoxan) in lupus GN, Wegener's granulomatosis, systemic vasculitis

b. Rapidly progressive glomerulonephritis (RPGN)

    (1) Definition: rapidly progressive renal failure with BUN and creatinine rising incrementally over the course of days to weeks, in association with an active urinary sediment (including RBC casts); pathologically RPGN is characterized by the presence of crescents (usually over 80%) on light microscopy

    (2) Etiology

        (a) PSGN, in rare cases; more likely in adults

        (b) Associated with chronic infectious processes (SBE, abdominal sepsis, hepatitis B)

        (c) Associated with systemic vasculitis (SLE, Wegener's granulomatosis, hypersensitivity angiitis, polyarteritis)

        (d) Antiglomerular basement membrane syndromes (Goodpasture's syndrome with lung hemorrhage)

        (e) Idiopathic

    (3) Clinical manifestations

        (a) May be dominated by the systemic manifestations of the associated disorder

        (b) Renal manifestations: hypertension, hematuria, proteinuria, active sediment (including RBC casts and broad tubular casts) indicating widespread renal damage, progressive increases in BUN and creatinine

    (4) Diagnosis: The above clinical manifestations require a renal biopsy to confirm the diagnosis and exclude unusual presentations of alternative diseases (including interstitial nephritis, ATN, and multiple myeloma)

    (5) Treatment: aggressive therapy with immunosuppressive regimens is indicated

        (a) Plasmapheresis and immunosuppression in early cases of Goodpasture's syndrome

        (b) Pulse steroids or cyclophosphamide for SLE and vasculitic syndromes

c. Nephrotic syndrome

    (1) Definition: protein excretion exceeding 3 g/24 hours, associated with edema, hypoalbuminemia, and hyperlipidemia, with or without the findings of acute glomerular diseases

        (2) Etiology

           (a) Children: 90% Nil disease, with steroid responsiveness

           (b) Adults: membranous nephropathy, focal sclerosis, amyloid disease, underlying malignancy, DM, drug induced (penicillamine, gold, NSAID, captopril, anticonvulsants, probenemid, chlorpropamide), and in addition, nephrotic range proteinuria can be part of all the ''acute glomerular syndromes''

4. Chronic intrinsic renal disease or interstitial disease

    a. Etiology

        (1) May represent the later stages of any acute glomerulonephritis that has progressed to a predominantly sclerotic or ''burned out'' phase

        (2) Nephrosclerosis secondary to longstanding hypertension

        (3) Diabetic glomerulosclerosis

        (4) Hereditary renal disease

           (a) Polycystic kidney disease

           (b) Alport's syndrome

    b. Diagnosis

        (1) Generally small renal outlines on ultrasound

        (2) Stable (over short periods) BUN and creatinine

        (3) Urine volumes that remain greater than 1L until end stage

        (4) Potassium levels that remain normal with stable urine volumes despite substantial elevations of creatinine

        (5) Evidence of retained uremic poisons (see p. 357)

        (6) Hypertension is frequently present

    c. Treatment

        (1) Before dialysis is necessary

           (a) Low-protein diet (40 g/day) may prolong remaining renal life

           (b) Avoid dehydration with overuse of diuretics

           (c) Strict control of hypertension; emphasis should be on vasoactive drugs with judicious diuretic use

           (d) Adjust drug doses to correct for prolonged half-lives (particularly digoxin and aminoglycosides)

           (e) Start PO_4 binder and vitamin D therapy when serum calcium and phosphorus levels become abnormal

        (2) Initiation of dialysis

           (a) Urgent indications: pericarditis, neuropathy, and neuromuscular abnormalities (asterixis, seizures)

           (b) Judgmental indications: creatinine clearance below 10-15 ml/minute; progressive anorexia, weight loss, reversal of sleep pattern, pruritus, uncontrolled fluid gains with hypertension and signs of congestive failure

5. Acute or chronic renal failure secondary to vascular disorders

    a. Atheromatous emboli

        (1) Most commonly seen following aortic catheterization, but can occur spontaneously

        (2) Characteristic livido reticularis pattern seen in the lower extremities

        (3) Likely acute and progressive

   b. Major renal vascular occlusive disease
      (1) Associated with renal vascular hypertension
      (2) Bruits likely to be present
      (3) Susceptibility to acute renal failure with captopril
      (4) Arteriography needed for definitive diagnosis
      (5) In selected cases, vascular repair or percutaneous angioplasty have
          slowed the progressive course
   c. Disseminated coagulopathy with acute renal failure
      (1) Hemolytic-uremic syndrome
      (2) Thrombotic thrombocytopenia
      (3) Malignant hypertension
   d. Nephrosclerosis secondary to chronic essential hypertension: charac-
      teristic benign sediment and minimum proteinuria
6. Toxic nephropathies have variable presentations; examples include:
   a. Ethylene glycol, acetaminophen, lysis nephropathy: acute renal failure
   b. Tubular disorders: chronic lead intoxication
   c. Cisplatinum use: electrolyte abnormalities (low magnesium, low po-
      tassium)
   d. Analgesic abuse (phenacetin, ASA): chronic renal failure
7. Myeloma kidney
   a. Tubular light chain deposition with acute renal failure
   b. Monoclonal light chains in the urine
   c. Must be differentiated from hypercalcemic nephropathy, ATN, and
      amyloid disease
8. Primary tubular disorders (when to suspect renal tubular acidosis):
   a. Electrolyte picture on non–anion gap acidosis without renal insuffi-
      ciency and in the absence of respiratory alkalosis, or hyperkalemia out
      of proportion to GFR decrement (occasional ''hyporeninemic hypoal-
      dosteronism'' presentation of patients with distal RTA)
   b. A patient presenting with severe hypokalemia
   c. Finding unexplained osteomalacia
   d. Finding nephrocalcinosis
   e. In paraproteinemic states
   f. After implicatable drug administration (amphotericin)
   g. Finding proximal amino acid and glucose urinary losses
   h. Urine pH and pCO_2
      (1) pH never below 6 in distal RTA; HCO_3 wasting in proximal RTA
      (2) Urinary pCO_2 low in distal RTA when HCO_3 is given

Diagnostic methods
1. Determine if renal failure is acute or chronic (Tables 16-1 and 16-2)
   a. Rate of rise in BUN and creatinine
   b. Urine/plasma creatinine ratios
   c. Renal size by ultrasonography
   d. Historic lab data if available
   e. Anemia can occur early in renal failure and correlates poorly with the
      duration of the disease

Table 16-1 Serum and radiographic abnormalities in renal failure

	Prerenal	Postrenal (Acute)	Intrinsic Renal (Acute)	Intrinsic Renal (Chronic)
BUN	↑ 10:1 > Creatinine	↑ 20-40/day △ rise	↑ 20-40/day △ rise	Stable, ↑ varies with protein intake
Serum creatinine	N/slight ↑	↑ 2-4/day △ rise	↑ 2-4/day △ rise	Stable ↑ (production = excretion)
Serum potassium	N/slight ↑	↑; varies with urine volume	↑ (particularly when the patient is oliguric) ↑↑↑ with rhabdomyolysis	Normal until end-stage, unless tubular dysfunction (Type IV RTA)
Serum phosphorus	N/slight ↑	Moderately ↑ ↑↑ with rhabdomyolysis	Poor correlation with duration of renal disease	Becomes significantly elevated when serum creatinine surpasses 3 mg/100 ml
Serum calcium	N	N/↓ with PO_4 retention	↓ (poor correlation with duration of renal failure) N/↑	Usually ↓
Renal size by ultrasound	N/↑	↑ and dilated calyces	N/↑	↓ and with ↑ echogenicity
FE_{Na}*	<1	<1 → >1	>1	>1

KEY: ↑, increase; ↓, decrease; N, normal; ↑↑, large increase.

*$FE_{Na} = \dfrac{U_{Na}}{P_{Na}} \bigg/ \dfrac{U_{creat}}{P_{creat}} \times 100$

Table 16-2 Urine abnormalities in renal failure

	Prerenal	Postrenal (Acute)	Intrinsic Renal (Acute)	Intrinsic Renal (Chronic)
Urine volume	↓	Absent-to-wide fluctuation	Oliguric or nonoliguric	1000 ml+ until end stage
Urine creatinine	↑ (U/P creat >40)	↓ (U/P creat >20)	↓ (U/P creat <20)	↓ (U/P creat <20)
Osmolarity	↑ (>400 mOsm/kg)	(<350 mOsm/kg)	(<350 mOsm/kg)	(<350 mOsm/kg)
Degree of proteinuria	Minimum	Absent	Varies with etiology of renal failure: Minimum with ATN Nephrotic range with interstitial nephritis secondary to NSAIDs	Varies with etiology of renal disease (from 1-2 g/day to nephrotic range)
Urine sediment	Negative, or occasional hyaline cast	Negative or hematuria with stones or papillary necrosis Pyuria with infectious prostatic disease	ATN: muddy brown Interstitial nephritis: lymphocytes, eosinophils (in stained preparations) and WBC casts RPGN: RBC casts Nephrosis: oval fat bodies	Broad casts with variable renal "residual" acute findings

KEY: ↑, increased; ↓, decreased; U/P, urine/plasma; clearance = $\dfrac{\text{Urine concentration} \times \text{Urine volume}}{\text{Plasma concentration}}$

2. Clinical correlates from history and physical exam
   a. Purpura: Henoch-Schoenlein purpura, vasculitis
   b. Pulmonary disease: Wegener's granulomatosis, Goodpasture's syndrome, SLE, vasculitis
   c. Connective tissue abnormalities: SLE, scleroderma, mixed connective tissue disease (MCTD)
   d. Heart murmur: SBE with glomerulonephritis
   e. Fever and abdominal pain: consider abdominal sepsis with glomerulonephritis
   f. Drug abuse: focal sclerosis, amyloidosis
   g. Amyloidosis: chronic infection, enteritis, rheumatoid arthritis
   h. Diabetes: glomerulosclerosis, pyelonephritis, papillary necrosis
   i. Sickle cell disease: papillary necrosis, type IV RTA
   j. Chemotherapy: lysis with uric acid nephropathy
   k. Hearing loss: Alport's syndrome
3. Diagnostic supports from serum analysis
   a. Consider SLE if positive ANA or anti-Sm antibody
   b. C_3: if decreased, suspect infectious etiology (post-streptococcal infection, SBE, visceral sepsis, primary mesangiocapillary disease)
   c. C_4: decreased in SLE
   d. Hepatitis B_sAg positive: consider nephritis with vasculitis, membranous nephropathy
   e. Cryoglobulins present: consider SLE, systemic vasculitis, postinfectious streptococcal infection, visceral sepsis, myeloma, Waldenstrom's macroglobulinemia, hepatitis B infection, mixed essential cryoglobulinemia
   f. Abnormal protein electrophoresis: myeloma
   g. Abnormal immuno-electrophoresis: myeloma, IgA nephropathy (Berger's disease), Waldenstrom's macroglobulinemia
   h. Rheumatoid factor positive: polyarteritis, connective tissue disease
   i. ASO titer: post-streptococcal, acute glomerulonephritis
4. Major diagnoses established by renal biopsy
   a. Differential diagnosis of the nephrotic syndrome: amyloid, focal sclerosis, membranous glomerulopathy, or diabetes (if not otherwise established)
   b. Separation of lupus vasculitis from other vasculitis (employing EM deposit pattern) and of lupus membranous from idiopathic membranous
   c. Confirmation of hereditary nephropathies on the basis of their ultrastructure
   d. Diagnosis of RPGN (crescenteric) with the finding of extracapillary cresent formation
   e. Separation of interstitial nephritis from ATN in cases of prolonged renal failure
   f. Separation of the primary glomerulonephritis syndromes: post streptococcal infection, mesangiocapillary types 1-4, membranous, focal vs diffuse, IgG or IgA (done by using immunofluorescence and electron microscopy to visualize varying deposit patterns)
   g. Finding focal segmental necrosis to suggest an underlying vasculitis not otherwise apparent

Postrenal failure

1. Etiology
   a. Urethral obstruction (prostatic hypertrophy, urethral stricture)
   b. Bladder calculi or neoplasms
   c. Pelvic or retroperitoneal neoplasms
   d. Bilateral ureteral obstruction (neoplasm, calculi)
   e. Retroperitoneal fibrosis
2. Diagnosis
   a. History of dysuria
   b. Evidence of prostatic hypertrophy in men and pelvic pathology in women
   c. Catheterization after voiding to assess residual volume
   d. Ultrasound of abdomen, pelvis, and kidney
3. Therapy: catheter drainage, ureteral stints, percutaneous nephrostomy following urologic consultation

Effects of retained uremic toxins and of uremic milieu

1. General
   a. Anorexia, early satiety
   b. Nausea and vomiting
   c. Pruritus
   d. Fatigue, weakness
2. Cardiovascular
   a. Cardiomyopathy: with chronic fluid overload; concentric hypertrophy is common
   b. Pericarditis: the clinical presentation varies from small pericardial effusions to acute pericarditis with tamponade
   c. Accelerated atherogenesis: elevated triglycerides, decreased HDL
   d. Hypertension: multifactorial (sodium retention, disturbances of renin-angiotension axis)
3. CNS: Abnormalities range from neuromuscular irritability (e.g., "restless legs") to asterixis and coma (metabolic encephalopathy)
4. Endocrine
   a. Abnormal glucose metabolism secondary to
      (1) Increased insulin resistance
      (2) Prolonged insulin half-life
      (3) Decreased gluconeogenesis with lower amino acid pool
      (4) Increased renal threshold for glucose
   b. Decreased T_4: secondary to decreased protein binding; normal free T_4
5. Hematopoietic
   a. Anemia: usually normochromic, normocytic; multifactorial:
      (1) Chronically depressed erythropoietin levels
      (2) Hemolysis
      (3) Blood loss
      (4) Folate deficiency
   b. Iron overload from transfusions
   c. Coagulopathy
      (1) Platelet count is normal, but thromboasthenia is present with decreased platelet aggregation and adhesiveness
      (2) Prolonged bleeding time improved with DDAVP or cryoprecipitate

6. Gastrointestinal
   a. Increased incidence of duodenitis (increased gastrin levels)
   b. Increased incidence of angiodysplasia of stomach and proximal intestine[3]
   c. Autonomic neuropathy in diabetics
7. Divalent ion disturbances
   a. Increased PTH: measurement is complicated by inactive fragments present in the assay; the midportion C-terminal or N-terminal are most reflective of the active compound
   b. Decreased production of calcitriol
   c. High phosphorus, low calcium, and bone disease: osteitis fibrosa cystica, osteomalacia
   d. Retained aluminum: from prolonged phosphorus binder therapy or dialysate levels; it can lead to bone disease and CNS abnormalities
8. Miscellaneous
   a. Trace metal deficiency: zinc-hypogusia
   b. Increased incidence of carpal tunnel syndrome: amyloid deposits
   c. Acquired cystic degeneration in reminant kidneys with hemorrhage and rarely neoplastic transformation
   d. Renal oxalate deposition

Considerations when evaluating the patient on chronic hemodialysis

1. Fluid overload caused by excessive interdialytic weight gain
2. Acute hyperkalemia
3. Pericarditis with tamponade
4. Spontaneous hypoglycemia
5. Hyperosmolarity and hyperkalemia (frequent in diabetics)
6. Infection and sepsis (vascular access site, SBE)
7. Subdural hematoma secondary to heparin use during dialysis
8. Seizures secondary to osmotic shifts produced by dialysis
9. Dysrhythmias caused by electrolyte shifts
10. GI bleeding secondary to coagulopathy, duodenitis, angiodysplasia
11. Hypercalcemia caused by excessive vitamin D replacement
12. Bone fractures secondary to osteodystrophy
13. Dementia possibly caused by elevated CNS aluminum concentrations
14. Rupture of CNS and aortic aneurysm in patients with polycystic kidneys
15. Higher incidence of pancreatitis, diverticular disease, carpal tunnel syndrome
16. Psychosocial disturbances (depression, loss of independence, denial)
17. Hepatitis and carrier state

| 16.2 |

DISORDERS OF SODIUM HOMEOSTASIS

Hyponatremia[1,6,7,10]

1. Definition: plasma sodium concentration <134 mEq/L
2. Etiology and classification
   a. Hypotonic hyponatremia (decreased serum osmolality)
      (1) Isovolemic
         (a) SIADH
         (b) Water intoxication (e.g., schizophrenic patients)

      (c) Renal failure

      (d) Reset osmostat (e.g., chronic active TB, carcinomatosis)

      (e) Glucocorticoid deficiency

      (f) Hypothyroidism

      (g) Thiazide diuretics

    (2) Hypovolemic

      (a) Renal losses (diuretics, partial urinary tract obstruction, salt-losing renal disease)

      (b) Extrarenal losses: GI (vomiting, diarrhea), extensive burns, third spacing (peritonitis, pancreatitis)

      (c) Adrenal insufficiency

    (3) Hypervolemic

      (a) CHF

      (b) Nephrosis

      (c) Cirrhosis

  b. Isotonic hyponatremia (normal serum osmolality)

    (1) Pseudohyponatremia (increased serum lipids, and serum proteins)

    (2) Isotonic infusions (e.g., glucose, mannitol)

  c. Hypertonic hyponatremia (increased serum osmolality)

    (1) Hyperglycemia: each 100 ml/dl increment in blood sugar above normal decreases plasma sodium concentration by 1.6 mEq/L[8]

    (2) Hypertonic infusions (e.g., glucose, mannitol)

3. Clinical manifestations of hyponatremia vary with the degree of hyponatremia and the rapidity of onset

  a. Moderate hyponatremia or gradual onset: confusion, muscle cramps, lethargy, anorexia, nausea

  b. Severe hyponatremia or rapid onset: seizures, coma

4. Diagnostic approach: refer to Fig. 16-1

5. Management

  a. Isovolemic hyponatremia

    (1) SIADH: fluid restriction (refer to section 12.7)

    (2) Acute symptomatic water intoxication: hypertonic (3%) saline infusion; generally half of the serum sodium deficit should be corrected in the initial 8-12 hours to prevent complications from rapid correction (cerebral edema, pontine myelinolysis, seizures)

  b. Hypovolemic hyponatremia: 0.9% saline infusion

  NOTE: In symptomatic patients with hyponatremia an increase in the serum sodium concentration of 2 mmol/L per hour to a level of 120-130 mmol is considered adequate by most experts,[11] however, less rapid correction may be indicated in patients with severe hyponatremia

  c. Hypervolemic hyponatremia: sodium and water restriction

  NOTE: The combination of captopril and furosemide is effective in patients with hyponatremia secondary to CHF

Hypernatremia[1,7,10]

1. Definition: plasma sodium concentration >144 mEq/L

2. Etiology and classification

  a. Isovolemic (decreased total body water [TBW], normal total body sodium [TBNa] and ECF)

    (1) Diabetes insipidus (neurogenic and nephrogenic)

    (2) Skin loss (hyperthermia), iatrogenic, reset osmostat

Text continued on p. 363.

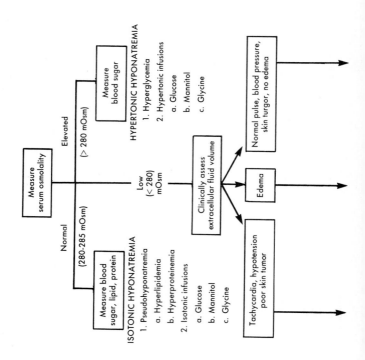

Hypovolemic hypotonic hyponatremia

Causes	BUN/Creat	Uric acid	Urinary Osm.	Urinary (Na)
GI losses	↑↑/↑	↑	↑↑	↓↓
Skin losses	↑↑/↑	↑	↑↑	↓↓
Lung losses	↑↑/↑	↑	↑↑	↓↓
Third space	↑↑/↑	↑	↑↑	↓↓
Renal losses				
Diuretics	↑↑/↑	↑	ISO	↑
Renal damage	↑↑/↑↑	↑	ISO	↑
Partial urinary tract obstruction	↑↑/↑	↑	ISO (↓)	↑
Adrenal insufficiency	↑↑/↑	↑	↑	↑

Hypervolemic hypotonic hyponatremia

Causes	BUN/Creat	Uric acid	Urinary Osm.	Urinary (Na)
CHF	↑↑/↑	↑	↑	↓
Liver damage	↑↑/↑	↑	↑	↓
Nephrosis	↑↑/↑ (↑↑/↑↑)	↑	↑	↓ (ISO↑)

Isovolemic hypotonic hyponatremia

Causes	BUN/Creat	Uric acid	Urinary Osm.	Urinary (Na)
H_2O intoxication	↓/↓	↓	↑,(↓)	↓
Renal failure	↑↑/↑↑	↑	ISO	↑
K^+ loss	↑/↑(N)	↑	↑	↓
SIADH	↓/↓	↓↓	↑	↑
Reset osmostat	N	N	V	V

Figure 16-1
Diagnostic approach to hyponatremia. ↑, Increases; ↓, decreases; N, normal; V, variable. From Narins, R.G., Jones, E.R., Stom, M.C., Rudnick, M.R., and Bastl, C.P.: Diagnostic strategies in disorders of fluid, electrolyte, and acid-base homeostasis, Am. J. Med. 72:498, 1982.

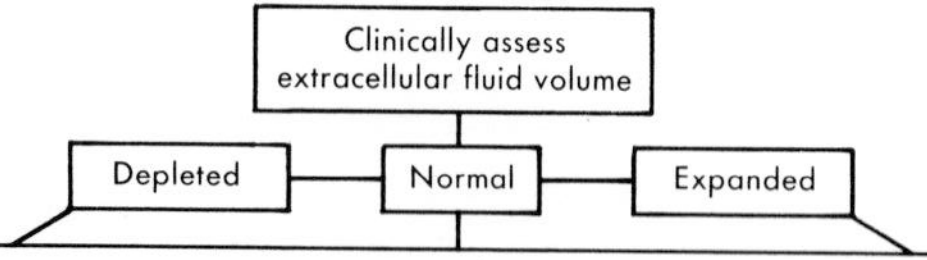
Clinically assess extracellular fluid volume
Depleted
Normal
Expanded

Hypovolemic hypernatremia

Loss of water + Na (H_2O loss > Na)

Causes	BUN/Creat	Urinary (Na)	Urinary Osm
Renal			
Diuretics	↑↑/↑	↑	↓
Glycosuria	↑/N,↑	↑	↓
Urea diuresis	↑↑/N,↑	↑	↓
Acute/chronic renal failure	↑↑/↑↑	↑	↓
Partial obstruction	↑↑/↑↑	↑	↓
Adrenal			
Congenital or acquired deficiencies	↑↑/↑	↑	±↑
GI losses	↑↑/↑	↓	↑
Respiratory losses	↑↑/↑	↓	↑
Skin losses	↑↑/↑	↓	↑

Isovolemic hypernatremia

Loss of water

Causes	BUN/Creat	Urinary (Na)	Urinary Osm
Diabetes insipidus			
Central	↑/N	N	↓
Nephrogenic	↑/N	N	↑
Reset osmostat	N/N	N	V
Skin loss	↑/N	↓	↑
Iatrogenic	N/N	V	↑

Hypervolemic hypernatremia

Gain water + Na (Na gain > H_2O)

Causes	BUN/Creat	Urinary (Na)	Urinary Osm
Iatrogenic	V	↑,(V)	V
Mineralocorticoid excess			
First-degree aldosteronism	N	N	V
Cushing's syndrome	N	N	V
Congenital adrenal hyperplasia	N	N	V
Exogenous	N	N	V

Figure 16-2

Dignostic approach to hypernatremia. ↑, Increases; ↓, decreases; N, normal; V, variable. From Narins, R.G., Jones, E.R., Stom, M.C., Rudnick, M.R., and Bastl, C.P.: Diagnostic strategies in disorders of fluid, electrolyte, and acid-base homeostasis, Am. J. Med. 72:501, 1982.

   b. Hypervolemic (increased TBW, and markedly increased TB_{Na} and ECF)
      (1) Iatrogenic (administration of hypernatremic solutions)
      (2) Mineralocorticoid excess (Conn's syndrome, Cushing's syndrome)
      (3) Salt ingestion
3. Clinical manifestations vary with degree of hypernatremia and rapidity of onset; they range from confusion and lethargy to seizures and coma
4. Diagnostic approach (refer to Fig. 16-2)
5. Management
   a. Isovolemic hypernatremia
      (1) Fluid replacement with D_5W
         (a) Correct only half of estimated volume deficit in initial 24 hours
         (b) The rate of correction of serum sodium should not exceed 1 mEq/L/hour
      (2) Water deficit in liters $= 0.6 \times$ body weight (kg) $\times$
         $$\left(\frac{\text{Measured serum sodium}}{140} - 1 \right)$$
   b. Hypovolemic hypernatremia:
      (1) Fluid replacement with hypotonic saline
      (2) The rate of correction of plasma osmolarity should not exceed 2 mOsm/kg/hour
   c. Hypervolemic hypernatremia: fluid replacement with D_5W (to correct hypertonicity) is instituted following use of diuretics (to increase sodium excretion)

16.3 DISORDERS OF POTASSIUM HOMEOSTASIS

Hypokalemia[1,4,10]

1. Definition: plasma potassium concentration <3.3 mEq/L
2. Etiology and classification
   a. Cellular shift (redistribution) and undetermined mechanisms
      (1) Alkalosis (each 0.1 increase in pH decreases serum potassium by 0.4-0.6 mEq/L)
      (2) Insulin administration
      (3) Vitamin B_{12} therapy for megaloblastic anemias, acute leukemias
      (4) Hypokalemic periodic paralysis: rare familial disorder manifested by recurrent attacks of flaccid paralysis and hypokalemia
      (5) β adrenergic agonists (e.g., terbutaline)
      (6) Barium poisoning, toluene intoxication
   b. Increased renal excretion
      (1) Drugs
         (a) Diuretics, including carbonic anhydrase inhibitors (e.g., acetazolamide)
         (b) Amphotericin B
         (c) High-dose sodium penicillin or carbenicillin
         (d) Cisplatinum
         (e) Aminoglycosides
         (f) Corticosteroids
      (2) Renal tubular acidosis: seen with proximal (Type II) or distal (Type I) RTA

      (3) DKA, ureteroenterostomy

      (4) Magnesium deficiency

      (5) Postobstruction diuresis, diuretic phase of ATN

      (6) Osmotic diuresis (e.g., mannitol)

      (7) Bartter's syndrome: hyperplasia of JG cells leading to increased renin and aldosterone, metabolic alkalosis, hypokalemia, muscle weakness, and tetany (seen in young adults)

      (8) Interstitial nephritis

      (9) Increased mineralocorticoid activity (primary or secondary aldosteronism), Cushing's syndrome

     (10) Chronic metabolic alkalosis from loss of gastric fluid (increased renal potassium secretion)

  c. GI loss

      (1) Vomiting, nasogastric suction

      (2) Diarrhea

      (3) Laxative abuse

      (4) Villous adenoma

      (5) Fistulae

  d. Inadequate dietary intake (e.g., anorexia nervosa)

  e. Cutaneous loss (excessive sweating)

6. Clinical manifestations

  a. Depending on the level of hypokalemia and the rate of decrease, manifestations range from mild muscle weakness to overt paralysis (including respiratory paralysis) and rhabdomyolysis

  b. Atrial and ventricular dysrhythmias may develop (particularly in patients receiving digitalis); ventricular dysrhythmias are one of the leading causes of death in patients with anorexia nervosa and severe potassium deficiency

7. ECG manifestations

  a. Mild hypokalemia: flattening of T waves, ST segment depression, PVCs, prolonged QT interval

  b. Severe hypokalemia: prominent U waves, AV conduction disturbances, ventricular tachycardia or fibrillation

8. Diagnostic approach

  a. Distinguish true hypokalemia from redistribution (e.g., alkalosis, insulin administration)

  b. Measure 24-hour urinary potassium excretion while patient is on a regular dietary sodium intake

      (1) <20 mEq: consider extrarenal potassium loss

      (2) >20 mEq: renal potassium loss

  c. If renal potassium wasting is suspected, the following steps are indicated:

      (1) Measure 24-hour urine chloride

         (a) >10 mEq: diuretics, Bartter's syndrome, mineralocorticoid excess

         (b) <10 mEq: vomiting, gastric drainage

      (2) Measure blood pressure; if elevated, consider mineralocorticoid excess (see section 12.11)

      (3) Measure serum bicarbonate (HCO_3): a low level is suggestive of renal tubular acidosis (RTA)

Table 16-3   Common potassium supplements

Product	Brand Name	Potassium Content
Potassium chloride		
Slow-release tab	Klotrix	10 mEq/tab
	K-Tab	10 mEq/tab
	Slow-K	8 mEq/tab
	Kaon-Cl	6.7 mEq/tab
Effervescent tab	K-Lyte/Cl	25 mEq/tab
	Klorvess	20 mEq/tab
Slow-release cap	Micro-K	8 mEq/cap
Powder	K-lyte/Cl	25 mEq/packet
	K-Lor	15 or 20 mEq/ packet
Liquid	Kaon-Cl 20%	40 mEq/15 ml
	Rum K	30 mEq/15 ml
	K-Lor	20 mEq/15 ml
	Potassium chloride oral solution	10 mEq/15 ml
Potassium acetate/bi-carbonate/citrate	Tri-K	45 mEq/15 ml
Potassium bicarbonate	K-Lyte	25 mEq/packet
Potassium gluconate	Kaon	20 mEq/15 ml

9. Management
   a. Potassium replacement; Table 16-3 describes commonly available products
      (1) PO potassium replacement is preferred
      (2) IV infusion should not exceed 40 mEq/hour
   b. Monitor ECG and urine output
   c. Identify underlying cause and treat accordingly[1]

Hyperkalemia[1,4,5,10]

1. Definition: plasma potassium concentration >4.9 mEq/L
2. Etiology and classification
   a. Pseudohyperkalemia
      (1) Hemolyzed specimen
      (2) Severe thrombocytosis (platelet count $>10^6$/ml)
      (3) Severe leukocytosis (WBC $>10^5$/ml)
   b. Excessive potassium intake
      (1) Potassium replacement therapy
      (2) High-potassium diet
      (3) Salt substitutes
      (4) Potassium salts of antibiotics
   c. Decreased renal excretion
      (1) Potassium-sparing diuretics (e.g., spironolactone, triamterene, amiloride)
      (2) Renal insufficiency
      (3) Mineralocorticoid deficiency

     (4) Hyporeninemic hypoaldosteronism (DM)
     (5) Tubular unresponsiveness to aldosterone (e.g., SLE, multiple my-
         eloma, sickle cell disease)
     (6) Type IV RTA
     (7) ACE inhibitors
     (8) Heparin administration
  d. Redistribution (excessive cellular release)
     (1) Acidemia (each 0.1 decrease in pH increases serum potassium by
         0.4-0.6 mEq/L)
     (2) Insulin deficiency
     (3) Drugs (e.g., succinylcholine, markedly increased digitalis level,
         arginine, β-adrenergic blockers)
     (4) Hypertonicity
     (5) Hemolysis
     (6) Tissue necrosis, rhabdomyolisis, burns
     (7) Hyperkalemic periodic paralysis
3. Clinical manifestations: weakness (generalized), irritability, paresthesias,
   decreased DTR, paralysis, cardiac dysrhythmias (ventricular ectopy,
   bradycardia, asystole)

Table 16-4   Therapy of acute hyperkalemia associated with
ECG changes or clinical manifestations

Treatment options	Onset of Action	Duration of Action
Glucose 50 g IV bolus or IV infusion of 500 ml of 10% dextrose solution, *plus* insulin 10 U regular insulin IV	Approximately 30 min	3 hr
Calcium gluconate* (10% solution) 5-10 ml IV over 3 min	5 min	Less than 1 hr
Dialysis (hemodialysis or peritoneal)	5 min after start of dialysis	3 hr after end of dialysis
Sodium bicarbonate (NaHCO₃) 1 ampul (44 mEq) over 5 min	Approximately 30 min	3 hr
Sodium polystyrene sulfonate (Kayexelate) PO or via NG tube: 20-50 g Kayexelate plus 100-200 ml of 20% sorbitol Retention enema: 50 g Kayexelate in 200 ml of 20% sorbitol	1-2 hr	3 hr

*Use with caution in patients receiving digitalis.

4. ECG manifestations
   a. Mild hyperkalemia: peaking or tenting of T waves, PVCs
   b. Severe hyperkalemia: peaking of T waves, widening of QRS complex, depressed ST segments, prolongation of PR interval, sinus arrest, deep S wave, PVCs, ventricular tachycardia or fibrillation
5. Diagnostic and therapeutic approach
   a. Rule out pseudohyperkalemia or lab error
      (1) Obtain ECG; in patients with pseudohyperkalemia secondary to hemolyzed specimen or thrombocytosis, the ECG will not show any manifestations of hyperkalemia
      (2) Repeat serum potassium level
      (3) In patients with thrombocytosis or severe leukocytosis, an accurate serum potassium can be determined by drawing a heparinized sample
   b. Stop all potassium intake (IV and PO)
   c. In patients with true hyperkalemia and ECG or clinical manifestations, immediate intervention is indicated with one or more measures depending on the severity of hyperkalemia (see Table 16-4)
   d. Monitor ECG
   e. Check pH, correct acidosis (if present)
   f. Check calcium, magnesium, electrolytes, BUN, creatinine levels
   g. Identify underlying cause of hyperkalemia and treat if possible
      (1) Dialysis for renal failure
      (2) Exogenous mineralocorticoids in mineralocorticoid deficiency
      (3) Stop any potassium-sparing diuretics

16.4 DISORDERS OF MAGNESIUM METABOLISM

Hypomagnesemia[1,9]

1. Definition: plasma magnesium concentration <1.8 mg/dl
2. Etiology
   a. Gastrointestinal and nutritional
      (1) Defective GI absorption (malabsorption)
      (2) Inadequate dietary intake (e.g., alcoholics)
      (3) Parenteral therapy without magnesium
   b. Excessive renal losses
      (1) Diuretics
      (2) Renal tubular acidosis
      (3) Diuretic phase of ATN
      (4) Endocrine disturbances (DKA, hyperaldosteronism, hyperthyroidism, hypoparathyroidism)
      (5) Cisplatinum therapy
3. ECG manifestations: prolonged QT interval
4. Clinical and lab manifestations
   a. Neuromuscular: muscle weakness, hyperreflexia, muscle fasciculations, tremors
   b. Cardiovascular: cardiac dysrhythmias
   c. Hypokalemia refractory to potassium replacement
   d. Hypocalcemia refractory to calcium replacement

5. Management
   a. Correct magnesium deficiency
      (1) Mild: 600 mg magnesium oxide PO provides 35 mEq of magnesium; dosage is 1-2 tab/day
      (2) Moderate: 50% solution magnesium sulfate (each 2 ml ampul contains 8 mEq or 96 mg of elemental magnesium); dosage is one 2 ml ampul of 50% magnesium solution q6h prn
      (3) Severe (serum magnesium level <1.0 mg/dl) and symptomatic patient (seizures, tetany): 2 g magnesium in 20 ml D_5W IV over 15 minutes; monitor ECG, blood pressure, pulse, respiration, deep tendon reflexes, and urine output
   b. Identify and correct underlying disorder

Hypermagnesemia

1. Definition: plasma magnesium concentration >2.3 mg/dl
2. Etiology
   a. Renal failure (decreased GFR)
   b. Decreased renal excretion secondary to salt depletion
   c. Abuse of antacids and laxatives containing magnesium
   d. Endocrinopathies (deficiency of mineralocorticoid or thyroid hormone)
   e. Increased tissue breakdown
3. ECG manifestations: shortened QT and QRS interval, heart block
4. Clinical manifestations: paresthesias, hypotension, confusion, decreased DTR, paralysis, apnea
5. Management
   a. Identify and correct underlying disorder
   b. Intracardiac conduction abnormalities can be treated with IV calcium gluconate
   c. Dialysis for severe hypermagnesemia

References

1. Arieff, A.I., and DeFronzo, R.A.: Fluid, electrolyte and acid base disorders, New York, 1985, Churchill-Livingstone.
2. Berkseth, R.O., and Kjellstrandt, C.M.: Radiologic contrast induced nephropathy, Med. Clin. North Am. **68**:351, 1984.
3. Clouse, R.E., et al.: Angiodysplasia as a cause of upper gastrointestinal bleeding, Arch. Intern. Med. **145**:458, 1985.
4. Cox, M.: Potassium homeostasis, Med. Clin. North Am. **65**:363, 1981.
5. DeFronzo, R.A., et al.: Clinical disorders of hyperkalemia, Ann. Rev. Med. **33**:521, 1982.
6. DeFronzo, R.A., and Thier, S.O.: Pathophysiologic approach to hyponatremia, Arch. Int. Med. **140**:897, 1980.
7. Goldberg, M.: Hyponatremia, Med. Clin. North Am. **65**:251, 1981.
8. Katz, M.A.: Hyperglycemia-induced hyponatremia: calculation of expected serum sodium depression, N. Engl. J. Med. **289**:843, 1973.
9. Levin, R.M.: The role of magnesium in cardiovascular disorders, Cardiovasc. Med. **10**:37-42, 1985.
10. Narins, R.G., et al.: Diagnostic strategies in disorders of fluid, electrolyte and acid-base homeostasis, Am. J. Med. **72**(3):496, 1982.
11. Narins, R.G.: Therapy of hyponatremia: does haste make waste? N.Engl. J. Med. **314**:1574, 1986.
12. Reeves, W.B., Foley, R.J., and Weinman, E.J.: Renal dysfunction from nonsteroidal anti-inflammatory drugs (editorial), Arch. Intern. Med. **144**:1943-441, 1984.
13. Zarich, S., Fang. L.S., and Diamond, Jr.: Fractional excretion of sodium: exceptions to its diagnostic value, Arch. Intern. Med. **145**:108, 1985.

Neurology

17

17.1 GENERALIZED TONIC-CLONIC SEIZURES
Kenneth Siegel

General approach

1. The diagnosis of a seizure disorder is made on clinical grounds
   a. Most seizures stop in 30-90 seconds
   b. The most important diagnostic tool is an adequate history obtained from the patient and other observers of the event
   c. A telephone call is frequently the most important diagnostic tool
2. History
   a. Recent head trauma
   b. Alcohol ingestion (ethanol withdrawal seizure)
   c. Diabetic patient on insulin or sulfonylureas: consider drug-induced hypoglycemia
   d. Previous neurologic insults (e.g., CVA)
   e. History of meningitis or encephalitis
   f. Were others present during the seizure?
   g. Were eyes tonically deviated during the seizure (e.g., eye deviation to the left during the seizure implies a lesion in the right hemisphere)
3. Approach varies with clinical presentation (e.g., alert patient after single convulsive episode vs patient with continuing seizure activity)

Evaluation of patient with single convulsive episode

1. Draw routine studies when an IV line is started
   a. Serum electrolytes: to rule out hyponatremia/hypernatremia
   b. Glucose: to rule out hypoglycemia
   c. Calcium: to rule out hypocalcemia/hypercalcemia
   d. Magnesium: to rule out hypomagnesemia
   e. CBC: to rule out infectious process (e.g., sepsis, meningitis, encephalitis)
   f. BUN and creatinine: to rule out renal failure
   g. Toxicology screen (blood and urine): to rule out suspected drug ingestion
2. If the patient has stopped convulsing, therapy with IV diazepam should not be instituted, nor should the patient be rushed into the CT scanner before being fully stabilized

3. Obtain a CT scan or MRI scan to rule out CNS hemorrhage/infarct, mass lesions, AVM, aneurysms
4. An electroencephalogram (EEG) is indicated in any patient with new-onset generalized tonic-clonic seizures
5. Perform a lumbar puncture only after visualizing the intracranial structures (CT scan or MRI scan) and in the absence of a demonstrable lesion
6. If there is suspicion of meningitis, perform a lumbar puncture immediately after ruling out increased intracranial pressure with a fundoscopic exam (without waiting for CT scan or MRI scan)

Treatment of a patient with a single tonic-clonic convulsive episode

1. Correct treatment is still very controversial
2. Focal abnormalities on neurologic exam, CT scan or MRI scan, or EEG serve as a guide; spike activity 24 hours after a seizure or a focal cerebral lesion on CT scan or MRI scan are reasons to institute therapy, since the risk of recurrence varies from 50%-90%
3. In the absence of abnormal EEGs, CT scan or MRI scan, observe patient; the chance of recurrence varies from 20%-30%
4. Pharmacologic therapy
   a. Oral anticonvulsants can achieve therapeutic levels in a short period of time in most patients
      (1) 24-28 hours with high dosages of phenytoin (Dilantin) 15-18 mg/kg PO in the first 24 hours or
      (2) 3-5 days with carbamazepine (Tegretol) 600 mg qd
   b. A single anticonvulsant should be tried and pushed to clinical toxicity level (if necessary) before considering a second drug
   c. The drug of choice in IV therapy is phenytoin 18 mg/kg at no more than 50 mg/minute (with ECG monitoring)

Management of status epilepticus

1. Aggressive treatment is required for patients with continuing seizures lasting 10 minutes or seizures without intervening consciousness
2. Seizure activity continuing for 30 minutes or intermittently over a 30-minute period without the patient regaining consciousness is termed *status epilepticus*[10]
3. Management of status epilepticus[7,10]
   a. Insert oral airway
   b. Start IV with normal saline solution
   c. Draw samples to evaluate ABG, electrolyte, glucose, BUN, creatinine, calcium, magnesium, and anticonvulsant levels
   d. Institute electrocardiographic, respiratory, and blood pressure monitoring
   e. Give 100 mg of thiamine IM
   f. Give 50 ml bolus injection of a 50% glucose solution
   g. Give diazepam (Valium) 2 mg IV push/minute to maximum of 20 mg
      (1) Monitor closely for respiratory depression and hypotension
      (2) Emergency intubation may be required
      (3) Increase saline infusion if patient becomes hypotensive
   h. Give phenytoin (Dilantin) simultaneously at a rate of 50 mg/minute until a loading dose of 18 mg/kg is given

4. Above measures will control 90% of all patients within 30-40 minutes; if seizures continue, *intubate patient* and proceed with the following measures:
   a. Give phenobarbital 100 mg/minute IV to maximum of 20 mg/kg, or
   b. Give diazepam (100 mg in 500 ml of D5W) infused at 40 ml/hour; this will result in diazepam serum levels of 0.2-0.8 μg/ml
   c. If seizure activity persists longer than 60 minutes, institute general anesthesia with isoflurane and neuromuscular blockade

| 17.2 | SYNCOPE |

Definition

Syncope is defined as a temporary loss of consciousness resulting from an acute, global reduction in cerebral blood flow.

Etiology[2,36]

1. Vasovagal (vasodepressor)
   a. Psychophysiologic
   b. Visceral reflex
   c. Carotid sinus
   d. Glossopharyngeal neuralgia
2. Orthostatic hypotension
   a. Hypovolemia
   b. Hypotensive drugs
   c. Neurogenic, idiopathic
   d. Pheochromocytoma
   e. Systemic mastocytosis
3. Cardiac
   a. Reduced cardiac output
      (1) Left ventricular outflow obstruction (aortic stenosis, hypertrophic cardiomyopathy)
      (2) Obstruction to pulmonary flow (pulmonary embolism, pulmonic stenosis, primary pulmonary hypertension)
      (3) MI with pump failure
      (4) Cardiac tamponade
   b. Dysrhythmias or asystole
      (1) Extreme tachycardia (>160-180/minute)
      (2) Severe bradycardia (<30-40/minute)
      (3) Sick sinus syndrome
      (4) AV block (second or third degree)
      (5) Ventricular tachycardia or fibrillation
4. Cerebrovascular
   a. Vertebrobasilar TIA, spasm
   b. Subclavian steal
   c. Basilar migraine
5. Other causes
   a. Mechanical reduction of venous return (Valsalva maneuver, cough, defecation, micturition, atrial myxoma, ball valve thrombus)
   b. Not related to decreased blood flow: hypoxia, hypoglycemia, anemia, hyperventilation, seizure disorder

Evaluation[23]

1. History
   a. Sudden loss of consciousness: consider cardiac dysrhythmias, vertebrobasilar TIA
   b. Gradual loss of consciousness: consider orthostatic hypotension, vasodepressor syncope, hypoglycemia
   c. Patient's activity at the time of syncope
      (1) Micturation, coughing, defecation: consider syncope secondary to decreased venous return
      (2) Turning his head while shaving: consider carotid sinus syndrome
      (3) Physical exertion in a patient with murmur: consider aortic stenosis
      (4) Arm exercise: consider subclavian steal syndrome
      (5) Assuming an upright position: consider orthostatic hypotension
   d. Associated events
      (1) Chest pain: consider MI, pulmonary embolism
      (2) Palpitations: consider dysrhythmias
      (3) History of aura, incontinence during episode, and transient confusion after ''syncope'': consider seizure disorder
   e. Current medications, particularly antihypertensive drugs
2. Physical exam
   a. Blood pressure: if low, consider orthostatic hypotension; if unequal in both arms (difference >20 mm Hg), consider subclavian steal or dissecting aneurysm
   b. Pulse: if patient has tachycardia, bradycardia, or irregular rhythm, consider dysrhythmia
   c. Mental status: if patient is confused after the syncopal episode consider postictal state secondary to seizure
   d. Heart: if there are murmurs present suggestive of AS or IHSS, consider syncope secondary to left ventricular outflow obstruction; if there is JVD and distant heart sounds, consider cardiac tamponade
3. Initial diagnostic tests
   a. CBC: rule out anemia
   b. Electrolytes, magnesium, and calcium: rule out electrolyte abnormalities, hypomagnesemia, and hypocalcemia
   c. ECG: rule out dysrhythmias
   d. Chest x-ray films: evaluate cardiac size, lung fields
   e. ABG: rule out pulmonary embolus, hyperventilation
4. Additional diagnostic tests may be indicated depending on the patient's history and physical exam
   a. If dysrhythmias are suspected, a 24-hour Holter monitor is indicated
   b. An echocardiogram is indicated in patients with a heart murmur to rule out AS or IHSS
   c. If a seizure is suspected, a CT scan of head and an EEG are indicated
   d. If pulmonary embolism is suspected, a ventilation/perfusion scan should be done
   e. Cardiac isoenzymes should be obtained if the patient gives a history of chest pain before the syncopal episode

Prognosis

The prognosis varies with the age of the patient and the etiology of the syncope. Various reports[9,13] indicate the following prognoses:

1. Benign prognosis (very low 1-year morbidity and mortality) in patients:
   a. Aged ≤ 30 and having noncardiac syncope
   b. Aged ≤ 70 and having vasovagal/psychogenic syncope or syncope of unknown cause
2. Poor prognosis (high morbidity and mortality) in patients with cardiac syncope

| 17.3 | DEMENTIA
Marvin Garrell

Definition

The American Psychiatric Association's diagnostic criteria for delirium and dementia are described in the following lists. Delirium is mainly differentiated from dementia from the history—short onset within hours to a few weeks, to chronic or gradual over time. The history must be substantiated by the caregivers.

DSM III diagnostic criteria for delirium*

1. Clouding of consciousness (reduced clarity of awareness of the environment), with reduced capacity to shift, focus, and sustain attention to environmental stimuli
2. At least two of the following:
   a. Perceptual disturbances, misinterpretations, illusions, or hallucinations
   b. Speech that is at times incoherent
   c. Disturbance of sleep-wakefulness cycle, with insomnia or daytime drowsiness
   d. Increased or decreased psychomotor activity
3. Disorientation and memory impairment (if testable)
4. Clinical features that develop over a short period of time (usually hours to days) and tend to fluctuate over the course of a day
5. Evidence from the history, physical examination, or laboratory tests, of a specific organic factor judged to be etiologically related to the disturbance

DSM-III diagnostic criteria for dementia†

1. A loss of intellectual abilities of sufficient severity to interfere with social or occupational functioning
2. Memory impairment
3. At least one of the following:
   a. Impairment of abstract thinking, as manifested by concrete interpretation of proverbs, inability to find similarities and differences between related words, difficulty in defining words and concepts, and other similar tasks

---

*From Diagnostic and statistical manual of mental disorders, p. 107, Washington, D.C., 1980, The American Psychiatric Association.
†Reprinted with permission from Diagnostic and Statistical Manual of Mental Disorders, ed. 3 Washington, D.C., 1980, American Psychiatric Association.

   b. Impaired judgment
   c. Other disturbances of higher cortical function, such as aphasia (disorder of language due to brain dysfunction), apraxia (inability to carry out motor activities despite intact comprehension and motor function), agnosia (failure to recognize or identify objects despite intact sensory function), "constructional difficulty" (e.g., inability to copy three-dimensional figures, assemble blocks, or arrange sticks in specific designs)
   d. Personality change, i.e., alteration or accentuation of premorbid traits
5. Either a or b:
   a. Evidence from the history, physical examination, or laboratory tests, of a specific organic factor that is judged to be etiologically related to the disturbance
   b. In the absence of such evidence, an organic factor necessary for the development of the syndrome can be presumed if conditions other than organic mental disorders have been reasonably excluded and if the behavioral change represents cognitive impairment in a variety of areas

Etiology

The boxed material on p. 375 describes the various causes of delirium and dementia.

Incidence and prevalence

The incidence and prevalence of physiologic dysfunction and psychiatric illness rise progressively with increasing age. Over 1 million Americans over 65 years old (and many others younger than 65) meet the criteria for dementia[29] (see the diagnostic criteria on p. 373 and 374).

Diagnosis

Gray hair with confusion is not synonymous with dementia!
1. The elderly person whose clinical presentation suggests neuromuscular or mental derangement, whether chronic or acute, must be evaluated as if he or she has a diagnostic state of delirium
2. Physical abnormalities or dysfunctions can have an impact on cognitive and neuromuscular function and disrupt psychiatric homeostasis; systemic and metabolic abnormalities must be ruled out with thorough history, physical exam, and lab evaluation
3. The diagnostic evaluation should include the following:
   a. An attempt at the Folstein Mini-Mental State test (see boxed material on p. 376 and 377) to screen for dementia and also to document the progression of disease over time by repeating the test at 3- to 6-month intervals
   b. One venipuncture for a profile of blood values:
      (1) Glucose
      (2) CBC
      (3) Electrolytes
      (4) pH
      (5) BUN, creatinine
      (6) VDRL
      (7) Calcium
      (8) Magnesium
      (9) Osmolarity
      (10) T_4, TSH
      (11) Vitamin B_{12} level

Confusion

Delirium

Drugs
Anticholinergics
Narcotics
Antidepressants
Anxiolytics
Methyldopa
β-blockers
Steroids
Non-steroidal antiinflammatory
  drugs
Phenytoin
Digoxin
Ethanol

Physical and Environmental
Stress of any type or source
Change in environment
Surgery
Anesthesia
Sleep loss
Pain
Fever or hypothermia

Fluids and Electrolytes
Hyponatremia
Hypernatremia
Hypovolemia
Hypervolemia
pH change
Hypercalcemia
Hypocalcemia
Hypomagnesemia

Systemic Changes
Infection (febrile or afebrile)
Vitamin deficiency
Fecal impaction
Urinary retention
Any abdominal disorders

Metabolic
Renal failure
Liver failure
Anemia
Thyroid dysfunction
Adrenal dysfunction
Hyperglycemia or hypogly-
  cemia

CNS
Strokes
Seizure
Hematoma
Infection
Severe hypertension
Superimposed on dementia

Chest
Congestive failure
Hypercapnea
Hypoxemia
Rhythm disturbance
Acute MI

Dementia

Degenerative
Alzheimer's-type disease
Parkinson's disease

Vascular
Multi-infarct
Arteritis

Infectious
Syphylis
Jakob Cruetzfeldt disease
Postencephalitic syndrome

Other
B_{12} deficiency
Vitamin deficiency
Chronic alcoholism
Subdural hematoma
Hydrocephalus
Chronic seizures
Hypothyroidism
Hearing loss
Blindness
Rule out depression

Mini-Mental State Examination

1. Orientation (maximum score 10)

   Ask, "What is today's date?" Then ask specifically for parts omitted; e.g., "Can you also tell me what season it is?"

   Ask, "Can you tell me the name of this hospital?"

   "What floor are we on?"

   "What town (or city) are we in?"

   "What county are we in?"

   "What state are we in?"

Date (e.g., January 21) . .	1 ___
Year	2 ___
Month	3 ___
Day (e.g., Monday)	4 ___
Season	5 ___
Hospital	6 ___
Floor	7 ___
Town/city	8 ___
County	9 ___
State	10 ___

2. Registration (maximum score 3)

   Ask the subject if you may test his/her memory. Then say, "ball," "flag," "tree" clearly and slowly, about one second for each. After you have said all three words, ask subject to repeat them. This first repetition determines the score (0-3) but keep saying them (up to six trials) until the subject can repeat all three words. If (s)he does not eventually learn all three, recall cannot be meaningfully tested.

"ball"	11 ___
"flag"	12 ___
"tree"	13 ___

   Record number of trials: _____

3. Attention and calculation (maximum score 5)

   Ask the subject to begin at 100 and count backward by 7. Stop after five subtractions (93, 86, 79, 72, 65). Score one point for each correct number.

   If the subject cannot or will not perform this task, ask him/her to spell the word "world" backwards (D, L, R, O, W). The score is one point for each correctly placed letter, e.g., DLROW = 5, DLORW = 3. Record how the subject spelled "world" backwards:

   _____

   D L R O W

"93"	14 ___
"86"	15 ___
"79"	16 ___
"72"	17 ___
"65"	18 ___

   OR

Number of correctly-placed letters	19 ___

4. Recall (maximum score 3)

   Ask the subject to recall the three words you previously asked him/her to remember (learned in registration)

"ball"	20 ___
"flag"	21 ___
"tree"	22 ___

Mini-Mental State Examination—cont'd

5. Language (maximum score 9)

   Naming: show the subject a wristwatch and ask, "What is this?" Repeat for pencil. Score 1 point for each item named correctly

   Watch . . . . 23 __

   Pencil . . . . 24 __

   Repetition: ask the subject to repeat, "No if, ands, or buts." Score 1 point for correct repetition.

   Repetition . . . . 25 __

   Three-stage command: give the subject a piece of blank paper and say, "Take the paper in your right hand, fold it in half, and put it on the floor." Score 1 point for each action performed correctly

   Takes in right hand . . . 26 __

   Folds in half . . . . . . 27 __

   Puts on floor . . . . . . 28 __

   Reading: on a blank piece of paper, print the sentence "Close your eyes." in letters large enough for the subject to see clearly. Ask subject to read it and do what it says. Score correct only if (s)he actually closes his/her eyes.

   Closes eyes . . . . 29 __

   Writing: give the subject a blank piece of paper and ask him/her to write a sentence. It is to be written spontaneously. It must contain a subject and verb and make sense. Correct grammar and punctuation are not necessary.

   Writes sentence . . . . . 30 __

   Copying: on a clean piece of paper, draw intersecting pentagons, each side about 1 inch, and ask subject to copy it exactly as it is. All 10 angles must be present and two must intersect to score 1 point. Tremor and rotation are ignored.

   e.g.

   Draws pentagons . . . . . 31 __

   Score: Add number of correct responses. In section 3 include items 14-18 or item 19, not both. (maximum total score 30)

   Total score ____

   Rate subject's level of consciousness: _____ (a) coma, (b) stupor, (c) drowsy, (d) alert

Reprinted with permission from Folstein, M.F., et al.: Mini-mental state: a practical method of grading the cognitive state of the patient for the physician, J. Psychiatr. Rev. **12:**189, 1975.

c. Depending on physical and historical findings, other tests may include CT scan of head and spinal tap
d. Of great importance is the identification of treatable causes of dementia (see the following list):[26,33]

(1) Drug induced
(2) Depression
(3) Hypothyroidism
(4) Hyperthyroidism
(5) Hypoglycemia
(6) Vitamin B_{12} or folate deficiency
(7) Subdural hematoma
(8) Liver failure
(9) Normal-pressure hydrocephalus
(10) Stroke
(11) CNS infections
(12) Generalized infections
(13) Cerebral neoplasms
(14) Renal failure
(15) Ethanol abuse
(16) Hypoxia
(17) Hypercalcemia
(18) Vasculitis
(19) Cardiopulmonary disorders
(20) Anemia

Management

1. Pursue the diagnosis
2. Avoid restraints, but use them for safety
3. Control hyperactivity of delirium with haloperidol in adequate doses (i.e., 2 mg q60min, IM or PO until calm)

| 17.4 | TRANSIENT ISCHEMIC ATTACK

Definition

Transient ischemic attack (TIA) is a sudden or rapid onset of neurologic deficit caused by cerebral ischemia. It may last for a few minutes or up to 24 hours and clears without residual signs.

Etiology[3,42]

1. Cardiac emboli
   a. Mural thrombi after MI (usually anterior wall MI)
   b. Atrial fibrillation
   c. Mitral valve disease (MS, MR, MVP)
   d. Prosthetic heart valves
   e. Bacterial and marantic endocarditis
   f. After MI, ventricular wall aneurysm (mural thrombus)
   g. Calcific aortic stenosis, calcification of mitral annulus
   h. Atrial myxoma
2. Carotid or vertebral artery disease
   a. Arteriosclerosis
   b. Artery-to-artery embolism
   c. Anterograde extension of embolus into cerebral arteries
   d. Fibromuscular hyperplasia
   e. Dissecting aortic aneurysm
   f. Arteritis (Takayasu's arteritis, giant cell arteritis)
   g. Vasculitis
   h. Meningovascular syphilis
   i. Other: traumatic and spontaneous carotid and vertebrobasilar artery dissection, granulomatous angiitis, vasculopathy from drug abuse, arteriolar spasm

3. Hematologic causes
   a. RBC disorders
      (1) Increased sludging (polycythemia vera, sickle cell anemia, erythrocytosis)
      (2) Decreased cerebral oxygenation (severe anemia)
   b. Platelet disorders: thrombocytosis, thombocytopenia
   c. Myeloproliferative disorders, leukemias with white cell counts > 150,000
   d. Increased viscosity (e.g., Waldenstrom's macroglobulinemia)
4. Other: transient hypotension, compression of neck vessels by osteophytes, kinking of neck vessels during rotation of the head

Risk factors[24]

1. Hypertension
2. Smoking
3. Obesity
4. Hyperlipidemias
5. Advanced age

General approach

1. Determine if the TIA involves the carotid or vertebrobasilar territory
   a. Prognosis and therapeutic approach depend on the vascular territory involved; the boxed material below describe the various characteristics of carotid and vertebrobasilar insufficiency
   b. In approximately 5%-10% of TIAs, patients experience symptoms that reflect abnormalities in both carotid and vertebrobasilar territories[3]

Characteristics of Carotid Artery Syndrome

1. Ipsilateral monocular vision loss (amaurosis fugax); the patient often feels as if "a shade" has come down over one eye
2. Episodic contralateral arm, leg, and face paresis and paresthesias
3. Slurred speech, transient aphasia
4. Ipsilateral headache of vascular type
5. Carotid bruit may be present over the carotid bifurcation
6. Microemboli, hemorrhages, and exudates may be noted in the ipsilateral retina

---

Characteristics of Vertebrobasilar Artery Syndome

1. Binocular visual disturbances (blurred vision, diplopia, total blindness)
2. Vertigo, nausea, vomiting, tinnitus
3. Sudden loss of postural tone of all four extremities (drop attacks) with no loss of consciousness
4. Slurred speech, ataxia, numbness around lips or face

2. Initial lab evaluation should include the following: CBC, platelet count, PT, PTT, glucose, VDRL, sedimentation rate, lipid profile, lytes, BUN, creatinine

3. Chest x-ray film: evaluate heart size and configuration; check for any lung masses (lung neoplasm can initially manifest only with neurologic findings secondary to cerebral metastases)

4. ECG: evaluate patient's baseline rhythm, rule out atrial fibrillation, rule out recent MI (mural thrombi)

5. CT scan of head: rule out hemorrhage/infarct and subdural hematoma; as many as 20% of patients with TIAs that resolve within 24 hours have evidence of cerebral infarction on CT scan of head[42]

6. Echocardiogram is indicated in young patients with cardiac murmurs to rule out an embolic focus from the heart

7. 24-hour Holter monitor is indicated in any patient with suspected dysrhythmias

8. Cerebral arteriography should be done only in patients whose symptoms suggest involvement of the carotid circulation and the patient is a candidate for carotid endoarterectomy; the morbidity associated with the retrograde femoral technique in patients with reasonable risk ranges from 0.2% to as much as 14%, and the incidence of serious complications (e.g., aortic dissection, embolic stroke) with permanent injury or even death is 0.5%-1.2%[42]

9. Digital subtraction angiography (DSA) is useful in demonstrating severe carotid stenosis; however, it often leaves the degree of stenosis difficult to judge, does not adequately delineate either intracranial arterial lesions or patterns of blood flow, and requires good patient cooperation (e.g., breath holding, cessation of swallowing)

10. Ultrasonic imaging of carotid bifurcation is useful in evaluating patients with asymptomatic bruits, following the progress of a known carotid stenosis,[24] and in selecting patients for cerebral arteriography

Treatment

1. Medical therapy
   a. Anticoagulation: initially with heparin, then followed by warfarin
      (1) Indications
         (a) TIA from emboli arising from mural thrombi after MI
         (b) TIA from suspected emboli in patients with mitral stenosis (with or without atrial fibrillation)
         (c) TIA in patients with prosthetic heart valves
         (d) Recurrent TIAs despite platelet antiaggregant agents
      (2) Duration of treatment
         (a) TIA secondary to mitral stenosis: prolonged treatment (years)
         (b) TIA secondary to mural thrombus: 2-6 months of anticoagulant therapy followed by an additional period of 6-12 months of aspirin therapy
      (3) General contraindications to oral anticoagulants: history of GI bleeding, bleeding tendencies, severe hypertension, elderly patients with frequent falls, uncooperative patient
   b. Antiplatelet therapy is indicated in patients who are not candidates for surgery or warfarin therapy (e.g., frequent falls, severe hypertension)

    (1) Aspirin decreases the risk of subsequent stroke in patients with TIA[18]; the optimum dosage is controversial,[45] but recommendations vary from ≤300 mg PO qd to 650 mg PO bid

    (2) Dipyridamole (Persantine) inhibits platelet aggregation through inhibition of platelet phosphodiesterase

        (a) Dosage is 75 mg PO bid or 50 mg PO tid

        (b) Its efficacy in patients with TIA is controversial

    (3) Combined use of ASA and dipyridamole: there is no proven added benefit to patients with TIAs[4]

2. Surgical therapy: carotid endoarterectomy is indicated in patients with TIAs within the carotid distribution, with documented significant stenosis (>70% stenosis), and no contraindications to surgery

 STROKE

Definition

Stroke can be defined as the rapid onset of a neurologic deficit involving a certain vascular territory and lasting longer than 24 hours.

Etiology and risk factors

For etiology and risk factors for stroke, refer to those given for TIA.

Classification

Ischemic strokes

1. Etiology: thrombosis or embolism; although the clinical distinction between them is often impossible, the major distinguishing factors are described in Table 17-1

Table 17-1 Characteristics of cerebral thrombosis and embolism

	Thrombosis	Embolism
Onset of symptoms	Progression of symptoms over hours to days	Very rapid (seconds)
History of prior TIA	Common	Uncommon
Time of presentation	Often during night hours while the patient is sleeping	The patient is usually awake and is involved in some type of activity
	Classically the patient awakes with a slight neurologic deficit that gradually progresses in a step-wise fashion	
Predisposing factors	Atherosclerosis, hypertension, diabetes, arteritis, vasculitis, hypotension, trauma to head and neck	Atrial fibrillation, mitral stenosis, and regurgitation, endocarditis, mitral valve prolapse

Table 17-2   Selected stroke syndromes

Artery Involved	Neurologic Deficit
Middle cerebral artery	Hemiplegia (upper extremity and face are usually more involved than lower extremities)
	Hemianesthesia (hemisensory loss)
	Hemianopsia (homonymous)
	Aphasia (if dominant hemisphere is involved)
Anterior cerebral artery	Hemiplegic (lower extremities more involved than upper extremities and face)
	Primitive reflexes (e.g., grasp and suck reflexes)
	Urinary incontinence
Vertebral and basilar arteries	Ipsilateral cranial nerve findings
	Controlateral (or bilateral) sensory or motor deficits
Deep penetrating branches of major cerebral arteries (lacunar infarction)	Usually seen in elderly hypertensive patients
	Four characteristic syndromes are possible[42]:
	1. Pure motor hemiplegia (66%)
	2. Dysarthria–clumsy hand syndrome (20%)
	3. Pure sensory stroke (10%)
	4. Ataxic hemiplegia syndrome with pyramidal tract signs

2. Clinical presentation varies with the cerebral vessel involved (see Table 17-2 for description of common stroke syndromes)
3. Management of ischemic strokes[8]
   a. CT scan of head
      (1) Indications
         (a) To rule out cerebral hemorrhage when considering anticoagulation
         (b) When signs and symptoms cannot be explained by one lesion
         (c) Any patient on anticoagulant therapy presenting with a stroke
         (d) To rule out brain abscess, tumor, and subdural hematoma
      (2) Diagnosis: cerebral infarction is seen on CT scan as an area of decreased density; initial CT scan may be negative and infarct may not be evident for 2-3 days after the infarction
   b. Blood pressure control:[27] lowering systemic blood pressure in patients with acute cerebral infarction is contraindicated since it may produce clinical deterioration (secondary to spontaneous fluctuations in blood pressure and impaired cerebral autoregulation); antihypertensive therapy is indicated only if:

(1) Diastolic blood pressure is ≥130 mm Hg
(2) Hypertensive encephalopathy is present
(3) Vital organs (heart, kidney) are compromised

  c. Anticoagulation: initially with heparin followed by warfarin
    (1) Indications
      (a) Worsening neurologic deficits (stroke in evolution)
      (b) Suspected cerebral embolism from
- Mural thrombus, after MI
- Mitral stenosis (with or without atrial fibrillation)
- Atrial fibrillation

    (2) Contraindications
      (a) Absolute: CT scan or lumbar puncture evidence of cerebral hemorrhage, tumor
      (b) Relative: history of GI bleeding, bleeding tendencies, severe hypertension

  d. Rehabilitation should be a combined effort by the attending physician, physical therapist, speech therapist, nursing staff, social service, and the patient's family

Hemorrhagic strokes

Subarachnoid hemorrhage (SAH)[42]

1. Etiology: ruptured congential aneurysm or AV malformation
2. Clinical manifestations
  a. Generalized excruciating headache that radiates into the posterior neck region, and is worsened by neck and head movements
  b. Coma
  c. Diplopia, dilated pupil, pain above or behind an eye, neck stiffness
3. Physical exam
  a. Focal neurologic signs may be absent
  b. Level of consciousness varies from normal to deeply comatose
  c. Fever and nuchal rigidity are present or usually develop within 24 hours
  d. Fundi may show papilledema and/or retinal hemorrhage
  e. Cranial nerve abnormalities may be noted (e.g., pupillary dilatation secondary to oculomotor nerve dysfunction)
4. Diagnosis
  a. CT scan of head confirms the presence of subarachnoid blood localized to the basal cisterns or extending intracerebrally or in the ventricles; a fresh hemorrhage produces an area of increased density
  b. Lumbar puncture is indicated if CT scan of head is not available
    (1) A good fundoscopic exam to rule out papilledema must be done before LP
    (2) In SAH the CSF will be uniformly grossly bloody, whereas in a traumatic LP, the number of RBC decreases progressively from tube 1 to tube 4
    (3) More reliable is the presence of xanthochromia in the CSF (see p. 62)
  c. Angiography is necessary to determine the best therapeutic approach (medical vs. surgical)

Table 17-3 Grading of cerebral AV malformations and surgical recommendations[28]

Grade	Size of AVM (Diameter)	Surgical Recommendations
I	≤2 cm	The natural risk (morbidity and mortality) ex-
II	2-4 cm	ceeds surgical risk in most circumstances, therefore, surgical excision is nearly always indicated
III	4-6 cm	The surgical risk probably exceeds the natural
IV	>6 cm	risk in most circumstances for patients after the fourth to fifth decade of life

5. Management of SAH varies with the patient's clinical status and the location and surgical accessibility of the aneurysm
   a. Medical management
      (1) Strict bed rest in a quiet, private room with cardiac monitoring (frequent dysrhythmias)
      (2) Control of headache with acetaminophen and codeine
      (3) Have patient avoid all forms of straining (stool softeners and mild laxatives are indicated to prevent constipation)
      (4) Maintain systolic blood pressure in the range 143-158 mm Hg[34]
      (5) Reduce cerebral edema with mannitol and dexamethasone
      (6) Antifibrinolytic therapy with epsilon-aminocaproic acid is controversial[1]; initial dosage is 18 g in 400 ml of D_5W infused over 12 hours followed by a total daily dosage of 36 g/day in six divided doses PO or by continuous IV infusion
   b. Surgical management: the indications for surgery and the patient's prognosis depend on the size of the aneurysm, the patient's age and clinical condition, and on the experience of the neurosurgeon; Table 17-3 describes general surgical recommendations for patients with cerebral AV malformations

Intracerebral hemorrhage
1. Etiology: generally associated with hypertension
2. Clinical manifestations
   a. The hemorrhage usually occurs during periods of activity, often manifesting with headache, vomiting, and sudden onset of neurologic deficits that can rapidly progress to coma and death; the neurologic deficits vary with the area involved
   b. The boxed material on p. 385 describes localizing signs in patients with intracerebral hemorrhage
   c. In addition to the focal deficits, the patient may also show signs of increased intracranial pressure (e.g., bradycardia, decreased respiratory rate, third nerve palsy)
3. Diagnosis: on a CT scan of the head, the area of hemorrhagic infarct appears as an area of increased density; shifts of intracranial contents and compression of the ventricles may be present

Localizing Signs in Patients with Intracerebral Hemorrhage[15]

Location of Intracerebral Hemorrhage	Common Neurologic Signs	Examples
Putamen	Both eyes deviate conjugately to the side of the lesion (away from hemiparesis)	Left putaminal hemorrhage
	Pupils are normal in size and react normally	
	Contralateral hemiplegia is present	
	Hemisensory defect is noted	
Thalamus	Both eyes deviate downward and look at the nose	Thalamic hemorrhage
	Impairment of vertical eye movements is present	
	Pupils are small in size (approximately 2 mm) and nonreactive	
	Contralateral hemisensory loss is present	
Pons	Both eyes are in midposition	Pontine hemorrhage
	There are absent doll's eye movements	
	Pupils are pinpoint but reactive (use magnifying glass)	
	Coma is common	
	Flaccid quadriplegia is noted	
Cerebellum	Ipsilateral paresis of conjugate gaze (inability to look at the side of lesion)	Cerebellar hemorrhage
	Pupils are normal in size and react normally	
	Inability to stand or walk	
	Vertigo and dysarthria are present	

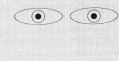

4. Management
   a. Medical therapy
      (1) Control of severe hypertension: lower blood pressure may reduce cerebral edema, but it risks promoting border zone ischemia[27]; blood pressure reduction, if indicated, should not exceed 20%[22] and should be achieved with short-acting agents (e.g., sodium nitroprusside)
      (2) Treatment of cerebral edema: mannitol, 1-1.5 g/kg of a 20% solution given IV over 30 minutes is generally effective
      (3) Maintain a clear airway
      (4) Supportive measures
         (a) Careful IV fluid administration; excessive fluid administration can worsen cerebral edema
         (b) Phenytoin if seizure activity is noted
         (c) Frequent turning of comatose patients to prevent decubitus ulcers
         (d) Nutritional support
         (e) Physical therapy
   b. Surgical evacuation of hematomas is indicated[46] in:
      (1) Noncomatose patients with cerebellar hemorrhage
      (2) Patients with surgically accessible cerebral hematomas that produce progressive signs of temporal lobe herniation

| 17.6 | CEREBRAL NEOPLASMS

Classification and prevalence[5, 48]

1. Primary CNS neoplasms
   a. Gliomas (33%-42%)
   b. Meningiomas (13%-18%)
   c. Pituitary adenoma (8%-17.8%)
   d. Acoustic neuroma (7.6%-8.7%)
   e. Craniopharyngioma (2.5%-4.6%)
   f. Miscellaneous (17.9%-18.2%)
2. Metastatic CNS neoplasms (4%-4.2%): lung, breast, melanoma, kidney, thyroid (other tumors metastasize to brain less frequently)

Clinical manifestations

Clinical manifestations depend on:
1. Type of tumor: e.g., patients with an ACTH-secreting pituitary adenoma will have symptoms of Cushing's disease (see p. 196)
2. Location of tumor: e.g., a tumor compressing the optic chiasm will result in bitemporal hemianopsia; Fig. 17-1 shows the visual field defects produced by lesions along the optic pathway
3. Size of tumor: large tumors often present with signs of increased intracranial pressure (headache, nausea, vomiting, bradycardia, papilledema, third nerve palsy, and hypoventilation)

Diagnosis

1. History
   a. Inquire about symptoms of visual disturbances, hearing loss, localized weakness, headaches, seizures, behavioral changes

b. Duration of symptoms

c. Family history of "brain tumors" (MEN)

2. Physical exam: perform careful neurologic exam, note any signs of increased intracranial pressure or evidence of focal motor or sensory deficits

3. Lab results: an elevated prolactin level is suggestive of a pituitary tumor (see p. 170)

4. Radiographic evaluation

    a. CT scan of head or MRI scan:

        (1) CT scan identifies approximately 90% of intraparenchymal lesions[17]

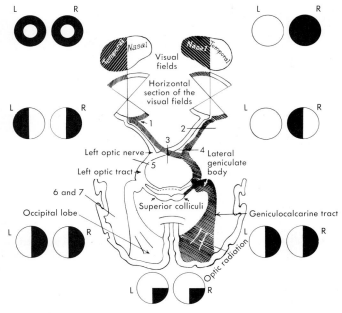

Figure 17-1

Visual field defects associated with lesions of the visual system. **1,** Circumferential blindness ("tubular vision") may be caused by hysteria, or optic or retrobulbar neuritis. **2,** Total blindness of right eye caused by complete lesion of right optic nerve, such as trauma. **3,** Bitemporal hemianopia because of chiasmal lesions, such as pituitary tumors. **4,** Right nasal hemianopia resulting from a lesion involving perichiasmal area, such as calcified right internal carotid artery. **5,** Right homonymous hemianopia caused by lesion of left parietal or temporal lobes with pressure on left optic tract. **6,** Right homonymous inferior quadrarantanopia because of partial involvement of optic radiation (upper portion of left optic radiation in this case). **7,** Right homonymous hemianopia with no pupillary change as a result of complete involvement of the left optic radiation. From Chusid, J.G.: Correlative neuroanatomy and functional neurology, ed. 19, Los Altos, Calif., 1985, Lange Medical Publications.

    (2) MRI is superior to CT scan in identifying cerebral neoplasms, particularly in the diagnosis of posterior fossa tumors.[30]
- b. Angiography is indicated in the following:[25]
  - (1) Detection of vascular lesions (AVM, meningioma)
  - (2) Preoperative evaluation of surgically relevant tumor vasculature
  - (3) Differentiation of hemorrhage secondary to tumor from hemorrhage due to aneurysm
  - (4) Aid in diagnosis of poorly visualized lesions by CT scan
- c. EEG: Nonspecific; useful in the evaluation of new onset seizure activity in a patient with suspected cerebral neoplasm
- d. Skull x-ray film: limited value; may show bone erosion, abnormal calcifications, or abnormalities in the shape of the sella turcica

Treatment

1. Medical management
   - a. Phenytoin (Dilantin) is indicated for prevention and treatment of seizures
   - b. Reduction of cerebral edema[6]
     - (1) Mannitol: 1-1.5 g/kg as a 20% solution infused over 30 minutes is indicated in an emergency situation
     - (2) Dexamethasone: 10 mg IV loading dose followed by 4 mg IV q6h until the effects of cerebral edema are controlled, then change to PO dexamethasone; the cerebral edema-reducing effect of dexamethasone is generally delayed for several hours
2. Surgery, radiotherapy, and chemotherapy: the use of these modalities depends on the type of tumor (benign vs. malignant), location (surgically accessible), and radiosensitivity (e.g., medulloblastomas are generally radiosensitive)

| 17.7 | PARKINSON'S DISEASE

Definition

Parkinson's disease is progressive neurologic disorder. It is characterized pathologically by cytoplasmic eosinophilic inclusions (Lewy bodies) in neurons of the substantia nigra and locus cerealus and by depigmentation of the brainstem nuclei. Parkinson's disease is part of the clinical syndrome of parkinsonism, an extrapyramidal disorder characterized by rigidity, tremor at rest, bradykinesia, and loss of postural reflexes.

Classification of Parkinsonism[14]

1. Primary (Parkinson's disease)
2. Secondary (acquired parkinsonism)
   - a. Iatrogenic (e.g., phenothiazines, butyrophenones)
   - b. Postencephalitic (sequela of encephalitis lethargica)
   - c. Toxins (e.g., manganese, carbon monoxide)
   - d. Hypoparathyroidism (e.g., postparathyroidectomy)
   - e. Vascular insufficiency (e.g., after CVA)
3. Parkinsonism-plus: symptoms and signs of parkinsonism occurring in association with other multisystem degenerative diseases (e.g., Wilson's disease, Alzheimer's disease, normal-pressure hydrocephalus)

Table 17-4 Initial symptoms in Parkinson's disease[47]

Symptoms	Percent of Cases
Tremor	70
Stiffness or slowness of movement	20
Loss of dexterity or handwriting disturbance	13
Gait disturbance	12
Muscle pain, cramps, aching	8
Other: depression, nervousness, psychiatric disturbance, speech disturbances, drooling	1-5

Clinical manifestations

The disease often begins insidiously and can manifest itself with a slight loss of motor dexterity, generalized slowness, or a decrease in overall motor activity. Table 17-4 describes the various initial presentations of Parkinson's disease. The classic manifestations of Parkinson's disease are:

1. Rigidity: increased muscle tone
   a. It involves both agonist and antagonist muscle groups
   b. The resistance to passive movement is widespread and more prominent at large joints ("cog-wheeling" rigidity is noted)
2. Tremor: resting tremor, with a frequency of 4-7 movements/second
   a. The tremor is usually noted in the hands and often involves the thumb and forefinger ("pill-rolling" tremor)
   b. Parkinsonian tremor is often confused with essential senile tremor; their major distinguishing characteristics are described in Table 17-5
3. Akinesia: inability to initiate or execute a movement
   a. The patient often sits immobile since even the simple task of getting up from a chair becomes impossible
   b. The face shows a marked absence of movement (masked facies); the mouth is usually open and the patient drools
4. Gait disturbance
   a. The patient assumes a stooped posture (head bowed, trunk bent forward, shoulders are drooped, knees and arms are flexed)
   b. There is difficulty initiating the first step and this is followed by small shuffling steps that increase in speed (festinating gait), as if the patient is chasing his or her center of gravity (the patient's steps become progressively faster and shorter while the trunk inclines further forward)
5. Abnormal reflexes
   a. Palmomental reflex: stroking the palm of the hand near the base of the thumb results in contraction of the ipsilateral mentalis muscle causing wrinkling of the skin of the chin
   b. Glabellar reflex: repeated gentle tapping on the glabella evokes repeated blinking of both eyes

Table 17-5   Distinguishing characteristics of parkinsonian tremor and essential senile tremor

Type of Tremor	Family History	Characteristics	Effect of Ethanol	Therapy
Parkinsonian tremor	Negative	Tremor present at rest Tremor improves or disappears with purposeful function Supination-pronation type of tremor	No effect	Levodopa Anticholinergics Bromocriptine
Essential senile tremor	Positive	Tremor present during maintenance of a posture (postural tremor) Flexion extension type of tremor	Decreases tremor	Propranolol 60-240 mg/day in 3-4 divided doses

Management

1. General principles: physical therapy, encouragement, reassurance, and treatment of possible associated conditions (e.g., depression)
2. Drug therapy[12,32] should be delayed until symptoms significantly limit the patient's daily activities, since tolerance and side effects to anti-parkinsonian agents are common
   a. Therapy is usually started with anticholinergics (alone or in combination); commonly used agents are:
      (1) Trihexyphenidyl (Artane): initial dosage is 1 mg PO tid after meals; side effects include dry mouth, blurred vision, urinary retention, and anhydrosis
      (2) Amantidine (Symmetrel): antiviral agent with antiparkinsonian effect; dosage is 100 mg PO qd or bid initially; side effects include livido reticularis, ankle edema, and visual hallucinations
   b. Levodopa therapy is indicated when the anticholinergics fail to control the parkinsonian symptoms or if the patient develops significant side effects; levodopa is commonly used in combination with a peripheral dopa decarboxylase inhibitor (Carbidopa) to minimize peripheral side effects
      (1) The combination of the two drugs is marketed under the trade name Sinemet
      (2) Carbidopa/levodopa is available in tablets of 10/100 mg, 25/100 mg, 25/250 mg
      (3) Therapy can be started with 10/100 mg PO tid
      (4) The best therapeutic approach is to minimize the patient's symptoms with the lowest possible dose
   c. Common side effects of long-term levodopa therapy are:
      (1) ''On-off effect'': sudden fluctuation of the patient's clinical status from good mobility to stiffness
      (2) Dyskinesia: choreic movements, more frequently seen when higher doses of levodopa are used
      (3) Development of tolerance: loss of efficacy, requiring higher dose of levodopa to achieve the previous therapeutic effect
   d. Reduction of side effects can be achieved with:
      (1) Addition of bromocriptine (Parlodel): dopamine receptor agonist
         (a) May be useful in minimizing the ''on-off effect''
         (b) Initial dosage is 1.25 mg PO qd in AM (following breakfast)
         (c) Side effects include anorexia, nausea, vomiting, and orthostatic hypotension
      (2) Concomitant use of anticholinergics: see above
      (3) Use of ''drug holiday:''[16] withdrawal of levodopa for a variable period (e.g., 4-11 days)
         (a) Proponents state that it permits the use of lower doses of levodopa/carbidopa for prolonged periods
         (b) Opponents[31] state that the risks and side effects (immobility, depression, difficulty swallowing, increased risk and pulmonary embolism, fatal hyperpyrexia)[40] outweigh any possible benefits

| 17.8 | MULTIPLE SCLEROSIS

Definition

Multiple sclerosis is a chronic demyelinating disease of unknown cause. It is characterized pathologically by zones of demyelinization (plaques) scattered throughout the white matter.

Clinical manifestations

The clinical signs vary with the location of the plaques. The more common manifestations are:

1. Weakness: usually involving the lower extremities; the patient may complain of difficulty ambulating, tendency to drop things, easy fatigability
2. Sensory disturbances: numbness, tingling, "pins and needles" sensation
3. Visual disturbances: diplopia, blurred vision, visual loss
4. Incoordination: gait impairment, clumsiness of upper extremities
5. Other: vertigo, incontinence, loss of sexual function, slurred speech

Physical exam

1. Visual abnormalities
   a. Paresis of medial rectus muscle on lateral conjugate gaze (internuclear ophthalmoplegia) and horizontal nystagmus of the adducting eye
   b. Central scotoma, decreased visual acuity (optic neuritis)
   c. Nystagmus
2. Abnormalities of reflexes
   a. Increased deep tendon reflexes
   b. Positive Hoffman's sign, positive Babinski's sign
   c. Decreased abdominal skin reflex, decreased cremasteric reflex
3. Lhermitte's phenomenon: flexion of the neck while the patient is laying down elicits an electrical sensation extending bilaterally down the arms, back, and lower trunk
4. Charcot's triad consists of nystagmus, scanning speech, and intention tremor

Diagnostic evaluation

1. Lumbar puncture
   a. In multiple sclerosis the CSF may show increased gamma globulin (mostly IgG, but often contains IgA and IgM)
   b. Agarose electrophoresis discloses separate discrete "oligoclonal" bands in the gamma region in approximately 90% of patients, including some with normal IgG levels[41]
   c. Other possible CSF abnormalities are: increased total protein, increased mononuclear white cells, and presence of myelin basic protein (elevated in acute attacks, it indicates active myelin destruction)
2. Measurement of visual evoked response (VER) is useful to assess nerve fiber conduction (myelin loss or destruction will slow conduction velocity)
3. CT scan may demonstrate hypodense areas; however, it is usually normal
4. MRI is more sensitive than CT scan; it can identify lesions as small as 3-4 mm

Therapy

1. Specific treatment: there is no proven treatment that will significantly alter the course of multiple sclerosis; some of the more common therapeutic attempts are listed below:
   a. Corticosteroids: short-term administration of ACTH or prednisone may shorten the duration of an acute attack[43]
   b. Immunosuppressants: a short course of high doses of cyclophosphamide has been reported to temporarily halt progression of multiple sclerosis[44]
2. Supportive measures
   a. Control of spasticity: diazepam (Valium) or baclofen (Lioresal) may be useful
   b. Control of paresthesias: carbamazepine (Tegretol) may be helpful
   c. Control of action tremor: isoniazid may be effective[38]
   d. Physical therapy, social counseling, and psychiatric support

Clinical course

The majority of patients experience clinical improvement in weeks to months following the initial manifestations. The course of the disease is generally characterized by exacerbations and remissions. The average interval from the initial clinical presentation to death is 35 years. Premature death is usually secondary to infection.[41]

| 17.9 | PERIPHERAL NERVE DYSFUNCTION

Definitions[39]

1. Peripheral neuropathy: any disorder involving the peripheral nerves
2. Polyneuropathy (symmetric polyneuropathy): generalized process resulting in widespread and symmetric effects on the peripheral nervous system
3. Focal or multifocal neuropathy (mononeuropathy, mononeuropathy multiplex): local involvement of one or more individual peripheral nerves
4. Paresthesia: spontaneous aberrant sensation (e.g., pins and needles)

Classification and characteristics[35]

1. Hereditary neuropathies
   a. Charcot-Marie-Tooth syndrome
      (1) Most common familial motor and sensory abnormality
      (2) Foot deformity is common
      (3) Braces for correction of foot drop are useful
      (4) Surgical management is generally necessary for stability and cosmetic appearance of the feet[11]
   b. Others: Dejerine-Sottas' disease, Refsum's disease, Riley-Day's syndrome
2. Acquired neuropathies
   a. Neuropathy associated with systemic disease
      (1) Diabetes mellitus (see p. 151)
      (2) Myxedema: distal sensory neuropathy manifested by burning and paresthesias of the limbs; delayed relaxation phase of deep tendon reflexes is common

    (3) Uremia: symmetric distal mixed motor and sensory disturbances
    (4) Sarcoidosis: cranial nerve palsies, (most common is facial nerve),
        polyneuropathy
    (5) Alcohol: pain, numbness, and weakness of extremities
    (6) Neoplasms: sensory and sensory-motor neuropathies
    (7) Others: nutritional deficiencies (thiamine, folic acid, vitamin B_{12}),
        collagen-vascular diseases, amyloidosis
  b. Guillain-Barré neuropathy see p. 395
  c. Toxic neuropathies[39]
    (1) Drugs: chloramphenicol, lithium, isoniazid, pyridoxine, nitrofur-
        antoin, disulfiram, dapsone, ethionamide, cisplatinum, vincristine,
        metronidazole, gold, hydralazine
    (2) Toxic chemicals: lead, arsenic, cyanide, thallium, carbon disul-
        fide, mercury, organophosphates, trichloroethylene
  d. Neuropathies associated with infection: leprosy, herpes zoster, diph-
     theria

Approach to patient with a peripheral neuropathy

1. History
   a. Family history of neuropathies: to rule out hereditary neuropathies
   b. Current and past employment: to rule out exposure to toxic agents
   c. Current or recent medications: to rule out neuropathy secondary to
      drugs
   d. Any systemic disease, such as diabetes, renal failure, hypothyroidism
   e. Ethanol abuse: alcoholic neuropathy
   f. Any special diets (e.g., food faddists): to rule out nutritional deficien-
      cies
   g. History of trauma: to rule out compression entrapment neuropathies
   h. Duration and progression of symptoms
2. Physical exam
   a. Define type of neuropathy present
      (1) Sensory vs. motor vs. mixed neuropathy
      (2) Number of nerves involved (e.g., mononeuropathy, polyneuropa-
          thy, mononeuropathy multiplex)
   b. Determine territory of neurologic deficit (see Figs. 2-3 and 2-4 for
      segmental distribution of cutaneous nerves)
   c. Evaluate deep tendon reflexes (DTR); they are decreased in root and
      peripheral nerve disease
3. Initial lab evaluation
   a. CBC, electrolytes, BUN, creatinine, glucose, liver function tests, cal-
      cium, magnesium, phosphorus
   b. If toxic neuropathy is suspected, heavy metal screening should be or-
      dered; in suspected lead poisoning, blood lead concentration, urinary
      tests for coproporphyrin and δ-aminolevulinic acid, and bone marrow
      aspirates (to evaluate the presence of basophilic stippling in normo-
      blasts) are indicated
   c. TSH level in suspected hypothyroidism
   d. Vitamin B_{12} and folate levels in suspected nutritional deficiencies
   e. Chest x-ray film to rule out sarcoidosis

   f. Lumbar puncture in suspected Guillain Barré syndrome

   g. X-ray films in suspected trauma or peripheral nerve compression

4. Electromyography (EMG): in neurogenic lesions there are spontaneous fibrillation potentials and positive sharp waves at rest

5. Nerve conduction studies

Treatment

1. Specific treatment (e.g., combination treatment with BAL-CaEDTA in patients with lead poisoning)

2. Supportive measures (e.g., physical therapy, emotional support)

17.10 GUILLAIN-BARRÉ SYNDROME

Definition

Guillain-Barré syndrome is an acute, rapidly progressing symmetric polyradiculoneuropathy, predominantly affecting motor function.[21]

Incidence

There are bimodal peaks of occurrence in the 15-35 year and 50-75 year age groups.

Clinical manifestations

1. Rapid progression of symmetric weakness manifested initially in the lower extremities
    a. The patient often reports difficulty in ambulating, getting up from a chair, or climbing stairs
    b. In some patients the initial manifestations may involve the cranial musculature or the upper extremities (e.g., tingling of the hands)

2. Two-thirds of all patients give a history of respiratory or gastrointestinal illness within 30 days of onset of neurologic symptoms[37]

Physical exam

1. Symmetric weakness, involving both proximal and distal muscles

2. Depressed or absent reflexes bilaterally

3. Minimum to moderate glove and stocking anesthesia

4. Ataxia and pain in a segmental distribution may be seen in some patients (caused by involvement of posterior nerve roots)

5. Autonomic abnormalities (bradycardia/tachycardia, hypotension/hypertension)

6. Respiratory insufficiency (caused by weakness of intercostal muscles)

7. Facial paresis, difficulty swallowing (secondary to cranial nerve involvement)

Diagnostic evaluation

1. Rule out other causes of neuropathy (e.g., metabolic; toxic, or nutritional deficiencies, spinal cord lesions, infections, porphyria, collagen-vascular disease)

2. Lumbar puncture
    a. Typical findings include elevated CSF protein (especially IgG) and presence of few mononuclear leukocytes

  b. Normal values may be seen at beginning of illness
  c. If the diagnosis is strongly suspected, repeat lumbar puncture is indicated
3. Electromyography reveals slowed conduction velocities; prolonged motor, sensory, and F wave latencies are also present

Therapy

1. Supportive measures
   a. Close monitoring of respiratory function (frequent measurements of vital capacity and pulmonary toilet) because respiratory failure is the major potential problem in Guillain-Barré syndrome; approximately 10%-20% of patients will require respiratory support[37]
   b. Frequent repositioning of patient to minimize formation of pressure sores
   c. Prevention of thrombophlebitis with antithrombotic stockings and SC heparin (5000 U q12h)
   d. Active physical therapy program
   e. Emotional support and social counseling
2. Plasmapheresis: Results from the Guillain-Barré Study Group[19] show that although plasmapheresis is not effective for all patients, it is particularly effective for patients who receive this treatment within 7 days of onset of symptoms and for patients who require mechanical ventilation
3. Use of corticosteroids is controversial; major studies[20] have shown that there is no benefit from corticosteroid therapy

References

1. Adams, H.P., Jr., et al.: Antifibrinolytic therapy in patients with aneuyrsmal subarachnoid hemorrhage: a report of the cooperative aneurysm study, Arch. Neurol. **38:**25, 1981.
2. Adams, R.D., and Martin, J.B.: Faintness, syncope, and seizures. In Petersdorf, R.G., et al. (editors): Harrison's principles of internal medicine, ed. 10, New York, 1983, McGraw-Hill Book Co.
3. Barnett, H.J.M.: Cerebrovascular diseases. In Wyngaarden, J.B., and Smith, L.H., (editors): Cecil's textbook of medicine, vol. 1, ed. 17, Philadelphia, 1985, W.B. Saunders Co.
4. Baussen, M.G., et al.: "AICLA" controlled trial of aspirin and dipyridamole in the secondary prevention of athero-thrombotic cerebral ischemia, Stroke, **14:**5, 1983.
5. Cushing, H.: Intracranial tumors: notes upon a series of two thousand verified cases with surgical mortality percentages pertaining thereto, Springfield, Ill., 1932, Charles C Thomas, Publisher.
6. Cutler, R.W.P.: Neoplastic disorders, Sci. Am. Med. **11**(6):4, 1985.
7. Dalessio, D.J.: Seizure disorders and pregnancy, N. Engl. J. Med. **312:**559, 1985.
8. Dawson, D.M.: Stroke and TIA: solutions to the Dx and Rx dilemmas, Modern Medicine, **53:**30, 1985.
9. Day, S.C., et al.: Evaluation and outcome of emergency room patients with transient loss of consciousness, AM. J. Med. **73:**15, 1982.
10. Delgado-Escueta, A.V., et al.: Management of status epileptieus N. Engl. J. Med. **306:**1337, 1982.
11. Drennan, J.: Orthopedic management of neuromuscular disorders, Philadelphia, 1983, J.B. Lippincott Co.
12. Duvoisin, R.C.: Parkinsonism. In Rakel, R.E., (editor): Conn's current therapy, Philadelphia, 1985, W.B. Saunders Co.

13. Eagle, K.A., et al.: Evaluation of prognostic classifications for patients with syncope, Am. J. Med. **79**:455, 1985.

14. Fahn, S.: The extrapyramidal disorders. In Wyngaarden, J.B., and Smith, L.H., (editors): Cecil's textbook of medicine, vol. 2, ed. 17, Philadelphia, 1985, W.B. Saunders Co.

15. Fisher, C.M.: Some neuro-ophthalmological observations, J. Neurol. Neurosurg. Psych. **30**:383, 1967.

16. Friedman, J.H.: "Drug holidays" in the treatment of Parkinson's disease, Arch. Intern. Med. **145**:913, 1985.

17. Greitz, T: Computer tomography for diagnosis of intracranial tumors compared with other neuroradiological procedures. In Lindgren T., (editor): Computer tomography of brain lesions, Acta Radiol. (suppl) **346**:14, 1975.

18. Grotta, J.C., Lemak, N.A., and Gary, H.: Does platelet antiaggregant therapy lessen the severity of a stroke? Neurol. **35**:632, 1985.

19. The Guillain-Barré Syndrome Study Group: Plasmapheresis and acute Guillan-Barré syndrome, Neurol. **35**:1096, 1985.

20. Hughes, R.A.C., Newsom-Davis, J.M., and Perkins, G.D.: Controlled trial of prednisolone in acute polyneuropathy, Lancet, **2**:750, 1978.

21. Jones, H.J., Jr.: Diseases of the peripheral motor-sensory unit, clinical symposia, vol. 37, no. 2, p. 12, CIBA-Geigy Corp., 1985.

22. Kaneko, T., Swada, T., and Niimi, T.: Lower limit of blood pressure in treatment of acute hypertension intracranial hemorrhage (AHCH), J. Cereb. Blood Flow Metabol **3** (suppl 1): S51, 1983.

23. Kapoor, W.N.: Evaluation of the patient with syncope, Cardiovasc. Med. p. 51, Oct., 1985.

24. Kistler, J.P., Ropper, A.H., and Heros, R.C.: Therapy of ischemic cerebral vascular disease due to atherothrombosis, N. Engl. J. Med. **311**:27, 1984.

25. Kornblith, P.L., Walker, M.D., and Cassady, Jr.: Neoplasms of the central nervous system. In DeVita, C.T., Jr., Hellman, S., and Rosenberg, S.A. (editors): Cancer principles and practice of oncology, vol. ed. 2, Philadelphia, 1985, J.B. Lippincott, Co.

26. Larson, E.B., and Reifler, B.V.: Dementia in elderly outpatients: a prospective study, Ann. Intern. Med. **100**:417, 1984.

27. Lavin, P.: Management of hypertension in patients with acute stroke, Arch. Intern. Med. **146**:66, 1986.

28. Leussenhop, A.J., and Rosa, L.: Cerebral arteriovenous malformations: indications for and results of surgery and the role of intravascular techniques, J. Neurosurg. **60**:14, 1984.

29. McEvoy, J.P.: Organic brain syndromes, Ann. Intern. Med. **95**:212, 1981.

30. McGinnis, B.D., Brady, T.J., and New, P.F.J.: Nuclear magnetic resonance (NMR) imagining of tumors in the posterior fossa, J. Comput. Assist. Tomogr. **7**:575, 1983.

31. Marsden, C.D., and Fahn, S.: Problems in Parkinson's disease, In Marsden, C.D., and Fahn, S., (editors): Movement disorders, vol. 2, 1982, Butterworth and Co.

32. Moses, H., III, and DeLong, M.R.: Parkinsonism and other disorders of extrapyramidal function, In Harvey, A.M. et al. (editors): The principles and practice of medicine, ed. 21, 1984, Appleton-Century Crofts.

33. National Institute of Aging Task Force: Senility reconsidered: Treatment possibilities for mental impairment in the elderly, JAMA, **244**:259, 1980.

34. Nibbelink, D.W.: Antihypertensive and antifibrinolytic therapy following subarachnoid hemorrhage from ruptured intracranial aneurysms. In Saks, A.L., Nibblelink, D.W., and Torner, (editors): Aneurysmal subarachnoid hemorrhage: report of the cooperative study, Baltimore, 1981, Urban and Schwarzenberg,

35. Pleasure, D.E., and Schotland, D.L.: Peripheral nerve disorders. In Rowland, L.P., (editor): Merritt's textbook of neurology, ed. 7, Philadelphia, 1984, Lea and Febiger.

36. Plum, F.: Brief loss of consciousness. In Wyngaarden, J.B., and Smith, L.A., Jr., (editors): Cecil's textbook of medicine, vol. 1, ed. 17, Philadelphia, 1985, W.B. Saunders, Co.
37. Riggs, J.E.: Adult-onset muscle weakness: how to identify the underlying cause, Postgrad. Med. 78(3):217, 1985.
38. Sabra, A.F., et al.: Treatment of action tremor in multiple sclerosis with isoniazid, Neurol. (NY) 32:912, 1982.
39. Schaumburg, H.: Diseases of the peripheral nervous system. In Wyngaarden, J.B., Smith, L.H., (editors): Cecil's textbook of medicine, vol. 1, ed. 17, Philadelphia, 1985, W.B. Saunders Co.
40. Sechi, G., Tanda, F., and Mutani, R.: Fatal hyperpyrexia after withdrawal of levodopa, Neurol. 34:249, 1984.
41. Silberg, D.H.: The demyelinating disease. In Wyngaarden, J.B. Smith, L.H., (editors): Cecil's textbook of medicine, ed. 17, vol. 2, Philadelphia, 1985, W.B. Saunders Co.
42. Toole, J.F.: Cerebrovascular disorders, ed. 3, New York, 1984, Raven Press.
43. Tourtellotte, W., et al.: Comprehensive management of multiple sclerosis. In Hall, Pike, J.F., Adams, C.W.M., and Tourtellotte, W., (editors): Multiple sclerosis: pathology, diagnosis and management, London, 1983, Chapman and Hall, Ltd.
44. Weiner, H.L., et al.: The use of cyclophosphamide in the treatment of multiple sclerosis: a randomized, placebo-controlled, double-blind study, N. Engl. J. Med. 308:181, 1983.
45. Weksler, B.B., et al.: Differential inhibition by aspirin of vascular and platelet prostaglandin synthesis in atherosclerotic patients, N.Engl. J. Med. 308:800, 1983.
46. Woolsey, R.M.: Intracerebral hemorrhage (non-traumatic). In Rakel, R.E., (editor): Conn's current therapy, Philadelphia, 1985, W.B. Saunders Co.
47. Yahr, M.D.: Parkinsonism. In Rowland, L.P. (editor): Merritt's textbook of neurology, ed. 7, Philadelphia, 1984, Lea & Febiger.
48. Zulch, K.J.: Brain tumors: their biology and pathology, American ed. 2, New York, 1965, Springer Publishing Co., Inc.

Pulmonary
Disease

USE AND INTERPRETATION OF PULMONARY FUNCTION TESTS[20]
George T. Kiss

Indications for pulmonary function testing
1. Physiologic assessment and diagnosis
2. Monitor disease process
3. Special applications
   a. Monitor response to therapy
   b. Exercise testing
   c. Bronchial provocation
   d. Pulmonary disability
   e. Preoperative assessment

Commonly available tests
1. Tests of ventilation
   a. Static lung volume: spirometry for vital capacity parameters and closed circuit helium equilibration to determine functional residual capacity; the patient is instructed to take a maximum inhalation and then exhale completely (Fig. 18-1 illustrates a normal tracing using a bell spirometer)
   b. Dynamic lung volumes
      (1) Forced expirogram (forced vital capacity or time-volume curve) to record a maximum rapid exhalation after a maximum inhalation against time (Fig. 18-2 demonstrates a normal curve using bellows or electronic spirometer)
      (2) Flow-volume curve: to directly measure maximum exhalation and flow with a pneumo tachograph or to calculate it from forced expirogram (Fig. 18-3 demonstrates the relationship between flow-volume and time-volume curves, i.e., $v = {volume}/{time}$)
   c. Arterial pCO_2 measurement is inversely proportional to alveolar ventilation in the absence of metabolic disturbances
   d. Radioactive xenon (inhaled) or krypton scan and washout to demonstrate and to quantitate regional alterations
   e. Single-breath nitrogen washout is a useful index of uneven distribution of air
   f. Body plethysmography to measure total thoracic gas and airway resistance; total lung capacity values are higher with this method

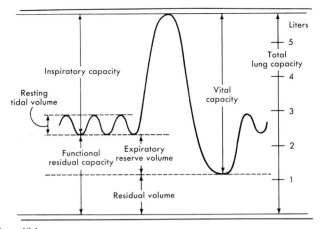

Figure 18-1
Basic spirometry. Lung volumes using a bell spirometer. From Kiss, G.T.: Diagnosis and treatment of pulmonary disease in primary practice, Baltimore, 1984, Williams and Wilkins Co.

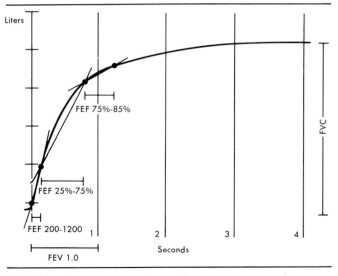

Figure 18-2
Timed vital capacity (or forced expirogram) using bellows or electronic spirometer. From Kiss, G.T.: Diagnosis and treatment of pulmonary disease in primary practice, Baltimore, 1984, Williams and Wilkins Co.

2. Test of pulmonary mechanics
   a. Maximum voluntary ventilation (MVV): maximum air movement extrapolated to 1 minute
   b. Inspiratory force: the negative force generated by a maximum inspiration against a closed airway
   c. Inspiratory pressure and compliance on ventilator patients (i.e., airway progressive per volume)

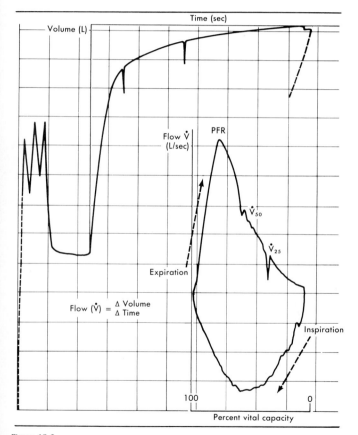

Figure 18-3
Relationship between flow-volume and time-volume curves. From Kiss, G.T.:
Diagnosis and treatment of pulmonary disease in primary practice, Baltimore, 1984,
Williams and Wilkins Co.

3. Measurement of perfusion: radioactive technetium (given intravenously) or krypton lung scan to localize and to quantitate changes in pulmonary flow
4. Measurement of diffusion (CO diffusing capacity): express transfer of gas into the blood; it is affected by ventilation, perfusion, hemoglobin level, surface area, thickness, and carbon monoxide concentration

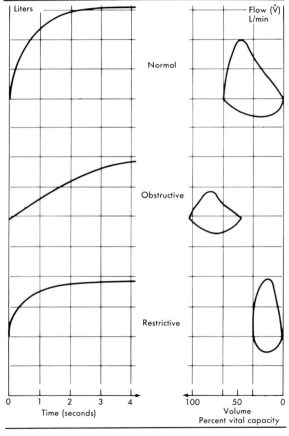

Figure 18-4
Ventilatory patterns of disease. From Kiss, G.T.: Diagnosis and treatment of pulmonary disease in primary practice. Baltimore, 1984, Williams and Wilkins Co.

5. Tests of oxygenation
   a. Arterial Pa_{O_2}
   b. Oxygen saturation is measured with co-oximeter (transcutaneous methods also available for a and b)
   c. Central venous Po_2 is sampled through pulmonary artery catheter
   d. Hemoglobin content
   e. Carbon monoxide (carboxy-hemoglobin level)
   f. Cardiac output

Physiologic assessments

Physiologic assessment tests are performed according to accepted protocols and the results are expressed as percents of established normals. Therapeutic bronchodilators should be withheld if possible before testing. Fig. 18-4 compares normal obstructive and restrictive ventilatory patterns. Table 18-1 summarizes pulmonary function testing abnormalities in common disorders.

1. The presence of obstructive disorders (e.g., bronchitis, asthma) is evidenced by reduced airflows:
   a. FEV_1/FVC: % predicted

>80	normal
65-79	mild obstructive disease
50-64	moderate obstructive disease
<50	severe obstructive disease

   b. FEF 25-75: indicates small airways
   c. Peak expiratory flow (PEFR): reflects mostly large airways
   d. FEF 50, 25: indicate small airways (flow-volume)
   e. Flow-volume tracing may also indicate extrathoracic obstruction, particularly in the inspiratory phase (Fig. 18-5 compares flow-volume curves in various disease states)
   f. Patients with COPD may have a mixture of reversible and irreversible airway obstruction
      (1) Improvement in FEV_1 >15% after inhaled bronchodilator demonstrates reversibility
      (2) Negative response does not exclude reversibility, however, since patients can still have improvement in pulmonary function on long-term bronchodilator therapy

Table 18-1   PFT abnormalities in common disorders

Disorder	FVC	FEV_1	FEV_1/FVC	RV	TLC	Diffusing Capacity
Asthma	↓	↓	↓	↑	N/↑	N
COPD	N/↓	↓	↓	↑	N/↑	N/↓
Kyphoscoliosis	↓	↓	N/↑	N/↓	↓	N
Interstitial fibrosis	↓	↓	N/↑	↓	↓	↓

KEY: ↓, Decreased; ↑, increased; N, normal; FVC, forced vital capacity; FEV_1, forced expiratory volume in 1 second; RV, residual volume; TLC, total lung capacity.

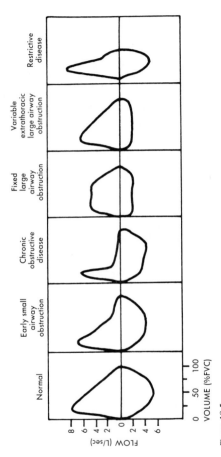

Figure 18-5
Flow-volume curves of restrictive disease and various types of obstructive diseases compared with normal curves.
FVC, Functional vital capacity.

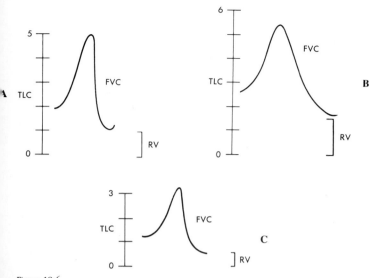

Figure 18-6
Spirometric patterns. TLC, total lung capacity; FVC, forced vital capacity; RV, residual volume. **A,** Normal person. **B,** Person with obstructive disease. **C,** Patient with restrictive disease. From Kiss, G.T.: Diagnosis and treatment of pulmonary disease in primary practice, Baltimore, 1984, Williams and Wilkins Co.

2. Increased residual volume (RV) on spirometry suggests hyperinflation (COPD, asthma); decreased RV occurs in restrictive disease (e.g., interstitial fibrosis) (Fig. 18-6 compares spirometric patterns in obstructive and restrictive disease)
3. Presence of restriction is manifested by a decrease in lung volumes, particularly VC and TLC; it occurs with neuromuscular, skeletal, pleural, and interstitial lung disorders
4. Diffusing capacity is reduced with interstitial disease, thickness of or loss of air exchange surface, and decreased ventilation or perfusion; useful as an early sign of emphysema or predictor of oxygen desaturation or poor exercise tolerance

Special applications of pulmonary function testing

1. Monitoring treatment
   a. Asthma or bronchospasm: follow peak flow (PEFR) or FEV_1 before and after inhalation treatments
   b. Interstitial lung disease (suspected or proven): perform periodic diffusing capacity
   c. Neuromuscular disorders: follow VC or inspiratory force

2. Exercise testing: indications
   a. To elicit bronchospasm
   b. To elicit hypoxemia
3. Bronchial provocation: done with inhalation of graded methacholine doses to demonstrate susceptibility to bronchospasm
4. Disability testing to compare levels of impairment with published levels
   a. Social security standards (reflect level of total disability)
   b. As part of comprehensive physiologic evaluation to assess degree of impairment
5. Preoperative assessment
   a. Spirometry is indicated for abdominal and thoracic surgery particularly when patient is more than 65 years old, has a history of smoking or other lung disease, or if obese
   b. When FEV_1 <2.0 L, FEV_1/FVC <50%, and MVV <50% there is a significantly increased incidence of postoperative complications
   c. If pneumonectomy is considered at above level, residual FEV_1 can be predicted by using quantified radionucleotide perfusion scanning; a residual FEV_1 of <800 ml is usually prohibitive
   d. Postoperative prognosis can be improved, however, by cessation of smoking and an appropriate program of preoperative and perioperative respiratory treatment

Practical approach to pulmonary function testing

1. Forced expirogram/flow volume loop in asymptomatic patient
2. Proceed to full lung volumes if abnormal
3. Determine ABGs for baseline or to assess abnormality
4. Do diffusing capacity for unexplained dyspnea and for evaluation/progress of interstitial disease; this is of little practical value in presence of severe obstructive disorder
5. Do exercise testing or bronchial provocation testing if airway disorder is suspected but not demonstrated

| 18.2 | PNEUMONIA

Etiology

1. Bacterial
   a. *Streptococcus pneumoniae*
   b. *Haemophilus influenzae*
   c. *Legionella pneumophila*
   d. *Klebsiella, Pseudomonas, E. coli*
   e. *Staphylococcus aureus*
2. *Mycoplasma pneumoniae* (atypical pneumonia)
3. Viruses: influenza viruses, adenovirus, CMV, respiratory syncytial virus, herpes
4. Fungi: histoplasmosis, coccidioidomycosis, cryptococcosis, aspergillus
5. Parasites: *Pneumocystis carinii*

Diagnostic considerations

1. History
   a. Evaluate predisposing factors
      (1) COPD: *H. influenzae, S. pneumoniae*
      (2) Recent seizures: aspiration pneumonia
      (3) Compromised host: *Pneumocystis carinii,* CMV, *Legionella,* gram-negative organisms, fungi
      (4) Alcoholism: *Klebsiella, S. pneumoniae, H. influenzae*
      (5) IV drug addict with bacterial endocarditis: *S. aureus*
   b. Distinguish between hospital-acquired vs. community-acquired pneumonia
      (1) Hospital-acquired: gram-negatives, *S. aureus*
      (2) Community-acquired: *S. pneumoniae, M. pneumoniae, H. influenzae*
   c. Consider patient's age
      (1) Infants: viral pneumonia
      (2) Young adults: *M. pneumoniae*
      (3) Adults: *S. pneumoniae*
   d. Rapidity of onset
      (1) Abrupt onset with fever, shaking chills, and copious amounts of rusty-colored sputum: *S. pneumoniae*
      (2) Insidious onset with gradual onset of fever and hacking cough with scant sputum: *M. pneumoniae*
2. Symptoms and physical exam: the presentation varies with the cause of the pneumonia and the patient's age and clinical condition
   a. A patient with *S. pneumoniae* classically presents with high fever, shaking chills, pleuritic chest pain, cough, and copious production of purulent sputum
   b. Patients with viral pneumonia usually present with generalized body aches, malaise, and dry, nonproductive cough
   c. Elderly or immunocompromised hosts may present with only minimal symptoms (e.g., low-grade fever, confusion)
3. Diagnostic methods
   a. Obtain an adequate sputum specimen for Gram stain and cultures
      (1) An expectorated sputum sample is often inadequate because of many false positives (secondary to contamination from oral flora), and many false negatives; a specimen may be considered adequate if the Gram stain shows >25 PMNs and <10 epithelial cells per low-power field
      (2) The diagnostic yield of a sputum can be increased by obtaining the sputum sample with the following methods, which are generally reserved for critically ill patients responding poorly to initial antimicrobial therapy:
         (a) Fiberoptic bronchoscopy
         (b) Percutaneous transtracheal aspiration
         (c) Transthoracic needle aspiration
         (d) Open lung biopsy
   b. Chest x-ray film: the findings vary with the stage and type of pneumonia and the hydration of the patient

(1) Classically, pneumococcal pneumonia presents with a segmental or lobar infiltrate, *Mycoplasma pneumoniae* shows patchy infiltrates, and viral pneumonia manifests radiographically with hazy infiltrates

(2) Diffuse infiltrates on chest x-ray film can be seen with any of the following: *Legionella* pneumonia, *M. pneumoniae,* viral pneumonia, *Pneumocystis carinii,* hypersensitivity pneumonitis, psittacosis, Q fever, aspergillosis, aspiration pneumonia, miliary TB, and ARDS associated with pneumonia

(3) An initial chest x-ray is also useful to rule out the presence of any complications (pneumothorax, empyema, abscesses)

c. Additional lab evaluation

(1) WBC with differential: a low WBC can be present with viral pneumonia or overwhelming bacterial pneumonias

(2) Blood cultures: positive in approximately 20% of cases of pneumococcal pneumonia

(3) Serologic studies

(a) Viral titers: A fourfold titer increase in paired acute and convalescent sera is considered diagnostic of viral pneumonia

(b) *Legionella* titer: a single titer of ≥ 1:256 or a fourfold rise in indirect fluorescent antibodies to a titer of at least 1:128 is diagnostic

(c) *Mycoplasma pneumoniae* complement fixation titer: a single, high titer ≥1:32 or a fourfold rise in titer from acute to convalescent is diagnostic of *M. pneumoniae*

(d) Direct immunofluorescent exam of sputum (e.g., direct fluorescent antibody (DFA) sputum evaluation for *Legionella*)

(e) Cold agglutinins: Nonspecific; positive in only about 50% of patients with *M. pneumoniae*

(f) Counter immunoelectrophoresis (CIE) can be done on sputum, blood, urine, and pleural fluid

(g) ABGs: useful to evaluate degree of hypoxia and need of oxygen therapy

Characteristics and therapy of common pneumonias

1. Pneumococcal pneumonia *(S. pneumoniae)*

a. Most common bacterial pneumonia

b. Predisposing factors are: splenectomy, COPD, sickle cell disease, CHF, cigarette smoking, lung cancer, cerebrovascular disease, dementia, institutionalization, seizure disorder, renal failure, cardiovascular disease, and immunosuppression

c. Gram stain of sputum shows lancet-shaped, gram-positive cocci

d. Treatment

(1) IV: aqueous penicillin G 600,000 U q6h; 2 million units IV q4-6h in life-threatening infections

(2) IM: procaine penicillin G 600,000 U q8-12h

(3) PO: penicillin V 250-500 mg PO q6h

(4) Erythromycin 500 mg PO/IV q6h is indicated in penicillin-allergic patients

(5) Duration of therapy is 10-14 days

2. *H. influenzae*
   a. Common in COPD, elderly patients, and children under 6 years of age
   b. Gram stain reveals pleomorphic, small, coccobacillary gram-negative organisms
   c. Treatment
      (1) IV
         (a) Ampicillin 1.0-1.5 g q4h in known ampicillin-susceptible strains
         (b) Cefuroxime in suspected or known ampicillin-resistant strains
         (c) Alternative antibiotics are trimethoprim-sulfamethoxazole or chloramphenicol
      (2) PO
         (a) Ampicillin 500 mg PO q6h in ampicillin-susceptible strains
         (b) Alternative antibiotics are trimethoprim-sulfomethoxazole (e.g., Bactrim-DS one tablet bid for 7-10 days) or cefaclor
3. *Mycoplasma pneumoniae* (atypical pneumonia)
   a. Generally involves young adults and children
   b. Characteristic finding on physical exam is bullous myringitis
   c. "Walking pneumonia": slow onset, nonproductive cough, myalgias, arthralgias
   d. Treatment: erythromycin 500 gm PO/IV q6h
   e. Duration of therapy is 14-21 days
4. *Legionella pneumophila* pneumonia
   a. Associated with water sources, air conditioning units
   b. Sporadic cases often involve immunocompromised patients
   c. Often associated with diarrhea, bradycardia, liver abnormalities, and mentation difficulties
   d. Treatment: erythromycin 500 mg-1 g IV q6h
   e. Duration of therapy is at least 3 weeks
5. Aspiration pneumonia
   a. Should be suspected in alcoholics, seizure disorders, repeated vomiting, excessive sedation
   b. X-ray films generally demonstrate infiltrates in the inferior segment of right upper lobe or apical segment of lower lobe
   c. Organisms commonly involved are: *Peptococcus, Fusobacterium, Bacteroides,* and other anaerobic organisms generally present in the mouth
   d. Treatment: penicillin G 2 million U IV q4-6 hours or clindamycin 600-900 mg IV q8h
6. *Staphylococcus aureus*
   a. High-risk groups are elderly patients recovering from influenza infection, narcotic abusers, and immunosuppressed patients
   b. Chest x-ray films often show a multicentric patchy appearance secondary to multiple abscess formation; pleural effusions and air fluid levels are often seen
   c. Treatment
      (1) Nafcillin 1.5-2.0 g IV q4h; alternatives are vancomycin 500 mg q6h or cephalotin 1.5-2.0 g q4h, IV
      (2) Penicillin susceptible strains should be treated with penicillin G, 2 million units IV q4h
   d. Duration of therapy is at least 3 weeks

7. *Klebsiella pneumonia* and other gram-negative pneumonias[18]
   a. *Klebsiella*
      (1) Common in alcoholics
      (2) Gram stain reveals encapsulated gram-negative bacilli
      (3) Treatment: aminoglycoside plus cephalosporin (e.g., Cefuroxime); antibiotic dosage must be adjusted for creatinine clearance and levels must be carefully monitored to avoid renal impairment
   b. Other gram-negative bacilli
      (1) Common in immunosuppressed, elderly, and hospitalized patients
      (2) Treatment: amikacin and azlocillin in immunocompromised patients with suspected *Pseudomonas aeruginosa;* adequate treatment of other gram-negative pneumonias is same as for *Klebsiella*

Initial antibiotic therapy

1. Initial antibiotic therapy should be based on clinical, radiographic, and lab evaluation; if the clinical diagnosis is substantiated by an adequate Gram stain (e.g., lancet-shaped, gram-positive cocci in a patient with suspected pneumococcal pneumonia) the choice of initial therapy is relatively simple
2. In otherwise healthy adult patients with community-acquired pneumonia and insidious presentation, erythromycin is the antibiotic of choice since it will adequately treat *Mycoplasma*, pneumococci, and *Legionella*
3. In immunocompromised patients with negative Gram stain, the initial antibiotic treatment should be broad spectrum but with emphasis on gram-negatives, *Legionella,* and *Pneumocystis;* the following antibiotics should be considered:[22]
   a. Patients with AIDS
      (1) Trimethoprim-sulfamethoxazole or pentamidine for *Pneumocystis carinii*
      (2) Erythromycin for *Legionella pneumophila*
   b. Neutropenic patients
      (1) Amikacin and azlocillin for *Pseudomonas aeruginosa*
      (2) Erythromycin for *Legionella*
      (3) Nafcillin for *S. aureus*
   c. Immunocomprised, non-AIDS, non-neutropenic patients
      (1) Aminoglycoside for gram-negative coverage
      (2) Erythromycin for *Legionella*
      (3) Nafcillin or oxacillin for *S. aureus*
      (4) Trimethoprim-sulfamethoxazole for *Pneumocystis* or *Nocardia*
   NOTE: Erythromycin should be part of the initial therapy because of the high prevalence of *Legionella pneumonia* in immunocompromised hosts[5]

18.3   TUBERCULOSIS

Diagnosis[28,30]

1. Clinical manifestations: many patients are asymptomatic at the time of diagnosis; others may complain of dry, nonproductive cough, nightsweats, fever, anorexia, fatigue, dyspnea, pleuritic chest pain, and hemoptysis

2. Physical exam may reveal rales near the lung apices
3. Tuberculin test
    a. Five tuberculin units (TU) of purified protein derivative (PPD) in 0.1 ml of solution is injected intracutaneously
    b. Sensitized individuals demonstrate a dermal reaction of redness, swelling, and induration
    c. A positive reaction is defined as ≥ 10 mm of induration at 48 hours
    d. Up to 25% of patients with newly diagnosed TB have a negative tuberculin skin test, particularly patients with renal failure, elderly patients, and patients on steroid therapy[29]
4. Acid-fast stain and cultures of sputum
5. Chest x-ray
    a. Initial chest x-ray film may show a variety of patterns; rarely, it may be completely normal
    b. Parenchymal infiltrates most commonly involve the upper lobes
    c. Hilar and paratracheal adenopathy, unilateral pleural effusion, and cavitary lesions may also be present

Treatment in adults[1]

1. Six-month regimen: indicated in compliant patients with fully susceptible organisms
    a. Initial 2 months
        (1) Isoniazid 5 mg/kg/day (up to 300 mg/day) PO qd, plus
        (2) Rifampin 10-20 mg/kg/day (up to 600 mg/day) PO qd, plus
        (3) Pyrazinamide 15-30 mg/kg (up to 2 g/day) PO qd
        (4) Ethambutol 15-25 mg/kg PO qd should be included in the initial 2 months if isoniazid resistance is suspected
    b. Remaining 4 months: isoniazid plus rifampin
2. Nine-month regimen
    a. Isoniazid plus rifampin
    b. When isoniazid resistance is suspected, ethambutol is added until susceptibility tests have been reported
    c. In cases of documented resistance to isoniazid, rifampin and ethambutol are given for a minimum of 12 months; initial supplementation with pyrazinamide is advisable
3. Patient compliance is an essential component of any therapeutic regimen

Prophylaxis[1]

1. General indications
    a. Household members and other close contacts of potentially infectious persons
    b. Newly infected persons (tuberculin skin test conversion within the past 2 years)
    c. Persons with past tuberculosis or those with a significant tuberculin reaction and abnormal chest x-ray films in whom current tuberculosis has been excluded
    d. Infected persons in the following clinical situations:
        (1) Silicosis
        (2) Diabetes mellitus
        (3) Adrenocorticosteroid therapy

(4) Immunosuppressive therapy or diseases
(5) AIDS or positive antibodies to HIV
(6) Reticuloendothelial malignancies (e.g., leukemia, Hodgkin's disease)
(7) End-stage renal disease
(8) Clinical conditions associated with rapid weight loss or chronic undernutrition (e.g., post-gastrectomy, chronic malabsorption, chronic peptic ulcer disease)
(9) Tuberculin skin reactors under 35 years of age

2. Therapy
   a. Isoniazid 300 mg PO qd
   b. Duration of therapy is 6-12 months
   c. Monitoring of adverse effects to isoniazid in patients 35 years of age and older consists or monthly symptom reviews and measurement of hepatic enzymes before starting isoniazid therapy and periodically throughout treatment; in patients younger than 35 years of age, a monthly symptom review is adequate

18.4 | CARCINOMA OF THE LUNG

Epidemiology

1. Leading cause of cancer deaths in both men (15% of cancer deaths) and women (18% of cancer deaths)
2. Increased incidence in cigarette smokers and exposure to certain environmental and industrial agents (e.g., ionizing radiation, asbestos, nickel, vinyl chloride)

Histologic classification

The World Health Organization distinguishes 12 types of pulmonary neoplasms,[13] among these the major types are squamous cell carcinoma, adenocarcinoma, small cell carcinoma, and large cell carcinoma. However, the crucial differential in the diagnosis of lung cancer is between small cell and non–small cell types, since the therapeutic approach is totally different[34] (see below).

Diagnosis

1. Characteristics and clinical manifestations
   a. Weight loss, fatigue, fever, anorexia
   b. Cough, hemoptysis, dyspnea
   c. Chest, shoulder, and bone pain
   d. Paraneoplastic syndromes
      (1) Eaton-Lambert's syndrome: myopathy characterized by increased strength and EMG amplitude with repeated effort, reversal with guanidine; this syndrome is often seen with small cell carcinoma
      (2) Endocrine manifestations
         (a) Ectopic ACTH, SIADH: small cell carcinoma
         (b) Hypercalcemia secondary to PTH-like substances: squamous cell carcinoma
      (3) Neurologic: subacute cerebellar degeneration, peripheral neuropathy, cortical degeneration

(4) Musculoskeletal: polymyositis, clubbing, hypertrophic pulmonary osteoarthropathy

(5) Hematologic/vascular: migratory thrombophlebitis, marantic thrombosis, anemia, thrombocytosis/thrombocytopenia

(6) Cutaneous: acanthosis nigricans, dermatomyositis

e. Pleural effusion, recurrent pneumonias (secondary to obstruction), localized wheezing

f. Superior vena cava syndrome
   (1) Obstruction of venous return in superior vena cava, most commonly caused by bronchogenic carcinoma
   (2) The patient usually complains of headache, nausea, dizziness, visual changes, syncope, and respiratory distress
   (3) Physical exam reveals distention of thoracic and neck veins, edema of face and upper extremities, facial plethora, and cyanosis
   (4) Chest x-ray film demonstrates a superior mediastinal mass
   (5) Treatment consists of irradiation and chemotherapy

g. Horner's syndrome: constricted pupil, ptosis, and facial anhidrosis caused by spinal cord damage between C8 to T1 secondary to a superior sulcus tumor (bronchogenic carcinoma at the extreme lung apex); a superior sulcus tumor associated with ipsilateral Horner's syndrome and shoulder pain is known as a "Pancoast tumor"

2. Cytologic exam of at least three sputum specimens unless a positive cytology is obtained in the first or second specimen

3. Chest x-ray films
   a. The radiographic presentation often varies with the cell type; for example, squamous cell and large cell carcinoma often present as a large peripheral mass, adenocarcinoma generally appears as a peripheral nodule, small cell anaplastic carcinoma can present as a perihilar mass or a peripheral nodule
   b. Pleural effusion, lobar atelectasis, and mediastinal adenopathy can accompany any of the above cell types
   c. Benign lesions which simulate thoracic malignancy are listed below[23]
      (1) Lobar atelectasis: pneumonia, tuberculosis, chronic inflammatory disease, allergic bronchopulmonary aspergillosis
      (2) Multiple pulmonary nodules: septic emboli, Wegener's granulomatosis, sarcoidosis, rheumatoid nodules, fungal disease, multiple pulmonary AV fistulas
      (3) Mediastinal adenopathy: sarcoidosis, lymphoma, primary tuberculosis, fungal disease, silicosis, pneumoconiosis, drug induced (e.g., diphenylhydantoin, trimethadione)
      (4) Pleural effusion: CHF, pneumonia with parapneumonic effusion, tuberculosis, viral pleuritis, ascites, pancreatitis, collagen-vascular disease

4. Thoracentesis of pleural effusions, with cytologic evaluation of the thoracentesis fluid

5. CT scan of chest: to evaluate mediastinal and pleural extension of suspected lung neoplasms

6. Establish tissue diagnosis of lung cancer
   a. Biopsy of any suspicious lymph nodes (e.g., supraclavicular node)
   b. Flexible fiberoptic bronchoscopy: brush and biopsy specimens are obtained from any visualized endobronchial lesions
   c. Transbronchial needle aspiration:[39] done via a special needle passed through the bronchoscope; this technique is useful to sample mediastinal masses or paratracheal lymph nodes
   d. Transthoracic fine needle aspiration biopsy[16] to evaluate peripheral pulmonary nodules
   e. Exploratory thoracotomy is particularly indicated in patients with high risk of having lung carcinoma (e.g., heavy smokers) who are being considered for surgical resection to cure a lung neoplasm

Staging

The most widely accepted staging system is the TNM system (tumor, node, metastasis) recommended by the American Joint Committee on Cancer.[3] However, in patients with small cell lung cancer, a more practical and widely accepted staging system was developed by the Veterans Administration Lung Cancer Study Group (VALG).[41] This staging system contains two stages:
1. Limited stage: disease is confined to the regional lymph nodes and to one hemithorax (excluding pleural surfaces)
2. Extensive stage: spread beyond the confines of limited state disease

Pretreatment staging procedures for lung cancer patients in addition to a complete history and physical exam generally include the following tests:
1. Chest x-ray films (PA and lateral), ECG
2. Lab evaluation: CBC, electrolytes, platelets, calcium, phosphorus, glucose, renal and liver function studies, ABG, and skin test for tuberculosis
3. Pulmonary function studies
4. CT scan of chest
5. Mediastinoscopy or anterior mediastinotomy in patients being considered for possible curative lung resection
6. Biopsy of any accessible suspicious lesions
7. CT scans of liver and brain, and radionuclide scans of bone in all patients with small cell carcinoma of the lung and all other patients with non–small cell lung neoplasms suspected of tumor involvement of these organs
8. Bone marrow aspiration and biopsy is indicated only in patients with small cell carcinoma of the lung

Treatment

1. Non–small cell carcinoma
   a. Surgery
      (1) Surgical resection is indicated in patients with limited disease* (approximately 15%-30% of newly diagnosed cases); the 5-year survival rate is approximately 30% in these patients
      (2) Preoperative evaluation includes review of cardiac status (e.g., recent MI, major dysrhythmias), and evaluation of pulmonary function (to determine if the patient can tolerate any loss of functional lung tissue)

*Not involving mediastinal nodes, ribs, pleura, or distant sites.

  (a) Pulmonary resection is possible if the patient has a preoperative FEV_1 ≥ 2 L, or if the MVV is $>50\%$ of predicted capacity[32]
  (b) In patients with equivocal results, a ventilation-perfusion lung scan provides information regarding the percentage of ventilation contributed by the non–tumor-bearing lung; if this value, when multiplied by the FEV_1 is ≥ 1 L, the pneumonectomy is functionally tolerable[26] (e.g., if the preoperative FEV_1 = 1.9 and a lung scan demonstrates that the percentage of ventilation of the non–tumor-bearing lung is equal to 60%, the product of these two values $(1.9 \times 0.6) = 1.14$, a value within the safe range)

  b. Treatment of unresectable non–small cell carcinoma of the lung
  (1) Radiotherapy can be used alone or combined with chemotherapy or surgery
  (2) Chemotherapy: there are various combination regimens available (e.g., MVP: combination of mitomycin, vinblastine, and cisplatin); however, the overall results are disappointing

2. Treatment of small cell bronchogenic carcinoma
  a. The main therapeutic approach consists of aggressive combination chemotherapy (e.g., combination cyclophosphamide, adriamycin, and vincristine rapidly alternating with combination cisplatin and VP-16, followed by prophylactic cranial radiotherapy[27])
  b. Thoracic radiotherapy generally plays only a secondary role in the treatment of these patients
  c. There is currently renewed interest in the role of surgery in the management of patients with limited disease;[34] however, present results are inconclusive and further studies are necessary

| 18.5 | MECHANICAL VENTILATION[35,36]

Indications for mechanical ventilation

The decision to initiate mechanical ventilation is generally based on the following:

1. Clinical assessment: presence of apnea, tachypnea (>40 breaths/minute), or respiratory failure that cannot be adequately corrected by any other means
2. ABGs: severe hypoxemia despite high-flow oxygen or significant CO_2 retention (e.g., P_{O_2} <50, P_{CO_2} >50)
3. Physiologic parameters are of limited use since many patients with respiratory insufficiency are unable to perform PFTs and their respiratory failure mandates immediate intervention; some of the commonly accepted physiologic parameters for intubation and respiratory support are:
  a. Vital capacity <15 ml/kg
  b. Inspiratory force < -25 cm H_2O
  c. FEV_1 <10 ml/kg
  NOTE: The clinical assessment is the most important determinant of the need for mechanical ventilation since both physiologic parameters and ABGs do not distinguish between acute and chronic respiratory insufficiency (e.g., a P_{CO_2} >60 mm Hg and a respiratory rate >30/minute may

be the ''norm'' for a patient with COPD, whereas the same values in a young otherwise healthy adult are indications for intubation and mechanical ventilation)

Common modes of mechanical ventilation

1. Intermittent mandatory ventilation (IMV): the patient is allowed to breathe spontaneously and the ventilator delivers a number of machine breaths at a preset rate and volume
   a. Advantages and indications
      (1) IMV is indicated in the majority of spontaneously breathing patients because it maintains respiratory muscle tone and results in less depression of cardiac output than assist/control
      (2) It is useful for weaning, because as the IMV rate is decreased the patient gradually assumes the bulk of the breathing work
   b. Disadvantages
      (1) The increased work of breathing results in increased oxygen consumption (deleterious to patients with myocardial insufficiency)
      (2) IMV is not useful in patients with depressed respiratory drive or impaired neurologic status
2. Assist/control: the patient breathes at his own rate and the ventilator senses the inspiratory effort and delivers a preset tidal volume with each patient effort; if the patient's respiratory rate decreases past a preset rate, the ventilator delivers tidal breaths at the preset rate
   a. Advantages/indications: useful in patients with neuromuscular weakness, or CNS disturbances
   b. Disadvantages
      (1) Tachypnea may result in significant hypocapnia and respiratory alkalosis
      (2) Improper setting of sensitivity to the negative pressure necessary to trigger the ventilator may result in ''fighting the ventilator'' when the sensitivity is set too low
      (3) Increased sensitivity may result in hyperventilation; sensitivity is generally set so that an inspiratory effort of 2-3 cm will trigger ventilation
      (4) The respiratory muscle tone is not well maintained in patients on assist/control and this may result in difficulty with weaning
3. Controlled ventilation: the patient does not breathe spontaneously; the respiratory rate is determined by the physician
   a. Advantages and indications
      (1) Useful in patients who are unable to make an inspiratory effort (e.g., severe CNS dysfunction), and in patients with excessive agitation or breathing effort
      (2) Patients with excessive agitation are often sedated with morphine or benzodiazepines and paralyzed with pancuronium bromide (Pavulon)
      (3) Initial pancuronium dose is 0.04-0.1 mg/kg IV in adults
      (4) Later incremental doses starting at 0.01 mg/kg may be used prn; pancuronium should be administered only by or under the supervision of experienced clinicians

b. Disadvantages: paralyzed patients on controlled ventilation must be closely monitored because ventilator malfunction or disconnection is rapidly fatal

Selection of ventilator settings

1. Tidal volume (TV): 10-15 ml/kg of ideal body weight
2. Rate (number of tidal breaths delivered/minute): 8-16 depending on the desired $PaCO_2$ or pH (increased rate = decreased $PaCO_2$)
3. Mode: IMV, assist/control, controlled ventilation
4. Oxygen concentration (FIO_2): the initial FIO_2 should be 100% unless it is evident that a lower FIO_2 will provide adequate oxygenation
5. Obtain ABGs 15 to 30 minutes after initiating mechanical ventilation
6. Immediate chest x-ray is indicated after intubation to evaluate for correct placement of endotracheal tube
7. Sedation orders (e.g., morphine, diazepam) may be necessary in selected patients
8. Positive end–expiratory pressure (PEEP)
   a. The application of positive pressure may prevent the closure of edematous small airways; it is indicated when arterial oxygenation is inadequate (saturation <90%) despite an FIO_2 >50%
   b. PEEP is generally started at 5 cm of H_2O and increased by increments of 2-5 cm to maintain the PaO_2 ≥60 mm Hg
   c. The use of PEEP can result in pulmonary barotrauma and hemodynamic compromise (secondary to decreased right ventricular filling)
   d. Patients receiving PEEP should have their cardiac output frequently monitored; the measurement of mixed venous oxygen saturation is useful to evaluate the effect of PEEP on cardiac output[17]
9. Adjust the initial ventilator setting depending on results of the ABGs and clinical response
   a. Use the lowest FIO_2 necessary to maintain a PaO_2 >60 mm Hg (90% hemoglobin saturation in patients with a normal pH)
   b. Adjust minute ventilation (tidal volume × rate) to normalize the pH and the $PaCO_2$
      (1) Increasing the TV or the rate will decrease $PaCO_2$ and increase the pH
      (2) Do not lower the patient's $PaCO_2$ below the "norm" for the patient (e.g., some patients with COPD should be allowed to maintain their usual mildly elevated $PaCO_2$ to avoid alkalosis and to provide stimulus for breathing)

Major complications of mechanical ventilation[19]

1. Pulmonary barotrauma (e.g., pneumomediastinum, pneumothorax, subcutaneous emphysema, emphysema, pneumoperitoneum): generally secondary to high levels of PEEP, excessive tidal volumes, high peak airway pressures, and coexistence of significant lung disease
2. Pulmonary thromboemboli can be prevented by vigorous leg care and use of prophylactic low-dose heparin (i.e., 5000 U SC q12h)
3. GI bleeding: prophylaxis with antacids or H_2 blockers is generally indicated in patients on mechanical ventilators; gastric pH should be kept >3.5

4. Dysrhythmias: avoid use of dysrhythmogenic drugs and prevent rapid acid-base shifts
5. Accumulation of large amount of secretions: frequent respiratory toilet is necessary in all patients on mechanical ventilators
6. Other: nosocomial infections, laryngotracheal injury, malnutrition, hypophosphatemia, oxygen toxicity, psychosis

Withdrawal of mechanical ventilatory support

1. Common criteria for ventilator weaning
   a. Improved clinical status (the patient is alert and hemodynamically stable)
   b. Adequate oxygenation (Pao_2 >60 mm Hg on 40% FIO_2)
   c. pH 7.33-7.48, with acceptable $Paco_2$
   d. Respiratory rate ≤25/minute
   e. Vital capacity ≥10 ml/kg
   f. Resting minute ventilation <10 L/minute, with ability to double the resting minute ventilation
   g. Maximum inspiratory pressure more negative than −20 cm H_2O
   NOTE: The above criteria are only guidelines; significant variation may be present (e.g., a respiratory rate of 30 breaths/minute may be acceptable in a patient with COPD)
2. Methods of weaning
   a. Weaning via IMV
      (1) Gradually decrease the IMV as tolerated (e.g., two breaths every 3-4 hours), monitoring ABGs after each adjustment
      (2) Do not change more than one parameter at a time
      (3) When the patient is tolerating an IMV of 4-6, a trial with a T-tube can be attempted; the T-tube is attached to the endotracheal tube and delivers humidified oxygen (FIO_2 40%)
      (4) If the patient tolerates the T-tube well, extubation may be attempted
         (a) Have adequate equipment and personnel available if reintubation is necessary (start early in the day)
         (b) Suction airway and oropharynx
         (c) Deflate cuff and extubate
         (d) Administer oxygen via facemask (FIO_2 40%-100%)
         (e) Auscultate lungs for adequate air movement
         (f) Closely monitor vital signs
         (g) Obtain ABGs approximately 15 to 30 minutes postextubation
         (h) Reintubate if extubation is poorly tolerated
   b. Stable patients without pulmonary disease and with a good probability of quick extubation (e.g., after uncomplicated cardiac surgery) may be given a direct trial of T-tube (bypassing gradual decreases of IMV)

Failure to wean from mechanical ventilator

Failure to wean usually results from premature attempts at weaning (e.g., patient is hemodynamically unstable). Other common reversible causes of failure to wean are:

1. Hypophosphatemia and nutritional deficiency
2. Drug toxicity (e.g., excessive CNS depression from sedatives)
3. Bronchospasm
4. Excessive secretions
5. Significant acid-base disturbances
6. Hypothyroidism

18.6   ACUTE BRONCHOSPASM

STATUS ASTHMATICUS

Definition

Status asthmaticus is characterized by severe continuous bronchospasm.

Clinical manifestations[11]

1. Usually there is a history of progressively worsening dyspnea, cough, tachypnea, chest tightness, and wheezing over a period of hours to days
2. The patient is generally sitting forward, is diaphoretic, and may be unable to speak because of severe dyspnea
3. Physical exam may reveal
   a. Tachycardia and tachypnea
   b. Use of accessory respiratory muscles
   c. Pulsus paradoxus (inspiratory decline in systolic blood pressure >10 mm Hg)
   d. Wheezing; the absence of wheezing (silent chest) or decreased wheezing can indicate worsening obstruction
   e. Mental status changes; these are generally secondary to hypoxia and hypercapnia and constitute an indication for urgent intubation
   f. An important sign of impending respiratory crisis is paradoxic abdominal and diaphragmatic movement on inspiration (detected by palpation over the upper part of the abdomen in a semirecumbent position) indicates diaphragmatic fatigue;[4] aminophylline infusion is effective in improving diaphragmatic contractility in these patients

Lab and radiographic evaluation

1. Arterial blood gases can be used in staging the severity of the asthmatic attack
   a. Mild: decreased Pao_2 and $Paco_2$, increased pH
   b. Moderate: decreased Pao_2, normal $Paco_2$, normal pH
   c. Severe: markedly decreased Pao_2, increased $Paco_2$, and decreased pH
2. CBC: leukocytosis with ''left shift'' may indicate coexistence of bacterial infection (e.g., pneumonia)
3. Sputum: eosinophils, Charcot-Leyden crystals; PMNs and bacteria may be found on gram stain in patients with pneumonia
4. Chest x-ray films generally show only evidence of thoracic hyperinflation (e.g., flattening of diaphragm, increased volume of retrosternal airspace)

Additional evaluation

1. ECG: tachycardia and nonspecific ST-T wave changes; may also show cor pulmonale, RBBB, right axis deviation, counter-clockwise rotation

2. Pulmonary function tests: FEV_1 <1 L and peak expiratory flow rates (PEFR) <80 L/minute indicate severe bronchospasm

Treatment

1. Oxygen is available via nasal cannula (each L/minute of flow generally adds 2% to the FIO_2) or with Ventimask (24, 28, 31, 35, 40, 50%)
   a. It is generally started at 2-4 L/minute via nasal cannula or Ventimask at 40% FIO_2
   b. Further adjustments are made according to ABGs
2. Sympathomimetics: various agents and modalities are available
   a. Epinephrine (1:1000 dilution)
      (1) Dosage range is 0.3-0.5 ml SC, may repeat after 15-20 minutes
      (2) Onset of action is within 15 minutes
      (3) Duration is less than 1-4 hours
      (4) Use with caution in patients over the age of 40 or anyone with heart disease
   b. Terbutaline (Brethine)
      (1) May be given SC 0.25 mg
      (2) Clinically significant increase in FEV_1 occurs within 15 minutes and persists for 90 minutes to 4 hours
      (3) It generally has fewer cardiac stimulating effects than epinephrine, however, systemic vasodilatation with compensatory tachycardia can occur
   c. Metaproterenol (Alupent)
      (1) May be administered via aerosol nebulizer, bulb nebulizer or IPPB (e.g., 0.3 ml of metaproterenol in 3 ml of saline, given via nebulizer)
      (2) Onset of action is within 5 minutes, duration is approximately 3-4 hours
   d. Isoetharine (Bronkosol), Isoproterenol (Isuprel): they are also quick acting agents when administered via inhalation, however their duration of action is less than metaproterenol
3. Theophylline: refer to p. 550 for loading and maintenance doses
4. Corticosteroids
   a. Early administration is advised, particularly in patients receiving steroids at home
   b. Patients may be started on hydrocortisone (Solu-Cortef) 2.5-4 mg/kg or methylprednisolone (Solu-Medrol) 0.5-1 mg/kg IV loading and then q6h prn; higher doses may be necessary in selected patients (particularly those receiving steroids at home)
   c. Rapid but judicious tapering off corticosteroids will eliminate serious steroid toxicity
   d. The most common error regarding steroid therapy in acute bronchospasm is the use of ''too little, too late''
5. Atropine analogs (e.g., ipratropium bromide) via nebulizer may be useful in patients not responding well to β antagonists
   a. The recommended dose of atropine is 0.05 mg/kg in saline given via nebulizer; use with caution in cardiac patients
   b. Its duration of action is approximately 3 hours
   c. If the recommended dose is ineffective it should be doubled[37]

6. IV hydration: judicious use is necessary to avoid pulmonary edema
7. IV antibiotics are indicated when there is suspicion of bacterial infection (e.g., infiltrate on chest x-ray film, fever, or leukocytosis)
8. Intubation and mechanical ventilation are indicated when above measures fail to produce significant improvement
9. General anesthesia: halothane anesthesia may reverse bronchospasm in a severe asthmatic who cannot be ventilated adequately with mechanical ventilation

EXACERBATION OF COPD

Clinical manifestations

Patients with COPD are classically subdivided into two major groups based on their appearance:

1. "Blue bloaters" are patients with chronic bronchitis; they derive their name from the bluish tinge of their skin (secondary to chronic hypoxemia and hypercapnia), and from the frequent presence of peripheral edema (secondary to cor pulmonale); chronic cough with production of large amounts of sputum is characteristic
2. "Pink puffers" are patients with emphysema; they have a cachectic appearance but a pink skin color (adequate O_2 saturation); shortness of breath is manifested by pursed-lip breathing and use of accessory muscles for respiration

Chest x-ray films

Chest x-ray films usually demonstrate hyperinflation with flattened diaphragm, tenting of the diaphragm at the insertions to the ribs, and increased retrosternal air space. Decreased vascular markings and bullae may be evident in patients with emphysema.

Lab evaluation

1. CBC may reveal leukocytosis with "shift to the left"
2. Sputum may be purulent in patients with bacterial respiratory tract infections

Treatment of acute exacerbation

1. Aerosolized β agonists (e.g., metaproterenol, isoetharine)
2. Theophylline (see Chapter 21 for dosage)
3. Inhaled parasympatholitic agents (e.g., inhaled atropine 0.025 mg/kg q4-8h) may be effective in selected patients;[33] side effects (tachycardia, urinary retention) may occur even at low dosages
4. Judicious oxygen administration
   a. Hypercapnia and further respiratory compromise may occur after high-flow oxygen therapy
   b. The use of a Venturi-type mask delivering an inspired fraction of oxygen (24% or 28%) is preferred to nasal cannula
5. Corticosteroids (e.g., hydrocortisone, methylprednisolone) may be beneficial during acute exacerbation if bronchospasm is a significant factor, however, chronic steroid therapy should be avoided if possible
6. Antibiotics are indicated in suspected respiratory infection
   a. *H. influenzae* and *S. pneumonia* are frequent causes of acute bronchitis

    b. Oral antibiotics of choice are: ampicillin, trimethoprim/sulfamethoxa-
       zole, tetracycline, or cefaclor

    c. The use of antibiotics has been shown to be beneficial in exacerbations
       of COPD presenting with increased dyspnea, sputum, and sputum
       purulence[2]

7. Pulmonary toilet: careful nasotracheal suction is indicated in patients with
    excessive secretions and inability to expectorate them

8. Intubation and mechanical ventilation may be necessary if the above mea-
    sures fail to provide satisfactory improvement

| 18.7 |

DIFFUSE INTERSTITIAL PULMONARY DISEASE[7,8,9]

Definition

Diffuse interstitial pulmonary disease is a group of disorders involving the
lung interstitium and characterized by inflammation of the alveolar structures
and progressive parenchymal fibrosis.

Etiology

There are over 100 known disorders that can cause interstitial lung disease
(ILD). The more common causes are:

1. Occupational and environmental exposure: pneumoconiosis, asbestosis,
    organic dusts, gases, fumes

2. Granulomatous lung disease: sarcoidosis, hypersensitivity pneumonitis,
    infections (e.g., viral, *Pneumocystis carinii,* fungal, mycobacterial)

3. Drug-induced: bleomycin, busulfan, methotrexate, chlorambucil, cyclo-
    phosphamide, BCNU, gold salts, nitrofurantoin, amiodarone, tocainide,
    penicillin

4. Radiation pneumonitis

5. Connective tissue diseases: SLE, rheumatoid arthritis, dermatopolymyo-
    sitis

6. Idiopathic pulmonary fibrosis: DIP, bronchiolitis obliterans, interstitial
    pneumonitis

7. Infections: viral pneumonia, pneumocystis

8. Others: Wegener's granulomatosis, Goodpasture's syndrome, eosinophilic
    granuloma, lymphangitic carcinomatosis, chronic uremia, chronic gastric
    aspiration

Diagnosis

1. Clinical history: inquire about possible drug, occupational, and environ-
    mental exposure

2. Clinical manifestations and physical exam
    a. The patient generally has progressive dyspnea and nonproductive
       cough; other clinical manifestations vary with the underlying disease
       process
    b. Physical exam typically shows end-inspiratory dry rales (velcro rales);
       cyanosis, clubbing, and signs of right heart failure are generally late
       findings

3. Chest x-ray films may be normal in approximately 10% of patients; roent-
    genographic abnormalities usually reflect the underlying disease process
    and the stage of the disease.
    a. Ground glass appearance is often an early finding
    b. A coarse, reticular pattern is usually a late finding

   c. Additional findings on chest x-ray films may include the following:
     (1) Kerley B-lines: lymphangitic carcinomatosis, left ventricular dysfunction
     (2) Hilar and mediastinal adenopathy: sarcoidosis, pneumoconiosis
     (3) Lytic bone lesions: eosinophilic granuloma, lymphangitic carcinomatosis
   d. Congestive heart failure causing interstitial changes on chest x-ray film must always be ruled out

4. Arterial blood gases provide only limited information; initial ABGs may be normal, but with progression of the disease, hypoxemia may be present.
5. Pulmonary function tests: findings are generally consistent with restrictive disease (decreased VC, TLC, and diffusing capacity)
6. Bronchoscopy with bronchoalveolar lavage is useful to characterize the pulmonary inflammatory response; the effector cell population in patients with ILD consists of two major cell types:
   a. Lymphocytes (e.g., sarcoidosis, berylliosis, silicosis, hypersensitivity pneumonitis)
   b. Neutrophils (e.g., asbestosis, collagen-vascular diseases, idiopathic pulmonary fibrosis)
7. Biopsy (open lung biopsy or transbronchial biopsy) to identify the underlying disease process and exclude neoplastic involvement; transbronchial biopsy is less invasive but provides less tissue for analysis (this factor may be important in patients with irregular pulmonary involvement)
8. Gallium-67 scanning plays a limited role in the evaluation of ILD because it is nonspecific and a negative result does not exclude disease (e.g., patients with end-stage fibrosis may have negative scan)

Treatment

1. Removal of offending agent (e.g., environmental exposure)
2. Treatment of infectious process with appropriate antibiotic therapy
3. Supplemental oxygen in patients with significant hypoxemia
4. Corticosteroids are beneficial in patients with sarcoidosis; in patients with interstitial lung disease caused by an inflammatory process they may suppress alveolitis, however response to therapy is highly variable
5. Immunosuppressive therapy in selected cases (e.g., cyclophosphamide in patients with Wegener's granulomatosis)
6. Treatment of any complications (e.g., pneumothorax, pulmonary embolism)

| 18.8 | SARCOIDOSIS |

Definition

Sarcoidosis is a chronic systemic granulomatous disease of unknown cause, characterized histologically by the presence of nonspecific, noncaseating granulomas.

Characteristics and clinical manifestations

1. Increased incidence in blacks, females, and patients between the ages of 20-40

2. Clinical manifestations often vary with the stage of the disease and degree of organ involvement; patients may be asymptomatic, but their chest x-ray film may demonstrate findings consistent with sarcoidosis (see below)
3. Frequent presentations are:
   a. Pulmonary manifestations: dry, nonproductive cough, dyspnea, chest discomfort
   b. Constitutional symptoms: fatigue, weight loss, anorexia, malaise
   c. Visual disturbances: blurred vision, ocular discomfort, conjunctivitis, iritis
   d. Dermatologic manifestations: erythema nodosum, macules, papules, subcutaneous nodules, hyperpigmentation
   e. Myocardial disturbances: dysrhythmias, cardiomyopathy
   f. GI disturbances: hepatomegaly
   g. Rheumatologic manifestations: arthralgias, arthritis
   h. Neurologic manifestations: cranial nerve palsies, diabetes insipidus, meningeal involvement

Diagnosis

1. Chest x-ray films: hilar and mediastinal adenopathy are frequent findings; parenchymal changes may also be present, depending on the stage of the disease
2. Lab abnormalities
   a. Hypergammaglobulinemia
   b. Liver function test abnormalities
   c. Hypercalcemia, hypercalciuria (secondary to increased GI absorption, abnormal vitamin D metabolism and increased calcitriol production by sarcoid granuloma[21])
   d. Cutaneous anergy to trichophytoin, *Candida,* or mumps
   e. Angiotensin converting enzyme (ACE): elevated in approximately 60% of patients with sarcoidosis; may be useful in following the course of the disease[38]
3. Pulmonary function studies may be normal or may reveal a restrictive pattern (see pp. 399-406)
4. Gallium-67 scan: Gallium-67 will localize in areas of granulomatous infiltrates; however, it is nonspecific
5. Ophthalmologic exam[10] is indicated in all patients with suspected sarcoidosis since ocular findings (iridocyclitis, uveitis, conjunctivitis, and keratopathy) are found in over 25%[31] of patients with documented sarcoidosis
6. Biopsy should be done on accessible tissues suspected of sarcoid involvement (conjunctiva, skin, lymph nodes); bronchoscopy with transbronchial biopsy is the procedure of choice in patients without another readily accessible site
7. Bronchoalveolar lavage is useful to evaluate the cellularity of the lavaged fluid
   a. Patients with sarcoidosis generally manifest lymphocytic alveolitis
   b. The levels of helper T-cell lymphocytes in bronchoalveolar lavage fluid can be used as a marker for sarcoid activity[15]
   c. Patients with high levels of T-lymphocytes (>28%) have a higher incidence of pulmonary roentgenographic and physiologic deterioration

Treatment

The majority of patients with sarcoidosis have spontaneous remission within 2 years and do not require any treatment. Their course can be followed by periodic clinical evaluation, chest x-rays, PFTs, ACE levels, and gallium scans. Corticosteroids should be considered in patients with severe symptoms (e.g., dyspnea, chest pain), hypercalcemia, ocular, CNS or cardiac involvement, and progressive pulmonary disease.

[18.9]   PULMONARY THROMBOEMBOLISM

Risk factors

1. Prolonged immobilization
2. Postoperative state
3. Trauma to lower extremities
4. Estrogen-containing birth control pills
5. Prior history of DVT or PE
6. Congestive heart failure
7. Pregnancy and early puerperium
8. Visceral cancer[12] (lung, pancreas, alimentary and genitourinary tract)
9. Trauma, burns
10. Advanced age
11. Obesity
12. Hematologic disease (e.g., antithrombin III deficiency,[6] protein C deficiency, protein S deficiency, lupus anticoagulant, polycythemia vera, dysfibrinogenemia, paroxysmal nocturnal hemoglobinuria)
13. COPD, diabetes mellitus, atrial fibrillation

Clinical manifestations

1. Dyspnea is the most common symptom
2. Chest pain may be nonpleuritic or pleuritic (infarction)
3. Syncope (massive PE)
4. Fever, diaphoresis
5. Hemoptysis, cough

Physical exam

1. Evidence of DVT may be present
2. Cardiac exam may reveal tachycardia, increased pulmonic component of S_2, murmur of tricuspid insufficiency, right ventricular heave, right sided S_3
3. Pulmonary exam may demonstrate rales, localized wheezing, friction rub
4. Tachypnea is the most common physical finding

Diagnostic studies

1. Chest x-ray films may be normal; suggestive findings include elevated diaphragm, pleural effusion, dilatation of pulmonary artery, infiltrate or consolidation, abrupt vessel cutoff
2. ECG: sinus tachycardia, S_1 Q_3 T_3 pattern, T-wave inversion in V_1-V_4, acute RBBB, new-onset atrial fibrillation; ST segment depression in lead II, right ventricular strain
3. ABGs: generally reveal decreased PaO_2 and $PaCO_2$ and increased pH; normal results do not rule out pulmonary embolism

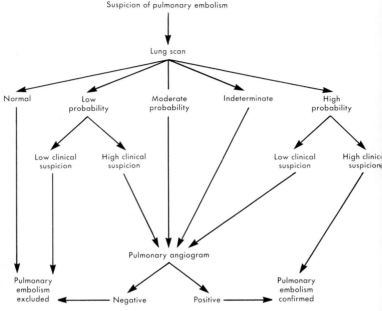

Figure 18-7
Evaluation of suspected pulmonary embolism.

4. Lung scan and arteriography[14]
   a. A normal lung scan rules out pulmonary embolism
   b. A ventilation/perfusion mismatch is suggestive of pulmonary embolism and a lung scan interpretation of high probability is confirmatory
   c. If the clinical suspicion of pulmonary embolism is high and the lung scan is interpreted as low probability, moderate probability, or indeterminate then a pulmonary arteriogram is indicated (see Fig. 18-7); a positive arteriogram confirms the diagnosis

Treatment[24,25]

1. Thrombolytic agents (urokinase, streptokinase): provide rapid resolution of clots; this is the treatment of choice in patients with massive pulmonary embolism who are hemodynamically unstable and with no contraindications to the use of thrombolytic agents
2. Heparin (see Chapter 21 for dosage)

3. Long-term treatment is generally carried out with warfarin therapy, but in some patients SC heparin is preferred (e.g., during pregnancy); in patients without persistent risk factors, therapy is generally discontinued after 6 months

4. If thrombolytics and anticoagulants are contraindicated (e.g., GI bleeding, recent CNS surgery, recent trauma) or if the patient is hypotensive (secondary to massive PE) and refractory to medical therapy, acute embolectomy is indicated; in these patients and in others with recurrent PE despite adequate anticoagulant therapy, vena caval interruption is indicated by transvenous placement of Greenfield filter, Hunter-Sessions occluding balloon or with surgical ligation or plication[40]

References

1. American Thoracic Society: Treatment of tuberculosis and tuberculosis infection in adults and children, Am. Rev. Resp. Dis. **134**:355, 1986.

2. Anthonisen, N.R., et al.: Antibiotic therapy in exacerbation of chronic obstructive pulmonary disease, Ann. Intern. Med. **106**:196, 1987.

3. Carr, D.T., and Mountain, C.F.: Staging of lung cancer, Semin. Resp. Med. **3**:154, 1982.

4. Cohen, C.A., et al.: Clinical manifestations of inspiratory muscle fatigue, Am. J. Med. **73**:308, 1982.

5. Cordonnier, C., et al.: Legionnaire's disease and hairy-cell leukemia: an unfortuitous association? **144**:2373, 1984.

6. Cosgriff, T.M., et al.: Familial antithrombin III deficiency: its natural history, genetics, diagnosis and treatment, Medicine (Baltimore) **62**:209, 1983.

7. Crystal, R.G., et al.: Interstitial lung disease of unknown cause: disorders characterized by chronic inflammation of the lower respiratory tract (part I), N. Engl. J. Med. **310**(3):154, 1984.

8. Crystal, R.G., et al.: Interstitial lung disease of unknown cause: disorders characterized by chronic inflammation of the lower respiratory tract (part II), N. Engl. J. Med. **310**(4):235, 1984.

9. Davis, W.B., and Crystal, R.G.: Chronic interstitial lung disease. In Simmons, D.H. (editor): Current pulmonology, vol. 5. New York, 1984, John Wiley and Sons.

10. Dresner, M.S., Brecher, R., and Henkind, P.: Opthalmology consultation in the diagnosis and treatment of sarcoidosis, Arch. Intern. Med. **146**:301, 1986.

11. Edelson, J.D., and Rebuck, A.S.: The clinical assessment of severe asthma, Arch. Intern. Med. **145**:321, 1985.

12. Gore, J.M., et al.: Occult cancer in patients with acute pulmonary embolism, Ann. Intern. Med. **96**:556, 1982.

13. Histologic typing of lung cancer, Tumor **67**:253, 1981.

14. Hull, R.D., et al.: Pulmonary angiography, ventilation lung scanning and venography for clinically suspected pulmonary embolism with abnormal perfusion lung scan, Ann. Intern. Med. **98**:891, 1983.

15. Hunninghake, G.W., and Crystal, R.G.: Pulmonary sarcoidosis: a disorder mediated by excess helper T-lymphocyte activity at sites of disease activity, N. Engl. J. Med. **305**:429, 1981.

16. Johnson, R.D., Gobien, R.P., and Valicenti, J.F., Jr.: Current status of radiologically directed pulmonary thin needle aspiration biopsy: an analysis of 200 consecutive biopsies and review of the literature, Ann. Clin. Lab. Sci. **13**:225, 1983.

17. Kandel, G., and Aberman, A.: Mixed venous oxygen saturation: its role in the assessment of the critically ill patient, Arch. Intern. Med. **143**:1400, 1983.

18. Karnad, A., and Alvarez, S.: Pneumonia caused by gram-negative bacilli, Am. J. Med. **79**(suppl 1A): 61, 1985.

19. Khan, F.A., Rajinder, K.C.: Complications of acute respiratory failure, Postgrad. Med. **79**(1):205, 1986.

20. Kiss, G.T.: Diagnosis and treatment of pulmonary disease in private practice, Baltimore, 1984, Williams and Wilkins.

21. Mason, R.S., et al.: Vitamin D conversion by sarcoid lymph node homogenate, Ann. Intern. Med. **36**:938, 1984.

22. Masur, H., Shelhamer, J., and Parrillo, J.E.: The management of pneumonias in immunocompromised patients, JAMA, **253**:1769, 1985.

23. Miller, W.R., et al.: Benign lesions which simulate thoracic malignancy, Primary Care and Cancer, p. 8, Sept., 1985.

24. Moser, K.M., and Fedullo, P.F.: Venous thromboembolism: three simple decisions (part I), Chest, **83**(1):117, 1983.

25. Moser, K.M., and Fedullo, P.F.: Venous thromboembolism: three simple decisions (part II), Chest, **83**(2):256, 1983.

26. Mountain, C.F.: Biologic, physiologic, and technical determinants in surgical therapy for lung cancer. In Straus, M.J. (editor): Lung cancer: clinical diagnosis and treatment 1977, Grune and Stratton.

27. Natale, R.B., et al.: Combination cyclophosphamide, adriamycin, and vincristine rapidly alternating with combination cisplatin and VP-16 in the treatment of small cell lung cancer, Am. J. Med. **79**:303, 1985.

28. National Consensus Conference on Tuberculosis: Preventive treatment of tuberculosis, Chest, **87**:128S, 1985.

29. National Consensus Conference of Tuberculosis: Public health issues in control of tuberculosis: surveillance techniques and the role of health care providers, Chest, **87**:135S, 1985.

30. National Consensus Conference on Tuberculosis: Standard therapy for tuberculosis, Chest, **87**:117S, 1985.

31. Obernauf, C.D., et al.: Sarcoidosis and its ophthalmic manifestations, Am. J. Ophthalmol. **86**:648, 1978.

32. Olsen, G.N., et al.: Pulmonary function evaluation of the lung resection candidate: a prospective study, Am. Rev. Respir. Dis. **111**:379, 1975.

33. Pak, C.C., et al.: Inhaled atropine sulfate:dose-response characteristics in adult patients with chronic airflow obstruction, Am. Rev. Resp. Dis. **125**(3): 331, 1984.

34. Perloff, M., Killen, J.Y., and Wittes, R.E.: Small cell bronchogenic carcinoma, Curr. Probl. Cancer, **10**(4):206, 1986.

35. Popovich, J., Jr.: The physiology of mechanical ventilation and the mechanical zoo: IPPB, PEEP, CPAP, Med. Clin. North Am. **67**(3):621, 1983.

36. Popovich, J., Jr.: Mechanical ventilation: keeping all systems "go," J. Respir. Dis. **6**(1):69, 1985.

37. Stibolt, T.B., Jr.: Asthma, Med. Clin. North Am. **70**(4): 909, 1986.

38. Studdy, P.R., Lapworth, R., and Bird, R.: Angiotensin-converting enzyme and its clinical significance, J. Clin. Pathol. **36**:938, 1983.

39. Wang, K.P., and Terry, P.B.: Transbronchial needle aspiration in the diagnosis and staging of bronchogenic carcinoma, Am. Rev. Resp. Dis. **127**:344, 1983.

40. West, J.W.: Pulmonary embolism, Med. Clin. North Am. **70**(4): 877, 1986.

41. Zelen, M.: Keynote address on biostatistics and data retrieval, Cancer Chemotherapy Rep. **4**(2):31, 1973.

Rheumatology

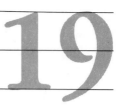

TEMPORAL ARTERITIS AND POLYMYALGIA RHEUMATICA[1]

Some authors consider temporal arteritis and polymyalgia rheumatica to be manifestations of the same disease, known as "giant cell arteritis."[6] Polymyalgia rheumatica occurs in 40%-60% of patients with temporal arteritis and the incidence of temporal arteritis in patients with polymyalgia rheumatica varies from 15%-78%.[18]

TEMPORAL ARTERITIS
Definition
Temporal arteritis is a systemic segmental granulomatous inflammation predominantly involving the arteries of the carotid system in patients over the age of 50. However, it can involve any large- and medium sized arteries.

Clinical manifestations
1. Headache, often associated with marked scalp tenderness
2. Tenderness, thickening, and nodulation of the temporal arteries
3. Constitutional symptoms (fever, weight loss, anorexia, fatigue)
4. Polymyalgia syndrome (aching and stiffness of the trunk and proximal muscle groups)
5. Visual disturbances (visual loss, blurred vision, amaurosis fugax)
6. Intermittent claudication of jaw and tongue upon mastication

Lab findings
1. Elevated ESR (usually >50 mm/h by the Westergren method); however, a normal ESR does not exclude the diagnosis[7]
2. Mild to moderate normochromic, normocytic anemia
3. Liver function test abnormalities (elevation of alkaline phosphatase is most common)

Diagnosis
The clinical diagnosis requires pathologic confirmation with multiple biopsies of the temporal artery. Overall reported sensitivity of temporal artery biopsy is 90.3%, specificity is 100%.[15] Pathologic confirmation is necessary because of significant toxicity associated with subsequent long-term steroid therapy.

Therapy

1. In stable patients without significant ocular involvement, therapy is usually started with prednisone 20-30 mg PO bid, continued for 4-6 weeks until symptoms resolve; the prednisone is gradually tapered over several months, the usual length of treatment is 6 months to 2 years[1]
2. In very ill patients and patients with significant ocular involvement (e.g., visual loss in one eye) rapid aggressive treatment with large doses of IV methylprednisolone is indicated to provide optimum protection to the uninvolved eye and offer any chance of visual recovery of the involved eye; the optimum dose of methylprednisolone ranges from 100 mg/day to 1000 mg q12h for 5 days[24]

POLYMYALGIA RHEUMATICA

Definition

Polymyalgia rheumatica (PMR) is a clinical syndrome predominantly involving individuals over the age of 50 and characterized by pain and stiffness involving mainly shoulder and hip girdle muscles.

Clinical manifestations

1. Symmetric polymyalgias and arthralgias involving back, shoulder, neck, and pelvic girdle muscles; duration of symptoms is generally longer than 1 month
2. Constitutional symptoms (fever, malaise, weight loss)
3. Symptoms of temporal arteritis (see above)
4. Symptoms are worse in the morning (difficulty getting out of bed)
5. Muscle strength is usually within normal limits

Lab findings

The lab findings for polymyalgia rheumatica are the same as for temporal arteritis.

Diagnosis

Diagnosis is based on clinical presentation and elevated ESR, although the latter is not essential for the diagnosis. There is controversy regarding the need for temporal artery biopsy in all patients with PMR. Proponents state that because of the high incidence of temporal arteritis (with associated risk of blindness), all patients who have an elevated ESR and aching muscles should undergo a temporal artery biopsy to rule out the presence of temporal arteritis. Opponents reason that biopsy is not indicated in patients without any signs or symptoms suggestive of cranial arteritis because the diagnostic yield is too low.

Treatment

1. Abolish symptoms
   a. Low-dose corticosteroids (e.g., prednisone 10-15 mg/day) will generally eliminate symptoms of PMR
   b. The dosage is then gradually tapered over several months based on repeated clinical observation
   c. In patients with mild symptoms NSAIDs may be used instead of corticosteroids

2. Monitor closely for possible development of temporal arteritis
    a. Instruct patient to immediately report any visual or neurologic symptoms
    b. As many as one third of patients with PMR can develop temporal arteritis within 1 year of onset of PMR[20]

19.2   SYSTEMIC LUPUS ERYTHEMATOSUS

Definition

Systemic lupus erythematosus (SLE) is a chronic multisystemic disease of unknown etiology, characterized by production of autoantibodies and protean clinical manifestations.

Clinical manifestations[23,25]

SLE generally affects women in the childbearing years and may present with any of the following manifestations:
1. Common cutaneous manifestations
    a. Butterfly rash: erythematous rash over the malar eminences, generally with sparing of the nasolabial folds
    b. Discoid lupus: raised erythematous patches with subsequent edematous plaques and adherent scales
    c. Symmetric erythematous lesions involving shoulders, chest, neck, and upper extremities
    d. Alopecia
    e. Raynaud's phenomenon
    f. Photosensitivity (particularly leg ulcerations)
    g. Nasal or oropharyngeal ulcerations
    h. Other: livedo reticularis, maculopapular eruptions, vasculitic ulcers
2. Joint disturbances: tenderness, swelling, or effusion generally involving peripheral joints
3. Renal disturbances: proteinuria, active renal sediment, renal insufficiency
4. Hematologic abnormalities: anemia (chronic disease, hemolysis), leukopenia, thrombotic events (secondary to lupus anticoagulant), immune thrombocytopenic purpura
5. Cardiac involvement: pericarditis, verrucous endocarditis (Libman-Sacks' endocarditis), myocarditis, coronary vasculitis, conduction abnormalities
6. Neurologic abnormalities: seizures, psychosis, depression, transverse myelitis, aseptic meningitis
7. Pulmonary involvement: pleural effusions, pleuritis, pulmonary infiltrates, vasculitis
8. GI manifestations: oral ulcers, abdominal pain, vomiting
9. Constitutional symptoms: fatigue, malaise, fever
10. Other: conjunctivitis, sicca syndrome

Lab diagnosis

1. Presence of anti-nuclear antibody (ANA): ANA is a generic term used to describe a variety of rheumatologic disorders. Distinctive profiles of ANA are associated with certain disorders. Antibodies to double-stranded DNA (anti-DNA) and to the Smith nuclear antigen (anti-Sm) are highly specific

Table 19-1 Anti-nuclear antibody

ANA Pattern	Corresponding Antibody	Found in
Rim and/or ho-mogeneous	Double-stranded DNA	SLE
Rim and/or ho-mogeneous	Double and single strand DNA	SLE and other rheu-matic diseases
Rim and/or ho-mogeneous	LE cell antibody	SLE drug induced LE
Homogeneous	Histones	Drug induced LE
Speckled	Sm (Smith)	SLE
Speckled	MA	SLE (severe)
Speckled	RNP	Mixed connective tissue disease
Atypical speckled	Sci-70 (Sci-1)	Scleroderma
Speckled	SS-B (La)	Sjogren's syndrome
Nucleolar	Nucleolar	Progressive systemic sclerosis

*Reproduced from Jacobs, D.S., Kasten, B.L., Jr., Dermott, W.R., and Wolffson, W.L.:
Laboratory test handbook with DRG index, St. Louis, 1984, Mosby/Lexi-Comp.

for SLE. Table 19-1 describes the ANA pattern and the corresponding antibody found in various rheumatologic disorders. ANA-negative SLE is very unusual; these patients generally have anti-SS-A and/or anti-SS-B antibodies.

2. Drug-induced lupus (DLE) can be caused by a variety of drugs (e.g., procainamide, hydralazine, isoniazid, hydantoins, quinidine, trimetha-dione). Its manifestations are similar to SLE. Distinguishing lab charac-teristics are:
   a. The virtual absence of anti-DNA and anti-Sm in DLE
   b. Higher frequency of antibodies to histones in patients with DLE
   NOTE: DLE does not have the same prognostic implications as SLE since it is reversible after discontinuation of the offending agent

3. Suggested initial lab evaluation of suspected SLE
   a. Immunologic evaluation: ANA, anti-DNA antibody, anti-Sm antibody
   b. Other lab tests: CBC with differential, platelet count, Coombs' test if anemia is detected, 24-hour urine collection for protein if proteinuria is detected, PTT in patients with thrombotic events, BUN, creatinine, urinalysis

4. Differentiation of DLE form SLE: general principles

Type of lupus	Immunologic tests	
	Anti-DNA Ab	**Anti-histone Ab**
DLE	(−)	(+)
SLE	(+)	(+)/(−)

Classification of SLE

The following list describes the 1982 revised criteria of the American Rheumatism Association for the classification of SLE.[27] A person is said to have systemic lupus erythematosus if any four or more of the 11 criteria are present, serially or simultaneously, during any interval of observation.

1. Butterfly rash
2. Discoid rash
3. Photosensitivity
4. Oral ulcers
5. Arthritis
6. Serositis
   a. Pleuritis
   b. Pericarditis
7. Renal disorder
   a. Persistent proteinuria greater than 0.5 g/day or greater than 3+ if quantitation not performed
   b. Cellular casts
8. Neurologic disorder
   a. Seizures (in the absence of offending drugs or known metabolic derangements)
   b. Psychosis (in the absence of offending drugs)
9. Hematologic disorder
   a. Hemolytic anemia with reticulocytosis
   b. Leukopenia (less than 4,000/mm^3 total on two or more occasions)
   c. Lymphopenia (less than 1,500/mm^3 on two or more occasions)
   d. Thrombocytopenia less than 100,000/mm^3 in the absence of offending drugs)
10. Immunologic disorder
    a. Positive LE cell preparation
    b. Anti-DNA (presence of antibody to native DNA in abnormal titer)
    c. Anti-Sm (presence of antibody to Sm nuclear antigen)
    d. False-positive STS known to be positive for at least 6 months and confirmed by TPI of FTA tests
11. Antinuclear antibody; an abnormal titer of antinuclear antibody by immunofluorescence or an equivalent assay at any point in time and in the absence of drugs known to be associated with ''drug-induced lupus'' syndrome

Treatment

Therapy of SLE should be individualized, based on the severity of the disease.

1. Joint pain and mild serositis is generally well controlled with nonsteroidal antiinflammatory drugs (NSAIDs)
2. Cutaneous manifestations are treated with
   a. Topical corticosteroids
   b. Antimalarials (e.g., hydroxychloroquinine [Plaquenil])
   c. Sunscreens that filter out ultraviolet B light
3. Renal disease
   a. Significant renal disease can be treated with corticosteroids, immunosuppressants (e.g., azathioprine [Imuran]), and alkylating agents (e.g.,

cyclophosphamide [Cytoxan]); recent studies have demonstrated that IV cyclophosphamide plus low dosages of prednisone result in better preservation of renal function than high dosages of prednisone alone[4]

b. Use of plasmapheresis in combination with immunosuppressive agents (to prevent rebound phenomenon of antibody levels after plasmapheresis) is an experimental therapy generally reserved for rapidly progressive renal failure or life-threatening systemic vasculitis

4. CNS involvement: treatment generally consists of corticosteroid therapy; anticonvulsants and antipsychotics are also indicated in selected cases

5. Hemolytic anemia: treatment of Coombs' positive hemolytic anemia consists of high doses of steroids; nonhemolytic anemia (secondary to chronic disease) does not require specific therapy

6. Thrombocytopenia
   a. Initial treatment consists of corticosteroids
   b. In patients with poor response to steroids encouraging results have been reported with the use of danazol[22]
   c. Splenectomy does not cure the thrombocytopenia of SLE[14]

Prognosis[3,5,12,29]

1. The leading cause of death in SLE is infection (one third of all deaths); active nephritis causes approximately 18% of deaths, and CNS disease 7% of deaths

2. The presence or absence of anti-Ro and anti-La antibodies is prognostically significant
   a. Presence of both anti-Ro and anti-La antibodies indicates decreased incidence of nephritis and anti-DNA antibodies
   b. Presence of anti-La antibody alone denotes absence of clinically apparent renal disease
   c. Presence of anti-Ro antibody alone is associated with increased incidence of nephritis and anti-DNA antibody

3. Renal histologic studies and evaluation of renal function are useful in predicting disease outcome in SLE (e.g., serum creatinine levels >3 mg/dl or evidence of diffuse proliferative involvement on renal biopsy are poor prognostic factors)

| 19.3 | RHEUMATOID ARTHRITIS |

Definition

Rheumatoid arthritis (RA) is a chronic systemic disorder characterized primarily by pain and inflammation in multiple joints.

Pathophysiology

The precise cause of RA is presently unknown. Current evidence shows that an undetermined stimulus (possibly an infectious agent) triggers an autoimmune response that through various mechanisms[9] results in destruction of cartilage and bone. There is evidence that the Epstein-Barr virus (EBV) may be involved in the pathogenesis of RA.[28] The role of genetic factors is unclear. It is known that the incidence of HLA-D_4 alloantigen occurs approximately four times more frequently in adult patients with RA than in the general population.[26]

Epidemiology and prognosis[31]

The incidence of RA is about 1% in the general population. Female to male ratio is approximately 3:1. Peak onset is between the ages of 20-45. The course of the disease is highly variable and characterized by exacerbations and remissions. Approximately 10% of patients will have severe destructive arthritis unresponsive to any therapeutic modalities, whereas 15% of all patients experience a complete remission. Latex positivity, persistently high ESR, and presence of subcutaneous nodules are generally associated with poorer prognosis.

Clinical manifestations[21]

The initial manifestations of RA are highly variable. In the majority of patients the onset is insidious, taking months or years to become clinically evident as a diagnosable entity. In other patients the onset is dramatic with rapid development of severe manifestations (see below). RA can present with any of the following articular and extraarticular manifestations:

1. Articular and periarticular manifestations
   a. Morning stiffness is often the initial complaint
   b. Symmetric polyarthritis
      (1) Joint swelling and tenderness to palpation, with significant limitation of motion of involved joints
      (2) Commonly involved joints in RA are metacarpophalangeal (MCP), metatarsophalangeal (MTP), proximal interphalangeal (PIP), wrist, knee, ankle, shoulder, and hip; however, any joint in the body can be affected
      (3) Joint deformities are generally secondary to hyperextension or flexion of the joints; for example:
         (a) Hyperextension of PIP joints and flexion of DIP joints (swan-neck deformity)
         (b) Flexion of PIP joints and extension of DIP joints (boutonniere deformity)
   c. Other: carpal tunnel syndrome, knee and ankle effusions, hoarseness secondary to cricoarytenoid arthritis
2. Extraarticular manifestations
   a. Pulmonary involvement consists of one or more of the following:
      (1) Pulmonary nodules; association of rheumatoid pulmonary nodules and interstitial pneumoconiosis is known as Caplan's syndrome
      (2) Pleural effusions
      (3) Pulmonary vasculitis
      (4) Pleuritis
   b. Ocular involvement: scleritis, episcleritis; RA is often associated with Sjögren's syndrome (characterized by dryness of eyes, mouth, and other mucous membranes secondary to lymphoplasmacytic infiltration of exocrine glands with destruction of mucus-generating glands)
   c. Vasculitis is generally seen in patients with elevated titers of rheumatoid factor (RF); it can involve any organ, and frequent manifestations are mononeuritis multiplex and digital arteritis
   d. Hematologic abnormalities
      (1) Normochromic, normocytic/microcytic anemia (multifactorial: chronic disease, blood loss secondary to salicylates and NSAIDs)

(2) Granulocytopenia; the presence of granulocytopenia and spleno-megaly in a patient with RA is known as Felty's syndrome[13]

(3) Hyperviscosity, cryoglobulinemia

  e. Cardiac involvement: pericarditis, conduction defects, myocarditis, arteritis

  f. Skin: subcutaneous nodules (caused by granulomatous inflammation of surrounding arteries) may be found over the olecranon process and any bony prominences

  g. Constitutional symptoms: fever, weight loss, anorexia, malaise

  h. Other: osteoporosis, myositis, compressive neuropathies, amyloidosis, mesangial glomerulonephrosis

Lab evaluation

There is no isolated lab test that can exclude or prove the diagnosis of RA. Any of the following lab abnormalities may be present:

1. Rheumatoid factor (RF): Latex positivity may be initially absent, but over the course of the disease approximately 85% of patients become latex positive; RF is not specific for RA and may be found in other conditions (e.g., osteomyelitis, SBE)

2. ESR: generally elevated during exacerbations

3. ANA: detected in approximately 15% of patients

4. Decreased hemoglobin/hematocrit, granulocytopenia

Arthrocentesis

See p. 67-71 for procedure and interpretation of results of arthrocentesis.

Radiographic evaluation

Initially, soft tissue swelling may be the only manifestation. As the disease progresses, there is periarticular osteopenia, cortical thinning, and marginal erosion. Subluxation and joint space diminution are late findings.

Diagnosis

RA is a clinical diagnosis. The 11 criteria of the American Rheumatism Association are described in the following list*:

1. Morning stiffness
2. Pain on motion or tenderness in at least one joint
3. Swelling in at least one joint
4. Swelling in at least one other joint
5. Symmetric joint swelling
6. Subcutaneous nodules
7. Radiographic changes typical of RA
8. Positive latex test (rheumatoid factor positive)
9. Poor mucin clot (inflammatory synovial fluid)
10. Characteristic histologic change in the synovial membrane
11. Characteristic histology of nodules

The presence of seven or more criteria indicates classic RA, the presence of five or six criteria denotes definite RA, and the presence of three or four

---

*From Ropes, M.W., Bennett, F.A., and Cobb, S.: 1958 revision of diagnostic criteria for rheumatoid arthritis, Arthritis Rheum. 2:16, 1959. Reproduced with permission.

criteria is associated with probable RA. The major value of the criteria lies not in diagnosing the individual patient but in epidemiologic and clinical research.

Treatment[10]

1. Improve the patient's quality of life with:
   a. Drug therapy to relieve pain and inflammation
   b. Active rehabilitation with adequate physical therapy programs
   c. Emotional support and social counseling
2. Arrest or retard the disease process with appropriate drug therapy
   a. Drug therapy of RA generally consists of a step-wise approach based on the severity of disease and clinical response
   b. There are two major categories of drugs:
      (1) Rapid acting: indicated for initial rapid relief of painful joint symptoms; examples are salicylates and NSAIDs
      (2) Remission-inducing agents
         (a) These agents are associated with significant toxicity
         (b) Their use is indicated in patients with severe, progressive disease
         (c) Examples are gold salts, penicillamine, and antimalarials
   c. Initial treatment of RA generally consists of high doses of salicylates (e.g., 3–6 g/day) or nonsteroidal antiinflammatory drugs (NSAIDs)
      (1) Frequent side effects of both consist of gastric irritation and GI bleeding
      (2) Patients responding poorly to salicylates or NSAIDs are generally treated with gold preparations; frequent complications of gold therapy are skin rashes and hematologic, pulmonary, and renal abnormalities
      (3) Penicillamine or antimalarials (e.g., hydroxychloraquinine) are generally used only after unsuccessful therapy with gold preparations
   d. Systemic corticosteroids are often used for brief periods in combination with slow-remitting agents to minimize symptoms in patients with significant disease but who need to continue full-time employment for socioeconomic reasons (e.g., head of household); intraarticular steroids are frequently used as adjunctive therapy to any of the previously described agents
   e. The use of cytotoxic agents is limited to severe, progressive disease unresponsive to the above measures; various studies have confirmed the effectiveness of methotrexate in the short-term treatment of refractory rheumatoid arthritis[2,30]
   f. The combined use of remittive agents is currently being evaluated in intractable rheumatoid arthritis[8]

| 19.4 |

OSTEOARTHRITIS (DEGENERATIVE JOINT DISEASE) [17,19]

Definition

Osteoarthritis is a common disease of the aging process, characterized pathologically by cartilage breakdown and bone remodeling and overgrowth. It can be primary (unrelated to other conditions) or secondary to various factors

(e.g., trauma, septic arthritis, inflammatory arthritis, congenital or developmental defects)

Clinical manifestations

Clinical manifestations are variable, depending on the joints involved and the stage of the disease. Onset is gradual with pain and stiffness of involved joints (generally more severe upon awakening in the morning or following a prolonged period of inactivity). Joints commonly involved are:

1. Hip: the patient generally complains of thigh or groin pain with motion or weight-bearing
2. Knee: significant restriction of movement, bony enlargement, and crepitation (with movement) may be present
3. Cervical spine: osteophyte formation along the margins of the vertebral bodies can result in cervical pain, headache, syncope (secondary to vertebral artery compression), and paresthesias of upper extremities (secondary to nerve compression); the areas most commonly involved are C4 to C6
4. Hands: osteoarthritis generally involves the DIP, PIP, and the carpometacarpal joints of the thumb; joint enlargement is known as Heberden's nodes for DIP joints and Bouchard's nodes for PIP joints

Lab evaluation

Generally noncontributory (normal ESR, negative ANA, absent RF, normal CBC)

Radiographic evaluation

Osteophytes may be detected in oblique views of the cervical spine in symptomatic patients; other involved joints may show thinning of joint space and subchondral bone sclerosis

Management

1. Relief of pain can be achieved with the following modalities:
   a. Medications
      (1) Salicylates or NSAIDs are generally used
      (2) Systemic corticosteroids are not indicated in osteoarthritis
      (3) Intraarticular injection of corticosteroids with local anesthetics is useful as adjunctive management of acutely inflamed joints refractory to other therapeutic modalities; frequent injections must be avoided (increased risk of steroid arthropathy)
   b. Local application of heat
   c. Periods of rest at selected times during the day
   d. Judicious exercise to maintain joint motion and muscle power; strenuous exercise or any activity which causes persistent pain should be avoided
   e. Weight reduction of painful joints with canes or crutches
   f. Surgical procedures may be necessary in patients with severe hip involvement or spinal nerve compression
2. Patient education and reassurance

ACUTE GOUTY ARTHRITIS[11,16]

Definition

Gout is a metabolic disease characterized by hyperuricemia and deposits of monosodium urate crystals in and about joints, with subsequent acute or chronic arthritis.

Epidemiology

Initial acute gouty arthritis occurs primarily in men aged 30-60. In women it usually occurs after menopause. Attacks can be precipitated by several factors (e.g., trauma, certain foods, ethanol intake, thiazide diuretics).

Clinical manifestations and diagnosis

1. The typical presentation is monoarticular and characterized by sudden severe pain involving the first metatarsophalangeal (MTP) joint (podagra), although the midtarsal and ankle are also frequently affected; acute asymmetric polyarthritis is uncommon
2. Physical exam reveals a warm, tender, swollen, erythematous joint; fever may be present, particularly if several joints are involved
3. Serum uric acid level is usually elevated, but may be normal (e.g., in patients taking antihyperuricemic agents)
4. Aspiration and analysis of synovial fluid from the inflamed joint confirms the diagnosis; examination of the fluid with a polarized light microscope with compensator reveals monosodium urate crystals (needle-shaped, strongly negative birefringent crystals) with synovial fluid leukocytes

Treatment of acute attack

Treatment options:
1. Colchicine can be given PO or IV; see Chapter 21 for dosages
2. Nonsteroidal antiinflammatory drugs (NSAIDs): indomethacin 50 mg q8h for 3-4 days, then gradually tapered off over approximately 1-2 weeks (depending on the patient's clinical response)
3. Glucocorticoids (IV): generally reserved for patients who cannot tolerate PO medication (e.g., postoperatively) and with contraindications to the use of IV colchicine
4. Corticotropin (IM): generally reserved for patients who cannot tolerate PO medication (e.g., postoperatively) and with contraindications to the use of IV colchicine

Prevention of recurrent attacks

Prevention is achieved through normalization of serum urate concentration with avoidance of foods high in purines (e.g., anchovies, sweet breads), alcohol, aspirin, and diuretics. Uricosuric agents (e.g., probenecid) or allopurinol are used in patients with recurrent attacks despite adequate dietary restrictions. However, hypouricemic therapy should not be started for at least 2 weeks after the acute attack has resolved because it may prolong the acute attack and can also precipitate new attacks by rapidly lowering the serum uric acid level. Colchicine 0.6 mg PO bid is indicated for acute gout prophylaxis before starting hypouricemic therapy. It is generally discontinued 6-8 weeks following normalization of serum urate levels.

References

1. Allen, N.B., Studenski, S.A.: Polymyalgia rheumatica and temporal arteritis, Med. Clin. North Am. **70**:369, 1986.
2. Andersen, P.A., et al.: Weekly pulse methotrexate in rheumatoid arthritis: clinical and immunologic effects in randomized, double-blind study, Ann. Intern. Med. **103**:489, 1985.
3. Austin, H.A., et al.: Prognostic factors in lupus nephritis: contribution of renal histologic data, Am. J. Med. **75**:382, 1983.
4. Austin, H.A., et al.: Therapy of lupus nephritis: controlled trial of prednisone and cytotoxic drugs, N. Engl. J. Med. **314**:614, 1986.
5. Ballou, SP, and Kushner, I.: Lupus patients who lack detectable anti-DNA: clinical features and survival, Arthritis Rheum. **25**:1126, 1982.
6. Bengtsson, B.A., and Malmvall, B.E.: The epidemiology of giant cell arteritis including temporal arteritis and polymyalgia rheumatica: incidences of different clinical presentations and eye complications, Arthritis Rheum. **24**:899, 1981.
7. Biller, J., et al.: Temporal arteritis associated with normal sedimentation rate, JAMA **247**:486, 1982.
8. Csuka, M., Carrera, G.F., and McCarthy, D.J.: Treatment of intractable rheumatoid arthritis with combined cyclophosphamide, asathioprine, and hydroxychloroquine: a follow-up study, JAMA **255**:2315, 255.
9. Decker, J.L., et al.: Rheumatoid arthritis: evolving concepts of pathogenesis and treatment, Ann. Intern. Med. **101**:810, 1984.
10. Dugowson, C.E., and Gilliland, B.C.: Management of rheumatoid arthritis, D.M. **32**(1):1, 1986.
11. German, D.C., and Holmes, E.W.: Hyperuricemia and gout, Med. Clin. North Am. **70**:419, 1986.
12. Ginzler, E.M., et al.: A multicenter study of outcome in systemic lupus erythematosus: entry variables as predictors of prognosis, Arthritis Rheum. **25**:601, 1982.
13. Goldberg, J., and Pinals, R.S.: Felty's syndrome, Semin. Arthritis Rheum. **10**:52, 1980.
14. Hall, S., et al.: Splenectomy does not cure the thrombocytopenia of systemic lupus erythematosus, Ann. Intern. Med. **102**:325, 1985.
15. Hedges, T.R., III, Gieger, G.L., and Albert, D.M.: The clinical value of negative temporal artery biopsy specimens, Arch. Ophthalmol. **101**:1251, 1983.
16. Holmes, E.W.: Clinical gout and the pathogenesis of hyperuricemia. In McCarthy, D.J. (editor): Arthritis and allied conditions, ed. 10, Philadelphia, 1985, Lee and Febiger.
17. Howell, D.S., Pita, J.C., and Woessner, J.F., Jr.: Discussion: which comes first—crystals, necrosis, or inflammation? J. Rheumatol. **10**(suppl 9):59, 1983.
18. Hunder, G.G., Rygvold, O., and Oystese, B.: Giant cell arteritis: a review, Bull. Rheum. Dis. **29**:980, 1978-1979.
19. Huskisson, E.C.: The drug treatment of osteoarthritis, Scand. J. Rheumatol. **43**(suppl):57, 1982.
20. Jones, J.G., and Hazelman, B.L.: Prognosis and management of polymyalgia rheumatica, Ann. Rheum. Dis. **40**:1, 1981.
21. Krane, S.M., and Simon, L.S.: Rheumatoid arthritis: clinical features and pathogenetic mechanisms, Med. Clin. North Am. **70**:263, 1986.
22. Marino, C., and Cook, P.: Danazol for lupus thrombocytopenia, Arch. Intern. Med. **145**:2251, 1985.
23. Pisetsky, D.S.: Systemic lupus erythematosus, Med. Clin. North Am. **70**:337, 1986.
24. Rosenfeld, S.I., et al.: Treatment of temporal arteritis with ocular involvement, Am. J. Med. **80**:143, 1986.
25. Rothfield, N.F.: Systemic lupus erythematosus: clinical aspects and treatment. In McCarthy, D.J., (editor): Arthritis and allied conditions, Philadelphia, 1985, Lea & Febiger.

26. Stastny, P.: Association of the B-cell alloantigen DRw$_4$ with rheumatoid arthritis, N. Engl. J. Med. **298:** 869, 1978.

27. Tan, E.M., et al.: The 1982 revised criteria for the classification of systemic lupus erythematosus, Arthritis Rheum. **25:**1271, 1982.

28. The viral etiology of rheumatoid arthritis, Lancet, **1:**772, 1984.

29. Wasicek, C.A., and Reichlin, M.: Clinical and serological differences between systemic lupus erythematosus patients with antibodies to Ro versus patients with antibodies to Ro and La, J. Clin. Invest. **69:**835, 1982.

30. Weinstein, A., et al.: Low-dose methotrexate treatment of rheumatoid arthritis, Am. J. Med. **79:**331, 1985.

31. Zwaifler, N.S.: Rheumatoid arthritis: a clinical perspective. In Lawrence, R.C., and Shulman, L.E., (editors): Current topics in rheumatology: epidemiology of the rheumatic diseases, New York, 1984, Gower Medical Publishing Ltd.

20 Laboratory Values and Interpretations of Results

This chapter covers over 150 of the most common laboratory tests. Each test is approached with the following format:

1. Laboratory test
2. Normal range in adult patients
3. Common abnormalities, such as positive test, increased or decreased value
4. Causes of abnormal result

The normal ranges may differ slightly, depending on the laboratory. The reader should be aware of the "normal range" of the particular laboratory performing the test. Every attempt has been made to present current laboratory test data with emphasis on practical considerations.

ACETONE (Serum or plasma)

Normal:
  Negative
Elevated in:
  Diabetic ketoacidosis, starvation, isopropanol ingestion

ACE LEVEL See ANGIOTENSIN CONVERTING ENZYME

ACID PHOSPHATASE (Serum)

Normal range:
  Male: 0.26-0.82 IU/L
  Female: 0.23-0.70 IU/L
Elevated in:
  Carcinoma of prostate, other neoplasms (breast, bone), Paget's disease, osteogenesis imperfecta, malignant invasion of bone, Gaucher's disease, multiple myeloma, myeloproliferative disorders, benign prostatic hypertrophy, prostatic palpation or surgery, hyperparathyroidism, liver disease, chronic renal failure

ACID SERUM TEST See HAM TEST

ALBUMIN (Serum)

Normal range:
  3.5-4.7 g/dl albumin/globulin ratio >1.0
Elevated in:
  Dehydration

Decreased in:
>   Liver disease, nephrotic syndrome, poor nutritional status, rapid IV hydration, protein-losing enteropathies (inflammatory bowel disease), severe burns, neoplasia, chronic inflammatory diseases, pregnancy, oral contraceptives, prolonged immobilization

ALDOLASE (Serum)

Normal range:
>   2-8 units/dl (Sibley-Lehninger)

Elevated in:
>   Muscular dystrophy, rhabdomyolysis, dermatomyositis/polymyositis, trichinosis, acute hepatitis and other liver diseases, MI, prostatic carcinoma, hemorrhagic pancreatitis, gangrene, delirium tremens

Decreased in:
>   Decreased muscle mass, late stages of muscular dystrophy

ALKALINE PHOSPHATASE (Serum)

Normal range:
>   25-70 IU/L

Elevated in:
>   Biliary obstruction, cirrhosis (particularly primary biliary cirrhosis), liver disease (hepatitis, infiltrative liver diseases, fatty metamorphosis), Paget's disease of bone, osteitis deformans, rickets, osteomalacia, hypervitaminosis D, hyperparathyroidism, hyperthyroidism, ulcerative colitis, bowel perforation, bone metastases, healing fractures, bone neoplasms, acromegaly, infectious mononucleosis, CMV infections, sepsis, pulmonary infarction, CHF, hypernephroma, leukemia, myelofibrosis, multiple myeloma, drugs (estrogens, albumin, erythromycin and other antibiotics, cholestasis-producing drugs [phenothiazines])

Decreased in:
>   Hypothyroidism, pernicious anemia, hypophosphatasia, hypervitaminosis D, malnutrition

ALPHA-1-FETOPROTEIN (Serum) See A-1-FETOPROTEIN

ALT See SERUM GLUTAMIC PYRUVATE TRANSANIMASE (SGPT)

AMMONIA (Serum)

Normal range:
>   11-35 mmol/L

Elevated in:
>   Hepatic failure, hepatic encephalopathy, Reye's syndrome, portacaval shunt, drugs (diuretics, polymyxin B, methicillin)

Decreased in:
>   Drugs (neomycin, lactulose, tetracycline), renal failure

AMYLASE (Serum)

Normal range:
>   80-160 Somogyi units/dl

Elevated in:
   Acute pancreatitis, pancreatic neoplasm, abscess, pseudocyst, ascites, macroamylasemia, perforated peptic ulcer, intestinal obstruction, intestinal infarction, acute cholecystitis, appendicitis, ruptured ectopic pregnancy, salivary gland inflammation, peritonitis, burns, diabetic ketoacidosis, renal insufficiency, drugs (morphine), carcinomatosis of lung, esophagus, ovary
Decreased in:
   Advanced chronic pancreatitis, hepatic necrosis

AMYLASE, URINE See **URINE AMYLASE**

ANA See **ANTINUCLEAR ANTIBODY**

ANGIOTENSIN CONVERTING ENZYME (ACE level)

Normal range:
   0-57 units/L
Elevated in:
   Sarcoidosis, primary biliary cirrhosis, alcoholic liver disease, hyperthyroidism, hyperparathyroidism, diabetes mellitus, amyloidosis, multiple myeloma, lung disease (asbestosis, silicosis, berylliosis, allergic alveolitis, coccidioidomycosis), Gaucher's disease, leprosy

ANION GAP

Normal range:
   8-16 mEq/L
Elevated in:
   Lactic acidosis
   Ketoacidosis (diabetic ketoacidosis, alcoholic starvation)
   Uremia (chronic renal failure)
   Ingestion of toxins (paraldehyde, methanol, salicylates, ethylene glycol)

ANTICOAGULANT See **CIRCULATING ANTICOAGULANT**

ANTI-DNA

Normal range:
   Absent
Present in:
   SLE, chronic active hepatitis, infectious mononucleosis, biliary cirrhosis

ANTIGLOMERULAR BASEMENT ANTIBODY See **GLOMERULO BASEMENT MEMBRANE ANTIBODY**

ANTIMITOCHONDRIAL ANTIBODY

Normal range:
   1:20 titer
Elevated in:
   Primary biliary cirrhosis (85%-95%), chronic active hepatitis (25%-30%), cryptogenic cirrhosis (25%-30%)

ANTINUCLEAR ANTIBODY (ANA)

Normal range:
   <1:20 titer
Positive test:
   SLE (more significant if titer >1:160), drugs (phenytoin, ethosuximide, primidone, methyldopa, hydralazine, carbamazepine, penicillin, procainamide, chlorpromazine, griseofulvin, thiazides), chronic active hepatitis, age over 60 (particularly age over 80), rheumatoid arthritis, scleroderma, mixed connective tissue disease, necrotizing vasculitis, Sjogren's syndrome, tuberculosis, pulmonary interstitial fibrosis

ANTI-RNP ANTIBODY See EXTRACTABLE NUCLEAR ANTIGEN

ANTI-Sm (Anti-Smith) ANTIBODY See EXTRACTABLE NUCLEAR ANTIGEN

ANTI-SMOOTH MUSCLE ANTIBODY See SMOOTH MUSCLE ANTIBODY

ANTI-STREPTOLYSIN-O-TITER (STREPTOZYME, ASLO titer)

Normal range for adults:
   <160 Todd units
Elevated in:
   Streptococcal upper airway infection, acute rheumatic fever, acute glomerulonephritis, increased levels of β-lipoprotein
   NOTE: A fourfold increase in titer between acute and convalescent specimens is diagnostic of streptococcal upper airway infection regardless of the initial titer

ANTITHROMBIN III

Normal range:
   81%-120% of normal activity; 17-30 mg/dl
Decreased in:
   Hereditary deficiency of antithrombin III, DIC, pulmonary embolism, cirrhosis, thrombolytic therapy, chronic liver failure, post-surgery, third trimester of pregnancy, oral contraceptives, nephrotic syndrome, IV heparin >3 days, sepsis
Elevated in:
   Warfarin drugs, post-MI

ARTERIAL BLOOD GASES

Normal range:
   PO_2: 75-100 mm Hg
   PCO_2: 35-45 mm Hg
   HCO_3: 24-28 mEq/L
   PH: 7.35-7.45
Abnormal values:
   Refer to Chapter 8

ASLO TITER See ANTI-STREPTOLYSIN-O-TITER

AST See SERUM GLUTAMIC OXALOACETIC TRANSAMINASE (SGOT)

BASOPHIL COUNT
Normal range:
  0.4%-1% of total white blood count; 40-100 mm^3
Elevated in:
  Leukemia, inflammatory processes, polycythemia vera, Hodgkin's lymphoma, hemolytic anemia, after splenectomy, myeloid metaplasia
Decreased in:
  Stress, hypersensitivity reaction, steroids, pregnancy, hyperthyroidism

BILE, URINE See URINE, BILE

BILIRUBIN, DIRECT (Conjugated bilirubin)
Normal range:
  0-0.5 mg/dl
Elevated in:
  Hepatocellular disease, biliary obstruction, drug-induced cholestasis, hereditary disorders (Dubin-Johnson's syndrome, Rotor's syndrome)

BILIRUBIN, INDIRECT (Unconjugated bilirubin)
Normal range:
  0-1.0 mg/dl
Elevated in:
  Hemolysis, liver disease (hepatitis, cirrhosis, neoplasm), hepatic congestion secondary to congestive heart failure, hereditary disorders (Gilbert's disease, Crigler-Najjar's syndrome)

BILIRUBIN, TOTAL
Normal range:
  0-1.0 mg/dl
Elevated in:
  Liver disease (hepatitis, cirrhosis, cholangitis, neoplasm, biliary obstruction, infectious mononucleosis), hereditary disorders (Gilbert's disease, Dubin-Johnson's syndrome), drugs (steroids, diphenylhydantoin, phenothiazines, penicillin, erythromycin, clindamycin, captopril, amphotericin B, sulfonamides, azathioprine, isoniazid, 5-aminosalicylic acid, allopurinol, methyldopa, indomethacin, halothane, oral contraceptives, procainamide, tolbutamide), hemolysis, pulmonary embolism or infarct, hepatic congestion secondary to CHF

BILIRUBIN, URINE See URINE, BILE

BLEEDING TIME (Modified Ivy Method—Mielke)
Normal range:
2 to 9½ min
Elevated in:
Thrombocytopenia, capillary wall abnormalities, platelet abnormalities (Von Willebrand's, Bernard-Soulier's, Glanzmann's), drugs (aspirin, warfarin, antiinflammatory medications, streptokinase, urokinase, dextran, β lactam antibiotics, moxalactam)

BUN See **UREA NITROGEN**

C3 See **COMPLEMENT C3**

C4 See **COMPLEMENT C4**

CALCITONIN (Serum)
Normal range:
Less than 150 pg/ml
Elevated in:
Medullary carcinoma of the thyroid (particularly if level >1500 pg/ml), carcinoma of the breast, APUDOMAS, carcinoids, renal failure, thyroiditis

CALCIUM (Serum)
Normal range:
8.6-10.6 mg/dl
Abnormal values:
Refer to Chapter 12, section 12.10

CALCIUM, URINE See **URINE, CALCIUM**

CARBON MONOXIDE See **CARBOXYHEMOGLOBIN**

CARBOXYHEMOGLOBIN
Normal range:
Saturation of hemoglobin <2%, smokers <9% (coma: 50%; death: 80%)
Elevated in:
Smoking, exposure to smoking, exposure to automobile exhaust fumes, malfunctioning gas-burning appliances

CARCINOEMBRYONIC ANTIGEN (CEA)
Normal range:
Nonsmokers <2.5 ng/ml, smokers <5 ng/ml
Elevated in:
Colorectal carcinomas, pancreatic carcinomas, and metastatic disease usually produce higher elevations (>20 ng/ml)
Carcinomas of the esophagus, stomach, small intestine, liver, breast, ovary, lung and thyroid usually produce lesser elevations
Benign conditions (smoking, inflammatory bowel disease, hypothyroidism, cirrhosis, pancreatitis, infections) usually produce levels <10 ng/ml

CAROTENE (Serum)

Normal range:
  50-200 µg/dl
Elevated in:
  Carotenemia, chronic nephritis, diabetes mellitus, hypothyroidism, nephrotic syndrome
Decreased in:
  Fat malabsorption, steatorrhea, pancreatic insufficiency, lack of carotenoids in diet

CATECHOLAMINES, URINE See URINE CATECHOLAMINES

CBC See COMPLETE BLOOD COUNT

CEA See CARCINOEMBRYONIC ANTIGEN

CEREBROSPINAL FLUID (CSF)

Normal range:
  Appearance: clear
  Glucose: 50-80 mg/dl
  Protein: 20-45 mg/dl
  Chloride: 118-132 mEq/L
  Pressure: 100-200 mm H_2O
  Cell count (cells/mm^3) and cell type: <6 lymphocytes, no polymorphonucleocytes
  NOTE: Refer to Chapter 9, section 9.1 for interpretation of abnormalities

CERULOPLASMIN (Serum)

Normal range:
  23-50 mg/dl
Elevated in:
  Pregnancy, estrogens, oral contraceptives, neoplastic diseases (leukemias, Hodgkin's lymphoma, carcinomas), inflammatory states, SLE, primary biliary cirrhosis, rheumatoid arthritis
Decreased in:
  Wilson's disease (values often <10 mg/dl), nephrotic syndrome, advanced liver disease, malabsorption, total parenteral nutrition, Menkes' syndrome

CHLORIDE (Serum)

Normal range:
  98-108 mEq/L
Elevated in:
  Dehydration, excessive infusion of normal saline
  Hyperparathyroidism, renal disease, metabolic acidosis
  Drugs (ammonium chloride administration, acetazolamide, boric acid, triamterene)
Decreased in:
  CHF, SIADH, Addison's disease, vomiting, gastric suction, salt-losing nephritis, continuous infusion of 5% dextrose, diuretic administration, diaphoresis, diarrhea, burns

CHLORIDE, URINE See URINE, CHLORIDE

CHOLESTEROL, TOTAL

Normal range:
120-240 mg/dl (varies with age)
Elevated in:
Primary hypercholesterolemia, biliary obstruction, diabetes mellitus, nephrotic syndrome, hypothyroidism, primary biliary cirrhosis, high cholesterol diet, third trimester of pregnancy, MI, drugs (steroids, phenothiazines, oral contraceptives)
Decreased in:
Starvation, malabsorption, sideroblastic anemia, thalassemia, abetalipoproteinemia, hyperthyroidism, Cushing's syndrome, hepatic failure, multiple myeloma, polycythemia vera, chronic myelocytic leukemia, myeloid metaplasia, Waldenstrom's macroglobulinemia, myelofibrosis

CHOLESTEROL, LOW-DENSITY LIPOPROTEIN See LOW-DENSITY LIPOPROTEIN CHOLESTEROL

CHOLESTEROL, HIGH-DENSITY LIPOPROTEIN See HIGH-DENSITY LIPOPROTEIN CHOLESTEROL

CIRCULATING ANTICOAGULANT (Lupus anticoagulant)

Normal:
Negative
Detected in:
SLE, drug-induced lupus, long-term phenothiazine therapy, multiple myeloma, ulcerative colitis, rheumatoid arthritis, postpartum, hemophilia, neoplasms, chronic inflammatory states

CK See CREATINE KINASE

CO See CARBOXYHEMOGLOBIN

COAGULATION FACTORS

Factor—Reference range
V: $>10\%$
VII: $>10\%$
VIII: 50%-170%
IX: 60%-136%
X: $>10\%$
XI: 50%-150%
XII: $>30\%$

COLD AGGLUTININS TITER

Normal range:
   <1:32

Elevated in:
   Primary atypical pneumonia (mycoplasma pneumonia), infectious mononucleosis, CMV infection

   Other: hepatic cirrhosis, acquired hemolytic anemia, frostbite, multiple myeloma, lymphoma, malaria

COMPLEMENT, C3 (Serum)

Normal range:
   83-177 mg/dl

Elevated in:
   Rheumatoid arthritis, neoplasms (GI tract, lungs, cervix, prostate), rheumatic fever, early SLE (acute phase reactant)

Decreased in:
   SLE, membranoproliferative and poststreptococcal infection glomerulonephritis, chronic active hepatitis, DIC (hemolytic-uremic syndrome), hereditary C3 deficiency, celiac disease, anorexia nervosa, bacterial endocarditis (subacute), chronic liver disease, gram-negative sepsis, fungemia, cryoglobulinemia

COMPLEMENT, C4 (Serum)

Normal range:
   15-45 mg/dl

Elevated in:
   Neoplasms (GI tract, lung, cervix, breast), juvenile rheumatoid arthritis, rheumatoid spondylitis, (acute phase reactant)

Decreased in:
   SLE, glomerulonephritis, chronic active hepatitis, hereditary angioneurotic edema, hereditary deficiency, hepatic cirrhosis, malaria, cryoglobulinemia

COMPLETE BLOOD COUNT (CBC)

   White blood count: $4.8\text{-}10.8 \times 10^3/\mu l$
   Red blood count:
      Male: $4.6\text{-}6.2 \times 10^6/\mu l$
      Female: $4.2\text{-}5.4 \times 10^6/\mu l$
   Hemoglobin:
      Male: 14-18 g/dl
      Female: 12-16 g/dl
   Hematocrit:
      Male: 42%-52%
      Female: 37%-47%
   MCV:
      Male: 80-94
      Female: 79-97
   MCH: 27-31 picogram/cell
   MCHC: 32-36 g/dl
   RDW: 11.5%-14.5%

Platelet count: 140,000-440,000/µl
Differential:
  2-6 stabs (bands, early mature neutrophils)
  60-70 segs (mature neutrophils)
  1-4 eosinophils
  0-1 basophils
  2-8 monocytes
  25-40 lymphocytes

CONJUGATED BILIRUBIN See BILIRUBIN, DIRECT

COOMBS' DIRECT

Normal:
  Negative
Positive:
  Autoimmune hemolytic anemia, erythroblastosis fetalis, transfusion re-
  actions, drugs (α-methyldopa, penicillins, tetracycline, sulfonamides,
  levodopa, cephalosporins, quinidine, insulin)
False positive:
  May be seen with cold agglutinins

COOMBS' INDIRECT

Normal:
  Negative
Positive:
  Acquired hemolytic anemia, incompatible cross-matched blood, anti-Rh
  antibodies, drugs (methyldopa, mefenamic acid, levodopa)

CPK See CREATINE KINASE

COPPER (Serum)

Normal range:
  0.75-1.5 µg/ml
Decreased in:
  Wilson's disease, Menkes' syndrome, malabsorption, malnutrition, nephrosis, TPN

COPPER, URINE See URINE, COPPER

CORTISOL (Plasma)

Normal range:
  Varies with time of collection (circadian variation):
    AM (8-10 AM) 5-25 µg/dl
    PM (4-6 PM) 2-9 µg/dl
Elevated in:
  Ectopic ACTH production (i.e., oat cell carcinoma of lung), loss of nor-
  mal diurnal variation
  Iatrogenic, stress, adrenal or pituitary hyperplasia or adenomas
Decreased in:
  Primary adrenocortical insufficiency, anterior pituitary hypofunction, sec-
  ondary adrenocortical insufficiency, adrenogenital syndromes

C-REACTIVE PROTEIN

Normal range:
 <8 μg/ml
Elevated in:
 Rheumatoid arthritis, rheumatic fever, inflammatory bowel disease, bacterial infections, MI, oral contraceptives, third trimester of pregnancy (acute phase reactant)

CREATINE KINASE (CK, CPK)

Normal range:
 Male: 0-85 IU/L
 Female: 0-50 IU/L
Elevated in:
 MI, myocarditis, rhabdomyolysis, myositis, crush injury/trauma, polymyositis, dermatomyositis, vigorous exercise, muscular dystrophy, myxedema, seizures, malignant hyperthermia syndrome, IM injections, CVA, pulmonary embolism and infarction
Decreased in:
 Steroids, decreased muscle mass, connective tissue disorders, alcoholic liver disease, metastatic neoplasms

CREATINE KINASE ISOENZYMES

 CK-MB
 Elevated in: MI, myocarditis, pericarditis, muscular dystrophy, cardiac defibrillation, cardiac surgery, extensive rhabdomyolysis, strenuous exercise (marathon runners), mixed connective tissue disease, cardiomyopathy
 CK-MM
 Elevated in: crush injury, seizures, malignant hyperthermia syndrome, rhabdomyolysis, myositis, polymyositis, dermatomyositis, vigorous exercise, muscular dystrophy, IM injections
 CK-BB
 Elevated in: CVA, subarachnoid hemorrhage, neoplasms (prostate, GI tract, brain, ovary, breast, lung) severe shock, bowel infarction, hypothermia

CREATININE (Serum)

Normal range:
 Male: 0.3-1.3 mg/dl
 Female: 0.7-1.1 mg/dl
Elevated in:
 Renal insufficiency (acute and chronic), decreased renal perfusion (hypotension, dehydration, CHF), urinary tract infection, rhabdomyolysis, ketonemia
 Drugs (antibiotics [aminoglycosides, cephalosporins], hydantoin, diuretics, methyldopa)
Falsely elevated in:
 Diabetic ketoacidosis, administration of some cephalosporins (e.g., cefoxitin, cephalothin)

Decreased in:
    Decreased muscle mass (including amputees and older persons), pregnancy, prolonged debilitation

CREATININE CLEARANCE

Normal range:
    70-157 ml/min
Elevated in:
    Pregnancy, exercise
Decreased in:
    Renal insufficiency, drugs (cimetidine, procainamide, antibiotics, quinidine)

CREATININE, URINE See URINE CREATININE

CRYOGLOBULINS (Serum)

Normal range:
    Not detectable
Present in:
    Collagen-vascular diseases, CLL, hemolytic anemias, multiple myeloma, Waldenstrom's macroglobulinemia, chronic active hepatitis, Hodgkin's disease

CSF See CEREBROSPINAL FLUID

ELECTROLYTES (Serum)

    Sodium: 134-144 mEq/L
    Potassium: 3.3-4.9 mEq/L
    Bicarbonate: 23-31 mEq/L
    Chloride: 98-108 mEq/L
    For interpretation of abnormal values refer to individual electrolytes and to Chapters 8 and 16

ELECTROLYTES, URINE See URINE, ELECTROLYTES

ELECTROPHORESIS, HEMOGLOBIN See HEMOGLOBIN ELECTROPHORESIS

ELECTROPHORESIS, PROTEIN See PROTEIN ELECTROPHORESIS

ENA-COMPLEX See EXTRACTABLE NUCLEAR ANTIGEN

EOSINOPHIL COUNT

Normal range:
    1%-4% eosinophils (0-440/mm^3)
Elevated in:
    Allergy, parasitic infestations (trichinosis, aspergillosis, hydatidosis), angioneurotic edema, drug reactions, warfarin sensitivity, collagen-vascular diseases, acute hypereosinophilic syndrome, eosinophilic nonallergic rhinitis, myeloproliferative disorders, Hodgkin's lymphoma, radiation therapy

ERYTHROCYTE SEDIMENTATION RATE (Westergren)

Normal range:
  Male: 0-15 mm/hr
  Female: 0-20 mm/hr
Elevated in:
  Collagen-vascular diseases, infections, MI, neoplasms, inflammatory
  states (acute phase reactant)

EXTRACTABLE NUCLEAR ANTIGEN (ENA complex, Anti-RNP antibody, Anti-Sm, Anti-Smith)

Normal:
  Negative
Present in:
  SLE, rheumatoid arthritis, Sjogren's syndrome, MCTD

FDP See FIBRIN DEGRADATION PRODUCTS

FECAL FAT, QUANTITATIVE, (72-hour collection)

Normal range:
  2-7 g/24 hrs
Elevated in:
  Malabsorption syndrome (refer to Chapter 13, section 13.5)

FERRITIN (Serum)

Normal range:
  Male: 35-260 ng/ml for all ages
  Female: (age 18-45) 10-65 ng/ml; (over 45) 25-155 ng/ml
Elevated in:
  Hyperthyroidism, inflammatory states, liver disease (ferritin elevated
  from necrotic hepatocytes), neoplasms (neuroblastomas, lymphomas,
  leukemia, breast carcinoma), iron replacement therapy, hemochroma-
  tosis
Decreased in:
  Iron deficiency anemia

α-1 FETOPROTEIN

Normal range:
  <25 ng/ml
Elevated in:
  Hepatocellular carcinoma (usually values >1000 ng/ml), germinal neoplasms (testis, ovary, mediastinum, retroperitoneum), liver disease (alcoholic cirrhosis, acute hepatitis, chronic active hepatitis), fetal anen-
  cephaly, spina bifida

FIBRIN DEGRADATION PRODUCTS (FDP)

Normal Range:
   <10 µg/ml
Elevated in:
   DIC, primary fibrinolysis, pulmonary embolism, severe liver disease
   NOTE: The presence of rheumatoid factor may cause falsely elevated FDP

FIBRINOGEN

Normal range:
   200-400 mg/dl
Elevated in:
   Tissue inflammation/damage (acute-phase protein reactant), oral contraceptives, pregnancy
Decreased in:
   DIC, hereditary afibrinogenemia, liver disease, primary or secondary fibrinolysis

FLUORESCENT TREPONEMAL ANTIBODY See FTA-ABS

FOLATE (FOLIC ACID)

Normal range:
   Plasma: 1.7-12.6 mg/ml
   Red cell: 153-602 mg/ml
Decreased in:
   Folic acid deficiency (inadequate intake, malabsorption), alcoholism, drugs (methotrexate, trimethoprim, phenytoin, oral contraceptives, azulfadine), vitamin B_{12} deficiency (defective red cell folate absorption)

FREE T_4 See T_4, FREE

FREE THYROXINE INDEX

Normal range:
   1.1-4.3
   (Refer to Chapter 12, section 12.9 for interpretation of abnormal values)

FTA-ABS (Serum)

Normal:
   Nonreactive
Reactive in:
   Syphilis, other treponemal diseases (yaws, pinta, bejel)

GAMMA-GLUTAMYL TRANSFERASE (GGTP) See γ-GLUTAMYL TRANSFERASE (GGTP)

GASTRIN (Serum)

Normal range:
40-200 pg/ml
Elevated in:
Zollinger-Ellison syndrome (gastrinoma), pernicious anemia, hyperparathyroidism, retained gastric antrum, chronic renal failure, gastric ulcer, chronic atrophic gastritis, pyloric obstruction, malignant neoplasms of the stomach, H_2 blockers

GLOMERULAR BASEMENT MEMBRANE ANTIBODY

Normal:
Negative
Present in:
Goodpasture's syndrome

GLUCOSE, FASTING

Normal range:
60-115 mg/dl
Elevated in:
Diabetes mellitus, stress, infections, MI, CVA, Cushing's syndrome, acromegaly, acute pancreatitis, glucagonoma, hemochromatosis, drugs (glucocorticoids, diuretics [thiazides, loop diuretics])
Decreased:
See Chapter 12, section 12.4

GLUCOSE 6-PHOSPHATE DEHYDROGENASE SCREEN (Blood)

Normal:
G-6-PD enzyme activity is detected
Abnormal:
If a deficiency is detected, quantitation of G-6-PD is necessary. A G-6-PD screen may be falsely interpreted as ''normal'' after an episode of hemolysis because most G-6-PD deficient cells have been destroyed.

GLUCOSE, POSTPRANDIAL

Normal range:
Age 0-50 yr–70-140 mg/dl
50-60 yr–70-150 mg/dl
60+ yr–70-160 mg/dl
Elevated in:
Diabetes mellitus, glucose intolerance
Decreased in:
Post-gastrointestinal resection, reactive hypoglycemia, hereditary fructose intolerance, galactosemia, leucine sensitivity

GLUCOSE TOLERANCE TEST

Elevated in:

Glucose intolerance, diabetes mellitus, Cushing's syndrome, acromegaly, pheochromocytoma

Gestational diabetes—two or more of the following results: FBS >105, one hour >190, 2 hours >165, 3 hours >145 mg/dl

Adult onset diabetes: FBS >140 more than once; or 2 hours >200, plus one or more of the following results: 30 minutes >200, 1 hour >200, 90 minutes >200

γ-GLUTAMYL TRANSFERASE (GGTP)

Normal range:

Male: 10-38 IU/L

Female: 5-25 IU/L

Elevated in:

Chronic alcoholic liver disease, neoplasms (hepatoma, metastatic disease to the liver, carcinoma of the pancreas), SLE, CHF, trauma, nephrotic syndrome, sepsis, cholestasis, drugs (phenytoin, barbiturates)

GLYCOSYLATED HEMOGLOBIN (HbA$_{1c}$)

Normal range:

4.0%-6.7%

Elevated in:

Uncontrolled diabetes mellitus (glycosylated hemoglobin levels reflect the level of glucose control over the preceding 120 days)

Decreased in:

Hemolytic anemias, decreased RBC survival, pregnancy, chronic blood loss, chronic renal failure, insulinoma

HAM TEST (Acid serum test)

Normal:

Negative

Positive in:

Paroxysmal nocturnal hemoglobinuria (PNH)

False positive in:

Hereditary or acquired spherocytosis, recent transfusion with aged RBC, aplastic anemia, myeloproliferative syndromes, leukemia, hereditary dyserythropoietic anemia type II (HEMPAS)

HAPTOGLOBIN (Serum)

Normal range:

27-134 mg/dl

Elevated in:

Inflammation (acute phase reactant), collagen-vascular diseases, infections (acute phase reactant), drugs (androgens)

Decreased in:

Hemolysis (intravascular > extravascular), megaloblastic anemia, severe liver disease, large tissue hematomas, infectious mononucleosis, drugs (oral contraceptives)

HEMATOCRIT

Normal range:
    Male: 42%-52%
    Female: 37%-47%
Elevated in:
    Polycythemia vera, smoking, COPD, high altitudes, dehydration, hypovolemia
Decreased in:
    Blood loss (GI, GU), anemia (refer to Chapter 14, sections 14.1-14.3), pregnancy

HEMOGLOBIN

Normal range:
    Male: 14-18 g/dl
    Female: 12-16 g/dl
Elevated in:
    Hemoconcentration, dehydration, polycythemia vera, COPD, high altitudes, false elevations (hyperlipemic plasma, WBC >50,000 mm^3)
Decreased in:
    Hemorrhage (GI, GU), anemia (refer to Chapter 14, sections 14.1-4.3)

HEMOGLOBIN ELECTROPHORESIS

Normal range:
    Hb A$_1$: 95%-98%
    Hb A$_2$: 1.5%-3.5%
    Hb F: <2%
    Hb C: absent
    Hb S: absent

HEMOGLOBIN, GLYCOSYLATED See GLYCOSYLATED HEMOGLOBIN

HEMOGLOBIN, URINE See URINE HEMOGLOBIN

HEMOSIDERIN, URINE See URINE, HEMOSIDERIN

HEPATITIS A ANTIBODY

Normal:
    Negative
Present in:
    Viral hepatitis A; can be IgM or IgG. (If IgM, acute hepatitis A; if IgG, previous infection with hepatitis A)

HEPATITIS B SURFACE ANTIGEN (HBsAg)

Normal:
    Not detected
Detected in:
    Acute viral hepatitis type B, chronic hepatitis B

HIGH-DENSITY LIPOPROTEIN CHOLESTEROL (HDL)

Normal range:
  Male: 30-65 mg/dl
  Female: 35-80 mg/dl
Elevated in:
  Estrogens (increased levels protect against coronary heart disease)
Decreased in:
  Deficiency of apoproteins, liver disease, uremia, Tangier's disease

5-HYDROXY-INDOLE-ACETIC ACID, URINE See URINE 5-HYDROXY-INDOLE-ACETIC ACID

IMMUNE COMPLEX ASSAY

Normal:
  Negative
Detected in:
  Collagen-vascular disorders, glomerulonephritis, neoplastic diseases, malaria, primary biliary cirrhosis, chronic acute hepatitis, bacterial endocarditis, vasculitis

IMMUNOGLOBULINS

Normal range:
  Ig A: 70-312 mg/dl
  Ig M: 56-352 mg/dl
  Ig G: 639-1349 mg/dl
Elevated in:
  IgA: lymphoproliferative disorders, Berger's nephropathy, chronic infections, autoimmune disorders
  IgM: primary biliary cirrhosis, infectious diseases (brucellosis, malaria, Waldenstrom's macroglobulinemia)
  IgG: chronic granulomatous infections, infectious diseases, inflammation, myeloma
Decreased in:
  IgA: congenital deficiency, lymphocytic leukemia, ataxia-telangiectasia, chronic sino-pulmonary disease, nephrotic syndrome, protein-losing enteropathy
  IgM: congenital deficiency, lymphocytic leukemia, protein-losing enteropathy
  IgM: congenital or acquired deficiency, lymphocytic leukemia

INDICAN See URINE, INDICAN

IRON (Serum)

Normal range:
  41-132 µg/dl
Elevated in:
  Hemochromatosis, liver disease, hemolytic anemias, sideroblastic anemias, thalassemia major, excessive iron supplements
Decreased in:
  Malabsorption, chronic blood loss, achlorhydria, gastrectomy, anemia of chronic disease, chronic renal failure, malnutrition

IRON-BINDING CAPACITY (TIBC)

Normal range:
220-368 μg/dl
Elevated in:
Iron deficiency anemia, pregnancy, polycythemia
Decreased in:
Anemia of chronic disease, hemochromatosis, chronic liver disease, hemolytic anemias, malnutrition (protein depletion)

LACTIC ACID (Blood)

Normal range:
0.5-2.2 mmol/L
Elevated:
See Chapter 8, section 8.2

LACTIC DEHYDROGENASE (LDH)

Normal range:
115-225 IU/L
Elevated in:
Infarction of myocardium, lung, kidney
Diseases of cardiopulmonary system, liver, collagen, CNS
Hemolytic anemias, megaloblastic anemias, transfusions, seizures, muscle trauma, muscular dystrophy, acute pancreatitis, hypotension, shock, infectious mononucleosis, inflammation, neoplasia, intestinal obstruction, hypothyroidism

LACTIC DEHYDROGENASE ISOENZYMES

Normal range:
LD_1: 22%-36% (cardiac, RBC)
LD_2: 35%-46% (cardiac, RBC)
LD_3: 13%-26% (pulmonary)
LD_4: 3%-10% (striated muscle, liver)
LD_5: 2%-9% (striated muscle, liver)
Normal ratios:
$LD_1 < LD_2$
$LD_5 < LD_4$
Abnormal values:
$LD_1 > LD_2$: MI (can also be seen with hemolytic anemias, pernicious anemia, folate deficiency, renal infarct)
$LD_5 > LD_4$: liver disease (cirrhosis, hepatitis, hepatic congestion)

LAP SCORE See LEUKOCYTE ALKALINE PHOSPHATASE

LDH See LACTIC DEHYDROGENASE

LEGIONELLA TITER

Normal:
Negative
Positive in:
Legionnaire's disease (presumptive: ≥ 1:256 titer; definitive: fourfold titer increase to ≥ 1:128)

LEUKOCYTE ALKALINE PHOSPHATASE (Lap Score)

Normal range:
11-95
Elevated in:
Leukemoid reactions, neutrophilia secondary to infections (except in sickle cell crisis—no significant increase in LAP score), Hodgkin's disease, polycythemia vera, hairy cell leukemia, aplastic anemia, Down's syndrome, myelofibrosis
Decreased in:
Acute and chronic granulocytic leukemia, thrombocytopenic purpura, paroxysmal nocturnal hemoglobinuria (PNH), hypophosphatemia, collagen disorders

LEUKOCYTE COUNT See COMPLETE BLOOD COUNT

LIPASE

Normal range:
4-24 IU/dl
Elevated in:
Acute pancreatitis, perforated peptic ulcer, carcinoma of pancreas (early stage), pancreatic duct obstruction

LIPOPROTEIN CHOLESTEROL, LOW-DENSITY See LOW-DENSITY LIPOPROTEIN CHOLESTEROL

LIPOPROTEIN CHOLESTEROL, HIGH-DENSITY See HIGH-DENSITY LIPOPROTEIN CHOLESTEROL

LOW-DENSITY LIPOPROTEIN CHOLESTEROL

Normal range:
110-200 mg/dl
Elevated in:
Primary hyperlipoproteinemia, diet high in saturated fats, acute MI, hypothyroidism, primary biliary cirrhosis, nephrosis, diabetes mellitus
Decreased in:
Abetalipoproteinemia, advanced liver disease, malabsorption, malnutrition

LUPUS ANTICOAGULANT See CIRCULATING ANTICOAGULANT

LYMPHOCYTES

Normal range:
15%-40%; 1500-4000/ml
Subsets:
T-helper lymphocyte percent: 37-62
T-suppressor lymphocyte percent: 16-44
T-helper lymphocyte count: 37-62/ml
T-suppressor lymphocyte count: 109-2088/ml
T-helper/T-suppressor ratio: 0.9:3.5

Elevated in:
   Chronic infections, infectious mononucleosis and other viral infections,
   CLL, Hodgkin's disease, ulcerative colitis, hypoadrenalism, ITP
Decreased in:
   AIDS, ARC, bone marrow suppression from chemotherapeutic agents or
   chemotherapy, aplastic anemia, neoplasms, steroids, adrenocortical
   hyperfunction, neurologic disorders (multiple sclerosis, myasthenia
   gravis, Guillain-Barré syndrome)

MAGNESIUM (Serum)
Normal range:
   1.8-2.3 mg/dl
   For interpretation of abnormal values refer to Chapter 16, section 16.4

MEAN CORPUSCULAR VOLUME (MCV)
Normal range:
   Male: 80-94 cubic micron
   Female: 79-97 cubic micron
Elevated in:
   Vitamin B_{12} deficiency, folic acid deficiency, liver disease, alcohol
   abuse, reticulocytosis, hypothyroidism, marrow aplasia, myelofibrosis
Decreased in:
   Iron deficiency, thalassemia syndrome and other hemoglobinopathies,
   anemia of chronic disease, sideroblastic anemia, chronic renal failure,
   lead poisoning

METANEPHRINES, URINE See URINE, METANEPHRINES

MONOCYTE COUNT
Normal range:
   2%-8%
Elevated in:
   Viral diseases, parasites, infections, neoplasms, inflammatory bowel dis-
   ease
Decreased in:
   Aplastic anemia, lymphocytic leukemia

MYOGLOBIN, URINE See URINE MYOGLOBIN

NEUTROPHIL COUNT
Normal range:
   50%-70%
   Subsets
      Stabs (bands, early mature neutrophils): 2%-6%
      Segs (mature neutrophils): 60%-70%
Elevated in:
   Acute bacterial infections, acute MI, stress, neoplasms, myelocytic leu-
   kemia
Decreased in:
   Viral infections, aplastic anemias, immunosuppressive drugs, radiation
   therapy to bone marrow, agranulocytosis, drugs (antibiotics, antithy-
   roid drugs), lymphocytic and monocytic leukemias

5′ NUCLEOTIDASE
Normal range:
   2-16 IU/L
Elevated in:
   Biliary obstruction, metastatic neoplasms to liver, primary biliary cirrhosis

OSMOLALITY, SERUM
Normal range:
   275-295 mOsm/kg
Elevated in:
   Dehydration, hypernatremia, diabetes insipidus, uremia, hyperglycemia, mannitol therapy, ingestion of toxins (ethylene glycol, methanol, ethanol)
Decreased in:
   SIADH, hyponatremia, overhydration

OSMOLALITY, URINE See URINE OSMOLALITY

PARTIAL THROMBOPLASTIN TIME (PTT)
Normal range:

Elevated in:
   Heparin therapy, coagulation factor deficiency (I, II, V, VIII, IX, X, XI, XII), liver disease, vitamin K deficiency, DIC, circulating anticoagulant, warfarin therapy, specific factor inhibition (PCN reaction, rheumatoid arthritis)

pH (Blood)
Normal values:
   Arterial: 7.35-7.45
   Venous: 7.32-7.42
   NOTE: For abnormal values refer to Chapter 8

PH, URINE See URINE PH

PHOSPHATASE, ACID See ACID PHOSPHATASE

PHOSPHATASE, ALKALINE See ALKALINE PHOSPHATASE

PHOSPHORUS (Serum)
Normal range:
   2-4 mg/dl
Elevated in:
   Renal failure, dehydration, Addison's disease, myelogenous leukemia, hypervitaminosis D, hypoparathyroidism, pseudohypoparathyroidism, bone metastases, sarcoidosis, milk-alkali syndrome, immobilization, magnesium deficiency, transfusions, hemolysis

Decreased in:
> Starvation (alcoholics), diabetic ketoacidosis, TPN, continuous IV dextrose administration, vitamin D deficiency, hyperparathyroidism, pseudohyperparathyroidism, antacids containing aluminum hydroxide, insulin administration, nasogastric suctioning, vomiting

PLATELET COUNT

Normal range:
> 150,000-450,000mm^3

Elevated in:
> Neoplasms (GI tract), CML, polycythemia vera, myelofibrosis with myeloid metaplasia, infections, after splenectomy, postpartum, after hemorrhage, hemophilia, iron deficiency, pancreatitis, cirrhosis

Decreased:
> See Chapter 14, section 14.11

POTASSIUM (Serum)

Normal range:
> 3.3-4.9 mEq/L
> For interpretation of abnormal values refer to Chapter 16, section 16.3

POTASSIUM, URINE See URINE POTASSIUM

PROLACTIN

Normal range:
> <20 ng/ml

Elevated in:
> Prolactinomas (level >200 highly suggestive), drugs (phenothiazines, cimetidine, tricyclic antidepressants, metoclopramide, estrogens, antihypertensives [methyldopa], verapamil, haloperidol), postpartum, stress, hypoglycemia, hypothyroidism

PROTEIN (Serum)

Normal range:
> 6.0-7.7 g/dl

Elevated in:
> Dehydration, multiple myeloma, Waldenstrom's macroglobulinemia, sarcoidosis, collagen-vascular diseases

Decreased in:
> Malnutrition, low-protein diet, overhydration, malabsorption, pregnancy, severe burns, neoplasms, chronic diseases, cirrhosis, nephrosis

PROTEIN ELECTROPHORESIS (Serum)

Normal range:
> Albumin: 58%-70%
> α 1: 2%-5%
> α 2: 6%-11%
> β: 8%-14%
> γ: 9%-18%

Elevated:
> Albumin: dehydration
> α-1: neoplastic diseases, inflammation
> α-2: neoplasms, inflammation, infection, nephrotic syndrome
> β: hypothyroidism, biliary cirrhosis, diabetes mellitus
> γ: see Immunoglobulins

Decreased:
> Albumin: malnutrition, chronic liver disease, malabsorption, nephrotic syndrome, burns, SLE
> α-1: emphysema (α-1 antitrypsin deficiency), nephrosis
> α-2: hemolytic anemias (decreased haptoglobin), severe hepatocellular damage
> β: hypocholesterolemia, nephrosis
> γ: see Immunoglobulins

PROTHROMBIN TIME (PT)

Normal range:
> 10-12 seconds

Elevated in:
> Liver disease, oral anticoagulants (Warfarin), heparin, factor deficiency (I, II, V, VII, X), DIC, vitamin K deficiency, afibrinogenemia, dysfibrinogenemia, drugs (salicylate, chloral hydrate, diphenylhydantoin, estrogens, antacids, phenylbutazone, quinidine, antibiotics, allopurinol, anabolic steroids)

Decreased in:
> Vitamin K supplementation, thrombophlebitis, drugs (gluthetimide, estrogens, griseofulvin, diphenhydramine)

PROTOPORPHYRIN (Free erythrocyte)

Normal range:
> <50 μg/dl

Elevated in:
> Iron deficiency, lead poisoning, sideroblastic anemias, anemia of chronic disease, hemolytic anemias, erythropoietic protoporphyria

PT See PROTHROMBIN TIME

PTT See PARTIAL THROMBOPLASTIN TIME

RDW See RED BLOOD CELL DISTRIBUTION WIDTH

RED BLOOD CELL COUNT

Normal range:
> Male: 4.6-6.2 × 10^6/μl
> Female: 4.2-5.4 × 10^6/μl

Elevated in:
> Polycythemia vera, smokers, high altitude, cardiovascular disease, renal cell carcinoma and other erythropoietin-producing neoplasms, stress, hemoconcentration/dehydration

Decreased in:
> Anemias, hemolysis, chronic renal failure, hemorrhage, failure of marrow production

RED BLOOD CELL FOLATE See **FOLATE, RBC**

RED BLOOD CELL MASS

Normal range:

Male: 24-32 ml/kg

Female: 21.6-26.8 ml/kg

Elevated in:

Polycythemia vera, hypoxia (smokers, high altitude, cardiovascular disease), hemoglobinopathies with high O_2 affinity, erythropoietin-producing tumors (renal cell carcinoma)

Decreased in:

Hemorrhage, chronic disease, failure of marrow production, anemias, hemolysis

RED BLOOD CELL DISTRIBUTION WIDTH (RDW)

Normal range:

11.5-14.5

Normal RDW and:

Elevated MCV: aplastic anemia, preleukemia

Normal MCV: normal, anemia of chronic disease, acute blood loss or hemolysis, CLL, CML, nonanemic enzymopathy or hemoglobinopathy

Decreased MCV: anemia of chronic disease, heterozygous thalassemia

Elevated RDW and:

Elevated MCV: vitamin B_{12} deficiency, folate deficiency, immune hemolytic anemia, cold agglutinins, CLL with high count

Normal MCV: early iron deficiency, early vitamin B_{12} deficiency, early folate deficiency, anemic globinopathy

Decreased MCV: iron deficiency, RBC fragmentation, Hb H, thalassemia intermedia

RETICULOCYTE COUNT

Normal range:

0.5%-1.5%

Elevated in:

Hemolytic anemia (sickle cell crisis, thalassemia major, autoimmune hemolysis, hemorrhage, postanemia therapy (folic acid, ferrous sulfate, vitamin B_{12})

Decreased in:

Aplastic anemia, marrow suppression (sepsis, chemotherapeutic agents, radiation), hepatic cirrhosis, blood transfusion, anemias of disordered maturation (iron deficiency anemia, megaloblastic anemia, sideroblastic anemia, anemia of chronic disease)

RHEUMATOID FACTOR

Normal:

Negative

Present in titer $>1:20$:

Rheumatoid arthritis, SLE, chronic inflammatory processes, old age

RNP See **EXTRACTABLE NUCLEAR ANTIGEN**

SEDIMENTATION RATE See ERYTHROCYTE SEDIMENTATION RATE

SERUM GLUTAMIC OXALOACETIC TRANSAMINASE (SGOT, AST, aminotransferase aspartate)

Normal range:
5-25 IU/L
Elevated in:
Liver disease (hepatitis, cirrhosis, Reye's syndrome), hepatic congestion, infectious mononucleosis, MI, myocarditis, severe muscle trauma, dermatomyositis/polymyositis, muscular dystrophy, drugs (antibiotics, narcotics, antihypertensive agents, heparin), malignancy, renal and pulmonary infarction, convulsions, eclampsia

SERUM GLUTAMIC PYRUVATE TRANSAMINASE (SGPT, ALT, aminotransferase alanine)

Normal range:
3-20 IU/L
Elevated in:
Liver disease (hepatitis, cirrhosis, Reye's syndrome), alcoholic liver disease (SGPT is less sensitive than SGOT), muscle trauma, rhabdomyolysis, polymyositis/dermatomyositis, heparin therapy

SGOT See SERUM GLUTAMIC OXALOACETIC TRANSAMINASE

SGPT See SERUM GLUTAMIC PYRUVATE TRANSANIMASE

SMOOTH MUSCLE ANTIBODY

Normal:
Negative
Present in:
Chronic active hepatitis (≥1:80), primary biliary cirrhosis (≤1:80), infectious mononucleosis

SODIUM (Serum)

Normal range:
134-144 mEq/L
NOTE: For interpretation of abnormal values refer to Chapter 16, section 16.2

STREPTOZIME See ANTI-STREPTOLYSIN-O-TITER

SUCROSE HEMOLYSIS TEST (Sugar water test)

Normal:
Absence of hemolysis
Positive in:
Paroxysmal nocturnal hemoglobinuria (PNH)
False positive: autoimmune hemolytic anemia, megaloblastic anemias
False negative: may occur with use of heparin or EDTA

SUGAR WATER TEST See SUCROSE HEMOLYSIS TEST

T_3 (by RIA)

Normal range:
 50-21 ng/100 ml
 NOTE: For interpretation of abnormal values refer to Chapter 12, section 12.9

T_3 RESIN UPTAKE (T_3RU)

Normal range:
 35%-45%
 NOTE: For interpretation of abnormal values refer to Chapter 12, section 12.9

T_4, FREE (Free thyroxine by RIA)

Normal range:
 0.8-2.3 ng/ml
 NOTE: For interpretation of abnormal values refer to Chapter 12, section 12.9

THROMBIN TIME (TT)

Normal range:
 10-15 seconds
Elevated in:
 Heparin therapy, DIC, hypofibrinogenemia, dysfibrinogenemia, streptokinase, urokinase

THYROID-STIMULATING HORMONE (TSH)

Normal range:
 Up to 10 µU/ml
 NOTE: For interpretation of abnormal values refer to chapter 12, section 12.9

THYROXINE (T_4 by RIA)

Normal range:
 4.5-12.5 µg/dl

TIBC See IRON BINDING CAPACITY

TRANSFERRIN

Normal range:
 200-400 mg/dl
Elevated in:
 Iron deficiency anemia, oral contraceptive administration, viral hepatitis
Decreased in:
 Nephrotic syndrome, liver disease, hereditary deficiency, protein malnutrition, neoplasms, chronic inflammatory states, chronic illness, thalassemia

TRIGLYCERIDES

Normal range:
35-135 mg/dl

Elevated in:
Hyperlipoproteinemias (types I, IIb, III, IV, V), hypothyroidism, pregnancy, estrogens, acute MI, pancreatitis, alcohol intake, nephrotic syndrome, diabetes mellitus, glycogen storage disease

Decreased in:
Malnutrition, congenital abetalipoproteinemias, drugs (e.g., clofibrate)

TRIIODOTHYRONINE See T_3 by RIA

TSH See THYROID-STIMULATING HORMONE

TT See THROMBIN TIME

UNCONJUGATED BILIRUBIN See BILIRUBIN, INDIRECT

UREA NITROGEN

Normal range:
9-19 mg/dl

Elevated in:
Drugs (aminoglycosides and other antibiotics, diuretics, lithium, corticosteroids), dehydration, gastrointestinal bleeding, decreased renal blood flow (shock, CHF, MI), renal disease (glomerulonephritis, pyelonephritis, diabetic nephropathy), urinary tract obstruction (prostatic hypertrophy)

URIC ACID (Serum)

Normal range:
Male: 3.7-8.6 mg/dl
Female: 2.4-6.0 mg/dl

Elevated in:
Renal failure, gout, excessive cell lysis (chemotherapeutic agents, radiation therapy, leukemia, lymphoma, hemolytic anemia), hereditary enzyme deficiency (hypoxanthine-guanine-phosphoribosyl transferase), acidosis, myeloproliferative disorders, diet high in purines or protein, drugs (diuretics, low doses of ASA, ethambutol, nicotinic acid), lead poisoning, hypothyroidism, Addison's disease, nephrogenic diabetes insipidus, active psoriasis

Decreased in:
Drugs (allopurinol, high doses of ASA, probenecid, warfarin, corticosteroid), deficiency of xanthine oxidase, SIADH, renal tubular deficits (Fanconi's syndrome), alcoholism, liver disease, diet deficient in protein or purines, Wilson's disease, hemochromatosis

URINALYSIS

Normal range:

Color: light straw	Protein: absent
Appearance: clear	Ketones: absent
pH: 4.5-8 (average—6)	Glucose: absent
Specific gravity: 1.005-1.030	Occult blood: absent

Microscopic exam:
RBC's: 0-5/high-power field
WBC's: 0-5/high-power field
Bacteria (spun specimen): absent
Casts: 0-4 hyaline cast/low-power field

URINE AMYLASE (2 hour)

Normal range:
30-350 amylase units/hr
Elevated in:
Pancreatitis, carcinoma of the pancreas

URINE BILE

Normal:
Absent
Abnormal:
Urine bilirubin:
Hepatitis (viral, toxic, drug-induced), biliary obstruction
Urine urobilinogen:
Hepatitis (viral, toxic, drug-induced), hemolytic jaundice, liver cell
dysfunction (cirrhosis, infection, metastases)

URINE CALCIUM

Normal range:
<300 mg/24 h
Elevated in:
Primary hyperparathyroidism, hypervitaminosis D, bone metastases, multiple myeloma, increased calcium intake, steroids, prolonged immobilization, sarcoidosis, Paget's disease, idiopathic hypercalciuria, renal
tubular acidosis
Decreased in:
Hypoparathyroidism, pseudohypoparathyroidism, vitamin D deficiency,
vitamin D-resistant rickets, diet low in calcium, drugs (thiazide diuretics, oral contraceptives), familial hypocalciuric hypercalcemia, renal
osteodystrophy

URINE CATECHOLAMINES

Normal range:
Norepinephrine: 15-80 μg/24 h
Epinephrine: 0-20 μg/24 h
Dopamine: 65-400 μg/24 h
Elevated in:
Pheochromocytoma, neuroblastoma, severe stress

URINE CHLORIDE

Normal range:
110-250 mEq/L
Elevated in:
Corticosteroids, Bartter's syndrome
Decreased in:
Chloride depletion (vomiting, diuretics), colonic villous adenoma

URINE COPPER

Normal range:
   <60 μg/24 h
Elevated in:
   Primary biliary cirrhosis, chronic active hepatitis, Wilson's disease, nephrotic syndrome

URINE CREATININE (24 hour)

Normal range:
   Male: 1.5-2.0 g/24 h
   Female: 0.8-1.5 g/24 h
   NOTE: Useful test as an indicator of completeness of 24-hour urine collec-
   tion

URINE ELECTROLYTES

Normal range:
   Sodium: 40-210 mEq/24 h
   Potassium: 30-90 mEq/24 h
   Chloride: 110-250 mEq/24 h
   NOTE: Refer to specific electrolyte for evaluation of abnormality

URINE GLUCOSE (Qualitative)

Normal:
   Absent
Present in:
   Diabetes mellitus, renal glycosuria (decreased renal threshold for glu-
   cose), corticosteroids

URINE HEMOGLOBIN, FREE

Normal:
   Absent
Present in:
   Hemolysis (with saturation of serum haptoglobin binding capacity and
   renal threshold for tubular absorption of hemoglobin)

URINE HEMOSIDERIN

Normal:
   Absent
Present in:
   Paroxysmal nocturnal hemoglobinuria (PNH), chronic hemolytic anemia,
   hemochromatosis

URINE 5-HYDROXY-INDOLE-ACETIC ACID

Normal range:
   1-7 mg/24 h
Elevated in:
   Carcinoid tumors, after ingestion of certain foods (bananas, plums, to-
   matoes, avocados, pineapples, eggplant, walnuts), drugs (MAO inhibitors, phenacetin, methyldopa, glyceril guaiacolate, acetaminophen,
   salicylates, phenothiazines, imipramine, methocarbamol, reserpine,
   metamphetamine)

URINE INDICAN

Normal:
Absent
Present in:
Malabsorption secondary to intestinal bacterial overgrowth

URINE KETONES (Semiquantitative)

Normal:
Absent
Present in:
Diabetic or alcoholic ketoacidosis, starvation, isopropanol ingestion

URINE METANEPHRINES

Normal range:
0-1.2 mg/24 h
Elevated in:
Pheochromocytoma, neuroblastoma, drugs (caffeine, phenothiazines, MAO inhibitors), stress

URINE MYOGLOBIN

Normal:
Absent
Present in:
Severe trauma, hyperthermia, polymyositis/dermatomyositis, carbon monoxide poisoning

URINE NITRITE

Normal:
Absent
Present in:
Urinary tract infections, pyelonephritis, cystitis

URINE OCCULT BLOOD

Normal:
Negative
Positive in:
Trauma to urinary tract, renal disease (glomerulonephritis, pyelonephritis), renal or ureteral calculi, bladder lesions (carcinoma, cystitis), prostatitis, prostatic carcinoma, menstrual contamination, hematopoietic disorders (hemophilia, thrombocytopenia), anticoagulants, ASA

URINE OSMOLALITY

Normal range:
300-1090 mOsm/kg
Elevated in:
SIADH, dehydration, glycosuria, adrenal insufficiency, high-protein diet
Decreased in:
Diabetes insipidus, excessive water intake, IV hydration with D_5W, acute renal insufficiency, glomerulonephritis

URINE pH
Normal range:
4.6-8.0 (average 6.0)
Elevated in:
Bacteriuria, vegetarian diet, renal failure with inability to form ammonia, drugs (antibiotics, sodium bicarbonate, acetazolamide)
Decreased in:
Acidosis (metabolic, respiratory), drugs (ammonium chloride, methenamine mandelate), diabetes mellitus, starvation, diarrhea

URINE POTASSIUM
Normal range:
20-90 mEq/24 h
Elevated in:
Aldosteronism (primary, secondary), glucocorticoids, alkalosis, renal tubular acidosis, excessive dietary potassium intake
Decreased in:
Acute renal failure, potassium-sparing diuretics, diarrhea, hypokalemia

URINE PROTEIN (Quantitative)
Normal range:
Male: <0.06 g/24 h
Female: <0.09 g/24 h
Elevated in:
Renal disease (glomerular, tubular, interstitial), CHF, hypertension, neoplasms of renal pelvis and bladder, multiple myeloma, Waldenstrom's macroglobulinemia

URINE SODIUM (Quantitative)
Normal range:
40-210 mEq/24 h
Elevated in:
Diuretic administration, high sodium intake, salt-losing nephritis, acute tubular necrosis, vomiting, Addison's disease, SIADH, hypothyroidism, CHF, hepatic failure

URINE SPECIFIC GRAVITY
Normal range:
1.005-1.030
Elevated in:
Dehydration, excessive fluid losses (vomiting, diarrhea, fever), x-ray contrast media, diabetes mellitus, CHF, SIADH, adrenal insufficiency, decreased fluid intake
Decreased in:
Diabetes insipidus, renal disease (glomerulonephritis, pyelonephritis), excessive fluid intake or IV hydration

URINE VANILLYLMANDELIC ACID (VMA)

Normal range:
 1.8-7.5 mg/24 h
Elevated in:
 Pheochromocytoma, neuroblastoma, ganglioblastoma, drugs (isoproter-
  enol, methocarbamol, levodopa, sulfonamides, chlorpromazine), se-
  vere stress, after ingestion of bananas, chocolate, vanilla, tea, coffee
Decreased in:
 Drugs (MAO inhibitors, reserpine, guanethidine, methyldopa)

VDRL

Normal range:
 Negative
Positive test:
 Syphilis, other treponemal diseases (yaws, pinta, bejel)
 Note: A false positive test may be seen in patients with SLE and other
  autoimmune diseases, infectious mononucleosis, atypical pneumonia,
  malaria, leprosy

VISCOSITY

Normal range:
 1.4-1.8 relative to water
Elevated in:
 Monoclonal gammopathies (Waldenstrom's macroglobulinemia, multiple
  myeloma), hyperfibrinogenemia, SLE, rheumatoid arthritis, polycythemia, leukemia

WESTERGREN See ERYTHROCYTE SEDIMENTATION RATE

D-XYLOSE ABSORPTION

Normal range:
 16%-35% excretion of a 25 g dose at 5 hours
Decreased in:
 Malabsorption syndrome (refer to Chapter 13, section 13.5)

Medications

This section provides essential and concise information on more than 150 commonly prescribed medications. For the reader's convenience, the common synonyms are cross-indexed to the generic names. Each drug is listed by its principal generic name and is approached with the following format:

1. Generic name (common synonyms)
2. Preparations
3. Adult dosage
4. Indications
5. Action
6. Contraindications and precautions

Hypersensitivity or allergic reaction to a medication or any of its components is a definite contraindication to its use. When prescribing multiple medications for the same patient, all the possible drug interactions must be carefully considered.

Every attempt has been made to cover the most important aspects of each drug and to keep medication dosages in conformity with the latest practices of the general medical community. However, it is *strongly recommended that the reader become completely familiar with the manufacturer's product information before prescribing any of these medications*. This is particularly important when prescribing for patients with renal or hepatic impairment and for elderly or debilitated patients. THE USE OF ANY DRUG IN WOMEN WHO ARE PREGNANT OR OF CHILDBEARING AGE REQUIRES THAT THE ANTICIPATED BENEFIT BE WEIGHED AGAINST THE POSSIBLE HAZARD. PLEASE NOTE THAT THIS SECTION DOES NOT LIST PREGNANCY AS A CONTRAINDICATION TO THE USE OF ANY OF THESE MEDICATIONS. *REFER TO THE MANUFACTURER'S PRODUCT INFORMATION FOR POSSIBLE WARNINGS, CONTRAINDICATIONS, OR ADVERSE REACTIONS BEFORE PRESCRIBING ANY OF THESE MEDICATIONS FOR PREGNANT WOMEN.*

Fig. 21-1 shows the composition of a prescription order.

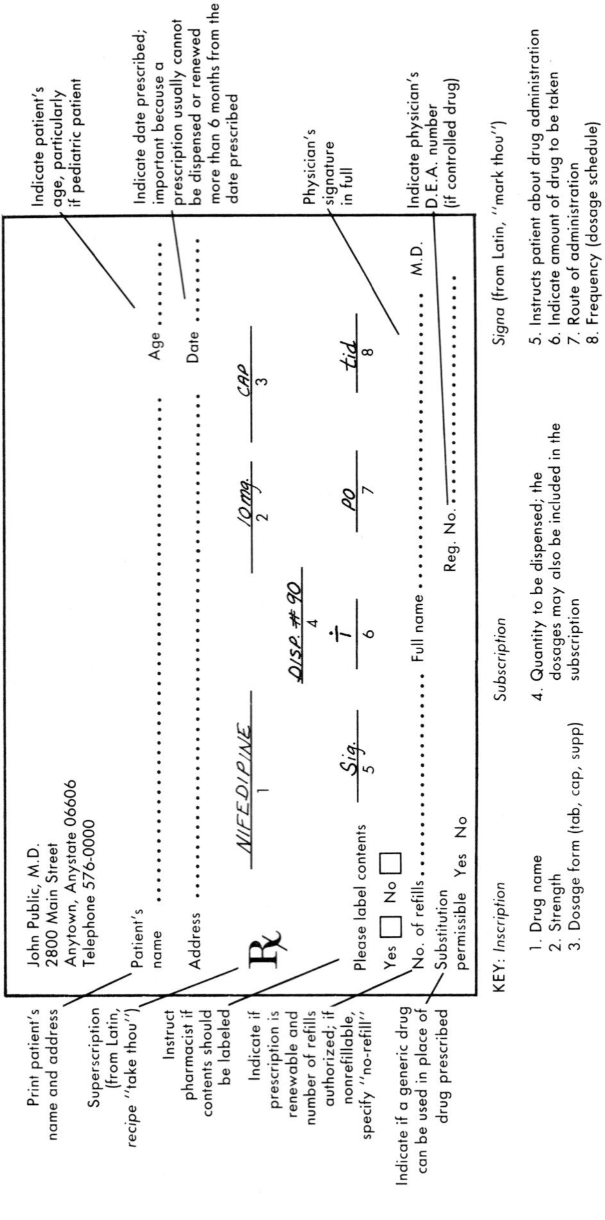

Figure 21-1
Composition of a prescription order.

Print patient's name and address

Superscription (from Latin, recipe "take thou")

Instruct pharmacist if contents should be labeled

Indicate if prescription is renewable and number of refills authorized; if nonrefillable, specify "no-refill"

Indicate if a generic drug can be used in place of drug prescribed

Indicate patient's age, particularly if pediatric patient

Indicate date prescribed; important because a prescription usually cannot be dispensed or renewed more than 6 months from the date prescribed

Physician's signature in full

Indicate physician's D.E.A. number (if controlled drug)

John Public, M.D.
2800 Main Street
Anytown, Anystate 06606
Telephone 576-0000

Patient's name ....

Address ....

Age ....

Date ....

℞

NIFEDIPINE — *10 mg.* — *CAP*
1 — 2 — 3

DISP # 90
4

Sig. — *i* — *po* — *tid*
5 — 6 — 7 — 8

Please label contents .... Full name .... M.D.

Yes ☐ No ☐

No. of refills .... Reg. No. ....

Substitution permissible Yes ☐ No ☐

KEY: *Inscription*

1. Drug name
2. Strength
3. Dosage form (tab, cap, supp)

Subscription

4. Quantity to be dispensed; the dosages may also be included in the subscription

Signa (from Latin, "mark thou")

5. Instructs patient about drug administration
6. Indicate amount of drug to be taken
7. Route of administration
8. Frequency (dosage schedule)

ACETAMINOPHEN (Tylenol)

Preparations: *Caplets* 325, 500 mg; *tab* 325, 500, 650 mg; *supp* 120, 125, 325, 650 mg
Adult dosage: 325-650 mg q4-6h prn
Indications: Relief of fever and pain
Action: Nonnarcotic analgesic and antipyretic
Contraindications and precautions: Hypersensitivity to acetaminophen; use with caution in patients with G-6-PD deficiency

ACETAZOLAMIDE (Diamox)

Preparations: *Tab* 125, 250 mg; *inj* 500 mg; *cap* 500 mg (Diamox sequels)
Adult dosage
1. Glaucoma: 250 mg-1 g/24h, in divided doses for amounts >250 mg
2. Drug-induced edema: 250-375 mg qod
3. Edema from CHF: 250-375 mg (5 mg/kg) qd or qod
4. Epilepsy: 8-30 mg/kg in divided doses

Indications
Adjunctive treatment of:
1. Chronic single glaucoma, secondary glaucoma, preoperatively in acute angle-closure glaucoma (Diamox sequels, Diamox)
2. Edema (drug-induced or from CHF) (Diamox)
3. Centrencephalic epilepsies (Diamox)

Action: Carbonic anhydrase inhibitor
Contraindications and precautions: Marked hepatic or renal disease, hyperchloremic acidosis, hyponatremia, hypokalemia, chronic noncongestive angle-closure glaucoma, suprarenal gland failure

ACHROMYCIN See TETRACYCLINE

ACYCLOVIR (Zovirax)

Preparations: *Cap* 200 mg; *ointment* 50 mg acyclovir/g, 15 g tube; *inj* 500 mg acyclovir/10 ml vial
Adult dosage:
1. Initial genital herpes: 200 mg PO q4h while awake (5 caps/day) × 10 days
2. Chronic suppressive therapy for recurrent disease: 200 mg PO tid for up to 6 mo
3. Apply ointment to affected areas 6 times/day × 7 days; not for use in the eye
4. *IV:* Herpes simplex infections in immunocompromised patient: 5 mg/kg IV infused slowly over 1 hr q8h (15 mg/kg day) × 7 days
5. Severe initial clinical episodes of genital herpes: same as above, except × 5 days
NOTE: Decrease dosage in patients with renal impairment

Indications: Treatment of initial episodes and management of recurrent episodes of genital herpes
Action: Antiviral nucleoside analog; competes for DNA polymerase
Contraindications and precautions: Hypersensitivity to any of its components

ADRENALIN See **EPINEPHRINE**

ALBUMIN

Preparations

5% solution: 50, 250, 500, 1000 ml bottles containing respectively 2.5, 12.5, 25, 50 g of albumin

25% solution (salt-poor albumin): 20, 50, 100 ml vials containing respectively 5, 12.5, 25 g of albumin

Adult dosage

1. 5% solution: Used for patients who are in shock with acute plasma volume depletion
2. 25% solution: Used for albumin replacement in patients with hypoproteinemia

Contraindications and precautions: CHF

ALBUTEROL (Ventolin, Proventil)

Preparations

Inhaler: 17.0 g canister, 0.09 mg/metered dose; *syrup:* 2 mg/5 ml, bottles of 16 fl. oz.; *tab:* 2, 4 mg

Adult dosage

1. Inhaler: 2 inhalations q4-6h
2. Syrup: Initially 2 mg (1 tsp) to 4 mg (2 tsp) tid or qid
3. Tab: Initially 2-4 mg tid or qid

Indications: Relief of bronchospasm in patients with reversible obstructive airway disease and for prevention of exercise-induced bronchospasm

Action: Sympathomimetic bronchodilator

Contraindications and precautions

1. Hypersensitivity to any of its components
2. Use with caution in patients with cardiovascular disorders, hyperthyroidism, diabetes mellitus, hypertension, and coronary insufficiency
3. Avoid concomitant use of MAO inhibitors, tricyclic antidepressants, and other sympathomimetic aerosol bronchodilators or epinephrine

ALDACTONE See **SPIRONOLACTONE**

ALDOMET See **METHYLDOPA**

ALLOPURINOL (Zyloprim)

Preparations: *Tab* 100, 300 mg

Adult dosage

1. Initially 100 mg/day; increase by 100 mg at weekly intervals until serum uric acid of ≤ 6 mg/dl is attained or a total dose of 800 mg/day
2. Maintenance (average dosages)
   a. Mild gout: 200-300 mg/day
   b. Severe gout: 400-600 mg/day in divided doses
3. A prophylactic dose of colchicine (0.5 mg bid) is also recommended by some to prevent an increase in attacks of gout when allopurinol is started
4. Secondary hyperuricemia associated with therapy of malignancies: 600-800 mg/day in divided doses for 3 days

NOTE: Reduce dosage in patients with renal insufficiency and in patients receiving mercaptopurine or azathioprine

Indications: Gout, hyperuricemia associated with treatment of malignancies, management of patients with recurrent calcium oxalate calculi whose daily uric acid excretion is >800 mg/day in male patients and >750 mg/day in female patients

Action: Xanthine oxidase inhibitor; it decreases both serum and urine uric acid levels

Contraindications and precautions
1. Allopurinol hypersensitivity
2. Use with caution in patients with renal insufficiency (decrease dosage), patients receiving dicumarol (prolonged prothrombin time), thiazide diuretics (increased allopurinol toxicity), ampicillin or amoxicillin (increased frequency of skin rash), chlorpropamide (increased risk of hypoglycemia), cyclophosphamide and other cytotoxic agents (possible enhanced bone marrow suppression)

ALPRAZOLAM (Xanax)

Preparations: *Tab* 0.25, 0.5, 1 mg
Adult dosage
1. Initially 0.25-0.5 mg tid
2. Maximum daily dose is 4 mg
3. Use 0.25 mg bid or tid in elderly or debilitated patients

Indications: Management of anxiety disorders and anxiety associated with depression

Action: Benzodiazepine; exact mechanism of action is unknown

Contraindications and precautions: Hypersensitivity to benzodiazepines, acute narrow-angle glaucoma, use during activities requiring complete mental alertness, concomitant use of ethanol and other CNS depressants

ALUMINUM HYDROXIDE AND/OR MAGNESIUM HYDROXIDE

Preparations
Suspension:
1. 320 mg/5 ml aluminum hydroxide (Amphojel)
2. 200 mg/5 ml aluminum hydroxide plus 200 mg/5 ml magnesium hydroxide and 20 mg/5 ml simethicone (Mylanta)
3. 400 mg/5 ml aluminum hydroxide with 400 mg/5 ml magnesium hydroxide and 40 mg/5 ml simethicone (Mylanta II)
Chewable tab:
1. 325, 650 mg aluminum hydroxide with 200 mg/5 ml magnesium hydroxide (Maalox)
2. 200 mg aluminum hydroxide with 200 mg magnesium hydroxide (Maalox #1)
3. 400 mg aluminum hydroxide with 200 mg magnesium hydroxide and 20 mg simethicone (Mylanta)
4. 400 mg aluminum hydroxide with 400 mg magnesium hydroxide and 40 mg simethicone (Mylanta II)

Adult dosage: 2 tsp or 2 tabs 2-4 hr between meals and hs

Indications: Symptomatic relief of hyperacidity associated with peptic ulcer disease, pyrosis, peptic esophagitis, and gastritis

Action: Neutralizes gastric acid

Contraindications and precautions

1. Do not use in patients taking tetracycline
2. Do not use any combination containing magnesium hydroxide in patients with renal insufficiency

ALUPENT See **METAPROTERENOL**

AMANTIDINE (Symmetrel)

Preparations: *Cap* 100 mg; *syrup* 10 mg/ml

Adult dosage

1. Drug-induced extrapyramidal reactions: 100 mg bid
2. Parkinsonism: 100 mg/day initially, may increase gradually to maximum of 400 mg/day in divided doses
3. Prophylaxis and treatment of Influenza A: 200 mg/day

NOTE: Decrease dosage in renal insufficiency, CHF, peripheral edema, or orthostatic hypotension

NOTE: Parkinsonian crisis may be caused by abrupt discontinuation of the drug

Indications: Parkinsonism, drug-induced extrapyramidal reactions, prophylaxis and treatment of Influenza A

Action: Antiviral agent with ability to release dopamine

Contraindications and precautions

1. Hypersensitivity to the drug, lactation
2. Use with caution in patients with history of seizures (increased risk of seizure activity), CHF, peripheral edema, liver disease, recurrent eczematous rash, psychosis or psychoneurosis not controlled by chemotherapeutic agents

AMIKACIN SULFATE (Amikin)

Preparations: *Inj* 50, 250 mg/ml

Adult dosage

1. 15 mg/kg/day in 2 or 3 divided doses (5 mg/kg q8h or 7.5 mg/kg q12h); do not exceed 1.5 g/day total dose
2. Dosage for uncomplicated UTI is 250 mg bid

NOTE: Decrease dosage in renal insufficiency

Indications: Infections caused by susceptible bacterial organisms

Action: Bacterial aminoglycoside; it attaches to the 30 S and 50 S ribosomal subunits

Contraindications and precautions

1. Hypersensitivity to amikacin
2. Avoid concurrent use of diuretics and concurrent or sequential use of neurotoxins or nephrotoxins

AMIKIN See **AMIKACIN SULFATE**

AMINOPHYLLINE See **THEOPHYLLINE PREPARATIONS**

AMITRIPTYLINE (Elavil)

Preparations: *Tab* 10, 25, 50, 75, 100, 150 mg; *inj* 10 mg/ml
Adult dosage
1. Initially 50-75 mg PO/day in divided doses or given as a single dose qhs
2. Usual maintenance dosage is 50-100 mg/day
3. IM dosage is 20-30 mg qid
NOTE: Use lower dosages in elderly and adolescent patients
Indications: Relief of symptoms of depression
Action: Antidepressant with sedative effects; it interferes with reuptake of norepinephrine and serotonin
Contraindications and precautions
1. Hypersensitivity to amitryptiline
2. Concomitant use of MAO inhibitors, disulfiram; use during acute recovery phase from MI; concomitant use of ethanol or other CNS depressants
3. Use with caution in patients with history of: seizures, urinary retention, angle-closure glaucoma, increased intraocular pressure, cardiovascular disorders, hyperthyroidism
4. Avoid concomitant use of ethchlorvynol, cimetidine, anticholinergic agents, sympathomimetic drugs, electroshock therapy
5. Use with caution in patients with suicidal tendencies

AMOXICILLIN (Amoxil)

Preparations: *Cap* 250, 500 mg; *suspension* 125, 250 mg/5 ml
Adult dosage
1. Infections of the lower respiratory tract: 500 mg q8h
2. Infections of ear, nose, throat, GU, skin, soft tissues: 250 mg q8h
3. Acute uncomplicated gonorrhea: 3 g PO (single dose) plus probencid 1 g PO (single dose) and tetracycline 500 mg PO qid for 7 days
Indications: Infections caused by susceptible bacterial organisms
Action: Semisynthetic broad-spectrum penicillin; it inhibits biosynthesis of cell wall mucopeptide
Contraindications and precautions: Hypersensitivity to penicillins

AMOXICILLIN POTASSIUM CLAVULANATE (Augmentin)

Preparations: *Tab* 250, 500 gm; *chewable tabs* 125, 250 mg; *oral suspension* 125, 250 mg/5 ml
Adult dosage: 250-500 mg q8h
Indications: Infections caused by susceptible bacterial organisms
Action: Same as amoxicillin; the addition of clavulinic acid provides protection against β-lactamase producing strains of *Staphylococcus aureus*
Contraindications and precautions: Allergy to penicillins

AMOXIL See AMOXICILLIN

AMPHOJEL See ALUMINUM HYDROXIDE

AMPHOTERICIN B (Fungizone)

Preparations: *Cream* 30 mg/g, 20 g tube; *lotion* 30 mg/ml, 30 ml bottle; *ointment* 30 mg/g, 20 g tube; *inj* 5 mg/ml (after reconstitution)

Adult dosage
1. Cream/lotion/ointment: apply to candidal lesions bid or qid
2. IV: initially 0.25 mg/kg in a concentration of 0.1 mg/ml infused slowly over 6 hr; total daily dosage should not exceed 1.5 mg/kg

Indications
1. Cream/lotion/ointment: cutaneous and mucocutaneous mycotic infections caused by *Candida* sp.
2. IV: progressive, potentially fatal fungal infections

Action: It binds to sterols in the fungal cytoplasmic membrane; it increases membrane permeability with resultant leakage of molecules

Contraindications and precautions
1. Hypersensitivity to any of its components
2. Caution when using nephrotoxic antibiotics or antineoplastic agents concomitantly
3. Avoid concomitant use of corticosteroids (unless necessary to control drug reactions)
4. Perform frequent renal and hepatic function tests; discontinue therapy if BUN >40 mg/dl, creatinine >3.0 mg/dl, or if liver function test abnormalities are noted

AMPICILLIN

Preparations: *Cap* 250, 500 mg; *suspension* 125, 250, 500 mg/5 ml; *inj* 125, 250, 500 mg, 1 g, 2 g vials

Adult dosage
1. Infections of the respiratory tract and soft tissues:
   a. PO: 250 mg q6h
   b. IM/IV: 250-500 mg q6h
2. Infections of the GI or GU tracts:
   a. PO: 500 mg q6h
   b. IM/IV: 500 mg q6h
3. Urethritis caused by *Neisseria gonorrhoeae* in males or females: PO: 3.5 g with 1 g of probenecid administered simultaneously followed by tetracycline 500 mg PO qid for 7 days
4. Urethritis caused by *Neisseria gonorrhoeae* in males: 500 mg IM/IV repeated once after 8-12h
5. Bacterial meningitis or septicemia: 150-200 mg/kg/day IV in equally divided doses q3-4h

Indications: Infections caused by susceptible bacterial organisms
Action: Semisynthetic penicillin; it inhibits cell wall synthesis
Contraindications and precautions: Penicillin hypersensitivity

AMYL NITRATE

Preparations: *Ampul* 0.3 ml
Indications:
Identification of cardiac murmurs
1. Increased murmur: AS, IHSS, PS, MS, TS, TR
2. Decreased murmur: MR, VSD, Austin-Flint murmur
Action: Vasodilating agent

ANAPROX See NAPROXEN

ANCEF See CEFAZOLIN

ANTIVERT See MECLIZINE

APRESOLINE See HYDRALAZINE

ASCORBIC ACID

Preparations: 50-2000 mg PO/IV
Adult dosage: Recommended daily dietary allowance is 60 mg
Indications: Treatment of scurvy and other deficiency states

ASPIRIN

Preparations: *Tab* 1 grain (65 mg), 1¼ grain (81 mg), 5 grain (325 mg), 7.7 grain (500 mg), 10 grain (650 mg); *supp* 65, 130, 195, 325, 650, 1200 mg
Adult dosage
  1. Minor pain and antipyretic action: 325-650 mg q4h
  2. Rheumatoid arthritis: 3-12 g/day in divided doses
  3. Reduction of risk of stroke: dosage varies from 650 mg bid to 325 mg qd
Indications: Relief of minor pains, fever, recurrent TIA in male patients
Action: Analgesic, antipyretic, antiinflammatory, antiplatelet agent
Contraindications and precautions
  1. Salicylate hypersensitivity
  2. Use with caution in patients with history of peptic ulcer disease, asthma, bleeding tendencies

ATARAX See HYDROXYZINE

ATENOLOL (Tenormin)

Preparations: *Tab* 50, 100 mg
Adult dosage: Initially 50 mg qd, may increase to 100 mg qd if no significant effect is noted after 2 weeks
Indications: Hypertension
Action: β-1 (cardioselective) adrenergic-receptor blocking agent
Contraindications and precautions
  1. Bradycardia, second- or third-degree heart block, CHF, cardiogenic shock
  2. Use with caution in patients with bronchospastic disease; if dosages greater than 50 mg/day are needed, divide the dose to achieve lower peak blood levels
  3. β blockage may mask tachycardia associated with hypoglycemia and thyrotoxicosis
  4. Use with caution in patients with impaired renal function and in patients receiving catecholomine-depleting drugs
  5. Abrupt cessation of atenolol therapy in patients with CAD can result in exacerbation of angina

ATIVAN See LORAZEPAM

ATROPINE

Preparations: *Inj* 0.3, 0.4, 0.5, 0.6, 1.0, 1.3 mg; *tab* 0.4 mg
Adult dosage
1. Bradycardia: 600 μg to 1 mg q5 min prn to maximum total dose of 2 mg
2. Preanesthesia: 400-600 μg SC/IM/IV 1 hr before induction

Indications: Bradycardia, asystole, preanesthesia
Action: Anticholinergic agent
Contraindications and precautions: Acute glaucoma, GI obstruction, obstructive uropathy, prostatism

AUGMENTIN See AMOXICILLIN/POTASSIUM CLAVULANATE

AZULFADINE See SULFASALAZINE

BACTRIM See TRIMETHOPRIM

BECLOMETHASONE DIPROPIONATE (Vanceril)

Preparations: *Oral inhaler* 16.8 canister; each metered-dose canister provides at least 200 inhalations of 42 μg/inhalation
Adult dosage: 2 inhalations (84 μg) tid or qid; maximum number of inhalations daily is 20 (840 μg)
Indications: Therapy of inflammatory component of asthma in patients requiring chronic treatment with corticosteroids in conjunction with other asthmatic therapy; patient's asthma should be reasonably stable before treatment with beclomethasone
Action: Antiinflammatory steroid
Contraindications and precautions: Do not use for primary treatment of status asthmaticus or other acute episode of asthma where intensive measures are required

BENADRYL See DIPHENHYDRAMINE

BENEMID See PROBENECID

BENZTROPINE MESYLATE (Cogentin)

Preparations: *Tab* 0.5, 1, 2 mg; *inj* (IM/IV) 2 ml ampul (1 mg/ml)
Adult dosage
1. Postencephalitic and idiopathic parkinsonism: 1-2 mg/day to maximum of 6 mg/day in two divided doses; initiate at low dosage and then increase by 0.5 mg increments at 6-day intervals
2. Drug-induced extrapyramidal symptoms: 1-4 mg qd

Indications: Control of extrapyramidal disorders caused by neuroleptic drugs and as an adjunct in the therapy of parkinsonism
Action: Competitive antagonist of acetylcholine; antihistaminic
Contraindications and precautions
1. Narrow-angle glaucoma
2. Use with caution in patients with prostatic hypertrophy, hypertension, GI or GU obstructive disease, hot climate (can cause anhidrosis)

BETAMETHASONE VALERATE (Valisone)

Preparations:
Concentration:
1. 0.1%: 15, 45, 110 g tubes, 430 g jar (cream)
2. 0.01%: 15, 60 g tubes (reduced strength)
3. 0.1%: 20 ml (18.7 g), 60 ml (56.2 g) bottles
4. 0.1%: 15, 45 g tubes (ointment)

Adult dosage
1. Cream, ointment: apply thin film to affected area 1-3 times/day
2. Lotion: apply few drops to affected area bid and massage lightly

Indications: Relief of pruritic and inflammatory manifestations of corticosteroid-responsive dermatosis

Action: Synthetic adrenocorticoid

Contraindications and precautions: Use with caution in pregnant patients and pediatric patients

BICILLIN See PENICILLIN-G BENZATHINE

BISACODYL (Dulcolax)

Preparations: *Enteric-coated tab* 5 mg; *supp* 10 mg

Adult dosage
1. Tab: 2 tabs to maximum of 6 tabs in preparation for special procedures
2. Supp: 1 supp at time of required bowel movement (usually effective in 15 min)

Indications: Acute or chronic constipation, preparation for radiography, surgery, and sigmoidoscopy

Action: Laxative; it acts directly on the colonic mucosa to increase peristaltic contractions

Contraindications and precautions
1. Acute abdominal condition requiring surgery
2. Hypersensitivity to any of its components

BLOCADREN See TIMOLOL

BRETHINE See TERBUTALINE

BRETYLIUM TOSYLATE (Bretylol)

Preparations: *Inj* 50 mg/ml

Adult dosage: 5-10 mg/kg IV over 5-10 min with additional doses of 10 mg/kg prn to maximum of 40 mg/kg total; maintenance IV infusion is 1-2 mg/min

NOTE: Reduce dosage in patients with impaired renal function

Indications
1. Prophylaxis and therapy of ventricular fibrillation
2. Life-threatening ventricular dysrhythmias that have failed to respond to adequate doses of a first-line antidysrhythmic agent

Action: Suppression of ventricular dysrhythmias; precise mechanism of action has not been clearly defined

Contraindications and precautions
1. Suspected digitalis-induced ventricular dysrhythmias
2. Use with caution in patients with fixed cardiac output (severe aortic stenosis or severe pulmonary hypertension)

BRETYLOL See BRETYLIUM TOSYLATE

BROMOCRIPTINE MESYLATE (Parlodel)

Preparations: *Tab* 2.5 mg; *cap* 5 mg
Adult dosage
1. Parkinson's disease: initial dose is 1.25 mg (half of a 2.5 mg tab) bid
2. Female infertility: initial dose is 2.5 mg bid or tid
3. Prevention of physiologic lactation: 2.5 mg bid × 14 days; do not start treatment sooner than 4 hr after delivery
4. Amenorrhea/galactorrhea: 2.5 mg qd × 1 wk then increase to bid; maximum duration of therapy is 6 mo

Indications: Parkinson's disease, prevention of physiologic lactation, amenorrhea/galactorrhea, female infertility associated with hyperprolactinemia (in absence of demonstrable pituitary tumor)
Action: Dopamine receptor agonist; it inhibits prolactin secretion
Contraindications and precautions
1. Sensitivity to ergot alkaloids
2. Use with caution in patients with renal and hepatic disease
3. Avoid use of phenothiazines during bromocriptine therapy
4. Evaluate the sella turcica in patients with amenorrhea/galactorrhea and infertility to rule out pituitary tumors before starting therapy with bromocriptine

BRONKOSOL See ISOETHARINE

BUMETANIDE (Bumex)

Preparations: *Tab* 0.5, 1, 2 mg; *inj* 2 ml ampul (0.25 mg/ml) and 2, 4, 10 ml vial (0.25 mg/ml)
Adult dosage: 0.5-2 mg/day PO/IV/IM given as a single dose; if the diuretic response is not adequate, may give a second or third dose at 4-5 hr intervals (maximum daily dose is 10 mg)
Indications: Treatment of edema associated with CHF, hepatic, and renal disease (including nephrotic syndrome)
Action: Loop diuretic; its major site of action is the ascending limb of the loop of Henle
Contraindications and precautions
1. Anemia, hepatic coma, severe electrolyte depletion, allergy to sulfonamides
2. Serum potassium should be measured periodically and hypokalemia should be corrected
3. Hypocalcemia and hyperuricemia may occur in some patients
4. Use with caution in patients receiving lithium, probenecid, indomethacin, antihypertensives, nephrotoxic or ototoxic agents

BUMEX See **BUMETANIDE**

BUSPAR See **BUSPIRONE**

BUSPIRONE (Buspar)
Preparations: *Tab* 5, 10 mg
Adult dosage: Initial dosage is 5 mg PO tid, may increase dosage by 5 mg/day q3d prn; optimal daily dosage is 20-30 mg; maximum daily dose is 60 mg
Indications: Management of anxiety disorders
Action: Azaspirodecanedione anxiolitic agent; mechanism of action is unknown
Contraindications and precautions: Avoid concurrent use of other CNS agents; concomitant use of a monoamine oxidase inhibitor (MAOI) may be hazardous (elevation of blood pressure)

CAFERGOT See **ERGOTAMINE TARTRATE**

CALAN See **VERAPAMIL**

CALCIMAR See **CALCITONIN SALMON**

CALCITONIN SALMON (CALCIMAR)
Preparations: *Inj* 2 ml vial (200 IU/ml)
Adult dosage
  1. Paget's disease: 100 IU/day SC/IM
  2. Hypercalcemia: 4 IU/kg q12h SC/IM initially; may increase dosage to 8 IU/kg q12h SC/IM after 24-48 hr if response is unsatisfactory; if response still remains unsatisfactory, may increase dose to 8 IU/kg SC/IM q6h after 2 more days
  3. Postmenopausal osteoporosis: 100 IU/day SC/IM
Indications: Symptomatic Paget's disease of bone, hypercalcemia, postmenopausal osteoporosis (in addition to supplemental calcium, adequate vitamin D intake, and adequate diet)
Action: Synthetic polypeptide with the same amino acid sequence as salmon calcitonin; it acts primarily on bone to inhibit the ongoing bone resorptive process
Contraindications and precautions
  1. Clinical allergy to synthetic salmon calcitonin
  2. Periodic examination of urine sediment is recommended for patients on chronic therapy

CALCITRIOL (Rocaltrol)
Preparations: *Cap* 0.25 μg, 0.5 μg
Adult dosage
  1. Dialysis patients: initial dose is 0.25 μg/day; may increase dosage by 0.25 μg/day at 4-8 wk intervals if a satisfactory response is not obtained
  2. Hypothyroidism: initial dose is 0.25 μg/day given in AM; may increase dose at 2-4 wk intervals
Indications: Hypocalcemia secondary to chronic renal dialysis, postsurgical and idiopathic hypoparathyroidism, pseudohypoparathyroidism
Action: Synthetic vitamin D analog; it is the most potent metabolite of vitamin D available

Contraindications and precautions
1. Hypercalcemia, evidence of vitamin D toxicity
2. Monitor serum calcium level frequently, particularly during titration period
3. Use with caution in patients on digitalis (hypercalcemia may precipitate cardiac dysrhythmias in these patients)
4. In patients with normal renal function maintain adequate fluid intake

CALCIUM CARBONATE (OS-CAL)

Preparations
Tab
1. Os-Cal 250 = 625 mg calcium carbonate (each tab contains 250 mg of elemental calcium and 125 USP units of vitamin D)
2. Os-Cal 500 = 1250 mg calcium carbonate (each tab contains 500 mg of elemental calcium
3. Os-cal Forte = 250 mg elemental calcium plus vitamins and minerals

Adult dosage: 1 tab tid
Indications: Calcium replacement therapy
Contraindications and precautions: Hypercalcemia, vitamin D intoxication

CAPOTEN See CAPTOPRIL

CAPTOPRIL (Capoten)

Preparations: *Tab* 12.5, 25, 50, 100 mg
Adult dosage
1. Hypertension: 25 mg PO, bid or tid initially; maximum dose is 150 mg tid
2. Heart failure: 6.25-12.5 mg tid initially; maximum daily dose is 450 mg
3. Decrease dosage in patients with renal insufficiency

Indications: Hypertension; heart failure not adequately controlled with diuretics and digitalis
Action: Angiotension I converting enzyme inhibitor
Contraindications and precautions
1. Bilateral or unilateral renal artery stenosis
2. Use with caution in patients with renal impairment and collagen-vascular disease
3. A CBC and urinalysis should be done before initiation of therapy with captopril

CARAFATE See SUCRALFATE

CARBENICILLIN (Geocillin, Geopen)

Preparations: *Tab* (Geocillin) 500 mg (382 mg of carbenicillin base equivalent); *inj* (Geopen) 1, 2, 5, 10 g
Adult dosage
1. Uncomplicated UTI: 500 mg tab PO q6h or 1-2 IM/IV q6h
2. Serious UTI: 200 mg/kg/day by continuous infusion
3. Serious infections outside of urinary tract: 300-500 mg/kg/day in divided doses or by continuous infusion

Indications: Infections caused by susceptible bacterial strains; particularly useful against *Pseudomonas* and *Proteus* sp.
Action: Broad-spectrum semisynthetic penicillin
Contraindications and precautions
1. Penicillin allergy; severely impaired renal function
2. High sodium content of parenteral carbenicillin may produce fluid overload
3. Monitor serum potassium frequently (severe hypokalemia can occur)

CARDIOQUIN See **QUINIDINE**

CARDIZEM See **DILTIAZEM**

CATAPRES See **CLONIDINE**

CECLOR See **CEFACLOR**

CEFACLOR (Ceclor)
Preparations: *Oral suspension* 125, 250 mg/5 ml; *cap* 250, 500 mg
Adult dosage: Usual dose is 250 mg PO q8h; may double dose in severe infections
Indications: Infections caused by susceptible bacterial strains
Actions: Semisynthetic cephalosporin; its bactericidal action results from inhibition of cell wall synthesis
Contraindications and precautions
1. Known allergy to cephalosporins
2. Administer with caution in patients with a history of allergy to penicillin

CEFADROXIL (Duricef)
Preparations: *Tab* 1 g; *cap* 500 mg; *oral suspension* 125, 250, 500 mg/5 ml
Adult dosage
1. Uncomplicated UTI: 1-2 g/day in single (qd) or divided doses (bid)
2. Moderate-severe UTI: 2 g/day in divided doses bid
3. Skin and skin structure infections: 1 g/day in single dose qd or divided doses bid
4. Group A β-hemolytic streptococcal pharyngitis and tonsillitis: 500 mg bid × 10 days
   NOTE: Decrease dosage in renal insufficiency
Indications: Infections caused by susceptible bacterial strains
Action: Semisynthetic cephalosporin; it exerts its bactericidal action via inhibition of cell wall synthesis
Contraindications and precautions
1. Allergy to cephalosporins
2. Use with caution in patients with a history of penicillin allergy

CEFADYL See **CEPHAPIRIN**

CEFAMANDOLE (Mandol)

Preparations: *Inj* 500 mg, 1 g, 2 g vial
Adult dosage: 500 mg-1 g IV/IM q4-6h to maximum of 12 g/day (2 g q4h); usual dosage is 1 g q6h
NOTE: Decrease dosage in patients with impaired renal function
Indications: Infections caused by susceptible bacterial strains
Action: Semisynthetic broad-spectrum cephalosporin; its bactericidal action results from inhibition of cell wall synthesis
Contraindications and precautions
1. Known allergy to cephalosporins
2. use with caution in patients with known allergy to penicillin

CEFAZOLIN (Ancef, Kefzol)

Preparations: 250 mg, 500 mg, 1 g vials
Adult dosage
1. Treatment of infections: 250 mg-1 g q8h IV/IM
2. Surgical prophylaxis: 1 g IM/IV 30-60 min before surgery and 500 mg-1 g q6-8h × 24h
NOTE: Decrease dosage in patients with impaired renal function
Indications: Infections caused by susceptible bacterial strains and for surgical prophylaxis
Action: Semisynthetic cephalosporin
Contraindications and precautions
1. Use with caution in patients allergic to penicillin
2. Do not use in patient allergic to cephalosporins

CEFIZOX See CEFTIZOXIME

CEFONICID (Monocid)

Preparations: *Inj* 500 mg, 1 g vials
Adult dosage
1. Uncomplicated UTI: 500 mg qd IV/IM
2. Mild to moderate infections: 1 g qd IV/IM
3. Severe infections: 2 g qd IV/IM
4. Surgical prophylaxis: 1 g 1 hour preoperatively
NOTE: Decrease dosage in patients with impaired renal function
Indications: Infections caused by susceptible bacterial strains; surgical prophylaxis
Action: Semisynthetic cephalosporin; its bactericidal action results from inhibition of cell wall synthesis
Contraindications and precautions
1. Allergy to cephalosporins
2. Use with caution in patients allergic to penicillin

CEFOTAXIME (Claforan)

Preparations: *Inj* 1 g, 2 g vials
Adult dosage
1. Treatment of gonorrhea: 1 g IV single dose
2. Uncomplicated infections: 1 g IV/IM q12h
3. Moderate to severe infections: 1-2 g IV/IM q8h

4. Septicemia and other life-threatening infections: 2 g IV q4h
5. Prevention of postoperative infection: single 1 g IV/IM dose 30-90 min before start of surgery
NOTE: Decrease dosage in patients with impaired renal function

Indications: Infections caused by susceptible bacterial strains; surgical prophylaxis

Action: Semisynthetic cephalosporin; its bactericidal action results from inhibition of cell wall synthesis

Contraindications and precautions: Allergy to cephalosporins; use with caution in patients allergic to penicillin, and patients with a history of GI disease, particularly colitis

CEFOXITIN (Mefoxin)

Preparations: *Inj* 1 g, 2 g vials
Adult dosage
1. Treatment of infections: 1-2 g q6-8h IV to maximum of 12 g/day (2 g q4h)
2. Surgical prophylaxis: 2 g IV/IM 30 min before surgery then 2 g q6h for 24 hr (72 hr for prosthetic arthroplasty)
NOTE: Decrease dosage in patients with impaired renal function

Indications: Infections caused by susceptible organisms; surgical prophylaxis

Action: Semisynthetic cephalosporin; its bactericidal action results from inhibition of cell wall synthesis

Contraindications and precautions: Hypersensitivity to cephalosporins; use with caution in patients allergic to penicillin

CEFTAZIDIME (Fortaz)

Preparations: *Inj* 0.5, 1, 2 g vials
Adult dosage
1. Uncomplicated UTI: 250 mg IV/IM q12h
2. Complicated UTI: 500 mg-1 g IV/IM q8-12h
3. Uncomplicated pneumonia and mild skin infections: 500 mg-1 g q8h
4. Bone and joint infections: 2 g IV q12h
5. Meningitis, serious gynecologic and intraabdominal infections, and severe life-threatening infections: 2 g IV q8h
6. Pseudomonal lung infections in patients with cystic fibrosis: 30-50 mg/kg IV q8h, up to 6 g/day
7. Usual recommended dosage: 1 g IV/IM q8-12h
NOTE: Decrease dose in patients with impaired renal function

Indications: Infections caused by susceptible bacterial strains; useful in infections caused by *Pseudomonas* strains

Action: Semisynthetic cephalosporin; its bactericidal action results from inhibitions of cell wall synthesis

Contraindications and precautions: Hypersensitivity to cephalosporins; use with caution in patients allergic to penicillin

CEFTIZOXIME (Cefizox)

Preparations: *Inj* 1, 2 g vials
Adult dosage
1. Uncomplicated urinary tract infection: 500 mg q12h IM/IV
2. Uncomplicated infection in other sites: 1 g q8-12h IM/IV
3. Severe or refractory infections: 1 g q8h IM/IV or 2 g q8-12h IM/IV
4. Life threatening infections: 3-4 g q8h IV
   NOTE: Decrease dosage in patients with impaired renal function
Indications: Infections caused by susceptible bacterial organisms
Action: Semisynthetic cephalosporin; its bactericidal action results from inhibition of cell wall synthesis
Contraindications and precautions: Hypersensitivity to cephalosporins; use with caution in patients allergic to penicillin and in patients with a history of GI diseases (particularly colitis)

CEFUROXIME (Zinacef)

Preparations: *Inj* 750 mg, 1.5 g vials
Adult dosage: 750 mg-1.5 g q6-8h depending on the severity of infection
   NOTE: Decrease dosage in patients with renal impairment
Indications: Infections caused by susceptible bacterial organisms
Action: Semisynthetic cephalosporin; its bactericidal action results from inhibition of cell wall synthesis
Contraindications and precautions: Hypersensitivity to cephalosporins; use with caution in patients allergic to penicillin

CEPHALEXIN (Keflex)

Preparations: *Cap* 250, 500 mg; *suspension* 125, 250 mg/5 ml; *tab* 1 g
Adult dosage: 250 mg-1 g q6h depending on severity of infection
   NOTE: Decrease dosage in patients with renal impairment
Indications: Infections caused by susceptible bacterial organisms
Action: Semisynthetic cephalosporin; its bactericidal action results from inhibition of cell wall synthesis
Contraindications and precautions: Hypersensitivity to cephalosporins; use with caution in patients allergic to penicillin

CEPHALOTHIN (Keflin)

Preparations: *Inj* 1, 2, 4 g vials
Adult dosage: 500 mg-1 g IV/IM q4-6h depending on severity of infection
   NOTE: Decrease dosage in patients with impaired renal function
Indications: Infections caused by susceptible bacterial organisms
Action: Semisynthetic cephalosporin; its bactericidal action results from inhibition of cell wall synthesis
Contraindications and precautions: Hypersensitivity to cephalosporins; use with caution in patients allergic to penicillin

CEPHAPIRIN (Cefadyl)

Preparations: *Inj* 500 mg, 1, 2, 4 g vials
Adult dosage
1. Treatment of infections: 500 mg-1 g IV/IM q4-6h; may use doses up to 12 g/day in serious of life-threatening infections
2. Perioperative prophylaxis to prevent postoperative infections in potentially contaminated surgery: 1-2 g IM/IV 30 min-1 hr before start of surgery, 1-2 g during surgery, 1-2 g IM/IV q6h × 24h postoperatively
NOTE: Decrease dosage in patients with renal insufficiency
Indications: Treatment of infections caused by susceptible bacterial organisms
Action: Semisynthetic cephalosporin; its bactericidal action results from inhibition of cell wall synthesis
Contraindications and precautions: Hypersensitivity to cephalosporins; use with caution in patients with known allergy to penicillin

CEPHULAC See LACTULOSE

CHARCOAL, ACTIVATED

Preparations: Bottles containing 30 g of activated charcoal, USP, suspended in 4 oz of water
Adult dosage: 30-120 g; usually followed by the administration of a cathartic to hasten the elimination of charcoal-absorbed drugs
Indications: Drug overdose or poisoning

CHLORAL HYDRATE

Preparations: *Cap* 500 mg; *syrup* 500 mg/10 ml 1 g/10 ml; *inj* when reconstituted, each vial contains 100 mg/ml (1 g/10 ml)
Adult dosage
1. Usual hypnotic dose: 500 mg-1 g, 15-30 min before bedtime or 30 min before surgery
2. Usual sedative dose: 250 mg tid after meals
Indications: Nocturnal sedation; preoperative sedative
Action: Sedative and hypnotic agent; mechanism of action is undertermined
Contraindications and precautions
1. Marked hepatic or renal impairment, severe cardiac disease
2. Do not use PO forms in patients with gastritis
3. Use with caution in patients receiving oral anticoagulants (potentiation of anticoagulant effect when chloral hydrate is stopped)
4. Abrupt withdrawal of this drug may result in delirium
5. Concomitant or recent ingestion of ethanol or other CNS depressants is contraindicated

CHLORAMPHENICOL (Chloromycetin)

Preparations: *Cap* 250 mg; *oral suspension* 30 mg/ml; *inj* when reconstituted, each vial contains 100 mg/ml (1 g/10 ml)
Adult dosage: IV/PO: 50 mg/kg/day divided in four doses at 6h intervals
NOTE: Decrease dosage in patients with impaired renal or hepatic function

Indications: Serious infections caused by organisms susceptible to its anti-microbial effects
Action: Broad-spectrum antibiotic; it inhibits protein synthesis by binding the 50 S ribosomal subunit
Contraindications and precautions
1. Treatment of trivial infections, lactation, preexisting bone marrow suppression
2. History of hypersensitivity or toxic reaction to chloramphenicol
3. Use with caution in patients with liver disease or impaired renal function
4. Avoid concomitant use of other drugs that may suppress bone marrow
5. Obtain baseline blood studies before starting therapy, and monitor CBC and platelet count q2d during therapy

CHLORDIAZEPOXIDE (Librium)

Preparations: *Cap* 5, 10, 25 mg; *tab* 5, 10, 25 mg; *inj* 100 mg/5 ml ampul
Adult dosage
1. Relief of mild and moderate anxiety disorders: PO 5-10 mg tid or qid
2. Relief of severe anxiety disorders: PO 20-25 mg tid or qid; IM/IV: 50-100 mg initially, then 25-50 mg tid or qid prn
3. Withdrawal symptoms of acute alcoholism: 50-100 mg IM/IV initially, repeat in 2-4h if necessary
4. Preoperative apprehension and anxiety: IM 50-100 mg 1 hr before surgery
   NOTE: Decrease dosage in elderly or debilitated patients
   NOTE: IV injection should be given slowly over 1 min
Indications: Management of anxiety disorders, short-term relief of symptoms of anxiety, withdrawal symptoms of acute alcoholism, preoperative apprehension and anxiety
Action: Benzodiazepine; exact mechanism of action is unknown, but it is believed to act on the limbic system of the brain
Contraindications and precautions
1. Do not use concomitantly with ethanol or other CNS depressants
2. Abrupt discontinuation can result in withdrawal symptoms
3. Do not use in patients in shock or comatose states
4. Use with caution in patients with renal or hepatic impairment, patients with a history of porphyria (possible exacerbation of symptoms)
5. Concomitant use of other psychotropic agents is not recommended

CHLOROMYCETIN See CHLORAMPHENICOL

CHLOROTHIAZIDE (Diuril)

Preparations: *Tab* 250, 500 mg; *suspension* 250 mg/5 ml; *inj* 0.5 g vial
Adult dosage
1. Edema states: 0.5-1 g qd-bid PO/IV; use smallest effective IV dosage (some patients respond well to alternate day therapy)
2. Hypertension: 0.5-1 g/day or a single or divided dose PO/IV (use smallest effective IV dosage; adjust dose according to blood pressure)

Indications: Hypertension, edema states
Action: Thiazide diuretic
Contraindications and precautions
1. Anuria, hypersensitivity to sulfanomide-derived drugs
2. Use with caution in patients with severe liver disease or renal disease
3. Concomitant use of lithium is not recommended (decreased renal clearance of lithium)
4. Patients should have periodic determinations of serum electrolytes
5. Use with caution in patients with SLE (exacerbation of lupus is possible)

CHLORPROMAZINE (Thorazine)

Preparations: *Tab* 10, 25, 50, 100, 200 mg; *syrup* 10 mg/5 ml; *inj* 25 mg/ml; *supp* 25, 100 mg
Adult dosage
1. Excessive anxiety, tension and agitation: 10-25 mg PO tid (in severe cases may increase dosage by 20-50 mg semiweekly until patient becomes calm and cooperative)
2. Prompt control of severe symptoms: 25 mg IM (if necessary repeat in 1 hr; subsequent doses should be oral, 25 mg to 50 mg tid)
3. Nausea and vomiting: 10-25 mg PO q4-6h prn; 25 mg IM, if no hypotension occurs, give 25-50 mg IM q3-4h prn until the vomiting stops, then switch to PO dosage; 100 mg supp PR q6-8h
4. Intractable hiccups: 25-50 mg PO tid or qid; if symptoms persist, give 25-50 mg IM
Indications: Management of manifestations of psychotic disorders, control of nausea and vomiting, relief of intractable hiccups
Action: Phenothiazine neuroleptic; the principal pharmacologic actions are psychotropic but it also exerts sedative and antiemetic activity
Contraindications and precautions
1. Comatose states, presence of large amounts of CNS depressants, bone marrow depression, Reye's syndrome, hypersensitivity to phenothiazines
2. Use with caution in patients with cardiovascular disease, COPD, severe asthma, patients exposed to extreme heat, organophosphorus insecticides, and patients receiving atropine or related drugs

CHLORPROPAMIDE (Diabinese)

Preparations: *Tab* 100, 250 mg
Adult dosage: Initial 100-250 mg qd; most patients do not require more than 250 mg/day; maximum daily dose is 750 mg
Indications: Hyperglycemia of non-insulin-dependent diabetes mellitus not adequately controlled with diet alone
Action: Sulfonylurea; it stimulates pancreatic insulin secretion (it is postulated that it enhances the postreceptor action of insulin and the number of insulin receptors)

Contraindications and precautions
1. Known hypersensitivity to the drug, diabetic ketoacidosis
2. Administration of oral hypoglycemic agents has been reported to increase the risk of cardiovascular mortality
3. Hypoglycemic effect of sulfonylureas can be potentiated by various drugs (coumarins, nonsteroidal antiinflammatory agents, salicylates); other drugs tend to produce hyperglycemia (diuretics, corticosteroids, phenytoin)

CHLORTHALIDONE (Hygroton)

Preparations: *Tab* 25, 50, 100 mg
Adult dosage
1. Hypertension: Initial dose is 25 mg qd; daily dosage range in 25-100 mg qd
2. Edema: Initial dose is 50-100 mg qd or 100 mg qod; daily dosage range is 50-200 mg qd or qod

Indications: Hypertension, edema states
Action: Thiazide diuretic
Contraindications and precautions
1. Anuria, hypersensitivity to sulfonamide-derived drugs
2. Use with caution in patients with impaired hepatic or renal function or SLE (exacerbation of lupus is possible)
3. Concomitant use of lithium is not recommended (decreased renal clearance of lithium)
4. Patients should have periodic determinations of serum electrolytes

CIMETIDINE (Tagamet)

Preparations: *Tab* 200, 300, 400, 800 mg; *liquid* 300 mg/5 ml syrup; *IV* 300 mg/2 ml vial or prefilled syringe
Adult dosage
1. Active duodenal ulcer:
   a. PO: 300 mg qid with meals and hs, 400 mg bid, or 800 mg qhs
   b. IV: 300 mg q6h (given over at least 2 min)
2. Prophylaxis of recurrent duodenal ulcer: 400 mg PO qhs
3. Active benign gastric ulcer: 300 mg PO qid or IV q6h (given over at least 2 min)
4. Pathologic hypersecretory conditions: 300 mg PO qid or IV q6h; some patients may require higher dosage (do not exceed 2400 mg/day)
   NOTE: Decrease dosage in patients with renal impairment

Indications: Short-term treatment of active duodenal ulcer; prophylactic use in duodenal ulcer patients to prevent ulcer recurrence; treatment of pathologic hypersecretory conditions (Zollinger-Ellison syndrome, multiple endocrine adenomas, systemic mastocytosis); short-term treatment of active benign gastric ulcer
Action: Histamine H_2 receptor antagonist; it inhibits gastric acid secretion
Contraindications
1. Nursing mothers (cimetidine is excreted in breast milk)
2. Use with caution in elderly patients and in patients with renal or hepatic impairment

3. Patients receiving warfarin-type anticoagulants, theophylline, phenytoin, lidocaine, propranolol, diazepam, and chlordiazepoxide may have increasing blood levels of these drugs from reduced hepatic metabolism

CLAFORAN See CEFOTAXIME

CLEOCIN See CLINDAMYCIN

CLINDAMYCIN (Cleocin)

Preparations: *Cap* 75, 150 mg; *inj* 150 mg/ml (2, 4, 6 mg vial); *granules* (pediatric) 75 mg/5 ml

Adult dosage

1. Serious infections: 150-300 mg PO q6h or 600-1200 mg/day IM/IV divided in two to four equal doses
2. More severe infections: 300-450 mg PO q6h or 1200-1700 mg/day IM/IV divided in two to four equal doses
3. Life threatening situations: Total daily doses up to 4800 mg may be used

NOTE: Decrease dosage in patients with severe renal or hepatic disease

Indications: Serious infections caused by susceptible bacterial organisms

Action: It inhibits bacterial protein synthesis by binding to the 50 S ribosomal subunit

Contraindications and precautions

1. Hypersensitivity to clindamycin or lincomycin
2. Use with caution in patients with a history of GI disease (particularly colitis), atopic individuals, patients receiving neuromuscular blocking drugs, patients with ASA hypersensitivity

CLINORIL See SULINDAC

CLONIDINE (Catapres)

Preparations: *Tab* 0.1, 0.2, 0.3 mg; *transdermal patches* 3.5 cm^2 (0.1 mg/ d), 7 cm^2 (0.2 mg/d), 10.5 cm^2 (0.3 mg/d)

Adult dosage

1. PO: 0.1 mg bid initially; usual dosage range is 0.2-0.8 mg/day; maximum daily dose is 2.4 mg
   a. Clonidine loading can be used to rapidly decrease blood pressure in severely hypertensive patients; loading dose is 0.2 mg, followed by 0.1 mg/hour (up to total dose of 0.6 mg)
   b. Blood pressure should be monitored q15min; when a satisfactory drop in blood pressure has been achieved, start clonidine 0.1 mg q8-12h and add a diuretic agent to decrease renal sodium and water retention
2. Transdermal: 3.5 cm^2 patch applied once weekly initially

Indications: Treatment of hypertension

Action: Central α-adrenergic receptor stimulant

Contraindications and precautions

1. Use with caution in patients with severe coronary insufficiency, recent MI, cerebrovascular disease, chronic renal failure
2. When discontinuing clonidine, the dose should be reduced gradually over several days to avoid significant rebound hypertension

CLORAZEPATE (Tranxene)

Preparations: *Cap* 3.75, 7.5, 15 mg; *tab* 3.75, 7.5 mg, 15 mg; 22.5 mg (Tranxene-SD), 11.25 mg (Tranxene-SD half-strength)

Adult dosage
1. For symptomatic relief of anxiety the usual daily dose is 30 mg in divided doses; Tranxene-SD and Tranxene-SD half-strength may be administered as a single dose
2. Dosage range is 15-60 mg/day
3. In elderly or debilitated patients initiate with 7.5-15 mg/day in divided doses

Indications: Management of anxiety disorders; adjunctive therapy in the management of partial seizures; symptomatic relief of acute alcohol withdrawal

Action: Benzodiazepine

Contraindications and precautions
1. Acute narrow-angle glaucoma, depressive neuroses, psychotic reactions
2. Use with caution in patients with impaired renal or hepatic function
3. Concomitant use of alcohol or other CNS depressants is contraindicated

CLOTRIMAZOLE (Mycelex)

Preparations: Topical cream 1% (15, 30, 45 g tubes); *topical solution* 1% (10, 30 ml bottles); *troche* 10 mg clotrimazole; *vaginal cream* (Mycelex-G) 1% 50 mg/applicatorful, 45, 90 g tubes; *vaginal tab* (Mycelex-G) 100, 500 mg

Adult dosage
1. Treatment of fungal skin infections: apply topical cream or solution to affected area bid
2. Prevention of oropharyngeal candidiasis: troche (10 mg) 5 times/day
3. Vulvovaginal candidiasis:
   a. 100 mg vaginal tab qd × 7 days; nonpregnant women may use 2 tabs bid × 3 days
   b. 500 mg vaginal tab inserted intravaginally 1 time only
   c. Apply vaginal cream intravaginally, one applicatorful qhs × 7-14 days

Indications: *Candida* or other dermatophyte skin infections; vulvovaginal candidiasis; prevention and treatment of oropharyngeal candidiasis

Contraindications: Ophthalmic use is contraindicated

COGENTIN See BENZTROPINE MESYLATE

COLACE See DIOCTYL SODIUM SULFOSUCCINATE

COLCHICINE

Preparations: *Tab* 0.5, 0.6 mg; *granules* 0.5 mg; *inj* 0.5 mg/ml

Adult dosage
1. Treatment of acute gout: *PO* 0.5-1.2 mg initially, then 0.5-0.6 mg q1-3h until the pain is relieved (maximum total dose is 8-10 mg); *IV* 1-2 mg diluted in 20 ml of 0.9 NaCl initially; additional doses are 0.5 mg q6-12h (maximum 24h dose is 4 mg)

NOTE: IV administration must be slow, and care must be taken to avoid extravasation

2. Prophylaxis of gout: 0.6 mg PO bid

Indications: Treatment and prophylaxis of gout

Action: Antiinflammatory; it impairs leukocyte chemotaxis and synovial cell phagocytosis of urate crystals

Contraindications and precautions: Use with caution in patients with GI, hepatic, renal, or cardiac disease and in elderly or debilitated patients

COMPAZINE See PROCHLORPERAZINE

CONJUGATED ESTROGEN TABLETS See ESTROGENIC SUBSTANCES, CONJUGATED

COUMADIN See WARFARIN

CYCLOBENZAPRINE (Flexeril)

Preparations: *Tab* 10 mg

Adult dosage: Usual dosage is 10 mg PO tid; maximum daily dosage is 60 mg/day

Indications: Relief of spasm associated with acute painful musculoskeletal conditions; should not be used continuously for longer than 3 weeks

Action: Relief of muscle spasm by reduction of tonic somatic motor activity influencing both γ and α motor systems

Contraindications and precautions
1. Concomitant use of MAO inhibitors or within 14 days after their discontinuation; concomitant use of tricyclic antidepressants, use during acute recovery phase of MI,
2. Hyperthyroidism, CHF, dysrhythmias, heart block, conduction disturbances
3. Cyclobenzaprine may enhance the effects of barbiturates, alcohol, and other CNS depressants
4. Use with caution in patients with a history of urinary retention, angle-closure glaucoma, increased intraocular pressure and in patients taking anticholinergic medications

DALMANE See FLURAZEPAM

DECADRON See DEXAMETHASONE

DEMEROL See MEPERIDINE

DEXAMETHASONE (Decadron)

Preparations: *Tab* 0.25, 0.5, 0.75, 1.5, 4, 6 mg; *elixir* 0.5 mg/5 ml; *inj* 4, 10, 24 mg/ml

Adult dosage
1. Cerebral edema: 10 mg IV initially, followed by 4 mg IV/IM q6h
2. Acute allergic disorders:
   Day 1: 5-8 mg IM
   Days 2 and 3: 3 mg PO in divided doses (1.5 mg PO bid)
   Day 4: 1.5 mg PO in divided doses (0.75 mg PO bid)
   Days 5 and 6: 0.75 mg PO qd
   Day 7: No treatment

3. Intraarticular, intralesional or soft tissue injection: Usual dose is 0.2-6 mg

Indications: Cerebral edema, adrenocortical insufficiency, collagen-vascular diseases (SLE, acute rheumatic arthritis), allergic states (contact dermatitis, bronchial asthma), diagnosis of Cushing's syndrome, hematologic disorders (ITP, acquired hemolytic anemias), inflammatory bowel disease, palliative management of leukemias, lymphomas, nephrotic syndrome (from SLE or idiopathic type), dermatologic disease (severe erythema multiforme, pemphigus), respiratory diseases (symptomatic sarcoidosis, berylliosis)

Action: Synthetic adrenocortical steroid

Contraindication and precautions
1. Systemic fungal infections, hypersensitivity to any of its components (sodium bisulfite)
2. Use with caution in patients with ocular herpes simplex
3. Immunization procedures should not be undertaken in patients receiving corticosteroids

DIABETA See **GLYBURIDE**

DIABINESE See **CHLORPROPAMIDE**

DIAMOX See **ACETAZOLAMIDE**

DIAZEPAM (Valium)

Preparations: *Tab* 2, 5, 10 mg; *inj* 5 mg/ml

Adult dosage
1. Anxiety disorders and relief of symptoms of anxiety: 2-10 mg PO bid to qid; 2-10 mg IV, may repeat in 3-4 hr if necessary
2. Acute alcohol withdrawal: 10 mg PO tid or qid during initial 24 h, then decrease dose to 5 mg tid or qid; 10 mg IV/IM initially, then 5-10 mg in 3-4 hr if necessary
3. Endoscopic procedures: 2-10 mg IV immediately before procedure, or 5-10 mg IM 30 min before procedure
4. Muscle spasm: 2-10 mg PO tid or qid; 5-10 mg IM/IV initially, then 5-10 mg in 3-4 hr if necessary (larger doses may be required for tetanus)
5. Preoperative: 5-15 mg IV 5-10 min before procedure
6. Status epilepticus: 5-10 mg IV initially; may repeat in 10-15 min intervals up to total maximum dose of 30 mg

NOTE: Use lower doses in elderly and debilitated patients

Indications: Management of anxiety disorders or short-term relief of the symptoms of anxiety, acute alcohol withdrawal, muscle spasm, status epilepticus

Action: Benzodiazepine

Contraindications and precautions: Acute narrow-angle glaucoma, concomitant ingestion of alcohol or other CNS depressants

DIGOXIN (Lanoxin)

Preparations: *Tab* 0.125, 0.25, 0.5 mg; *elixir* 0.05 mg/ml; *inj* 0.1, 0.25 mg/ml; *cap* 0.05, 0.1, 0.2 mg (Lanoxicaps)

Adult dosage
1. Loading dose 10-15 μg/kg IV/PO in divided doses over 12-24 hr (e.g., 0.5 mg initially then 0.25 mg q6h × 4 doses)
2. Maintenance dosage: range is 0.125-0.5 mg/day; maintenance dosage should be monitored by clinical response and serum digoxin levels; however, serum levels are greatly influenced by other factors (e.g., hypokalemia) and therefore do not consistently reflect therapeutic response or toxicity

NOTE: Dosage must be reduced in patients with impaired renal function

NOTE: Concomitant use of quinidine and/or verapamil increases serum digoxin levels

NOTE: Digoxin requirements are reduced in patients with hypothyroidism

Indications: Low output CHF, atrial fibrillation, atrial flutter, paroxysmal atrial tachycardia (PAT)

Action: Positive inotropic effect, negative chronotropic effect, decreased conduction velocity through the AV node

Contraindications and precautions
1. Ventricular fibrillation, second-or third-degree AV block (in absence of mechanical pacemaker), idiopathic hypertrophic subaortic stenosis (IHSS) (use of digoxin may result in worsening of outflow obstruction)
2. Patients with Wolff-Parkinson-White (WPW) syndrome and atrial fibrillation (use of digoxin can result in enhanced transmission of impulses through accessory pathway)
3. Sick sinus node disease (digoxin may worsen sinus bradycardia or sinoatrial block)
4. Hypokalemia, hypomagnesemia, and hypercalcemia predispose to digoxin toxicity
5. Patients with atrial dysrhythmias secondary to hyperthyroidism, heart failure from amyloid heart disease, or constrictive cardiomyopathies respond poorly to digoxin

DILANTIN See PHENYTOIN

DILAUDID See HYDROMORPHONE HYDROCHLORIDE

DILTIAZEM (Cardizem)

Preparations: *tab* 30, 60 mg

Adult dosage: 30 mg qid initially; dosage range is 180-360 mg/day in 3-4 divided doses

Indications: Angina pectoris resulting from coronary artery spasm, angina pectoris caused by atherosclerotic coronary artery disease

Action: Calcium channel antagonist

Contraindications and precautions
1. Sick sinus syndrome (except in the presence of a functioning pacemaker), hypotension, second- or third-degree AV block
2. Use with caution in patients with impaired renal or hepatic function
3. Concomitant use of diltiazem, β-blockers, or digitalis may result in additive effects on cardiac conduction

DIOCTYL SODIUM SULFOSUCCINATE (Colace)

Preparations: *Cap* 50, 100 mg; *syrup* 20 mg/5 ml
Adult dosage: 50-200 mg qd
Indications: Constipation because of hard stools, painful anorectal conditions, cardiac or other conditions in which ease of defecation is desirable
Action: Stool softener; surface-active agent
Contraindications and precautions: None

DIPHENHYDRAMINE (Benadryl)

Preparations: *Cap* 25, 50 mg; *elixir* 12.5 mg/5 ml; *inj* 10, 50 mg/ml
Adult dosage
  1. PO: 25-50 mg tid or qid; for motion sickness give first dose 30 min before exposure to motion
  2. IV: 10-50 mg IM/IV tid or qid; maximum total daily dosage is 400 mg
Indications: Allergic reactions (urticaria, anaphylaxis), allergic rhinitis, motion sickness, parkinsonism, nighttime sleep aid
Action: Antihistamine with anticholinergic and sedative effects
Contraindications and precautions
  1. Avoid concomitant use of MAO inhibitors, alcohol, or other CNS depressants
  2. Use with caution in elderly patients and patients with narrow-angle glaucoma, stenotic peptic ulcer, pyloroduodenal obstruction, symptomatic prostatic hypertrophy, bladder neck obstruction, increased intraocular pressure, hypertension, cardiovascular disease, bronchial asthma, and hyperthyroidism

DIPHENOXYLATE WITH ATROPINE (Lomotil)

Preparations: *Tab* 2.5 mg of diphenoxylate and 0.025 mg of atropine; *liquid* each 5 ml contains 2.5 mg of diphenoxylate and 0.025 mg of atropine
Adult dosage: Two tabs qid or 10 ml (2 regular tsp) qid until initial control of diarrhea is achieved, then decrease dosage to meet individual requirements
Indications: Adjunctive therapy in the management of diarrhea
Action: Antidiarrheal action from increased contact of the intraluminal contents with the intestinal mucosa (secondary to enhanced intestinal segmentation)
Contraindications and precautions
  1. Hypersensitivity to diphenoxylate or atropine, obstructive jaundice, diarrhea associated with pseudomembranous enterocolitis
  2. Correct severe dehydration and electrolyte imbalance before starting Lomotil
  3. Use with caution in patients with ulcerative colitis
  4. May potentiate the action of alcohol, tranquilizers, and barbiturates
  5. Avoid concomitant use of MAO inhibitors
  6. Avoid use in any patient with contraindications to use of atropine

DIPYRIDAMOLE (Persantine)

Preparations: *Tab* 25, 50, 75 mg
Adult dosage: 50 mg tid or 75 mg bid, taken at least 1 hr before meals

Indications: Adjunct to coumarin anticoagulants to prevent postoperative thromboembolic complications of cardiac valve replacement

Contraindications and precautions: Use with caution in patients with hypotension (may produce peripheral vasodilation)

DISOPYRAMIDE PHOSPHATE (Norpace)

Preparations: *Cap* 100, 150 mg, sustained release cap (Norpace CR) 100, 150 mg

Adult dosage

1. Loading dose: 300-400 mg; maintenance dosage: 150 mg q6h (100 mg q6h if body weight is <50 kg), 300 mg q12h (Norpace CR)
2. Avoid loading dose in patients with possible cardiac decompensation or cardiomyopathy and decrease maintenance dose to 100 mg q6-8h
3. Decrease dosage in hepatic or renal insufficiency

Indications: Suppression and prevention of recurrence of: unifocal or multifocal premature (ectopic) ventricular contractions (PVC), paired PVC or episodes of ventricular tachycardia

Action: Type I antidysrhythmic agent

Contraindications and precautions

1. Cardiogenic shock, congenital Q-T prolongation, preexisting second- or third-degree AV block (in absence of pacemaker), glaucoma, myasthenia gravis, urinary retention
2. Do not use in patients with hypotension or CHF (unless secondary to cardiac dysrhythmia)
3. Discontinue use if patient develops QT prolongation >25%, QRS widening >25%, heart block > first-degree (decrease dosage if patient develops first-degree heart block), hypoglycemia secondary to disopyramide
4. Concomitant use of other type I antidysrhythmic agents or propranolol can result in serious negative inotropic effects and may severely prolong conduction
5. Use with caution in patients with myocarditis, cardiomyopathy, WPW syndrome, sick sinus syndrome, or bundle branch block
6. Digitalize patients with atrial flutter or fibrillation before administering disopyramide

DIURIL See CHLOROTHIAZIDE

DIULO See METOLAZONE

DOBUTAMINE (Dobutrex)

Preparations: *Vial* 250 mg/20 ml

Adult dosage: Rate of infusion needed to increase cardiac output usually ranges from 2.5-10 µg/kg/min (Table 21-1); the starting dose is 1-2 µg/kg/minute

Indications: Inotropic support in short-term treatment of cardiac decompensation caused by depressed contractility (secondary to organic heart disease or cardiac surgical procedures)

Continued on p. 508.

Table 21-1 Dobutamine infusion (dosage = μg Dobutrex/kg/min)

Flow Rate (μgtt/min)	Quantity of Dobutrex* (μg/min)†	Body Weight															
		(lb) 77 (kg) 35	88 40	99 45	110 50	121 55	132 60	145 65	154 70	165 75	176 80	187 85	198 90	209 95	220 100	231 105	242 110
2	66.7	1.9	1.7	1.5	1.3	1.2	1.1	1.0	1.0	0.88	0.83	0.78	0.74	0.70	0.67	0.63	0.60
3	100	2.9	2.5	2.2	2.0	1.8	1.7	1.5	1.4	1.3	1.3	1.2	1.1	1.1	1.0	1.0	0.90
4	133.3	3.8	3.3	3.0	2.7	2.4	2.2	2.1	1.9	1.8	1.7	1.6	1.5	1.4	1.3	1.3	1.2
5	166.7	4.8	4.2	3.7	3.3	3.0	2.8	2.6	2.4	2.2	2.1	2.0	1.9	1.8	1.7	1.6	1.5
6	200	5.7	5.0	4.4	4.0	3.6	3.3	3.1	2.9	2.7	2.5	2.4	2.2	2.1	2.0	1.9	1.8
7	233.3	6.7	5.8	5.2	4.7	4.2	3.9	3.6	3.3	3.1	2.9	2.7	2.6	2.5	2.3	2.2	2.1
8	266.7	7.6	6.7	5.9	5.3	4.9	4.5	4.1	3.8	3.6	3.3	3.1	3.0	2.8	2.7	2.5	2.4
9	300	8.6	7.5	6.7	6.0	5.5	5.0	4.6	4.3	4.0	3.8	3.5	3.3	3.2	3.0	2.9	2.7
10	333.3	9.5	8.3	7.4	6.7	6.1	5.6	5.1	4.8	4.4	4.2	3.9	3.7	3.5	3.3	3.2	3.0

12	400	11.4	10.0	8.9	8.0	7.3	6.7	6.2	5.7	5.3	5.0	4.7	4.4	4.2	4.0	3.8	3.6
14	466.7	13.3	11.7	10.4	9.3	8.5	7.8	7.2	6.7	6.2	5.8	5.5	5.2	4.9	4.7	4.4	4.2
16	533.3	15.2	13.3	11.9	10.7	9.7	8.9	8.2	7.6	7.1	6.7	6.3	5.9	5.6	5.3	5.1	4.9
18	600	17.1	15.0	13.3	12.0	10.9	10.0	9.2	8.6	8.0	7.5	7.1	6.7	6.3	6.0	5.7	5.5
20	667	19.1	16.7	14.8	13.3	12.1	11.1	10.3	9.5	8.9	8.3	7.8	7.4	7.0	6.7	6.3	6.1
22	733	21.0	18.3	16.3	14.7	13.3	12.2	11.3	10.5	9.8	9.2	8.6	8.1	7.7	7.3	7.0	6.7
24	800	22.9	20.0	17.8	16.0	14.5	13.3	12.3	11.4	10.7	10.0	9.4	8.9	8.4	8.0	7.6	7.3
26	867	24.8	21.7	19.3	17.3	15.8	14.4	13.3	12.4	11.6	10.8	10.2	9.6	9.1	8.7	8.3	7.9
28	933	26.7	23.3	20.7	18.7	17.0	15.6	14.4	13.3	12.4	11.7	11.0	10.4	9.8	9.3	8.9	8.5
30	1000	28.6	25.0	22.2	20.0	18.2	16.7	15.4	14.3	13.3	12.5	11.8	11.1	10.5	10.0	9.5	9.1

From Purcell, J.A.: Am. J. Nurs. 82(6):965, 1982.

*Dobutamine (Dobutrex) solution 2,000 µg/ml (1,000 mg Dobutrex/500 ml or 500 mg Dobutrex/250 ml).

†Based on 60 µgtt/ml, each µgtt of this solution contains 33.3 µg Dobutrex.

Table 21-2　Dopamine infusion (dosage = μg dopamine/kg/min)

Flow Rate (μgtt/min)	Quantity of Dopamine* (μg/min)†	Body Weight															
		(lb) 77	88	99	110	121	132	143	154	165	176	187	198	209	220	231	242
		(kg) 35	40	45	50	55	60	65	70	75	80	85	90	95	100	105	110
5	133	3.8	3.4	2.9	2.6	2.4	2.2	2.0	1.9	1.8	1.6	1.6	1.5	1.4	1.3	1.3	1.2
10	267	7.6	6.7	5.9	5.3	4.9	4.5	4.1	3.8	3.6	3.3	3.1	3.0	2.8	2.7	2.5	2.4
15	400	11	10	8.9	8.0	7.3	6.6	6.1	5.7	5.3	5.0	4.7	4.4	4.2	4.0	3.8	3.6
20	533	15	13	12	11	9.7	8.9	8.2	7.6	7.1	6.7	6.3	5.9	5.6	5.3	5.1	4.9
25	667	19	17	15	13	12	11	10	9.5	8.9	8.4	7.8	7.4	7.0	6.6	6.3	6.0
30	800	23	20	18	16	15	13	12	11	11	10	9.4	8.9	8.4	8.0	7.6	7.3
35	933	27	23	21	19	17	16	14	13	12	12	11	10	9.8	9.3	8.9	8.5
40	1067	31	27	24	21	19	18	16	15	14	13	13	12	11	11	10	9.7
45	1200	34	30	27	24	22	20	18	17	16	15	14	13	13	12	11	11
50	1333	38	33	30	27	24	22	21	19	18	17	16	15	14	13	13	12

55	1467	13	14	15	15	16	17	18	20	21	23	24	27	29	33	37	42
60	1600	15	15	16	17	18	19	20	21	23	25	27	29	32	36	40	46
65	1733	16	17	17	18	19	20	22	23	25	27	29	32	35	39	43	50
70	1867	17	18	19	20	21	22	23	25	27	29	31	34	37	42	47	53
75	2000	18	19	20	21	22	24	25	27	29	31	33	36	40	45	50	57
80	2133	19	20	21	23	24	25	27	28	31	33	36	39	43	47	53	61
85	2267	21	22	23	24	25	27	28	30	32	35	38	41	45	50	57	65
90	2400	22	23	24	25	27	28	30	32	34	37	40	44	48	53	60	69
95	2533	23	24	25	27	28	29	32	34	36	39	42	46	51	56	63	72
100	2667	24	25	27	28	30	31	33	36	38	41	45	49	53	59	67	76

From Purcell, J.A.: Am. J. Nurs. 82(6):965, 1982.

*Dopamine solution (Intropin) 1,600 µg/ml (800 mg Intropin/500 ml or 400 mg Intropin/250 ml).

†Based on 60 µgtt/ml, each µgtt of this solution contains 26.7 µg Dopamine.

Action: Direct-acting inotropic agent; primary activity results from stimulation of β receptors of heart. Refer to Fig. 11-2 for a graphic representation of dobutamine's effects on systemic vascular resistance, renal blood flow, pulmonary capillary wedge pressure, and cardiac output.

Contraindications and precautions

1. Idiopathic hypertrophic subaortic stenosis (IHSS)
2. Correct hypovolemia before starting dobutamine
3. Dobutamine may be ineffective and peripheral vascular resistance may increase if patient has recently received a β-blocking agent

DOBUTREX See **DOBUTAMINE**

DOPAMINE (Intropin)

Preparations: *Ampul* 200 mg/5 ml; *syringe* 200, 400, 800 mg

Adult dosage

1. Initial 2-5 μg/kg/min; increase gradually until hemodynamic response is obtained, generally up to a maximum of 50 μg/kg/minute
2. Constantly evaluate patient's blood pressure, volume status, myocardial contractability, peripheral perfusion, and note development of new dysrhythmias
3. Use decreased dosage in patients who have been receiving MAO inhibitors

Indications: Shock syndrome as a result of MI, endotoxins, trauma, open heart surgery, renal failure, chronic cardiac decompensation

Action: Inotropic agent (refer to Fig. 11-2 for a graphic representation of the effects of dopamine on systemic vascular resistance, renal blood flow, pulmonary capillary wedge pressure, and cardiac output)

Contraindications and precautions: Pheochromocytoma, uncorrected hypovolemia, tachydysrhythmias, or ventricular fibrillation

DULCOLAX See **BISACODYL**

DURICEF See **CEFADROXIL**

EDECRIN See **ETHACRYNIC ACID**

ELAVIL See **AMITRIPTYLINE**

ENAPRIL (Vasotec)

Preparations: *Tab* 5, 10, 20 mg

Adult dosage: Initially 5 mg daily; use 2.5 mg daily in patients taking diuretics or with renal Cr Cl <30 ml/min; usual dosage range is 10-40 mg daily in single or divided doses

Indications: Hypertension

Action: Angiotensin-converting enzyme inhibitor

Contraindications and precautions

1. Use with caution in patients with impaired renal function or renal artery stenosis
2. Discontinue product immediately if laryngeal edema or angioedema occurs

EPINEPHRINE (Adrenalin)

Preparations: *Ampul* 1 mg/ml (1:1000)
Adult dosage
1. SC/IM for bronchial asthma and allergic reactions: 0.2-1 mg
2. IV/Intracardiac for cardiac resuscitation: 0.5 ml (0.5 mg) diluted to 10 ml with sodium chloride
3. For use with local anesthetics: Concentration should be 1:100,000 (0.01 mg/ml) to 1:20,000 (0.05 mg/ml)

Indications: Bronchospasm, hypersensitivity reactions, prolongation of action of infiltration anesthetics, cardiac resuscitation
Action: Sympathomimetic; it acts on both α and β-receptors (most potent α receptor activator)
Contraindications and precautions
1. Narrow-angle glaucoma, shock, organic brain damage, use during anesthesia with halogenated hydrocarbons or cyclopropane, labor, cardiac dilation, coronary insufficiency
2. Do not use with local anesthesia in fingers and toes (vasoconstriction may cause necrosis)
3. Use with caution in patients receiving digitalis or other drugs that sensitize the heart to dysrhythmias, antihistamines, tricyclic antidepressants, patients with cardiovascular disease, hypertension, elderly patients, diabetics, patients with hyperthyroidism

ERGOTAMINE TARTRATE (Cafergot)

Preparations: *Tab* 1 mg ergotamine and 100 mg caffeine; *Supp* 2 mg of ergotamine and 100 mg caffeine
Adult dosage
1. PO: 2 tabs at beginning of vascular headache, then 1 tab q30min prn (maximum of 6 tabs/attack, 10 tabs/week)
2. PR: 1 supp at beginning of vascular headache, then 1 additional supp after 1 hr if needed (maximum of 2 supp/attack, 5 supp/week)

Indications: Prevention or abortion of vascular headache (migraine, migraine variants)
Action: α-adrenergic blocking agent; it directly stimulates smooth muscle of peripheral and cranial vessels
Contraindications and precautions: Hypertension, coronary artery disease, sepsis, peripheral vascular disease, impaired renal or hepatic function, hypersensitivity to any of its components

ERYTHROMYCIN

Preparations: *Enteric-coated tab* (E-Mycin) 250, 333 mg; erythromycin lactobionate (Erythrocin) 500, 1000 mg vial; erythromycin ethyl succinate (EES) *Chewable tab* 200 mg; *tab* 400 mg; *granules* 200 mg/5 ml; *drops* 100 mg/2.5 ml; *liquid* 200, 400 mg/5 ml; *cap* (ERYC) 125,250 mg
Adult dosage
1. Erythromycin ethyl succinate (EES) 400 mg PO q6h (maximum of 4 g/day)
2. Enteric-coated tablets (E-Mycin) 250-500 mg PO q6h (maximum of 4 g/day)

3. Erythromycin lactobionate (Erythrocyn) 15-20 mg/kg/day in four divided doses (maximum of 4 g/day)
4. Erythromycin cap (ERYC) 250 mg q6h

Indications: Infections caused by susceptible bacterial organisms

Action: Bacteriostatic macrolide antibiotic; it inhibits protein synthesis by binding to the 50 S ribosomal subunit

Contraindications and precautions

1. Use with caution in patients with hepatic insufficiency
2. Increase in serum theophylline levels and prothrombin time may be seen in patients receiving concomitant theophylline or warfarin

ESKALITH See LITHIUM CARBONATE

ESTROGENIC SUBSTANCES, CONJUGATED (Premarin)

Preparations: *Tab* 0.3, 0.625, 0.9, 1.25, 2.5 mg; *vaginal cream* 0.625 mg conjugated estrogens/g; each tube contains 42.5 g

Adult dosage

1. Decrease progression of postmenopausal osteoporosis: 1.25 mg/day PO cyclically (3 weeks on, 1 week off)
2. Dysfunctional uterine bleeding: 2.5-5 mg/day for 7-10 days, then decrease to 1.25 mg/day for 2 wks with addition of progesterone the third week
3. Female castration and primary ovarian failure: 1.25 mg/day PO cyclically (3 weeks on, 1 week off)
4. Inoperable progressing prostatic carcinoma: 1.25-2.5 mg PO tid
5. Inoperable progressing breast cancer in selected men and postmenopausal women: 10 mg PO tid for at least 3 mo
6. Emergency postcoital contraception: 10 mg PO tid, starting within 72 hours of intercourse and continued for 5 days
7. Atrophic vaginitis and kraurosis vulvae: 2-4 g/day intravaginally or topically
8. Postmenopausal symptoms and prevention of osteoporosis: 0.3-1.25 mg/day cyclically (3 weeks on, 1 week off)

Indications: See above

Action: Mixture of estrogens

Contraindications and precautions

1. Pregnancy, known or suspected estrogen dependent neoplasia, undiagnosed abnormal genital bleeding, active thrombophlebitis or thromboembolic disorders, past history of thromboembolic disorders associated with previous estrogen use, known or suspected cancer of the breast except in appropriately selected patients being treated for metastatic disease
2. Estrogens have been reported to increase the risk of endometrial carcinoma

ETHACRYNIC ACID (Edecrin)

Preparations: *Tab* 25, 50 mg; *inj* 50 mg/vial

Adult dosage: IV 0.5-1.0 mg/kg of body weight; PO 50-100 mg/day initially; adjust dose to produce desired diuresis (minimal effective dosage range is 50-200 mg/day given in a continuous or intermittent schedule)

Indications: Edema resulting from CHF, cirrhosis, nephrosis; short-term management of ascites caused by malignancy, lymphedema, or idiopathic edema

Action: Diuretic; it acts on the ascending limb of the loop of Henle and on the proximal and distal tubules

Contraindications and precautions
1. Anuria
2. Use with caution in patients with advanced cirrhosis, elderly patients, and cardiac patients (avoid rapid volume loss and hypokalemia)
3. Concomitant use of lithium is not recommended

FAMOTIDINE (Pepcid)

Preparations *Tab* 20, 40 mg

Adult dosage
1. Duodenal ulcer: Acute therapy is 40 mg PO qhs or 20 mg PO bid; maintenance dosage is 20 mg PO qhs
2. Pathologic hypersecretory conditions: Dosage should be adjusted according to patient's needs; usual adult starting dose is 20 mg PO q6h

Indications: Duodenal ulcer and pathologic hypersecretory conditions

Action: It inhibits histamine H_2 receptors

Contraindications and precautions: Decrease dose in patients with renal insufficiency

FELDENE See PIROXICAM

FEOSOL See FERROUS SULFATE

FERROUS SULFATE (Feosol)

Preparations: *Tab* 325 mg of ferrous sulfate USP; *cap* 250 mg of ferrous sulfate USP; *elixir* 220 mg of ferrous sulfate/5 ml (tsp)

Dosage: *Tab:* 1 tab tid or qid (after meals and at hs)
elixir: 1-2 tsp tid between meals; cap: qd or bid

Indications: Iron deficiency anemia

Action: Iron replacement

Contraindications and precautions
1. Hemochromatosis
2. Do not take within 2 hours of oral tetracycline

FLAGYL See METRONIDAZOLE

FLECAINIDE (Tambocor)

Preparations: *Tab* 100 mg

Adult dosage: Starting dosage is 100 mg PO bid; dosage may be increased by 50 mg bid q4d until maximum efficacy is achieved; maximum dose is 400 mg/day; however, up to 600 mg/day may be used in patients with symptomatic nonsustained ventricular tachycardia and plasma levels <0.06 μg/ml

Indications: Significant ventricular ectopy

Action: Class I_C antidysrhythmic agent

Contraindications and precautions

1. Flecainide is contraindicated in patients with preexisting second-or third-degree AV block or bifascicular block (unless pacemaker is present)
2. Use with extreme caution in patients with sick sinus syndrome, cardiomiopathy, CHF, ejection fraction <30%, pacemakers (may increase endocardial pacing thresholds and suppress ventricular escape rhythm)
3. Avoid concurrent use of other antidysrhythmic drugs
4. Therapy should be initiated in the hospital setting, with rhythm monitoring
5. Plasma trough levels should be monitored and kept below 0.7-1.0 μg/ml
6. Correct existing electrolyte abnormalities before initiating flecainide
7. Decrease dosage in patients with renal insufficiency

FLEXERIL See CYCLOBENZAPRINE

FLUOCINONIDE (Lidex)

Preparations: *Cream* (0.5%) tubes of 15, 30, 60, 120 g; *gel* (0.05%) tubes of 15, 30, 60, 120 g; *ointment* (0.05%) tubes of 15, 30, 60, 120 g; *topical solution* (0.05%) bottles of 20, 60 ml

Adult dosage: Apply as a thin film to affected area bid to qid

Indications: Inflammatory and pruritic manifestations of corticosteroid-responsive dermatoses

Action: Topical corticosteroid (antiinflammatory and antipruritic action)

Contraindications and precautions: History of hypersensitivity to any of its components

FLURAZEPAM (Dalmane)

Preparations: *Cap* 15, 30 mg

Adult dosage: 15-30 mg at hs (use lower dosage [15 mg] in elderly or debilitated patients)

Indications: Insomnia

Action: Benzodiazepine

Contraindications and precautions

1. Pregnancy, hypersensitivity to flurazepam
2. Avoid concomitant use of alcohol or other CNS depressants

FOLIC ACID

Preparations: *Tab* 1 mg

Adult dosage: 1 mg PO qd

Indications: Megaloblastic anemia from folic acid deficiency

Action: Acts on the bone marrow to correct megaloblastic changes secondary to folic acid deficiency

Contraindications and precautions: Do not use for treatment of vitamin B_{12} deficiency

FORTAZ See CEFTAZIDIME

FUNGIZONE See AMPHOTERICIN B

FUROSEMIDE (Lasix)

Preparations: *Tab* 20, 40, 80 mg; *oral solution* (10 mg/ml) 60, 120 ml; *inj* (10 mg/ml) 2, 4, 10 ml ampul or prefilled syringe

Adult dosage
1. Edema
    a. PO: 20-80 mg initially; if insufficient response after 8-12h, increase dose by 20-40 mg (maximum daily dosage is 600 mg/day); best response is achieved by intermittent dosage (2-4 consecutive days/week)
    b. IV: 20-40 mg (given over 1-2 min) if insufficient response, increase this dose by 20 mg increments at least 2 hours after initial dose; adequate dose can be given qd or bid
2. Hypertension: initial dosage is 40 mg PO bid; adjust dose according to blood pressure response
3. Acute pulmonary edema: 40 mg IV slowly; may double the dose after 1 hour if insufficient response

Indications: Edema, hypertension, acute pulmonary edema

Action: Diuretic; acts on loop of Henle and distal and proximal tubules; onset of diuresis is 5 min following IV injection, 1 hour following PO dose

Contraindications and precautions
1. Anuria
2. Use with caution in elderly patients and in patients receiving lithium, salicylates, or succinylcholine (increased toxicity)

GARAMYCIN See GENTAMICIN

GENTAMICIN (Garamycin)

Preparations: *Inj* 40 mg/ml

Adult dosage
1. Loading dose: 2 mg/kg of adjusted lean body weight; maintenance dose: 3 mg/kg/day administered in 3 equal doses q8h; in patients with life-threatening infections dosages up to 5 mg/kg/day may be administered
2. On the morning of the third day of treatment obtain peak levels 30 min after administration of the drug and trough level right before the next dose; therapeutic peak level is 5-8 µg/ml, toxic level is >10 µg/ml; therapeutic trough level is 1-2 µg/ml, toxic level is >2 µg/ml
3. In elderly patients and in patients with renal insufficiency maintenance dose is modified according to ealculated corrected creatinine clearance (CC Cr)
    a. Male: CC Cr = (140 − age of patient) / serum creatinine
    b. Female: CC Cr = 0.85 × CC Cr of male
4. Table 21-3 shows dose intervals and percent of calculated weight-related maintenance dose

Indications: Infections by susceptible bacterial organisms

Action: Aminoglycoside antibiotic; inhibits protein synthesis in susceptible organisms

Table 21-3 Dose intervals and percent of calculated weight-related maintenance dose

CC Cr	8 hr (%)	12 hr (%)	24 hr (%)
Normal	100	—	—
50	75	—	—
25	50	65	—
10	20	30	50
<10	10	20	40

NOTE: In every patient reevaluate renal status with serum creatinine q48h, and readjust dose administered according to trough and peak levels

Contraindications and precautions
1. Concurrent or sequential use of other nephrotoxic/neurotoxic drugs is contraindicated
2. Use with caution in patients with impaired renal function

GEOCILLIN See **CARBENICILLIN**

GEOPEN See **CARBENICILLIN**

GLIPIZIDE (Glucotrol)
Preparations: *Tab* 5, 10 mg
Adult dosage: Initially 5 mg PO qd before breakfast; in geriatric patients and patients with hepatic impairment initial dosage is 2.5 mg PO qd
Indications: Control of hyperglycemia in non–insulin-dependent diabetics inadequately controlled with diet alone
Action: Second-generation sulfonylurea; lowers serum glucose primarily by stimulating insulin secretion from pancreatic β cells
Contraindications and precautions
1. Diabetic ketoacidosis
2. Use with caution in patients with renal and hepatic disease.
3. Hypoglycemic action of glipizide may be potentiated by drugs that are highly protein bound; β-adrenergic blocking agents may mask symptoms of hypoglycemia

GLUCOTROL See **GLIPIZIDE**

GLYBURIDE (Diabeta, Micronase)
Preparations: *Tab* 1.25, 2.5, 5 mg
Adult dosage: Usual starting dosage is 2.5-5 mg qd; may use lower dosages in elderly patients
Indications: Control of hyperglycemia in non-insulin-dependent diabetics inadequately controlled with diet alone
Action: Second-generation sulfonylurea; lowers serum glucose primarily by stimulating insulin secretion from pancreatic β cells
Contraindications and precautions
1. Diabetic ketoacidosis
2. Hypoglycemic action of glyburide may be potentiated by drugs that are highly protein bound; β-adrenergic blocking agents may mask symptoms of hypoglycemia

Table 21-4 Preparation of NTG infusion

Solution Concentration*	Preparation†
100 μg NTG/ml (common initial solution)	25 mg NTG (5 ml Tridil) in 250 ml D₅W or normal saline
200 μg NTG/ml	50 mg NTG (10 ml Tridil) in 250 ml D₅W or normal saline
400 μg NTG/ml (maximum recommended solution concentration)	100 mg NTG (20 ml Tridil) in 250 ml D₅W or normal saline

From Purcell J.A., and Holder K.C.: Am. J. Nurs. **82**(2):254, 1982.
*These recommendations only apply to Tridil; if using other products, consult package insert for correct solution concentrations.
†Only glass or polyolefin bottles may be used.

GLYCERYL TRINITRATE (Nitroglycerin)

Preparations: *SL tab* 150 μg (1/400 grain), 300 μg (1/200 grain), 400 μg (1/150 grain), 600 μg (1/100 grain); *cap* 2.5, 6.5, 9 mg; *tab* 1.3, 2.6, 6.5 mg; *inj* 100, 200, 400 mg/ml; *topical ointment (2%)* 60 g tube; *transdermal infusion* 2.5, 5, 10, 15 mg; *transmucosal tab* 1, 2, 3 mg

Adult dosage

1. IV infusion: start at 5-10 μg/min and titrate dose based on blood pressure and clinical response (if polyvinyl chloride tubing is used, a higher starting dose may be needed because a large amount of nitroglycerin will be absorbed by the tubing); Tables 21-4 and 21-5 show preparation and infusion of IV NTG; maximum dosage is 200 μg/minute
2. SL: 0.3-0.6 mg prn for chest pain
3. Topical ointment: 2.5-12.5 cm q4-6h
4. Transdermal infusion: 2.5-15 mg or 5-30 cm² q24h
5. Cap: 2.5-9 mg q8-12h
6. Tab: 1.3-6.5 mg q8-12h
7. Transmucosal tab: 1-2 mg tid

Indications: Angina pectoris; CHF associated with acute myocardial infarction (IV NTG); production of controlled hypotension during surgical procedures and control of blood pressure in perioperative hypertension (IV NTG)

Action: Venodilation and relaxation of vascular smooth muscle

Contraindications and precautions: Hypotension, idiopathic hypertrophic subacute aortic stenosis (IHSS); increased intracranial pressure; inadequate cerebral circulation; pericardial tamponade, constrictive pericarditis; uncorrected hypovolemia; known idiosyncratic reaction to organic nitrates

GOLITELY See POLYETHYLENE GLYCOL 3350 SOLUTION

HALCION See TRIAZOLAM

HALDOL See HALOPERIDOL

Table 21-5 Conversion table for NTG solution 100 µg/ml (dosage of NTG in µg/kg/min)

Flow Rate (µgtt/min*)	Quantity of NTG (µg/min)	Body Weight															
		(lb) 77 (kg) 35	88 40	99 45	110 50	121 55	132 60	143 65	154 70	165 75	176 80	187 85	198 90	209 95	220 100	231 105	242 110
3	5	0.14	0.13	0.11	0.10	0.09	0.08	0.08	0.07	0.07	0.06	0.06	0.06	0.05	0.05	0.05	0.05
5	8.35	0.24	0.21	0.19	0.17	0.15	0.14	0.13	0.12	0.11	0.10	0.10	0.09	0.09	0.08	0.08	0.08
10	16.7	0.48	0.42	0.37	0.33	0.30	0.28	0.26	0.24	0.22	0.21	0.20	0.19	0.18	0.17	0.16	0.15
15	25.0	0.71	0.63	0.56	0.50	0.45	0.42	0.38	0.36	0.33	0.31	0.29	0.28	0.26	0.25	0.24	0.23
20	33.3	0.95	0.83	0.74	0.67	0.61	0.56	0.51	0.48	0.44	0.42	0.39	0.37	0.35	0.33	0.32	0.30
25	41.7	1.2	1.0	0.93	0.83	0.76	0.70	0.64	0.60	0.56	0.52	0.49	0.46	0.44	0.42	0.40	0.38
30	50.0	1.4	1.3	1.1	1.0	0.91	0.83	0.77	0.71	0.67	0.63	0.59	0.56	0.53	0.50	0.48	0.45
35	58.4	1.7	1.5	1.3	1.2	1.1	0.97	0.90	0.83	0.78	0.73	0.69	0.65	0.61	0.58	0.56	0.53
40	66.7	1.9	1.7	1.5	1.3	1.2	1.1	1.0	0.95	0.89	0.83	0.78	0.74	0.70	0.67	0.64	0.61

		2.1	1.9	1.7	1.5	1.4	1.3	1.2	1.1	1.0	0.94	0.88	0.83	0.79	0.75	0.71	0.68
45	75.0	2.1	1.9	1.7	1.5	1.4	1.3	1.2	1.1	1.0	0.94	0.88	0.83	0.79	0.75	0.71	0.68
50	83.3	2.4	2.1	1.9	1.7	1.5	1.4	1.3	1.2	1.1	1.0	0.98	0.93	0.88	0.83	0.79	0.76
55	91.7	2.6	2.3	2.0	1.8	1.7	1.5	1.4	1.3	1.2	1.2	1.1	1.0	0.97	0.92	0.87	0.83
60	100	2.9	2.5	2.2	2.0	1.8	1.7	1.5	1.4	1.3	1.3	1.2	1.1	1.1	1.0	0.95	0.91
65	108	3.1	2.7	2.4	2.2	2.0	1.8	1.7	1.6	1.4	1.4	1.3	1.2	1.14	1.1	1.0	0.98
70	117	3.3	2.9	2.6	2.3	2.1	1.9	1.8	1.7	1.6	1.5	1.4	1.3	1.2	1.2	1.1	1.1
75	125	3.6	3.1	2.8	2.5	2.3	2.1	1.9	1.8	1.7	1.6	1.5	1.4	1.3	1.3	1.2	1.14
80	133	3.8	3.3	3.0	2.7	2.4	2.2	2.1	1.9	1.8	1.7	1.6	1.5	1.4	1.33	1.3	1.2
85	142	4.1	3.5	3.2	2.8	2.6	2.4	2.2	2.0	1.9	1.8	1.7	1.6	1.5	1.4	1.4	1.3
90	150	4.3	3.8	3.3	3.0	2.7	2.5	2.3	2.1	2.0	1.9	1.8	1.7	1.6	1.5	1.43	1.4
95	158	4.5	4.0	3.5	3.2	2.9	2.6	2.4	2.3	2.1	2.0	1.9	1.8	1.7	1.6	1.5	1.44

From Purcell J.A., and Holder K.C.: Am. J. Nurs. 82(2):254, 1982.

*Based on 60 μgtt/ml, each μgtt of this solution contains 1.67 μg NTG

HALOPERIDOL (Haldol)

Preparations: *Tab* 0.5, 1, 2, 5, 10, 20 mg; *Inj* 5 mg/ml; *oral concentrate* 2 mg/ml in 15 ml and 120 ml bottle

Adult dosage

1. Moderate symptomatology and use in geriatric or debilitated patients: 0.5-2.0 mg PO bid to tid
2. Severe symptomatology and use in chronic or resistant patients: 3-5 mg PO bid to tid
3. Acutely agitated patients with moderately severe to severe symptoms: 2.5 mg IM, may repeat q1h prn
4. Control of tics and utterances of Tourette's syndrome: 0.05-0.075 mg/kg/day

Indications: Management of psychotic disorders; control of tics and vocal utterances of Tourette's syndrome

Action: Neuroleptic of the butyrophenone series

Contraindications and precautions: CNS depression from any cause; Parkinson's disease

NOTE: Use with caution in patients receiving lithium (increased risk of neurologic toxicity), anticonvulsants (decreased convulsive threshold), anticoagulants (may cause interference), alcohol (additive CNS effects)

NOTE: Use with caution in patients with severe cardiovascular disorders (may precipitate angina and hypotension)

HEPARIN

Preparations: *Inj* 1000; 5000; 10,000; 40,000 U/ml

NOTE: Test for guaiac in stool and obtain baseline hematocrit, platelet count, prothrombin time (PT) and partial thromboplastin time (PTT) before starting heparin

Dosage: Full dose heparinization protocol

1. Initial loading dose is 50 U heparin/lb of lean body weight given as an undiluted IV injection (i.e., a 150 lb patient would receive a bolus of 7500 U)
2. Three hours following the initial IV bolus start continuous IV heparin infusion (10 U/lb/hr). To prepare the infusion, place 20,000 U heparin in 1000 ml of isotonic saline or D_5W (concentration = 20 U/ml). Rate of infusion varies with the patient's weight. For example, a 160 lb patient would receive 1600 U/hr (20,000 U heparin/1000 ml 0.9% Na Cl at 80 ml/hr). In patients necessitating strict fluid restriction higher concentration may be used (e.g. 10,000 U heparin/100 ml 0.9% NaCl $\rightarrow$ 100 U/ml); however, when very high concentrations are used, even a small change in the rate of infusion can result in a significant change in the amount of heparin infused.
3. Closely monitor rate of infusion:
   a. During the initial 24 hr (or until stable) obtain the first partial thromboplastin time (PTT) approximately 4 hr after initiation of continuous heparin infusion and then as often as necessary until stable (but no sooner than 4 hr after modification of the rate of heparin infusion)
   b. After stability has been achieved, monitor PTT once daily
   c. Maintain PTT at 1.5-2 times the patient's pretreatment PTT level, modifying the rate of infusion to achieve this result

4. Test for guaiac in all stools during heparin therapy
5. Obtain hematocrit and platelet count every third day during heparin therapy (increased risk of thrombocytopenia and GI bleeding)
6. Heparin can be neutralized by protamine sulfate; each mg of protamine sulfate neutralizes 100 USP units of heparin

Indications: Pulmonary embolism, prophylaxis of deep vein thrombosis, treatment of venous thrombosis, prevention of cerebral thrombosis in evolving stroke, adjunct therapy of coronary occlusion with acute MI

Action: Binds with antithrombin III (heparin cofactor); accelerates rate at which antithrombin III neutralizes activated forms of factors II, VII IX, X, XI, XII

Contraindications and precautions
1. Hypersensitivity to heparin, bleeding tendencies, active bleeding
2. Use with caution in conditions with increased danger of hemorrhage (e.g., dissecting aneurysm, severe hypertension, hemophilia, thrombocytopenia, ulcerative colitis, diverticulitis)

HYDRALAZINE (Apresoline)

Preparations: *Tab* 10, 25, 50, 100 mg; *Inj* 20 mg/ml ampul

Adult dosage
1. PO: Initially 10 mg qid for 2-4 days, then increase to 25 mg qid; may increase to 50 mg qid after 2 weeks; adjust dosage according to response
2. IM/IV: 20-40 mg prn; monitor blood pressure frequently; maximal hypotensive effect occurs within 20-80 min
   NOTE: Use lower doses in patients with renal impairment

Indications: Essential hypertension

Action: Causes peripheral vasodilation by direct relaxation of vascular smooth muscle

Contraindications and precautions
1. Coronary artery disease; mitral valve rheumatic heart disease (may increase pulmonary artery pressure)
2. Use with caution in patients with cerebrovascular accidents and in patients receiving MAO inhibitors

HYDROCHLOROTHIAZIDE (Hydrodiuril and others)

Preparations: *Tab* 25, 50, 100 mg hydrochlorothiazide (Hydrodiuril); *tab* 25 mg hydrochlorothiazide and 75 mg triamterene (Maxzide); *cap* 25 mg hydrochlorothiazide and 50 mg triamterene (Dyazide); *cap* 50 mg hydrochlorothiazide and 5 mg amiloride (Moduretic)

Adult dosage: Hydrodiuril: 25-100 mg PO qd to bid; Maxzide: 1 tab PO qd; Dyazide 1 cap PO qd to bid; Moduretic: 1 tab PO qd to bid

Indications: Edema states, hypertension

Action: Hydrochlorothiazide is a thiazide diuretic; it interferes with resorption of sodium and chloride in the cortical diluting segment of the nephron

Contraindications and precautions
1. Anuria; allergy to sulfonamide-derived drugs or to any of its components
2. Use with caution in patients with renal or hepatic disease
3. Concomitant use of lithium may result in lithium toxicity

HYDROCOLLOID MUCILLOID (Metamucil)

Preparations: *Powder containers* 3.7, 7.4, 11.1 oz.
Adult dosage: One tsp, stirred in an 8 oz glass of water or other liquid, taken PO qd to tid prn
Indications: Chronic constipation, irritable bowel syndrome
Action: Bulk laxative containing a dietary fiber derived from the psyllium seed
Contraindications and precautions: Intestinal obstruction, fecal impaction

HYDROCORTISONE SODIUM SUCCINATE (Solu-Cortef)

Preparations: *Inj* 100, 250, 500, 1000 mg vials
Adult dosage
1. IV/IM: Initial dose is 100-500 mg depending on severity of condition
2. Give IV slowly (e.g., 500 mg over 10 min)
3. Dosage may be repeated q2-6h prn
4. If hydrocortisone is continued >72 h, hyponatremia may occur; sodium retention may be minimized by switching to methylprednisolone

Indications: See dexamethasone; its indications are identical except (hydrocortisone is not indicated in cerebral edema)
Action: Synthetic adrenocortical steroid
Contraindications and precautions: See dexamethasone

HYDRODIURIL See HYDROCHLOROTHIAZIDE

HYDROMORPHONE HYDROCHLORIDE (Dilaudid)

Preparations: *Inj* 1, 2, 4 mg ampuls; *tab* 1, 2, 3, 4 mg; *suppository* 3 mg
Adult dosage
1. SC/IM: 1-2 mg q4-6h prn
2. IV (slowly over 3-5 min): 1-2 mg q4-6h prn
3. PO: 2-4 mg q6h prn
4. PR: 3 mg q6-8h prn

Indications: Relief of moderate to severe pain
Action: Narcotic analgesic; it is a hydrogenated ketone of morphine
Contraindications and precautions
1. Intracranial lesion associated with increased intracranial pressure; depressed ventilatory function
2. Use with caution in patients receiving other CNS depressants, elderly or debilitated patients, acute abdominal conditions, prostatic hypertrophy, Addison's disease, hypothyroidism, urethral stricture, patients with impaired renal or hepatic function

HYDROXYZINE (Atarax, Vistaril)

Preparations: *Tab* 10, 25, 50, 100 mg; *syrup* 10 mg/5 ml; *inj* 25, 50 mg/ml; *cap* 25, 50, 100 mg
Adult dosage
1. PO
   a. Relief of anxiety: 50-100 mg qid
   b. Treatment of pruritus from allergic conditions: 25 mg tid to qid
   c. Sedation before and after general anesthesia: 50-100 mg

2. IM
   a. Anxiety and agitation: 50-100 mg q4-6h prn
   b. Nausea and vomiting: 25-100 mg
   c. Preoperatively and postoperatively: 25-100 mg

Indications: Anxiety, pruritus secondary to allergic conditions, sedation pre-operatively and postoperatively, alcohol withdrawal symptoms, antiemetic

Action: H_1 histamine competive antagonist with antiemetic and sedative effects

Contraindications and precautions
1. Hydroxyzine will potentiate the CNS action of alcohol and other CNS depressants
2. Decrease meperidine dose when using concomitantly with hydroxyzine

HYGROTON See CHLORTHALIDONE

IBUPROFEN (Motrin and others)

Preparations: *Tab* 200, 300, 400, 600, 800 mg

Adult dosage: Mild to moderate pain: 400 mg q4-6h prn; osteoarthritis, rheumatoid arthritis: 400-800 mg tid to qid; dysmenorrhea: 400 mg q4h prn

Indications: Osteoarthritis, rheumatoid arthritis, mild to moderate pain, dysmenorrhea

Action: Nonsteroidal antiinflammatory agent with antipyretic and analgesic properties

Contraindications and precautions
1. Syndrome of nasal polyps, bronchospastic activity and angioedema following ingestion of aspirin and other nonsteroidal antiinflammatory agents.
2. Use with caution in patients with history of GI bleeding, cardiac decompensation, hypertension, impaired renal function, or bleeding disorders
3. Concomitant administered of coumarin-type anticoagulants may result in potentiation of their effects

IMIPENEM-CILASTIN SODIUM (Primaxin)

Preparations: *Inj* 250, 500 mg vial

Adult dosage
1. Mild infections 250-500 mg IV q6h
2. Severe infections 500 mg-1 g IV q6-8h
3. Maximum daily dose should not exceed 4 g/day or 50 mg/kg/day (whichever is lower)
4. Decrease dosage in patients with impaired renal function

Indications: Infections caused by susceptible bacterial organisms

Action: Thienamycin antibiotic; it inhibits cell wall synthesis

Contraindications and precautions
1. Hypersensitivity to any of its components
2. Use with caution in patients with a history of allergy to penicillin, cephalosporins, other β lactams, and other allergens

IMODIUM See LOPERAMIDE

INDAPAMIDE (Lozol)

Preparations: *Tab* 2.5 mg
Adult dosage: Initially 2.5 mg qd in AM; if insufficient response after 1 week, increase dose to 5 mg qd
Indications: Hypertension
Action: Indoline diuretic; it differs from the thiazides in that it does not possess the thiazide ring system and contains only one sulfonamide group
Contraindications and precautions
   1. Anuria; hypersensitivity to sulfonamide-derived drugs
   2. Concomitant use of lithium is not recommended
   3. Use with caution in patients with renal or hepatic insufficiency and in postsympathectomy patients (increased antihypertensive effect)

INDERAL See PROPRANOLOL

INDOCIN See INDOMETHACIN

INDOMETHACIN (Indocin)

Preparations: *Cap* 25, 50 mg; *SR cap* 75 mg; *suppository* 50 mg
Adult dosage
   1. Moderate to severe osteoarthritis, rheumatoid arthritis, ankylosing spondylitis: 25 mg PO bid to tid increasing dose at weekly intervals to maximum of 150-200 mg/day; if SR capsule is used, initial dose is 75 mg qd
   2. Shoulder bursitis/tendinitis: 25-50 mg PO tid; usual duration of therapy is 7-14 days
   3. Acute gouty arthritis: 50 mg PO tid initially, then taper off dosage gradually
   4. Administer capsules immediately after meals or with antacids
   5. Do not administer suppositories in patients with rectal bleeding or proctitis
Indications: See above
Action: Nonsteroidal anti-inflammatory agent with analgesic and antipyretic action
Contraindications and precautions
   1. Syndrome of nasal polyps, angioedema, or bronchospastic reaction to aspirin and other nonsteroidal anti-inflammatory agents; active GI bleeding or history of recurrent GI lesions
   2. Concomitant use of lithium may result in lithium toxicity
   3. Use with caution in patients with renal or hepatic insufficiency, bleeding disorders (inhibition of platelet aggregation), parkinsonism, depression, epilepsy, psychiatric disturbances (worsening of symptoms)
   4. Concomitant use of aspirin or other salicylates should be avoided

INH See ISONIAZID

INTROPIN See DOPAMINE

ISOETHARINE (Bronkosol)

Preparations: Isoetharine HCL (1.0%) 10, 30 ml bottle (Bronkosol); Iso-etharine mesylate inhalation aerosol (0.61%) 10, 15 ml vial with oral neb-ulizer (Bronkometer)

Adult dosage
1. Hand nebulizer: 1-2 inhalations q4h prn (Bronkometer); 3-7 inhala-tions q4h prn (Bronkosol)
2. Oxygen aerosolization (Bronkosol): 0.25-0.5 ml diluted 1:3 with sa-line q4h prn
3. IPPB (Bronkosol): 0.25-1.0 ml diluted 1:3 with saline q4h prn

Indications: Reversible bronchospasm caused by bronchial asthma, emphy-sema, or bronchitis

Action: Bronchodilator

Contraindications and precautions
1. Hypersensitivity to any of its components
2. Avoid concomitant administration of epinephrine or other sympatho-mimetic amines
3. Use with caution in patients with coronary insufficiency, hyperten-sion, cardiac asthma, or hyperthyroidism

ISONIAZID (INH)

Preparations: *Tab* 300 mg

Adult dosage
1. Treatment of active tuberculosis: 5 mg/kg (up to 300 mg) qd
2. Prophylaxis of tuberculosis: 300 mg qd

Indications: Treatment and prophylaxis of tuberculosis

Action: Inhibits the synthesis of mycolic acid (component of mycobacterial cell wall)

Contraindications and precautions
1. Acute liver disease; history of INH-associated liver damage or hyper-sensitivity reaction to INH
2. Use with caution in patients with chronic liver disease or severe renal impairment
3. Avoid concomitant use of alcohol (increased risk of isoniazid hepati-tis)
4. Concomitant use of phenytoin may result in phenytoin toxicity
5. Ophthalmologic exam (before and during therapy) is recommended

ISOPROTERENOL (Isuprel)

Preparations: *Inhalation solution* 0.25%,0.5%, 1%; *inhalation* (metered dose) 0.08, 0.12, 0.131 mg/spray; *inj* (1:5000 solution) 0.2 mg/ml

Adult dosage
1. Inhalation (metered-dose) for bronchospasm: 1-2 inhalations (there should be a 1-5 min interval between inhalations); may be repeat up to tid
2. Shock: Place 1 mg of isoproterenol in 500 ml of saline and infuse at 0.5-5 μg/min
3. Cardiac arrest and cardiac dysrhythmias: Dilute 0.2 mg (1 ml of 1:5000 solution) to 10 ml with 0.9% NaCl or D_5W, and inject IV 0.02-0.06 mg (1-3 ml); may repeat prn

Indications: Treatment of bronchospasm caused by bronchial asthma, emphysema, bronchitis, and bronchiectasis; adjunctive treatment of shock; cardiac arrest; cardiac dysrhythmias (ventricular dysrhythmias, Adams-Stokes syndrome, carotid sinus hypersensitivity)

Action: Synthetic sympathomimetic amine

Contraindications and precautions
1. Tachycardia caused by digitalis intoxication
2. Simultaneous administration of epinephrine is contraindicated
3. Correct hypovolemia before treatment with isoproterenol; maintain pulse <130/min
4. Use with caution in patients with hyperthyroidism, coronary insufficiency, elderly patients, patients sensitive to sympathomimetics, and diabetic patients
5. Do not use in patients with preexisting cardiac dysrhythmias associated with tachycardia (except ventricular dysrhythmias requiring inotropic support)

ISOPTIN See **VERAPAMIL**

ISORDIL See **ISOSORBIDE DINITRATE**

ISOSORBIDE DINITRATE (Isordil)

Preparations: *SL tab* 2.5, 5, 10 mg; *chew tab* 10 mg; *swallowed tab* 5, 10, 20, 30, 40 mg; *controlled-release tab* and *cap* (Tembids) 40 mg

Adult dosage
1. Initial dosage
   a. SL tab: 2.5-10 mg q2-3h
   b. Chew tab: 5-10 mg q2-3h
2. Swallowed tab: 5-40 mg q6h
3. Controlled-release cap or tab: 40-80 mg q8-12h
   NOTE: Titrate dosage to clinical response

Indications: Treatment and prevention of angina pectoris

Action: Organic nitrate; causes venodilation and relaxation of vascular smooth muscle

Contraindications and precautions: Allergic reaction to nitrates or nitrites; hypotension, volume depletion; idiopathic hypertrophic subacute aortic stenosis (IHSS)

ISUPREL See **ISOPROTERENOL**

KAOLIN AND PECTIN MIXTURE (Kaopectate)

Preparations: *Oral suspension* 90 ml bottle (hospital size) also 240 ml and 360 ml bottle

Adult dosage: PO: 30-60 ml q4-6h prn

Indications: Symptomatic treatment of mild diarrhea

Action: Absorbent antidiarrheal agent

Contraindications and precautions: Intestinal obstruction; undiagnosed abdominal pain

KAOPECTATE See **KAOLIN AND PECTIN MIXTURE**

KAYEXALATE See **SODIUM POLYSTYRENE SULFONATE**

KEFLEX See **CEPHALEXIN**

KEFLIN See **CEPHALOTIN**

KEFZOL See **CEFAZOLIN**

KETOCONAZOLE (Nizoral)

Preparations: *Tab* 200 mg
Adult dosage
1. 200 mg PO qd; if insufficient response may increase dose to 400 mg qd
2. Ketoconazole requires gastric acidity for absorption (if patient is receiving H_2 blockers, antacids, or anticholinergics, they should be administered at least 2 hours after ketoconazole administration)

Indications: Systemic fungal infections
Action: Broad-spectrum antifungal agent
Contraindications and precautions
1. Do not use for fungal meningitis (poor CNS penetratration)
2. Use with caution in patients with a history of liver disease, patients receiving warfarin-like drugs (increased prothrombin time), cyclosporin A (increased serum level), phenytoin (altered metabolism), oral hypoglycemic agents (increased risk of hypoglycemia), rifampin (decreased serum level)

KWELL See **LINDANE**

LABETOLOL (Trandate, Normodyne)

Preparations: *Tab* 100, 200, 300 mg; *inj* 20 ml ampul (5 mg/ml)
Adult dosage
1. PO: Initial dosage is 100 mg bid; may increase by 100 mg bid q3 days; usual maintenance dose is 200-400 mg PO bid
2. IV: 20 mg (by slow injection over 2 min); may repeat with 40-80 mg q10 min until desired supine blood pressure is achieved or a total of 300 mg IV has been given; maximum effect occurs within 5 min of IV injection; half-life of labetolol is 5-8 hours

NOTE: Decrease dosage in patients with hepatic dysfunction.
Indications: Hypertension
Action: β-Blocker and α-1 vasodilator
Contraindications and precautions
1. Bronchial asthma, severe bradycardia, second- or third-degree heart block, overt cardiac failure, cardiogenic shock
2. Use caution when administering to patients with pheochromocytoma (increased risk of paradoxical hypertensive response), diabetes (blunted signs of hypoglycemia), patients receiving cimetidine (increased bioavailability of labetolol), tricyclic antidepressants (increased tremor), nitrates (blunting of reflex tachycardia associated with hypotension)

LACTULOSE (Cephulac)

Preparations: *Syrup* supplied in containers of 30 ml (20 g lactulose), 473 ml (315 g lactulose), 1.89 L (1260 g lactulose)

Adult dosage

1. 2-3 tablespoons (20-30 g lactulose) tid to qid; adjust dose to produce 2-3 soft stools/day
2. In hepatic encephalopathy may use 30-45 ml of lactulose q1h until clinical improvement occurs
3. May be given as a retention enema in patients in hepatic coma (mix 300 ml of lactulose with 700 ml of NS and retain for 30-60 min, may repeat q4-6h)

Indications: Prevention and treatment of hepatic encephalopathy

Action: Decreases blood ammonia concentration by acidification of colon contents (facilitating conversion of ammonia into ammonium ion) and expulsion of the ammonium ion with its laxative action

Contraindications and precautions

1. Patients requiring a low-galactose diet
2. Use with caution in diabetics (contains galactose)
3. Do not use in patients with possible bowel obstruction or ileus

LANOXIN See DIGOXIN

LASIX See FUROSEMIDE

LEVOPHED See NOREPINEPHRINE

LIBRIUM See CHLORDIAZEPOXIDE

LIDEX See FLUOCINONIDE

LIDOCAINE

Preparations: *Inj* 10, 20, 40, 100 mg/ml

Adult dosage

1. Loading dose: 50-100 mg (0.70-1.4 mg/kg) administered at rate of 25-50 mg/min; if no response, may rebolus after 5 min; do not administer >300 mg over 1 hour
2. *IV infusion:* Place 1-2 g of lidocaine in 1000 ml of D_5W and infuse at a rate of 2 mg/min (20-50 μg/kg/minute)
   a. Constant ECG monitoring is essential
   b. Reduce dosage in patients with severe liver or kidney impairment and in elderly or debilitated patients

Indications: Acute management of ventricular dysrhythmias

Action: Antidysrhythmic agent

Contraindications and precautions

1. Stokes-Adams syndrome, Wolff-Parkinson-White (WPW) syndrome; severe degrees of intraventricular, atrioventricular, or sinoatrial block; hypersensitivity to local anesthetics of the amide type
2. Use with caution in patients with a genetic predisposition to malignant hyperthermia and in elderly patients
3. Liver disease, CHF, and hypotension prolong the half-life of lidocaine and increase the risk of developing lidocaine toxicity

LINDANE (Kwell)

Preparations: *Lotion (1%)* 60 ml, 472 ml, and 3.8 L bottle; *shampoo (1%)* 60 ml, 472 ml, and 3.8 L bottle; *cream (1%)* 60 g tube and 454 g jar
Adult dosage
1. Lotion and cream: Apply to infested area, rub scalp and hair, and leave in place for 8-12 hr, then wash out
2. Shampoo: Apply to infested area and leave in place for 4 min, then rinse thoroughly

Indications: Treatment of patients with *Sarcoptes scabei* (scabies), *Pediculus capitis* (head lice), and *Phthirus pubis* (crab lice)
Action: Scabicide and pediculocide
Contraindications and precautions
1. Hypersensitivity to the product or any of its components
2. Use with caution in children, infants, and pregnant women (can penetrate the skin and cause CNS toxicity)

LITHIUM CARBONATE (Eskalith)

Preparations: *Cap* 300 mg; *tab* 300 mg; *controlled-release tab* 450 mg
Adult dosage: Acute mania: 600 mg tid; maintenance: 300 mg tid
  NOTE: Closely monitor serum level (therapeutic is 0.5-1.5 mEq/L)
  NOTE: Some patients (particularly elderly patients) can experience signs of lithium toxicity at normally therapeutic levels. It is essential that patients receiving lithium maintain an adequate salt and fluid intake to avoid potential toxicity

Indications: Treatment of manic episodes of manic-depressive illness
Action: Antimanic drug; precise mechanism of action is unknown
Contraindications and precautions: Use with caution in sodium or volume-depleted patients, hypothyroid patients, patients with renal or cardiovascular disease (increased risk of toxicity), and in patients taking haloperidol (increased risk of encephalopathic syndrome), neuromuscular blocking agents (prolongation of their effect), indomethacin and other nonsteroidal antiinflammatory agents (increased serum lithium level)

LOMOTIL See DIPHENOXYLATE

LOPERAMIDE (Imodium)

Preparations: *Cap* 2 mg; *liquid* 1 mg/5 ml, 4 oz bottle
Adult dosage
1. Acute diarrhea: 4 mg initially, followed by 2 mg after each unformed stool; maximum daily dose is 16 mg
2. Chronic diarrhea: Same as for acute diarrhea; dosage should be based on individual requirements (average maintenance dose is 4-8 mg/day)

Indications: Control of acute nonspecific diarrhea; reduction of volume discharge from ileostomies; chronic diarrhea
Action: Inhibition of peristaltic activity by direct effect on the muscles of the intestinal wall
Contraindications and precautions
1. Pseudomembranous colitis; diarrhea from organisms that penetrate the intestinal mucosa
2. Use with caution in patients with ulcerative colitis and in patients with hepatic dysfunction

LOPRESSOR See **METOPROLOL**

LORAZEPAM (Ativan)

Preparations: Tab 0.5, 1, 2 mg; inj 2, 4 mg/ml
Adult dosage
1. Anxiety: 1 mg PO bid to tid
2. Premedicant: 0.05 mg/kg IM (maximum of 4 mg) given at least 2 hr before operative procedure
3. Sedation and relief of anxiety: 0.044 mg/kg (maximum of 2 mg) given 15-20 min before anticipated procedure
NOTE: Decrease dose in elderly and debilitated patients and in patients with renal, hepatic, or pulmonary disease
Indications: Anxiety, preanesthetic medication, sedation
Action: Benzodiazepine with sedative effects
Contraindications and precautions
1. Hypersensitivity to benzodiazepines or any of its components; acute narrow-angle glaucoma
2. Avoid concomitant use of alcohol or other CNS depressants
3. Use with caution in depressed patients
4. Do not use for primary depressive disorders or psychoses
5. Fetal damage may result when administered to pregnant women

LOZOL See **INDAPAMIDE**

MACRODANTIN See **NITROFURANTOIN**

MANDOL See **CEFAMANDOLE**

MANNITOL

Preparations: *Inj* 5%, 10%, 15%, 20%, 25% solution
Adult dosage: Cerebral edema: 25 g (100 ml of 20% solution) given over 15-30 min; may repeat q2-3h prn
Indications: Reduction of intracranial or intraocular pressure
Action: Osmotic diuretic; inhibits sodium and chloride reabsorption in the proximal tubule and ascending loop of Henle
Contraindications and precautions: Anuria, renal failure; severe pulmonary congestion; CHF; severe dehydration

MECLIZINE (Antivert)

Preparations: *Tab* 12.5, 25, 50 mg; *chew tab* 25 mg
Adult dosage
1. Motion sickness: 25-50 mg taken 1 hr before start of the journey
2. Vertigo: 12.5-50 mg bid
Indications: Motion sickness; vertigo caused by diseases of the vestibular system
Action: Antihistamine
Contraindications and precautions
1. Concomitant use of alcoholic beverages
2. Use with caution in patients with asthma, prostatic hypertrophy, glaucoma

MEDROL See **METHYLPREDNISOLONE**

MEFOXIN See **CEFOXITIN**

MELLARIL See **THIORIDAZINE**

MEPERIDINE (Demerol)

Preparations: *Inj* 50 mg/ml; *tab* 50, 100 mg; *syrup* 50 mg/5ml
Adult dosage
1. Relief of pain: 50-150 mg IM/SC/PO q3-4h prn
2. PO dose is less effective than parenteral administration
3. IV administration should be very slow, using a diluted solution
4. Concomitant administration of phenothiazines or other tranquilizers (e.g., hydroxyzine) will potentiate the action of meperidine

Indications: Relief of moderate to severe pain
Action: Narcotic analgesic
Contraindications and precautions
1. Current or recent use of MAO inhibitors; head injury, increased intra-cranial pressure
2. Use with caution in patients receiving other CNS depressants (additive effect) and in patients with asthma or other respiratory abnormalities (decreased respiratory drive), supraventricular tachycardias (increased ventricular response rate), acute abdominal conditions (masking of diagnosis), convulsive disorders (increased convulsions), hypothyroidism, impaired renal or hepatic function, prostatic hypertrophy, urethral stricture, Addison's disease, elderly or debilitated patients

METAMUCIL See **HYDROCOLLOID MUCILLOID**

METAPROTERENOL (Alupent)

Preparations: *Inhal* 0.65 mg/metered dose (300 doses/inhaler); *tab* 10, 20 mg; *syrup* 10 mg/5 ml; *vial* 2.5 ml (inhalant solution 0.6% unit dose vials)
Adult dosage
1. Inhaled (via nebulizer): 0.2-0.3 ml in 2-5 ml of normal saline q4-6h prn for bronchospasm
2. PO: 20 mg tid to qid
3. Metered-dose inhaler: 2-3 inhalations; do not repeat more often than q4h

Indications: Bronchial asthma, emphysema, bronchitis
Action: β-2 adrenergic agonist
Contraindications and precautions
1. Cardiac dysrhythmias associated with tachycardia
2. Use with caution in patients with coronary artery disease, CHF, hypertension, hyperthyroidism, history of hypersensitivity to sympathomimetic amines, diabetes

METHYLDOPA (Aldomet)

Preparations: *Tab* 125, 250, 500 mg; *susp* 250 mg/5 ml; *inj* 250 mg/5 ml
Adult dosage
1. PO: 250 mg bid to tid initially; may increase dose after 2-3 days if inadequate response; maximum daily dosage is 2 g; usual dosage is 250-500 mg bid to qid
2. IV: 250-500 mg q6h
NOTE: Use smaller doses in patients with renal impairment

Indications: Hypertension

Action: Antihypertensive; it is believed that its metabolites cause a reflex depression of sympathetic control of arterial blood pressure

Contraindications and precautions

1. Active hepatic disease (acute hepatitis, active cirrhosis); development of Coombs' positive hemolytic anemia while taking methyldopa
2. Use with caution in patients with a history of liver disease
3. Not recommended for treatment of patients with pheochromocytoma
4. Do not use Aldomet oral suspension in patients allergic to sulfites (contains sodium bisulfite)
5. Sudden withdrawal may result in significant rebound hypertension

METHYLPREDNISOLONE (Medrol, Solumedrol)

Preparations: *Tab* 2, 4, 8, 16, 24, 32 mg; *inj* 40, 125, 500, 1000 mg vial

Adult dosage

1. PO: 4-48 mg/day depending on disease and clinical response
2. IV: 30 mg/kg infused over 10-20 min for septic shock; dosage for severe bronchospasm is 0.5-1 mg/kg initially, followed by tapering doses q4-6h

Indications: See dexamethasone; its indications are identical except that methylprednisolone is not indicated in cerebral edema

Action: Synthetic adrenocortical steroid

Contraindications and precautions: See dexamethasone

METOCLOPRAMIDE (Reglan)

Preparations: *Tab* 10 mg; *syrup* 5 mg/5 ml; *inj* 5 mg/ml

Adult dosage

1. GI reflux: 10-15 mg PO 30 min before each meal and at hs; maximum duration of therapy is 12 wk
2. Diabetic gastroparesis: 10 mg PO 30 min before each meal and at qs.
3. Prophylaxis of nausea and vomiting in cancer chemotherapy: IV infusion 1-2 mg/kg diluted in 0.9% saline and given slowly (over 15 min) 30 min before beginning cancer chemotherapy and repeated q2h × 2 doses, then q3h × 3 doses
4. Facilitation of small bowel intubation: 10 mg IV (undiluted) given over 2 min

Indications: See above

Action: Antiemetic; stimulates motility of upper GI tract

Contraindications and precautions

1. GI obstruction, perforation, hemorrhage, or any other GI condition where increased GI motility is contraindicated; pheochromocytoma, epilepsy
2. Avoid concomitant use of other drugs likely to cause extrapyramidal reactions

METOLAZONE (Diulo, Zaroxolyn)

Preparations: *Tab* 2.5, 5, 10 mg

Adult dosage

1. Hypertension: 2.5-5 mg qd
2. Edema from renal disease: 5-20 mg qd
3. CHF 5-10 mg qd

Indications: Hypertension; edema
Action: Diuretic; inhibits sodium reabsorption at the cortical diluting site and in the proximal convoluted tubule
Contraindications and precautions
1. Anuria; hepatic coma or precoma
2. Use caution when administering metolazone to hyperuricemic patients, patients with severely impaired renal function, diabetics

METOPROLOL (Lopressor)

Preparations: *Tab* 50, 100 mg; *inj* 5 mg/5 ml ampul or prefilled syringe
Adult dosage
1. Hypertension: 100 mg PO qd in single or divided doses; may increase dosage q1-2 weeks until satisfactory response is achieved; usual range is 100-450 mg/day
2. Angina: 100 mg PO daily in two divided doses initially, increased prn at weekly intervals; effective dosage range is 100-400 mg/day
3. Acute MI: 5 mg IV boluses at 2 min intervals 3 times (total 15 mg IV), then 25-50 mg PO q6h × 48 hr, then 100 mg PO bid; start PO dosage 15 min after IV dose

NOTE: Patients with contraindications to IV treatment in the early phase of an acute MI may be started on 100 mg PO bid as soon as their condition permits
Indications: Hypertension; MI; angina pectoris
Action: β-adrenergic receptor blocking agent
Contraindications and precautions
1. Heart block greater than first degree; sinus bradycardia; cardiogenic shock; CHF
2. Use with caution in patients with bronchospastic disease (may exacerbate bronchospasm), diabetes (may mask tachycardia from hypoglycemia), impaired hepatic function
3. Avoid abrupt cessation of β blocker therapy

METRONIDAZOLE (Flagyl)

Preparations: *Tab* 250, 500 mg; *inj* 500 mg
Adult dosage
1. Anaerobic infections: IV loading dose of 15 mg/kg followed by maintenance dose of 7.5 mg/kg q6h; maximum daily dose is 4 g; IV administration should be by infusion over 1 hr
2. Trichomoniasis: 1-2 g PO as a single dose or 500 mg PO bid × 5 days
3. Giardiasis: 2 g PO qd as a single dose × 3 days or 250 mg bid to tid × 7-10 days
4. Decrease dosage in patients with severe liver disease
Indications: Anaerobic infections; trichomoniasis; giardiasis
Action: Disrupts DNA and inhibits nucleic acid synthesis
Contraindications and precautions: History of hypersensitivity to metronidazole or other nitroimidazole derivatives

MEXILETINE (Mexitil)

Preparations: *Cap* 150, 200, 250 mg

Adult dosage: Usual starting dose is 200 mg PO q8h, taken with food; dosage can be increased or decreased by 50-100 mg increments at intervals of at least 2-3 days; usual dosage range is 200-300 mg PO q8h; total daily dose >1200 mg is rarely tolerated

Indications: Treatment of symptomatic ventricular dysrhythmias

Action: It shortens the action potential duration and effective refractory period of Purkinje fibers

Contraindications and precautions
1. Contraindicated in cardiogenic shock, preexisting second- or third-degree AV block (unless pacemaker is present)
2. Use with caution in patients with hypotension, CHF, hepatic impairment, sinus node dysfunction, or intraventricular conduction defect

MEXITIL See MEXILETINE

MICONAZOLE (Monistat)

Preparations: *Cream (2%)* (Monistat-7) 45 g tube; *suppository* 100 mg (Monistat-7), 200 mg (Monistat-3)

Adult dosage
1. Vaginal cream (Monistat-7): one applicatorful intravaginally qhs × 7 days
2. Vaginal suppository (Monistat-7): one suppository intravaginally qhs × 7 days
3. Vaginal suppository (Monistat-3): one suppository intravaginally qhs × 3 days

Indications: Local treatment of vulvovaginal candidiasis

Action: Fungicidal

Contraindications: Hypersensitivity to miconazole

MICRONASE See GLYBURIDE

MINIPRESS See PRAZOSIN

MONISTAT See MICONAZOLE

MONOCID See CEFONICID

MORPHINE SULFATE

Preparations: *Inj* 8, 10, 15 mg/ml; *tab* 10, 15, 30 mg; *solution* 10, 20 mg/5 ml

Adult dosage
1. PO: 8-20 mg q4h, 30 mg (MS Contin) q12h for control of pain
2. SC/IM: 5-15 mg q4h for control of pain
3. IV: 4-10 mg, diluted and injected over a 5 min period
NOTE: Decrease dosage in patients with impaired renal or hepatic function, elderly or debilitated patients, and patients with urethral stricture, prostatic hypertrophy, hypothyroidism or Addison's disease

Indications: Relief of severe pain

Action: Narcotic analgesic
Contraindications and precautions
1. Respiratory depression or insufficiency, severe bronchial asthma, increased cerebrospinal or intracranial pressure, acute alcoholism, convulsive disorders, delirium tremens, brain tumor, cardiac failure caused by chronic pulmonary disease, suspected surgical abdomen, cardiac dysrhythmias, after biliary tract surgery and postsurgical anastomosis, use during or within 14 days of MAO inhibitor therapy
2. Avoid concurrent use with other CNS depressants

MOTRIN See **IBUPROFEN**

MYCELEX See **CLOTRIMAZOLE**

MYCOSTATIN See **NYSTATIN**

NAFCILLIN (Unipen)

Preparations: *Cap* 250 mg; *tab* 500 mg; *inj* 500 mg, 1, 2, 10g; *oral solution* 250 mg/5 ml
Adult dosage
1. IV: 500 mg-1 g q4h for severe infections
2. IM: 500 mg q4-6h for severe infections
3. PO: 250-500 mg q4-6h for mild-to-moderate infections, 1 g q4-6h for severe infections

Indications: Infections from penicillinase-producing staphylococci
Action: Semisynthetic antistaphylococcal penicillin
Contraindications and precautions: Allergy to any of the penicillins

NALOXONE (Narcan)

Preparations: *Inj* 0.02, 0.4, 1.0 mg/ml
Adult dosage: For narcotic overdose 0.4-2mg IV; may repeat q2min prn; if no response after 10 mg consider other diagnosis
Indications: Reversal of narcotic depression
Action: Narcotic antagonist
Contraindications and precautions: Hypersensitivity to naloxone

NAPROSYN See **NAPROXEN**

NAPROXEN (Naprosyn, Anaprox)

Preparations: *Tab* 250, 375, 500 mg (Naprosyn base); 275 mg (Anaprox-sodium)
Adult dosage
1. Primary dysmenorrhea, acute tendinitis and bursitis, mild to moderate pain: Naprosyn 500 mg PO initially, then 250 mg PO q6h or Anaprox 550 mg PO initially followed by 275 mg PO bid
2. Rheumatoid arthritis, osteoarthritis, ankylosing spondylitis: Naprosyn 250-375 mg PO bid, Anaprox 275 mg PO bid, or Anaprox 275 mg PO in AM 550 mg PO in evening
3. Acute gout: Naprosyn 750 mg PO initially, then 250 mg PO q8h until attack has subsided, or Anaprox 825 mg initially then 275 mg q8h until attack has subsided

Indications: See above
Action: Nonsteroidal anti-inflammatory drug (NSAID)
Contraindications and precautions
1. Allergic reactions to NSAIDs or aspirin
2. Use with caution in patients with history of GI disease, impaired renal function, liver disease, heart failure, elderly patients, and patients receiving diuretics

NARCAN See **NALOXONE**

NIFEDIPINE (Procardia)
Preparations: *Cap* 10, 20 mg
Adult dosage: Initially 10 mg PO tid; usual dosage range is 30-60 mg/day
Indications: Vasospastic angina; chronic stable angina
Action: Calcium channel blocker (inhibitor of calcium ion influx)
Contraindications and precautions: Hypotension, peripheral edema

NIPRIDE See **NITROPRUSSIDE**

NITROFURANTOIN (Macrodantin)
Preparations: *Cap* 25, 50, 100 mg
Adult dosage: 50-100 mg PO qid; therapy should be continued for at least 1 week and for at least 3 days after urine sterility has been documented
Indications: Urinary tract infections from susceptible bacterial organisms
Action: Interference with bacterial enzyme systems through covalent bonding to DNA
Contraindications and precautions: Impaired renal function, anuria, oliguria, hypersensitivity to nitrofurantoin preparations

NITROGLYCERIN See **GLYCERYL TRINITRATE**

NITROPRUSSIDE (Nipride)
Preparations: 5 ml vials containing 50 mg sodium nitroprusside to be reconstituted with sterile 5% dextrose in water (see Table 21-6)
Adult dosage
1. In patients not receiving antihypertensive drugs the dosage range is 0.5-10 μg/kg/min
2. Average dose of 3 μg/kg/min will usually lower diastolic pressure by 30%-40%
3. Smaller doses are required in hypertensive patients receiving concomitant antihypertensive medications and when used for therapy of CHF
Indications
1. Immediate reduction of blood pressure in hypertensive crises
2. Vasodilator therapy in refractory CHF
Action: Potent, immediately active hypotensive agent; its hypotensive effects occur as a result of peripheral vasodilatation
Contraindications and precautions
1. Do not use in compensatory hypertension
2. Do not use to produce controlled hypotension during surgery in patients with known inadequate cerebral circulation

3. Frequent monitoring of serum thiocyanate levels is indicated in patients with renal impairment, in any patient receiving large doses of nitroprusside, or during prolonged use; metabolic acidosis is the earliest and most reliable evidence of cyanide toxicity; thiocyanate levels should be kept less than 10 mg/dl

4. Use with caution in patients with hepatic insufficiency, hypothyroidism, or severe renal impairment

NIZORAL See KETOCONAZOLE

NORFLOXACIN (Noroxin)

Preparations: *Tab* 400 mg
Adult dosage
1. UTI, uncomplicated: 400 mg PO bid × 7-10 days
2. UTI, complicated: 400 mg PO bid × 10-21 days
NOTE: Administer 1 hr before or 2 hr after a meal

Indications: Urinary tract infections caused by susceptible organisms
Action: Fluoroquinolone broad-spectrum bactericidal agent; inhibits DNA synthesis
Contraindications and precautions
1. Contraindicated in pregnancy, in children, and in patients with hypersensitivity to quinolone antibiotics
2. Decrease dosage in patients with impaired renal function

NORMODYNE See LABETOLOL

NOROXIN See NORFLOXACIN

NORPACE See DISOPYRAMIDE

NYSTATIN (Mycostatin)

Preparations: *Tab* 500,000 U; *susp* 100,000 U/ml; *cream and oint* 100,000 U/g; *powd* 100,000 U/g; *vag tab* 100,000 U
Adult dosage
1. Cutaneous or mucocutaneous candidiasis: Apply cream, powder or ointment to affected area bid to tid
2. Oral candidiasis: Place 4-6 ml in the mouth and retain as long as possible before swallowing
3. Intestinal candidiasis: 1-2 tabs PO tid
4. Vulvovaginal candidiasis: Insert 1 tab intravaginally (with applicator) qhs × 2 weeks

Indications: Cutaneous or mucocutaneous candidiasis, candidiasis of the oral cavity, intestinal candidiasis, vulvovaginal candidiasis
Action: Antifungal antibiotic
Contraindications and precautions
1. Hypersensitivity to any of its components
2. Discontinue topical or vaginal. preparations if the patient develops signs of local irritation

OS-CAL See CALCIUM CARBONATE

Table 21-6 Nitroprusside infusion (dosage = µg Nipride/kg/min)

Flow Rate (µgtt/min)	Quantity of Nipride* (µg/min)†	Body Weight															
		(lb) 77 (kg) 35	88 40	99 45	110 50	121 55	132 60	143 65	154 70	165 75	176 80	187 85	198 90	209 95	220 100	231 105	242 110
5	16.7	0.48	0.42	0.37	0.33	0.30	0.28	0.26	0.24	0.22	0.21	0.20	0.19	0.18	0.17	0.16	0.15
10	33.3	0.95	0.83	0.74	0.67	0.61	0.56	0.51	0.48	0.44	0.42	0.39	0.37	0.35	0.33	0.32	0.30
15	50	1.4	1.25	1.1	1.0	0.91	0.83	0.77	0.71	0.67	0.63	0.59	0.56	0.53	0.50	0.48	0.45
20	67	1.9	1.7	1.5	1.3	1.2	1.1	1.0	0.95	0.89	0.84	0.79	0.74	0.70	0.67	0.64	0.61
25	83	2.4	2.1	1.8	1.7	1.5	1.4	1.3	1.2	1.1	1.0	0.98	0.93	0.88	0.83	0.79	0.76
30	100	2.9	2.5	2.2	2.0	1.8	1.7	1.5	1.4	1.3	1.3	1.2	1.1	1.1	1.0	0.95	0.91
35	117	3.3	2.9	2.6	2.3	2.1	2.0	1.8	1.7	1.6	1.5	1.4	1.3	1.2	1.2	1.1	1.1
40	133	3.8	3.3	3.0	2.7	2.4	2.2	2.0	1.9	1.8	1.7	1.6	1.5	1.4	1.3	1.3	1.2
45	150	4.3	3.8	3.3	3.0	2.7	2.5	2.3	2.1	2.0	1.9	1.8	1.7	1.6	1.5	1.4	1.4

50	167	4.8	4.2	3.7	3.3	3.0	2.8	2.6	2.4	2.2	2.1	2.0	1.9	1.8	1.7	1.6	1.5
55	183	5.2	4.6	4.1	3.7	3.3	3.1	2.8	2.6	2.4	2.3	2.2	2.0	1.9	1.8	1.7	1.7
60	200	5.7	5.0	4.4	4.0	3.6	3.3	3.1	2.9	2.7	2.5	2.4	2.2	2.1	2.0	1.9	1.8
65	217	6.2	5.4	4.8	4.3	3.9	3.6	3.3	3.1	2.9	2.7	2.6	2.4	2.3	2.2	2.1	2.0
70	233	6.7	5.8	5.2	4.7	4.2	3.9	3.6	3.3	3.1	2.9	2.7	2.6	2.5	2.3	2.2	2.1
75	250	7.1	6.3	5.6	5.0	4.5	4.2	3.8	3.6	3.3	3.1	2.9	2.8	2.6	2.5	2.4	2.3
80	267	7.6	6.7	5.9	5.3	4.8	4.5	4.1	3.8	3.6	3.3	3.1	3.0	2.8	2.7	2.5	2.4
85	283	8.1	7.1	6.3	5.7	5.1	4.7	4.3	4.0	3.8	3.5	3.3	3.1	3.0	2.8	2.7	2.6
90	300	8.6	7.5	6.7	6.0	5.5	5.0	4.6	4.3	4.0	3.8	3.5	3.3	3.2	3.0	2.9	2.7
95	317	9.1	7.9	7.0	6.3	5.8	5.3	4.9	4.5	4.2	4.0	3.7	3.5	3.3	3.2	3.0	2.9
100	333	9.5	8.3	7.4	6.7	6.1	5.6	5.1	4.8	4.4	4.2	3.9	3.7	3.5	3.3	3.2	3.0

From Purcell, J.A.: AM. J. Nurs. **82**(6):965, 1982.

*Nitroprusside (Nipride) solution 200 µg/ml (100 mg Nipride/500 ml or 50 mg Nipride/250 ml).

†Based on 60 µgtt/ml. each µgtt of this solution contains 3.33 µg Nipride

OXAZEPAM (Serax)

Preparations: *Cap* 10, 15, 30 mg; *tab* 15 mg
Adult dosage
1. Mild to moderate anxiety: 10-15 mg PO tid to qid
2. Severe anxiety, alcohol withdrawal: 15-30 mg PO tid to qid
3. Decrease dosage in elderly patients

Indications: Anxiety disorders, alcohol withdrawal
Action: Benzodiazepine
Contraindications and precautions
1. Psychoses
2. Avoid concomitant use of alcohol or other CNS depressant drugs

OXYCODONE (Percocet)

Preparations: Percocet contains oxycodone HC1 5 mg and acetaminophen 325 mg
Adult dosage: Usual dosage is 1 tab q6h prn for pain
Indications: Relief of moderate to severe pain
Action: Narcotic analgesic
Contraindications and precautions
1. Hypersensitivity to oxycodone or acetaminophen; head injury and increased intracranial pressure; acute abdominal conditions
2. Use with caution in patients with impaired renal or hepatic function, hypothyroidism, prostatic hypertrophy, Addison's disease, urethral stricture, and in elderly or debilitated patients
3. Avoid concomitant use of CNS depressants, anticholinergics with narcotics (increased risk of paralytic ileus), MAO inhibitors, or tricylic antidepressants

PARLODEL See BROMOCRIPTINE

PENICILLIN PREPARATIONS

Penicillin	Dosage forms	Route of administration
Penicillin G benza-thine (Bicillin L-A, Permapen)	300,000, 600,000 U/ml	IM
Penicillin G Procaine (Bicillin CR, Wycil-lin	300,000 U/ml 500,000, 600,000 U/ml	IM
Penicillin G sodium	5,000,000 U/vial	IV
Penicillin G potas-sium (Pentids)	200,000, 250,000, 400,000 U/5 ml *(Reconstituted susp/ syrup)*	*PO*

PENICILLIN PREPARATIONS—cont'd

Penicillin	Dosage forms	Route of administration
Penicillin G potassium (Pentids) —cont'd	*100,000, 200,000, 250,000, 400,000, 500,000, 800,000 U* (*Tab* 250 mg = 400,000 U)	PO
	200,000, 500,000, 1,000,000, 5,000,000, 10,000,000, 20,000,000 U	IM/IV (>5,000,000 U use IV only)
Penicillin V Potassium (V-Cillin K, Pen Vee K)	200,000, 400,000, 800,000 U (*Tab* 125 mg = 200,000 U)	PO
	200,000 U (125 mg/ 5ml) 400,000 U (250 mg/ 5ml) (*Solution/susp*)	PO

PENTAM 300 See PENTAMIDINE

PENTAMIDINE ISOTHIONATE (Pentam 300)

Preparations: *Inj* 300 mg vial
Adult dosage: IV/IM: 4 mg/kg qd × 14 days
Indications: *Pneumocystis carinii* pneumonia
Action: Antiprotozoal agent; inhibits synthesis of DNA, RNA, phospholipids, and proteins.
Contraindications and precautions
1. IV dose should be infused slowly (over 60 min) while the patient is lying down and the blood pressure is closely monitored (patients may develop severe hypotension)
2. Monitor metabolic parameters (BUN, creatinine, glucose, CBC, platelet count, liver function, calcium) frequently while the patient is receiving pentamidine therapy

PEPCID See FAMOTIDINE

PERCOCET See OXYCODONE

PERSANTINE See DIPYRIDAMOLE

PHENOBARBITAL

Preparations: *Tab* 8, 16, 32, 65, 100 mg; *inj* 30, 60, 130 mg/ml; *elixir* 4 mg/ml

Adult dosage
1. Control of epileptic seizures: Initial dose is 1–5 mg/kg/day; usual dose is 100-200 mg qhs
2. Status epilepticus: 4-6 mg/kg IM

NOTE: Decrease dosage in chronic liver disease or renal impairment

Indications: Epilepsy, sedation

Action: Barbiturate anticonvulsant

Contraindications and precautions
1. Respiratory disease with presence of dyspnea or obstruction
2. Use with caution in patients with cardiovascular, pulmonary, hepatic, or renal disease

PHENYTOIN (Dilantin)

Preparations: *Cap* 30, 100 mg; *suspension* 125 mg/5 ml; *inj* 50 mg/ml; *chew tab* 50 mg

Adult dosage
1. Usual PO dose is 4-6 mg/kg/day
   a. This can be given in divided doses (100 mg PO tid) or as one daily dose (300 mg PO qd of *extended* phenytoin sodium capsules [Dilantin Kapseals]) when patient compliance is a problem
   b. If an oral loading dose is necessary, patient should be given a total of 1 g divided into 3 doses (400, 300, 300 mg) and administered at 2 hour intervals; maintenance dose is then instituted 24 hours after the loading dose; periodic serum levels should be obtained (therapeutic range is 10-20 μg/ml)
2. Status epilepticus: Loading dose of 10-15 mg/kg by slow IV injection (≤50 mg/min) followed by 100 mg PO/IV q6-8h

Indications: Seizure disorders; digitalis-induced ventricular dysrhythmias

Action: Hydantoin anticonvulsant

Contraindications and precautions
1. Sinus bradycardia, AV block greater than first-degree, sinoatrial block, Stokes-Adams syndrome
2. Do not use for seizures secondary to hypoglycemia or other metabolic causes
3. Discontinue phenytoin if patient develops skin rash
4. Use with caution in elderly patients and in patients with impaired liver function
5. Continuous monitoring of ECG and BP is necessary when administering IV phenytoin loading dose
6. Phenytoin serum levels are affected by many common drugs (e.g., increased levels may be seen with concomitant use of cimetidine, dicumarol, salicylates, sulfonamides, tolbutamide, diazepam)

PIPERACILLIN (Pipracil)

Preparations: *Inj* 2, 3, 4 g vials or bottles

Adult dosage
1. Serious infections: 200-300 mg/kg/day given IV in 4-6 divided doses
2. Complicated UTI: 125-200 mg/kg/day given IV in 3-4 divided doses

3. Uncomplicated UTI and community-acquired pneumonia: 100-125 mg/kg IV in 2-4 divided doses

NOTE: Decrease dosage in patients with renal impairment

Indications: Infections caused by susceptible bacterial organisms

Action: Piperazine penicillin derivative with increased activity against many gram-negative bacteria and *S. faecalis*

Contraindications and precautions: History of allergic reaction to penicillin or cephalosporins

PIPRACIL See PIPERACILLIN

PIROXICAM (Feldene)

Preparations: *Cap* 10, 20 mg

Adult dosage: 20 mg PO qd

Indications: Osteoarthritis, rheumatoid arthritis, ankylosing spondylitis

Action: Nonsteroidal antiinflammatory agent

Contraindications and precautions

1. Patients with syndrome of bronchospasm, nasal polyps, and angioedema precipitated by aspirin or other NSAIDs
2. Use with caution in patients with a history of upper GI bleeding, heart failure, renal insufficiency, liver dysfunction, hypertension and in patients with other conditions predisposing to fluid retention

POLYETHYLENE GLYCOL (PEG) 3350 ELECTROLYTE SOLUTION (Go litely)

Preparations: Disposable jug containing: PEG 236 g, sodium sulfate 22.74 g sodium bicarbonate 6.74 g, sodium chloride 5.86 g, potassium chloride 2.97 g; water is added to jug until a 4 L volume is reached

Adult dosage: PO 8 oz (240 ml) q10min until 4 L are consumed (may be given via nasogastric tube); bowel exam is usually scheduled 4 hours after initiation of PO ingestion (3 hours for drinking and 1 hour for complete bowel evacuation)

Indications: Bowel cleansing before colonoscopy and barium enema x-ray exam

Action: Osmotic agent

Contraindications and precautions: GI obstruction, gastric retention, bowel perforation, megacolon, or toxic colitis

PRAZOSIN (Minipress)

Preparations: *Cap* 1, 2, 5 mg

Adult dosage

1. Initial: 1 mg PO bid to tid (the first dose is best given at hs while the patient is in bed to decrease the risk of syncope)
2. Maintenance: 6-15 mg/day given in 2-3 divided doses
3. Maximum daily dose: 20 mg/day

Indications: Hypertension

Action: Postsynaptic α-adrenergic receptor blockage and possible direct relaxant action on vascular smooth muscle

Contraindications and precautions: Syncope occurs in 1% of patients given an initial dose $\geq$ 2 mg; hypotension may occur with concomitant use of β blockers

PREDNISONE
Preparations: *Tab* 1, 2.5, 5, 10, 20, 50 mg; *syrup* 1 mg/ml
Adult dosage: Total daily dose varies with clinical disorder being treated and patient's response to therapy
Indications: See dexamethasone
Action: Synthetic glucocorticoid with minimal sodium-retaining activity
Contraindications and precautions: See dexamethasone

PREMARIN See ESTROGENIC SUBSTANCES, CONJUGATED

PRIMAXIN See IMIPENEM-CILASTIN SODIUM

PROBENECID (Benemid)
Preparations: *Tab* 500 mg
Adult dosage
   1. Gout: initially 250 mg PO bid × 1 wk, then increase to 500 mg bid
   2. Prolongation of penicillin action: 500 mg PO qid
   NOTE: Decrease dosage in elderly patients and in patients with renal impairment
Indications: Hyperuricemia associated with gout and gouty arthritis; prolongation of penicillin action
Action: Decreases serum uric acid levels by inhibiting its tubular reabsorption; increases penicillin plasma levels by inhibiting tubular secretion of penicillin
Contraindications and precautions
   1. Acute gouty attack (therapy should not be started until attack has subsided)
   2. Use with caution in patients with blood dyscrasias, uric acid kidney stones, or history of peptic ulcer
   3. Avoid concomitant use of penicillin in patients with renal impairment
   4. Salicylates antagonize the uricosuric action of probenecid
   5. Probenecid increases the serum levels of conjugated sulfonamides (increased action of oral sulfonylureas and indomethacin)
   6. Probenecid may not be effective when the glomerular filtration rate is ≤ 30 ml/min
   7. When probenecid is used for gout, patient should alkalinize urine with sodium bicarbonate (3-7.5 g qd) and have adequate fluid intake to avoid crystallization of uric acid in acid urine

PROCAINAMIDE (Procan-SR, Pronestyl)
Preparations: *Cap and tab* 250, 375, 500 mg; *inj* 100, 500 mg/ml; *SR tab* 250, 500, 750, 1000 mg
Adult dosage
   1. IV loading (two methods):
      a. 100 mg IV bolus q5 min (slow IV injection) until dysrhythmia is suppressed or a maximum dose of 1 g has been given
      b. Infusion of 1000 mg of procainamide in 50 ml of D_5W (concentration is 20 mg/ml) administered at a constant rate of 1 ml/min over 30 min

2. Maintenance infusion: 1000 mg of procainamide in 250 ml of D_5W (concentration is 4 mg/ml) administered at 0.5-1.5 ml/min (2-6 mg/min)
3. PO: 50 mg/kg/day initially given in divided doses q3-6h (e.g., 60-70 kg person would receive 375 mg q3h or 750 mg q6h); dosage must be individualized to maintain therapeutic blood levels
NOTE: Elderly patients and others with cardiac, renal or hepatic insufficiency require lower doses

Indications: Premature ventricular contractions, ventricular tachycardia, prevention of recurrence of paroxysmal supraventricular tachycardia, atrial fibrillation or flutter following conversion to normal sinus rhythm

Action: Class I antidysrhythmic agent

Contraindications and precautions

1. Complete heart block, torsades des pointes, lupus erythematosus, long QT syndrome, second-degree heart block or bifascicular bundle branch block, severe sinus node dysfunction
2. Use caution when using procainamide in dysrhythmias associated with digitalis intoxication and in patients receiving other group IA antidysrhythmic agents
3. Discontinue procainamide if the patient develops a positive antinuclear antibodies test (ANA), first-degree AV block, QRS or QT prolongation >35% of baseline measurement
4. Myasthenia gravis may be exacerbated by procainamide

PROCAN-SR See PROCAINAMIDE

PROCARDIA See NIFEDIPINE

PROCHLORPERAZINE (Compazine)

Preparations: *Tab* 5, 10 mg; *syrup* 5 mg/5 ml; *suppos* 2.5, 5, 25 mg; *inj* 5 mg/ml ampul; *cap (spansule)* 10, 15, 30 mg

Adult dosage

1. PO: 5-10 mg tid to qid; if using spansule, 10 mg bid or 15 mg qAM
2. IM: 5-10 mg q6h; do not exceed 40 mg day
3. PR: 25 mg suppository bid
NOTE: Decrease dosage in elderly or debilitated patients

Indications: Control of severe nausea and vomiting; manifestations of psychotic disorders

Action: Phenothiazine tranquilizer with antiemetic properties

Contraindications and precautions

1. Comatose states, bone marrow depression, children <9 kg or younger than 2 years, pediatric surgery
2. Prochlorperazine may mask the underlying disorder causing the nausea and vomiting (e.g., drug overdose, intestinal obstruction)
3. Parenteral administration in patients with impaired cardiovascular system may result in hypotension

PRONESTYL See PROCAINAMIDE

PROPRANOLOL (Inderal)

Preparations: *Tab* 10, 20, 40, 60, 80, 90 mg; *inj* 1 mg/ml; *cap (Inderal LA)* 80, 120, 160 mg

Adult dosage
1. Hypertension: 40 mg PO bid initially; usual maintenance dosage is 120-140 mg/day
2. Angina pectoris: 10-20 mg PO qid; increase dosage at 3-7 day intervals prn; average dose is 160 mg/day
3. Dysrhythmias: 10-30 mg PO qid
4. Hypertrophic subaortic stenosis: 20-40 mg qid
5. Migraine: 40 mg PO bid; usual range is 160-240 mg/day
6. Post-MI prophylaxis: 180-240 mg/day in 2-3 divided doses

Indications: See above

Action: Nonselective β-adrenergic blocker

Contraindications and precautions
1. Cardiogenic shock, sinus bradycardia, greater than first-degree AV block, bronchial asthma, CHF (unless secondary to dysrhythmia treatable with propranolol
2. Use with caution in diabetics (may mask the symptoms of hypoglycemia), impaired renal or hepatic function, Wolff-Parkinson-White syndrome (may cause severe bradycardia), concomitant MAO inhibitor therapy, or in patients receiving catecholamine-depleting drugs

PROTAMINE SULFATE

Preparations: *Inj* 5 ml/50 mg ampul; 25 ml/250 mg vial

Adult dosage
1. Each mg of protamine sulfate neutralizes approximately 100 USP units of heparin
2. Protamine sulfate should only be given by slow IV injection; do not exceed 50 mg in any 10 min period

Indications: Treatment of heparin overdosage

Action: Neutralizes action of heparin by forming a heparin-protamine complex; neutralization of heparin occurs within 5 min of IV administration

Contraindications and precautions: Very rapid administration of protamine can result in severe hypotension and anaphylactoid-like reactions; monitor neutralizing effect by determining the PTT few minutes after administration of protamine sulfate

PROVENTIL See ALBUTEROL

QUINAGLUTE See QUINIDINE

QUINIDEX EXTENTABS See QUINIDINE

QUINIDINE

Preparations
1. *Tab*
   a. Sulfate salt: 100, 200, 300 mg (Quinidine sulfate, Quinora)
   b. Polygalacturonate salt: 275 mg (Cardioquin)
2. *Inj*
   a. Gluconate salt: 80 mg/ml
   b. Sulfate salt: 200 mg/ml

3. *Slow-release tab*
    a. Gluconate salt: 324 mg (Quinidine gluconate SR, Quinaglute Dura-tabs)
    b. Sulfate salt: 300 mg (Quinidex Exentabs)

Adult dosage
1. Quinidine sulfate
    a. PAC, PVC: 200-300 mg PO tid to qid
    b. Paroxysmal supraventricular tachycardia: 400-600 mg PO q2-3h until paroxysm is terminated
    c. Conversion of atrial fibrillation: 200 mg PO q2-3h × 5-8 doses (do not exceed 4 mg/day); increase daily dose until sinus rhythm is restored or toxic effects occur
    d. Maintenance therapy is 200-300 mg tid to qid
2. Quinidine polygalacturonate: 1 to 3 tabs PO may be used to terminate dysrhythmia; this dose may be repeated in 3-4 hr; if normal sinus rhythm is not restored after 3-4 equal doses, dose may be increased by ½-1 tab (137.5-275 mg) and administered 3-4 times before any further dosage increase; maintenance dosage is 1 tab bid
3. Slow-release tabs (gluconate and sulfate salts) may be given q12h

Indications: Ventricular dysrhythmias (PVCs, paroxysmal ventricular tachycardia not associated with heart block), supraventricular dysrhythmias (atrial flutter, atrial fibrillation, PAC, paroxysmal atrial tachycardia), junctional dysrhythmias (AV junctional premature complexes, paroxysmal junctional tachycardia)

Action: Class I antidysrhythmic; decreases conduction velocity and automaticity and prolongs refractory period

Contraindications and precautions
1. Complete AV block; digitalis intoxication manifested by AV conduction disorders; complete bundle branch block or other severe intraventricular conduction defects, especially those exhibiting a marked grade of QRS widening; myasthenia gravis; aberrant impulses and abnormal rhythms caused by escape mechanisms
2. Quinidine will produce a doubling of the digitalis plasma level in patients receiving digitalis (consider reduction of digitalis dose when starting quinidine)
3. Use with caution in patients with incomplete AV block (asystole and complete AV block may be produced)
4. Closely monitor patients with cardiac, hepatic, or renal insufficiency (increased risk of toxicity)
5. In the treatment of atrial fibrillation or flutter, digitalization is indicated before starting quinidine in order to block AV nodal conduction; if quinidine is used before digitalization, it may increase AV nodal conduction and ventricular rate

RANITIDINE (Zantac)
Preparations: *Tab* 150, 300 mg; *inj* 25 mg/ml
Adult dosage
1. PO: 150 mg PO bid or 300 mg PO qhs
2. IV: 50 mg q8h
NOTE: Decrease dosage in patients with renal impairment

Indications Short-term management of duodenal and gastric ulcers, treatment of pathologic hypersecretory conditions
Action: Histamine H_2 receptor antagonist
Contraindications and precautions: Use with caution in patients with impaired hepatic function (metabolized in the liver)

REGLAN See **METOCLOPRAMIDE**

RESTORIL See **TEMAZEPAM**

RIFAMPIN

Preparations: *Cap* 150, 300 mg
Adult dosage
   1. Pulmonary tuberculosis: 600 mg PO qd
   2. Meningococcal carriers: 600 mg PO qd
   NOTE: Rifampin should be administered 1 hr before, or 2 hr after a meal
Indications: Primary tuberculosis; treatment of asymptomatic carriers of *N. meningitidis* to eliminate meningococci from the nasopharynx
Action: It inhibits bacterial DNA-dependent RNA polymerase activity
Contraindications and precautions
   1. History of hypersensitivity to any of the rifamycins
   2. Use with caution in patients receiving anticoagulants of the coumarin type (increases requirement) and in patients with liver disease or receiving concomitant hepatotoxic agents (increased risk of hepatotoxicity)

ROCALTROL See **CALCITROL**

SELDANE See **TERFENADINE**

SEPTRA See **TRIMETHOPRIM**

SERAX See **OXAZEPAM**

SILVADENE See **SILVER SULFADIAZINE**

SILVER SULFADIAZINE (Silvadene)

Preparations: 20, 400, 1000 g jars; 20 g tubes
Adult dosage: Apply qd to bid to burn area (dressings not required over burn area)
Indications: Prevention and treatment of wound sepsis in patients with second- and third-degree burns
Action: Topical bactericidal agent effective against many gram-negative and gram-positive bacteria as well as yeast
Contraindications and precautions
   1. Use with caution in patients with G-6-PD deficiency (increased risk of hemolysis)
   2. Accumulation of the drug may occur in patients with impaired renal or hepatic function

SODIUM POLYSTYRENE SULFONATE (Kayexalate)

Preparations *Jar* 1 lb (453.6 g)
Adult dosage
1. PO: 15-60 g q6h prn given as a suspension in water or syrup (3-4 ml/g of resin)
2. PR: 30-50 g q6h prn given with 100 ml of sorbitol as a retention enema

Indications: Treatment of hyperkalemia
Action: Cation exchange resin; as it passes through the GI tract, the partially released sodium ions are replaced by potassium ions; its efficiency is approx 33%
Contraindications and precautions
1. Use with caution in patients with congestive heart failure, marked edema, severe hypertension, and any other condition in which a sodium load may be detrimental
2. Closely monitor serum K, Mg, and Ca (severe hypokalemia, hypomagnesemia, hypocalcemia may occur)
3. Concomitant administration of magnesium hydroxide, nonabsorbable cation-donating antacids, and laxatives should be avoided

SOLUCORTEF See HYDROCORTISONE SODIUM SUCCINATE

SOLUMEDROL See METHYLPREDNISOLONE

SPIRONOLACTONE (Aldactone)

Preparations: Tab 25, 50, 100 mg
Adult dosage
1. Edema: 25-200 mg/day administered in single or divided doses; adjust dose after 5 days; if diuresis remains inadequate, add a second diuretic agent with action more proximally in the renal tubule
2. Essential hypertension: 50-100 mg/day initially; adjust dose after 2 weeks; consider adding a diuretic agent with action on the proximal renal tubule if the patient remains hypertensive
3. Hypokalemia: 25-100 mg/day

Indications: Primary hyperaldosteronism; edema states secondary to cirrhosis, nephrotic syndrome, CHF; essential hypertension; hypokalemia (diuretic-induced) when oral potassium supplements or other potassium-sparing regimens are inappropriate
Action: Aldosterone antagonist; acts through competitive binding of receptors at the aldosterone-dependent Na^+-K^+ exchange site in the distal convoluted renal tubule
Contraindications and precautions
1. Anuria, hyperkalemia, renal impairment
2. Avoid excessive potassium intake (increased risk of hyperkalemia)
3. Avoid concomitant administration of other potassium-sparing diuretics
4. Decrease dosage of other diuretics or antihypertensive agents when starting spironolactone (potentiation of their effect)

SUCRALFATE (Carafate)

Preparations: *Tab* 1 g
Adult dosage: 1 g qid
   NOTE: Sucralfate should be taken on an empty stomach
   NOTE: Do not take antacids within 30 min of sucralfate (before or after)
Indications: Short-term treatment of duodenal ulcer
Action: It forms an ulcer-adherent complex that covers the ulcer site and protects it against further attack by acid, pepsin, and bile salts
Contraindications and precautions: Simultaneous administration of sucralfate with tetracycline, phenytoin, digoxin, or H_2 blockers will result in a reduction in the bioavailability of these agents

SULFASALAZINE (Azulfadine)

Preparations: *Tab* 500 mg; *enteric-coated tab* 500 mg; *oral suspension* 250 mg/5 ml
Adult dosage: 500 mg PO qid initially
   NOTE: Azulfadine should be taken after meals to decrease adverse GI effects
Indications: Adjunctive therapy of ulcerative colitis
Action: Sulfasalazine is split in the colon into sulfapyridine and 5-aminosalicylic acid; the latter has antiinflammatory activity (inhibition of prostaglandin synthesis)
Contraindications and precautions
   1. Hypersensitivity to sulfonamides or salicylates, infants under 2 years of age, intestinal or urinary obstruction, porphyria
   2. Use with caution in patients with severe allergy, bronchial asthma, G-6-PD deficiency
   3. Concomitant administration of folic acid or digoxin will result in decreased absorption of these drugs

SULINDAC (Clinoril)

Preparations: *Tab* 150, 200 mg
Adult dosage: 150-200 mg PO bid
   NOTE: Sulindac should be administered with food
Indications: Osteoarthritis, rheumatoid arthritis, ankylosing spondylitis, acute gouty arthritis, acute subacromial bursitis/supraspinatus tendinitis
Action: Nonsteroidal antiinflammatory agent
Contraindications and precautions
   1. Patients with a history of asthmatic attacks, urticaria, or rhinitis precipitated by aspirin or other nonsteroidal antiinflammatory agents
   2. Peptic ulceration and GI bleeding can occur in patients taking sulindac; use with caution in patients with a history of PUD, hemorrhagic disorders, and in elderly patients
   3. Closely monitor patients with hypertension, impaired renal, hepatic, or cardiac function (or any other conditions predisposing to fluid retention)

SYMMETREL See **AMANTIDINE**

SYNTHROID See **THYROXINE**

TAGAMET See **CIMETIDINE**

TAMBOCOR See **FLECAINIDE**

TEMAZEPAM (Restoril)

Preparations: *Cap* 15, 30 mg
Adult dosage: 15-30 mg PO qhs
   NOTE: Use lower doses in elderly or debilitated patients
Indications: Insomnia
Action: Short-acting benzodiazepine
Contraindications and precautions: Avoid concomitant use of alcohol or
   other CNS depressants

TENORMIN See **ATENOLOL**

TERBUTALINE (Brethine)

Preparations: *Tab* 2.5, 5 mg; *inj* 1 mg/ml ampul
Adult dosage
   1. PO: 2.5-5 mg PO tid
   2. IM/SC: 0.25 mg; may repeat once after 30 min if no relief
   NOTE: Do not exceed a total PO dose 14 mg/24 h in adults
Indications: Bronchial asthma and reversible bronchospasm
Action: Bronchodilator
Contraindications and precautions
   1. Known hypersensitivity to sympathetic amines
   2. Avoid concomitant use of other sympathomimetic agents
   3. Use with caution in patients with cardiac disease, cardiac dysrhyth-
      mias, diabetes, hypertension, hyperthyroidism, or history of seizures

TERFENADINE (Seldane)

Preparations: *Tab* 60 mg
Adult dosage: 60 mg PO bid
Indications: Relief of symptoms associated with seasonal allergic rhinitis
Action: Peripheral specific histamine H_1 receptor antagonist
Contraindications and precautions: Known hypersensitivity to terfenadine

TETRACYCLINE (Achromycin)

Preparations: *Cap* and *tab* 250, 500 mg; *inj* 100, 250, 500 mg; *syrup* 125
   mg/5 ml
Adult dosage: 250-500 mg PO q6h (taken between meals)
Indications: Infections caused by susceptible bacterial organisms
Action: Inhibits protein synthesis at the 30S ribosomal subunit
Contraindications and precautions
   1. Hypersensitivity to any of the tetracyclines
   2. Use with caution in patients with impaired renal or hepatic function
   3. Concomitant therapy with antacids impairs tetracycline absorption
   4. Discontinue tetracycline if overgrowth of nonsusceptible organisms
      occurs
   5. Patients receiving anticoagulants should readjust the dose (tetracycline
      depresses plasma prothrombin activity)

Table 21-7 Theophylline preparations

Route of Administration	Trade Name	Preparations	Comments
PO	Slo-Phyllin	*Tab* 100, 200 mg *Syrup* 80 mg/15 ml *Capsules (Gyrocaps)* 60, 125, 250 mg	Rapidly absorbed for acute therapy Slow-release product for chronic asthma
PO	Theodur	*Tab* 100, 200, 300 mg *Cap* 50, 75, 125, 200 mg	Slow-release product for chronic asthma
PO	Theo-24	*Cap* 100, 200, 300 mg	Long-acting preparation requiring once/day dosage
PR	Somophyllin	*Rectal solution* 300 mg/ 5 ml	Rapidly absorbed for acute therapy
IV	Aminophyllin	*IV solution* 25 mg/ ml	Rapidly absorbed for acute therapy

THEODUR See **THEOPHYLLINE**

THEOPHYLLINE PREPARATIONS

Preparations: See Table 21-7

Adult dosage
1. Loading dose for acute bronchospasm: 5 mg/kg; 3 mg/kg if the patient is on theophylline but a level cannot be immediately obtained
2. Maintenance dose for acute symptoms: See Table 21-8
3. Maintenance for chronic asthma: 400 mg/day PO in divided doses (e.g., Theodur 200 mg bid); monitor theophylline plasma concentration (therapeutic is 10-20 μg/ml) and adjust dosage accordingly

Indications: Relief or prevention of symptoms of bronchial asthma; reversible bronchospasm associated with chronic bronchitis and emphysema

Action: Direct relaxation of the smooth muscle of the bronchial airway and pulmonary blood vessels (bronchodilator and smooth muscle relaxant); additional effects include diuresis, coronary vasodilation, cardiac, skeletal muscle, and cerebral stimulation

Contraindications and precautions
1. Use with caution in patients with severe cardiac disease, hypertension, hepatic or renal impairment, hyperthyroidism, dysrhythmias, and in elderly patients
2. Cimetidine and erythromycin may increase the serum theophylline level
3. Dilantin and phenobarbital decrease the serum theophylline level

Table 21-8 Theophylline maintenance dosage for acute symptoms

Population Group	IV Aminophylline (mg/kg/hr)	Oral Theophylline (mg/kg/hr)
Otherwise healthy adult smokers	0.9	0.83
Otherwise healthy nonsmoking adults; otherwise healthy elderly patients	0.3-0.5	0.53
Cardiac or hepatic decompensation; cor pulmonale	0.2-0.3	0.26

THIAMINE

Preparations: *Tab* 10, 50, 100 mg; *inj* 100 mg/ml
Adult dosage: Severe deficiency: 100 mg IM/PO qd
Indications: Thiamine deficiency

THIORIDAZINE (Mellaril)

Preparations: *Tab* 10, 15, 25, 50, 100, 150, 200 mg; *liq conc* 30, 100 mg/ml; *susp* 25, 100 mg/5 ml
Adult dosage
  1. Psychotic manifestations: Usual starting dose is 50-100 mg PO tid
  2. Treatment of depression anxiety: Usual starting dose is 25 mg PO tid
Indications: Management of manifestations of psychotic disorders; short-term treatment of depression, anxiety, agitation
Action: Phenothiazine
Contraindications and precautions: Severe CNS depression, hypertensive or hypotensive heart disease, hypersensitivity to phenothiazines

THORAZINE See CHLORPROMAZINE

THYROXINE (Synthroid)

Preparations: *Tab* 25, 50, 100, 125, 150, 175, 200, 300 μg; *inj* 100, 200, 500 μg
Adult dosage
  1. Hypothyroidism in otherwise healthy adult: 100 μg/day initially, increasing to a maintenance dose of 100-200 μg/day over a 3 wk period
  2. Hypothyroidism in elderly patients: 25 μg/day initially, increasing by 25 μg/day at 3-4 wk intervals depending on patient's response
  3. Myxedema coma: 200-500 μg IV initially; may give additional 100-300 μg in 24 hr if necessary; decrease dosage in patients with heart disease
Indications: Hypothyroidism
Action: Synthetic preparation of thyroid hormone T_4

Contraindications and precautions
1. Thyrotoxicosis; acute MI, uncorrected adrenal insufficiency are relative contraindications
2. Use with caution in elderly patients and in patients with cardiovascular disease

TICAR See **TICARCILLIN**

TICARCILLIN (Ticar)

Preparations: *Inj* - 1, 3, 6 g vials
Adult dosage
1. Serious systemic infections: 200-300 mg/kg/day IV in divided doses q3h, q4h, or q6h
2. Complicated urinary tract infections (UTI): 150-200 mg/kg/day IV in divided doses q4h or q6h
3. Uncomplicated UTI: 1 g IV/IM q6h
NOTE: Decrease dosage in renal or hepatic insufficiency

Indications: Treatment of susceptible bacterial organisms
Action: Semisynthetic penicillin; has activity similar to carbenicillin, less active against gram-positive organisms, more active against *Pseudomonas aeruginosa*
Contraindications and precautions: Hypersensitivity to penicillin

TIGAN See **TRIMETHOBENZAMIDE**

TIMOLOL (Blocadren)

Preparations: *Tab* 5, 10, 20 mg
Adult dosage
1. Hypertension: 10 mg PO bid initially; usual maintenance dose is 20-40 mg/day
2. Post-MI: 10 mg PO bid

Indications: Hypertension, post-MI
Action: Nonselective β-adrenergic receptor blocking agent
Contraindications and precautions
1. Bronchial asthma, severe COPD, sinus bradycardia, second- or third-degree AV block, overt cardiac failure, cardiogenic shock
2. Use with caution in patients subject to hypoglycemia or in diabetics receiving sulfonylureas or insulin therapy
3. Avoid abrupt withdrawal (increases risk of exacerbation of ischemic heart disease)
4. Use with caution in patients with impaired renal or hepatic function (partially metabolized in the liver and excreted mainly by the kidneys)

TOBRAMYCIN

Preparations: *Inj* 10, 40 mg/ml
Adult dosage
1. Adults with normal renal function and serious infection: 1 mg/kg q8h; for *life-threatening infection* may use 1.66 mg/kg q8h (reduce dose as soon as possible)

2. Patients with impaired renal function: Give initial loading dose of 1 mg/kg; additional doses should be adjusted based on the creatinine clearance (refer to gentamycin reduction schedule)

NOTE: Monitor serum tobramycin levels and adjust dosage accordingly

Indications: Treatment of serious infections caused by susceptible bacterial organisms

Action: Aminoglycoside antibiotic; inhibits protein synthesis in susceptible organisms

Contraindictions and precautions
1. Use with caution in patients with impaired renal function.
2. Concurrent or sequential use of other nephrotoxic or neurotoxic drugs should be avoided
3. Advanced age and dehydration increase the risk of toxicity
4. Eighth cranial nerve function should be closely monitored

TOCAINIDE (Tonocard)

Preparations *Tab* 400, 600 mg

Adult dosage: Initially 400 mg PO q8h; usual adult dosage is 400-800 mg tid

NOTE: Decrease dosage in patients with renal or hepatic impairment

Indications: Suppression of symtomatic ventricular dysrhythmias

Action: Primary amine analog of lidocaine; produces dose-dependent decreases in sodium and potassium conductance, thereby decreasing excitability of myocardial cells

Contraindications and precautions
1. Hypersensitivity to tocainide or to local anesthetics of the amide type, use in patients with second- or third-degree AV block in absence of an artificial ventricular pacemaker
2. Use with caution in patients with heart failure (tocainide can worsen the degree of failure); in patients with severe renal or hepatic disease, decreased elimination can lead to toxicity

TOLAZAMIDE (Tolinase)

Preparations: *Tab* 100, 250, 500 mg

Adult dosage: 100-250 mg PO qd initially; may gradually increase to 1 g daily in 1-2 doses

NOTE: Should be administered with breakfast

Indications: Hyperglycemia from non–insulin-dependent diabetes mellitus (type II) not satisfactorily controlled by diet alone

Action: First-generation sulfonylurea; lowers plasma glucose mainly by stimulating release of insulin from pancreas

Contraindications and precautions
1. Diabetic ketoacidosis
2. Use as sole therapy for type I diabetes

TOLINASE See TOLAZAMIDE

TONOCARD See TOCAINIDE

TRANDATE See LABETOLOL

TRANXENE See CLORAZEPATE

TRIAZOLAM (Halcion)

Preparations: *Tab* 0.125, 0.25, 0.5 mg

Adult dosage: Initially 0.125-0.25 mg at hs; usual dosage range is 0.25-0.5 mg at hs

NOTE: Use lower doses in geriatric or debilitated patients

Indications: Short-term management of insomnia

Action: Short-acting benzodiazepine

Contraindications and precautions

1. Hypersensitivity to triazolam or other benzodiazepines
2. Simultaneous ingestion of alcohol or other CNS depressant drugs is contraindicated

TRIMETHOBENZAMIDE (Tigan)

Preparations: *Cap* 100, 250 mg; *supp* 100, 200 mg; *inj* 100 mg/ml

Adult dosage

1. Cap: 250 mg PO tid to qid
2. Supp: 200 mg PR tid to qid
3. Inj: 200 mg IM tid to qid

Indications: Control of nausea and vomiting

Action: Antiemetic agent; exerts its action on chemoreceptor trigger zone in medulla oblongata

Contraindications and precautions

1. Do not use suppositories in patients allergic to benzocaine
2. Determine etiology of vomiting before using antiemetics

TRIMETHOPRIM AND SULFAMETHOXAZOLE (Bactrim, Septra)

Preparations: *Ampul* and *5 ml vial* 80 mg trimethoprim (16 mg/ml) and 400 mg sulfamethoxazole (80 mg/ml); *10 ml vial:* 160 mg trimethoprim (16 mg/ml) and 800 mg sulfamethoxazole (80 mg/ml); *Tab:* 80 mg trimethoprim and 400 mg sulfamethoxazole; 160 mg trimethoprim and 800 mg sulfamethoxazole (Bactrim DS); *suspension:* 40 mg trimethoprim and 200 mg sulfamethoxazole/5 ml teaspoonful

Adult dosage

1. *Pneumocystits carinii* pneumonitis: 20 mg/kg trimethoprim and 100 mg/kg sulfamethoxazole/24 h given by IV infusion in equally divided doses q6h $\times$ 14 days
2. Urinary tract infections, acute exacerbation of chronic bronchitis, shigellosis: 1 Bactrim DS tab bid or two regular Bactrim tabs bid; duration of therapy is 14 days for chronic bronchitis, 10-14 days for UTI, and 5 days for shigellosis

Indications: Urinary tract infections, acute exacerbation of chronic bronchitis, shigellosis, *Pneumocystis carinii* pneumonitis

Action: Sulfamethoxazole inhibits bacterial synthesis of dihydrofolic acid; trimethoprim blocks production of tetrahydrofolic acid from dihydrofolic acid; together they block two consecutive steps in the biosynthesis of nucleic acids and proteins

Contraindications and precautions

1. Hypersensitivity to trimethoprim or sulfonamides; documented megaloblastic anemia from folate deficiency

2. Use with caution in impaired renal or hepatic function, G-6-PD deficiency, and in patients with severe allergy or bronchial asthma

TYLENOL See **ACETAMINOPHEN**

UNIPEN See **NAFCILLIN**

VALISONE See **BETAMETHASONE**

VALIUM See **DIAZEPAM**

VANCERIL See **BECLOMETHASONE**

VANCOCIN See **VANCOMYCIN**

VANCOMYCIN (Vancocin)

Preparations: *Inj* 500 mg vial; *PO* mix a 1 g vial with 20 ml of H_2O (250 mg/5 ml); 10 g vial mix with 115 ml of H_2O (500 mg/ 6 ml)
Adult dosage
1. Pseudomembranous colitis: 125-500 mg PO q6h or 1 g PO q12h × 7 = 10 days
2. Potentially life-threatening infections: 500 mg IV q6h or 1 g IV q12h
NOTE: IV doses should be infused over one hour
NOTE: Dosage must be reduced in patients with renal insufficiency
Indications: Pseudomembranous colitis, infections caused by susceptible bacterial organisms
Action: Bactericidal against many gram-positive bacteria; exerts its action by inhibition of cell wall synthesis
Contraindications and precautions
1. Avoid concomitant use of ototoxic or nephrotoxic agents
2. Use with caution in patients with impaired renal function
3. Monitor auditory function and vancomycin serum levels in patients receiving vancomycin for prolonged duration; therapeutic peak levels are 20-35 μg/ml, trough levels 5-10 μg/ml

VASOTEC See **ENAPRIL**

VENTOLIN See **ALBUTEROL**

VERAPAMIL (Calan, Isoptin)

Preparations: *Tab* 80, 120 mg; *inj* 5 mg/2 ml; *sustained release tab* 240 mg
Adult dosage
1. PO: 80 mg tid to qid initially; increase dose gradually until optimal response is obtained; average total daily dose is 320-480 mg; do not exceed 480 mg/day in patients with angina; dose for hypertension is 240 mg (SR) qd
2. IV: Initial dose is 5-10 mg (0.075-0.15 mg/kg) given as slow IV bolus (>2 min); may repeat with 10 mg (0.15 mg/kg), given over 5 min approx 30 min after first dose if initial response is inadequate
Indications: PO: angina, hypertension; IV: rapid conversion of paroxysmal supraventricular tachycardia to sinus rhythm, temporary control of rapid ventricular rate in atrial flutter or atrial fibrillation (except when the atrial flutter or fibrillation is associated with accessory bypass tracts)
Action: Calcium channel antagonist

Contraindications and precautions: Severe hypotension or cardiogenic shock, second- or third-degree AV block (except in patients with functioning artificial pacemaker), sick sinus syndrome (in absence of artificial pacemaker), severe CHF (unless secondary to SVT amenable to verapamil therapy), ventricular tachycardia, atrial flutter or fibrillation and an accessory bypass tract, severe left ventricular dysfunction (negative inotropic effect); verapamil increases serum digoxin levels by 50%-75%

VISTARIL See **HYDROXYZINE**

WARFARIN (Coumadin)

Preparations: *Tab* 2, 2.5, 5, 7.5, 10 mg

Adult dosage: Initially 10-15 mg PO qd × 2-3 days; monitor prothrombin time and adjust dosage accordingly to maintain prothrombin time 1.3-1.5 times control prothrombin time (higher levels may be indicated in patients with mechanical prosthetic valves and patients with recurrent systemic embolism)

Indications: Prophylaxis and treatment of venous thrombosis, atrial fibrillation with embolization, prophylaxis and treatment of pulmonary embolism (following heparin therapy)

Action: Inhibits hepatic synthesis of coagulation factor (depression of factors II, VII, IX, X)

Contraindications and precautions: Hemorrhagic tendencies, pregnancy, severe hepatic or renal disease, severe hypertension, blood dyscrasias, vitamin K deficiency; vitamin K (Phytonadione) 10-50 mg SCIM or fresh frozen plasma (FFP) can be used to reverse the effect of warfarin

XANAX See **ALPRAZOLAM**

ZANTAC See **RANITIDINE**

ZAROXOLYN See **METOLAZONE**

ZINACEF See **CEFUROXIME**

ZOVIRAX See **ACYCLOVIR**

ZYLOPRIM See **ALLOPURINOL**

Bibliography and suggested reading

1. Girwood, R.H.: Clinical pharmacology, ed. 25, Philadelphia, 1985, W.B. Saunders Co.
2. Goth, A., and Vessell, E.S.: Medical pharmacology: principles and concepts, ed. 11, St. Louis, 1984, The C.V. Mosby Co.
3. Herfindal, E. and Hirschman J: Clinical pharmacy and therapeutics, ed. 3, Baltimore, 1984, Williams & Wilkins.
4. Knoben, J.E., and Anderson, P.O.: Handbook of clinical drug data, ed. 5, Hamilton, Ill., 1985, Drug Intelligence Publications, Inc.
5. Information obtained from individual drug manufacturer's product information package inserts.

Appendixes

APPENDIX I: ENTERAL NUTRITIONAL PRODUCTS

Routine oral or tube supplemental feeding (Ensure)

Intact protein, protein isolates, lactose-free product: each 100 ml contains:

Protein	3.65 g	Calcium	2.7 mEq
Carbohydrate	14.24 g	Chloride	3.0 mEq
Fat	3.65 g	Calories	106
Potassium	3.2 mEq	mOsm = 450	
Sodium	3.3 mEq		

This product also contains all known essential vitamins and minerals for adults and for children 4 or more years of age.

Routine tube feeding (Isocal)

Lactose-free and low in sodium; each 100 ml contains:

Protein	3.25 g	Calcium	3.00 mEq
Carbohydrate	12.50 g	Chloride	2.80 mEq
Fat	4.20 g	Calories	100
Potassium	3.20 mEq	mOsm = 300	
Sodium	2.20 mEq		

This product also contains all known essential vitamins and minerals for adults and for children 4 or more years of age.

Routine tube feeding (Osmolite HN)

Lactose-free and low in sodium; each 100 ml contains:

Protein	4.4 g	Calcium	76 mg
Carbohydrate	13.9 g	Chloride	4.1 mEq
Fat	3.6 g	Calories	106
Potassium	4.0 mEq	mOsm = 310	
Sodium	4.0 mEq		

This product also contains all known essential vitamins and minerals for adults and for children 4 or more years of age.

High-calorie supplemental feeding (Magnacal)

Lactose-free product; each 100 ml contains:

Protein	7.0 g	Calcium	5.0 mEq
Carbohydrate	25.0 g	Chloride	2.7 mEq
Fat	8.0 g	Calories	200
Potassium	3.2 mEq	mOsm = 590	
Sodium	4.3 mEq		

This product also contains all known essential vitamins and minerals for adults and for children 4 or more years of age.

Low-residue oral or tube feeding (Criticare)

High-nitrogen elemental diet; each 100 ml contains:

Protein	3.80 g
Carbohydrate	22.20 g
Fat	0.03 g
Calories	106

mOsm = 650

This product also contains all known essential vitamins and minerals for adults and for children 4 or more years of age.

Essential amino acid formulation (Amin-Aid)

Nutritional product for management of uremic patients; each 100 ml contains:

Protein	1.94 g
Carbohydrate	36.54 g
Fat	4.62 g
Calories	195.5

mOsm = 850

This product is low in electrolytes and contains no vitamins.

Branched-chain amino acid formulation (Hepatic-Aid)

Nutritional management of liver disease; each 100 ml contains:

Protein	4.26 g
Carbohydrate	28.80 g
Fat	3.62 g
Calories	164.7

mOsm = 900

This product contains negligible electrolytes and no vitamins or minerals.

Oral supplemental feeding (Citrotein)

Lactose-free, cholesterol-free, gluten-free; each 100 ml contains:

Protein	4.29 g
Carbohydrate	13.0 g
Fat	0.18 g
Potassium	1.9 mEq
Sodium	3.2 mEq
Calcium	5.6 mEq
Chloride	2.9 mEq
Calories	71

mOsm = 496

Routine oral supplemental feeding (Forta Pudding)

Each 150 g contains:

Protein	6.8 g
Carbohydrate	34.0 g
Fat	9.7 g
Potassium	7.7 mEq
Sodium	9.6 mEq
Calcium	10.0 mEq
Chloride	6.0 mEq
Calories	250

This product also contains all known essential vitamins and minerals for adults and for children 4 or more years of age.

Caloric additive product (Polycose)

Each 100 ml contains:

Carbohydrate	50.0 g
Potassium	0.5 mEq
Sodium	2.5 mEq
Calcium	1.5 mEq
Chloride	3.1 mEq
Calories	200
mOsm = 850	

Routine oral supplemental feeding (Instant Breakfast)

Each 100 ml contains:

Protein	6.25 g
Carbohydrate	12.10 g
Fat	3.40 g
Potassium	5.90 mEq
Sodium	4.70 mEq
Calcium	7.30 mEq
Chloride	n/a
Calories	103.6

Nutritionally complete supplement when mixed with 8 oz. whole milk.

High-protein clear liquid product (high-protein gelatin)

Each 150 ml contains:

Protein	17.0 g
Carbohydrate	18.0 g
Fat	0.0 g
Potassium	5.3 mEq
Sodium	10.8 mEq
Calories	140

This product may be used as a supplement on clear liquid diets.

APPENDIX II: NOMOGRAM FOR CALCULATION OF BODY SURFACE AREA

Place a straight edge from the patient's height in the left column to his weight in the right column. The point of intersection on the body surface area column indicates the body surface area (BSA). Reproduced from Behrman, R.E., and Vaughn, V.C. (editors): Nelson's textbook of pediatrics, ed. 12, Philadelphia, 1983, W.B. Saunders Co.

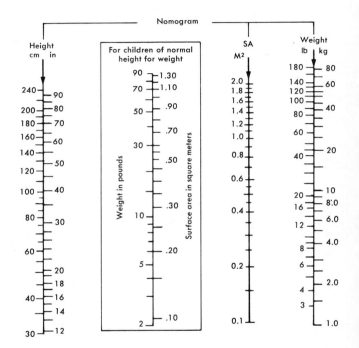

APPENDIX III: NARCOTIC ANALGESICS COMPARISON CHARTS

PO narcotic analgesics

Drug	Equivalent PO Dose (mg)	Duration of Analgesia (hr)
Codeine	200	4-6
Hydromorphone (Dilaudid)	7.5	4-6
Levorphanol (Levor-Dromoran)	4	4-7
Meperidine (Demerol)	300	4-6
Methadone (Dolophine)	20	3-5
Morphine	60	4-7
Oxycodone (Percodan)	30	3-5
Pentazocine (Talwin)	180	4-7
Propoxyphene (Darvon)	240	4-6

IM narcotic analgesics (conversion from PO to IM: codeine 200 mg PO = 130 mg IM)

Drug	Equivalent IM Dose (mg)	Duration of Analgesia (hr)
Codeine	130	4-6
Hydromorphone (Dilaudid)	1.5	4-5
Levorphanol (Levo-Dromoran)	2	4-6
Meperidine (Demerol)	75	4-6
Methadone (Dolophine)	10	3-5
Morphine	10	4-6
Nalbuphine (Nubain)	10	3-6
Pentazocine (Talwin)	60	4-6

APPENDIX IV: CORTICOSTEROID COMPARISON CHART

Drug	Equivalent Antiinflammatory Dosages (mg)	Glucocorticoid Potency	Mineralocorticoid Potency	Route of Administration
Prednisone	10	4	0.8	PO
Hydrocortisone (Solu-Cortef)	40	1.0	1.0	PO, IM, IV
Methylprednisolone (Solu-Medrol)	8	5.0	0.5	PO, IM, IV
Dexamethasone (Decadron)	1.5	30	0	PO, IV
Cortisone	50	0.8	0.8	PO, IM

APPENDIX V: CONVERSION FORMULAS

1. Temperature
   a. $°C = (°F - 32) \times 5/9$
   b. $°F = (°C \times 9/5) + 32$
2. Weight
   a. 1 lb = 0.454 kg
   b. 1 kg = 2.204 lb
3. Length
   a. 1 inch = 2.54 cm
   b. 1 cm = 0.3937 inch

APPENDIX VI: COMMONLY USED COMBINATION DRUG PREPARATIONS*

Trade Name	Therapeutic Category	Dosage Forms and Composition	Common Adult Dosage
Actifed	Decongestant-antihis-tamine	Tab: pseudoephedrine (60 mg), triprolidine (2.5 mg) Syrup: pseudoephedrine (30 mg), triprolidine (1.25 mg)/5 ml	1 tab tid or qid PO 10 ml tid or qid PO
Actifed-C expectorant (C5)	Antitussive-expecto-rant	Syrup: pseudoephedrine (30 mg), triprolidine (2 mg), codeine (10 mg), guaifenesin (100 mg)/5 ml	10 ml tid or qid PO
Aldactazide	Diuretic	Tab: spironolactone (25 mg), hydrochlorothiazide (25 mg)	1 tab bid or qid PO
Aldoril-15	Antihypertensive	Tab: hydrochlorothiazide (15 mg), methyldopa (250 mg)	1 tab bid or tid PO
Aldoril-30		Tab: hydrochlorothiazide (30 mg), methyldopa (250 mg)	1 tab bid or tid PO
Aldoril D30		Tab: hydrochlorothiazide (30 mg), methyldopa (500 mg)	1 tab bid or tid PO
Aldoril D50		Tab: hydrochlorothiazide (50 mg), methyldopa (500 mg)	1 tab bid or tid PO
Anusol-HC	Hemorrhoidal prepa-ration	Cream and supp: hydrocortisone (0.5%), bismuth subgallate (2.25%), bismuth resorcinol (1.75%), benzyl benzoate (1.2%), zinc oxide (11%), Peruvian balsam (1.8%)	Cream: topically prn Supp: 1 PR bid

KEY: C2: Controlled substance, schedule II; C3: Controlled substance, schedule III; C4: Controlled substance, schedule IV; C5: Controlled substance, schedule V.
*From DiGregorio G.J., Barbieri E.J., and Piraino A.J.: Handbook of commonly prescribed drugs, 1984, Medical Surveillance Inc.

Continued.

APPENDIX VI: COMMONLY USED COMBINATION DRUG PREPARATIONS—cont'd

Trade Name	Therapeutic Category	Dosage Forms and Composition	Common Adult Dosage
Bactrim	Antibacterial	Tab: trimethoprim (80 mg), sulfamethoxazole (400 mg)	2 tab q12h PO
		Susp: trimethoprim (40 mg), sulfamethoxazole (200 mg)/5 ml	20 ml q12H PO
		Inj: trimethoprim (80 mg), sulfamethoxazole (400 mg)/5 ml	Total daily dose: 8 to 20 mg/kg (based on trimethoprim) in 2-4 equally divided doses q6, 8 or 12 hr IV
Bactrim DS	Antibacterial	Tab: trimethoprim (160 mg), sulfamethoxazole (800 mg)	1 tab q12h PO
Combid	Antispasmodic	Cap:isopropamide (5 mg), prochlorperazine (10 mg)	1 cap q12h PO
Cortisporin otic	Steroid-antibiotic	Sol and susp: hydrocortisone (1%), neomycin (5 mg), polymyxin B (10,000 U/ml)	4 drops into ear tid or qid
Darvocet-N 100 (C4)	Narcotic analgesic	Tab: propoxyphene (100 mg), acetaminophen (650 mg)	1 tab q4h prn pain PO
Darvon compound-65 (C4)	Narcotic analgesic	Cap: propoxyphene (65 mg), aspirin (389 mg), caffeine (32.4 mg)	1 cap q4h prn pain PO
Deconamine	Decongestant-antihistamine	Tab: pseudoephedrine (60 mg), chlorpheniramine (4 mg)	1 tab q4-8h PO
		Syrup: pseudophedrine (30 mg), chlorpheniramine (2 mg)/5 ml	5-10 ml tid or qid PO
Demulen	Oral contraceptive	Tab: ethynodiol (1 mg), ethinyl estradiol (50 μg)	1 tab qd PO

Dimetapp	Decongestant-antihis- tamine	Elix: pseudoephedrine (5 mg), brompheniramine (4 mg), phenylpropanolamine (5 mg)/5 ml	5-10 ml tid or qid PO
		Tab: pseudoephedrine (15 mg), brompheniramine (12 mg), phenylpropanolamine (15 mg)	1 tab q12h PO
Donnatal	Antispasmodic	Cap and tab: atropine (19.4 μg), scopolamine (6.5 μg), hyoscyamine (0.1 mg), phenobarbital (16.2 mg)	1-2 cap or tab tid or qid PO
		Elix: atropine (19.4 μg), scopolamine (6.5 μg), hyoscyamine (0.1 mg), phenobarbital (16.2 mg), alcohol (23%)/5 ml	5-10 ml tid or qid PO
Drixoral	Decongestant-antihis- tamine	Tab: pseudoephedrine (120 mg), dextromphenira- mine (5 mg)	1 tab q12h PO
Dyazide	Diuretic	Cap: triamterene (50 mg), hydrochlorothiazide (25 mg)	1 cap qd or bid PO
Empirin w/codeine #2 (C3)	Narcotic analgesic	Tab: aspirin (325 mg), codeine (15 mg)	1-2 tab q4h prn pain PO
Empirin w/codeine #3 (C3)		Tab: aspirin (325 mg), codeine (30 mg)	1-2 tab q4h prn pain PO
Empirin w/codeine #4 (C3)		Tab: aspirin (325 mg), codeine (60 mg)	1 tab q4h prn pain PO
Entex LA	Expectorant	Tab: phenylpropanolamine (75 mg), guaifenesin (400 mg)	1 tab q12h PO
Equagesic (C4)	Nonnarcotic analgesic	Tab: aspirin (325 mg), meprobamate 200 mg)	1-2 tab tid or qid PO
Fiorinal (C3)	Nonnarcotic analgesic	Tab and cap: aspirin (325 mg), caffeine (40 mg), butalbital (50 mg)	1-2 tab or cap q4h PO

Continued.

APPENDIX VI: COMMONLY USED COMBINATION DRUG PREPARATIONS—cont'd

Trade Name	Therapeutic Category	Dosage Forms and Composition	Common Adult Dosage
Fiorinal w/codeine #1 (C3)	Narcotic analgesic	Cap: Fiorinal components + codeine (7.5 mg)	1-2 cap, repeat prn up to 6 caps per day PO
Fiorinal w/codeine #2 (C3)		Cap: Fiorinal components + codeine (15 mg)	
Fiorinal w/codeine #3 (C3)		Cap: Fiorinal components + codeine (30 mg)	
Hydropres 25	Antihypertensive	Tab: hydrochlorothiazide (25 mg), reserpine (0.125 mg)	1-2 tab qd or bid PO
Hydropres 50		Tab:hydrochlorothiazide (50 mg), reserpine (0.125 mg)	1 tab qd or bid PO
Inderide-40/25	Antihypertensive	Tab: propranolol (40 mg), hydrochlorothiazide (25 mg)	1-2 tab daily or bid PO
Inderide-80/25		Tab: propranolol (80 mg), hydrochlorothiazide (25 mg)	1-2 tab daily or bid PO
K-Lyte	Potassium supplement	Tab: potassium bicarbonate and potassium citrate (25 mEq)	1 tab, dissolved in cold water, bid to qid PO
Librax	Antispasmodic	Cap: clidinium (2.5 mg), chlordiazepoxide (5 mg)	1-2 cap tid or qid PO
Limbitrol 5-12.5 (C4)	Antianxiety-antidepressant	Tab: chlordiazepoxide (5 mg), amitriptylene (12.5 mg)	1 tab tid or qid PO
Limbitrol 10-25 (C4)		Tab: chlordiazepoxide (10 mg), amitriptylene (25 mg)	1 tab tid or qid PO

Lomotil (C5)	Antidiarrheal	Tab: diphenoxylate (2.5 mg), atropine (0.025 mg) Liq: diphenoxylate (2.5 mg), atropine (0.025 mg)/5 ml	2 tab qid PO 10 ml qid PO
Lo/Ovral	Oral contraceptive	Tab: norgestrel (0.3 mg), ethinyl estradiol (30 μg)	1 tab qd PO
Mycolog	Steroid-antibiotic	Cream and Oint: triamcinolone (0.1%), neomycin (0.25%), gramicidin (0.25 mg), nystatin (100,000 U)/g	Topically bid or tid
Naldecon	Decongestant-antihistamine	Tab: phenylpropanolamine (40 mg), phenylephrine (10 mg), chlorpheniramine (5 mg), phenyltoloxamine (15 mg)	1 tab tid PO
		Syrup: phenylpropanolamine (20 mg), phenylephrine (5 mg), chlorpheniramine (2.5 mg), phenyltoloxamine (7.5 mg)/5 ml	5 ml q3-4h PO
Neosporin	Antibiotic	Powder and Oint: polymyxin B (5000 U), neomycin (3.5 mg), bacitracin (400 U)/g	Topically 2-5 times daily
		Aero: polymyxin B (100,000 U), neomycin (70 mg), bacitracin (8000 U)/g	Spray topically prn
		Ophth Oint: polymyxin B (10,000 U), neomycin (3.5 mg), bacitracin (400 U)/g	Apply to eye(s) q3-4h
		Ophth Drop: polymyxin B (10,000 U), neomycin (1.75 mg), gramicidin (25 μg)/ml	2 drops to eye(s) bid to qid
		Cream: polymyxin B (10,000 U), neomycin (3.5 mg), gramicidin (0.25 mg)/g	Topically 2-5 times daily
Norgesic forte	Skeletal muscle relaxant	Tab: orphenadrine (50 mg), aspirin (770 mg), caffeine (60 mg)	1 tab tid or qid PO

Continued.

APPENDIX VI: COMMONLY USED COMBINATION DRUG PREPARATIONS—cont'd

Trade Name	Therapeutic Category	Dosage Forms and Composition	Common Adult Dosage
Ornade	Decongestant-antihistamine	Cap: phenylpropanolamine (75 mg), chlorpheniramine (12 mg)	1 cap q12h PO
Ortho-novum	Oral contraceptive	Tab: norethindrone (1 mg), mestranol (30 µg)	1 tab daily PO
Ovral	Oral contraceptive	Tab: norgestrel (0.5 mg), ethinyl estradiol (50 µg)	1 tab daily PO
Ovulen	Oral contraceptive	Tab: ethynodiol (1 mg), mestranol (100 µg)	1 tab daily PO
Parafon forte	Skeletal muscle relaxant	Tab: chlorzoxazone (250 mg), acetaminophen (300 mg)	2 tab qid PO
Percocet-5 (C2)	Narcotic analgesic	Tab: oxycodone (5 mg), acetaminophen (325 mg)	1 tab q6h prn pain PO
Percodan (C2)	Narcotic analgesic	Tab: oxycodone (5 mg), aspirin (325 mg)	1 tab q6h prn pain PO
Phenergan expectorant w/ codeine (C5)	Antitussive-expectorant	Syrup: promethazine (5 mg), codeine (10 mg), potassium guaiacolsulfonate (44 mg), sodium citrate (197 mg), citric acid (60 mg), ipecac fluidex: (0.17 min)/5 ml	5 ml q4-6h PO
Phenergan VC expectorant w/codeine (C5)	Antitussive-expectorant	Syrup: promethazine (5 mg), phenylephrine (5 mg), codeine (10 mg), potassium guaiacoisulfonate (44 mg), sodium citrate (197 mg), citric acid (60 mg)/5 ml	5 ml q4-6h PO
Septra, Septra DS	see Bactrim, Bactrim DS		
Synalgos-DC (C3)	Narcotic analgesic	Cap: dihydrocodeine (16 mg), aspirin (356 mg), caffeine (30 mg)	2 cap q4h prn pain PO

Triavil 2-10	Tranquilizer-antidepressant	Tab: perphenazine (2 mg), amitriptylene (10 mg)	1 tab bid to qid PO
Triavil 2-25		Tab: perphenazine (2 mg), amitriptylene (25 mg)	1 tab bid to qid PO
Triavil 4-10		Tab: perphenazine (4 mg), amitriptylene (10 mg)	1 tab bid to qid PO
Triavil 4-25		Tab: perphenazine (4 mg), amitriptylene (25 mg)	1 tab bid to qid PO
Triavil 4-50		Tab: perphenazine (4 mg), amitriptylene (50 mg)	1 tab bid PO
Trinalin	Decongestant-antihistamine	Tab: pseudoephedrine (120 mg), azatadine (1 mg)	1 tab q12h PO
Tussionex (C3)	Antitussive	Cap: phenyltoloxamine resin (10 mg), hydrocodone (5 mg)	1 cap q8-12h PO
		Susp: phenyltoloxamine resin (10 mg), hydrocodone (5 mg)/5 ml	5 ml q8-12h PO
Tuss-ornade	Antitussive	Cap: phenylpropranolamine (75 mg), caramiphen (40 mg)	1 cap q12h PO
		Liq: phenylpropranolamine (12.5 mg), caramiphen (6.7 mg)/5 ml	10 ml q4h PO
Tylenol w/codeine (C3)	Narcotic analgesic	Elix: acetaminophen (120 mg), codeine (12 mg), alcohol (7%)/5 ml	15 ml q4h prm pain PO
Tylenol w/codeine No. 1 (C3)		Tab: acetaminophen (300 mg), codeine (7.5 mg)	1-2 tab q4h prm pain PO
Tylenol w/codeine No.2 (C3)		Tab: acetaminophen (300 mg), codeine (15 mg)	1-2 tab q4h prm pain PO
Tylenol w/codeine No.3 (C3)		Tab: acetaminophen (300 mg), codeine (30 mg)	1-2 tab q4h prm pain PO
Tylenol w/codeine No. 4 (C3)		Tab: acetominophen (300 mg), codeine (60 mg)	1-2 tab q4h prm pain PO
Vicodin (C3)	Narcotic analgesic	Tab: acetaminophen (500 mg), hydrocodone (5 mg)	1 tab q6h prm pain PO

APPENDIX VII: RECEPTOR ACTIVITY AND MAIN CLINICAL USES OF SELECTED SYMPATHOMIMETIC DRUGS*

Drug	Use(s)				
	A	B	C	D	P
α-Receptor Activity					
Metaraminol					X
Methoxamine					X
Oxymetazoline				X	
Phenylephrine				X	X
Phenypropanolamine				X	
α- and β-Receptor Activity					
Dopamine			X		X
Ephedrine		X		X	X
Epinephrine	X	X	X		X
Pseudoephedrine				X	
β-Receptor Activity					
Albuterol (β$_2$-selective)		X			
Dobutamine (β$_1$-selective)			X		
Isoetharine (β$_2$-selective)		X			
Isoproterenol		X	X		
Metaproterenol (β$_2$-selective)		X			
Terbutaline (β$_2$-selective)		X			

KEY: A, allergic reactions; B, bronchospasm; C, cardiac inotropism; D, nasal decongestion; P, vasopressor.

*From DiGregorio, G.J., Barbieri, E.J., and Piraino, A.J.: Handbook of commonly prescribed drugs, 1984, Medical Surveillance Inc.

APPENDIX VIII: DIALYZABILITY OF SELECTED DRUGS*

Drug	Hemodialysis	Peritoneal Dialysis	Route of Elimination
Acetaminophen	+	−	Hepatic
Amitriptyline	−	−	Hepatic
Aspirin	+	+	Renal
Cephalexin	+	+	Renal
Cephalothin	+	+	Renal
Diazepam	−		Hepatic and renal
Digoxin	−	−	Renal
Gentamicin	+	+	Renal
Heparin	−		
Isoniazid	+	+	Hepatic and renal
Lithium	+	+	Renal
Methadone	−	−	Hepatic
Methaqualone	+		Hepatic
Nitroprusside	+	+	
Penicillin G	+	−	Renal
Pentazocine	+		Hepatic
Phenobarbital	+	+	Hepatic
Phenytoin	−		Hepatic
Propoxyphene	−	−	Hepatic
Propranolol	−		Hepatic
Quinidine	+	+	Hepatic and renal
Secobarbital	−	−	Hepatic
Tetracyline	−	−	Renal

KEY: +, Yes; −, no.

*From DiGregorio, G.J., Barbieri, E.J., and Piraino, A.J.: Handbook of commonly prescribed drugs, 1984, Medical Surveillance Inc.

APPENDIX IX: TOXIC AND THERAPEUTIC SERUM VALUES OF COMMONLY USED DRUGS

Drug	Therapeutic Level	Toxic Level
Acetaminophen	5-20 μg/ml	>70 μg/ml
Amikacin	Peak: 15-30 μg/ml	Peak: >35 μg/ml
	Trough: 5-10 μg	Trough: >10 μg/ml
Amitriptyline	125-250 ng/ml	>500 ng/ml
Barbiturates		
Short acting	1-5 μg/ml	>8 μg/ml
Long acting	15-40 μg/ml	>40 μg/ml
Carbamazepine	2-10 μg/ml	>12 μg/ml
Clonazepam	15-60 μg/ml	>100 ng/ml
Diazepam	100-1500 ng/ml	>3000 mg/ml
Digitoxin	10-30 ng/ml	>35 ng/nl
Digoxin	0.9-2 ng/ml	>2 ng/ml
Ethanol	—	Fatal: >450 mg/dl
Ethosuximide	40-100 μg/ml	>150 μg/ml
Gentamicin	Peak: 5-8 μg/ml	Peak: >10 μg/ml
	Trough: 1-2 μg/ml	Trough: >2 μg/ml
Glutethimide	2-6 μg/ml	>10 μg/ml
Kanamycin	Peak: 20-30 μg/ml	Peak: >35 μg/ml
	Trough: 5-10 μg/ml	Trough: >10 μg/ml
Lidocaine	2-5 μg/ml	>6 μg/ml
Lithium	0.5-1.5 mEq/L	>1.5 mEq/L
Nortriptyline	50-150 ng/ml	>500 ng/ml
Phenobarbital	15-35 μg/ml	>60 μg/ml
Phenytoin	10-20 μg/ml	>30 μg/ml
Primidone	5-10 μg/ml	>12 μg/ml
Procainamide and NAPA	10-30 μg/ml	>30 μg/ml
Quinidine	2-5 μg/ml	>6 μg/ml
Salicylate	2-29 mg/dl	>30 μg/dl
Streptomycin	Peak 15-20 μg/ml	Peak: >30 μg/ml
	Trough 5 μg/ml	Trough: >5 μg/ml
Theophylline	10-20 μg/ml	>20 μg/ml
Thiocyanate (nitroprus-side)	4-10 μg/ml	>10 μg/ml
Tobramycin	Peak: 5-8 μg/ml	Peak: >10 μg/ml
	Trough: 1-2 μg/ml	Trough: >2 μg/ml
Valproic acid	50-100 μg/ml	>200 μg/ml

APPENDIX X: MANAGEMENT OF SPECIFIC CARDIAC ARREST SEQUENCES*

Guidelines for treatment of asystole

> If rhythm is unclear and possibly ventricular
> fibrillation, defibrillate as for VF; if asystole is present[a]:
> ↓
> Continue CPR
> ↓
> Establish IV access
> ↓
> Epinephrine, 1:10,000, 0.5-1.0 mg IV push[b]
> ↓
> Intubate when possible[c]
> ↓
> Atropine, 1.0 mg IV push (repeat in 5 minutes)
> ↓
> (Consider bicarbonate)[d]
> ↓
> Consider pacing

This sequence was developed to assist in teaching how to treat a broad range of patients with asystole. Some patients may require care not specified herein. This algorithm should not be construed to prohibit such flexibility. Flow of algorithm presumes asystole is continuing. VF indicates ventricular fibrillation; IV, intravenous.

[a]Asystole should be confirmed in two leads.

[b]Epinephrine should be repeated every 5 minutes.

[c]Intubation is preferable; if it can be accomplished simultaneously with other techniques, then the earlier the better. However, cardiopulmonary resuscitation (CPR) and use of epinephrine are more important initially if patient can be ventilated without intubation. (Endotracheal epinephrine may be used.)

[d]Value of sodium bicarbonate is questionable during cardiac arrest, and it is not recommended for the routine cardiac arrest sequence. Consideration of its use in a dose of 1 mEq/kg is appropriate at this point. Half of original dose may be repeated every 10 minutes if it is used.

*From 1985 National conference on standards and guidelines for cardiopulmonary resuscitation and emergency cardiac care, JAMA, **255**:2933, 1986.

Guidelines for ventricular fibrillation and pulseless ventricular tachycardia

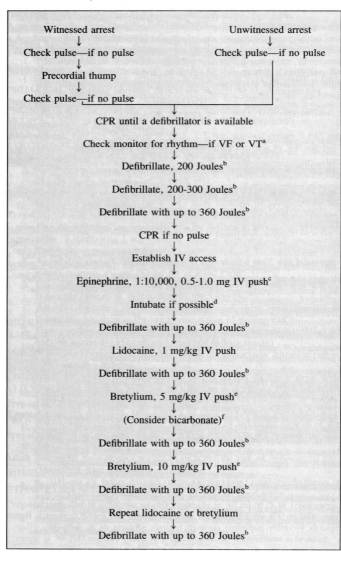

Witnessed arrest
↓
Check pulse—if no pulse
↓
Precordial thump
↓
Check pulse—if no pulse

Unwitnessed arrest
↓
Check pulse—if no pulse

CPR until a defibrillator is available
↓
Check monitor for rhythm—if VF or VT[a]
↓
Defibrillate, 200 Joules[b]
↓
Defibrillate, 200-300 Joules[b]
↓
Defibrillate with up to 360 Joules[b]
↓
CPR if no pulse
↓
Establish IV access
↓
Epinephrine, 1:10,000, 0.5-1.0 mg IV push[c]
↓
Intubate if possible[d]
↓
Defibrillate with up to 360 Joules[b]
↓
Lidocaine, 1 mg/kg IV push
↓
Defibrillate with up to 360 Joules[b]
↓
Bretylium, 5 mg/kg IV push[e]
↓
(Consider bicarbonate)[f]
↓
Defibrillate with up to 360 Joules[b]
↓
Bretylium, 10 mg/kg IV push[e]
↓
Defibrillate with up to 360 Joules[b]
↓
Repeat lidocaine or bretylium
↓
Defibrillate with up to 360 Joules[b]

This sequence was developed to assist in teaching how to treat a broad range of patients with ventricular fibrillation (VF) or pulseless ventricular tachycardia (VT). Some patients may require care not specified herein. This algorithm should not be construed as prohibiting such flexibility. Flow of algorithm presumes that VF is continuing. CPR indicates cardiopulmonary resuscitation.

[a]Pulseless VT should be treated identically to VF.

[b]Check pulse and rhythm after each shock. If VF recurs after transiently converting (rather than persists without ever converting), use whatever energy level has previously been successful for defibrillation.

[c]Epinephrine should be repeated every 5 minutes.

[d]Intubation is preferable. If it can be accomplished simultaneously with other techniques, then the earlier the better. However, defibrillation and epinephrine are more important initially if the patient can be ventilated without intubation.

[e]Some may prefer repeated doses of lidocaine, which may be given in 0.5-mg/kg boluses every 8 minutes to a total dose of 3 mg/kg.

[f]Value of sodium bicarbonate is questionable during cardiac arrest, and it is not recommended for routine cardiac arrest sequence. Consideration of its use in a dose of 1 mEq/kg is appropriate at this point. Half of original dose may be repeated every 10 minutes if it is used.

Guidelines for treatment of sustained ventricular tachycardia

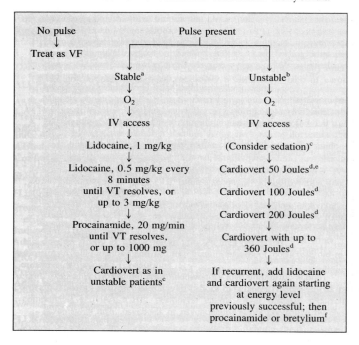

This sequence was developed to assist in teaching how to treat a broad range of patients with sustained VT. Some patients may require care not specified herein. This algorithm should not be construed as prohibiting such flexibility. Flow of algorithm presumes that VT is continuing. VF indicates ventricular fibrillation.

[a]If patient becomes unstable (see footnote b for definition) at any time, move to "unstable" arm of algorithm.

[b]Unstable indicates symptoms (e.g., chest pain or dyspnea), hypotension (systolic blood pressure <90 mm Hg), congestive heart failure, ischemia, or infarction.

[c]Sedation should be considered for all patients, including those defined in footnote b as unstable, except those who are hemodynamically unstable (e.g., hypotensive, in pulmonary edema, or unconscious.)

[d]If hypotension, pulmonary edema, or unconsciousness is present, unsynchronized cardioversion should be done to avoid delay associated with synchronization.

[e]In the absence of hypotension, pulmonary edema, or unconsciousness, a precordial thump may be employed before cardioversion.

[f]Once VT has resolved, begin intravenous (IV) infusion of antidys-rhthymic agent that has aided resolution of VT. If hypotension, pulmonary edema, or unconsciousness is present, use lidocaine if cardioversion alone is unsuccessful, followed by bretylium. In all other patients, recommended order of therapy is lidocaine, procainamide, and then bretylium.

Guidelines for treatment of electromechanical dissociation

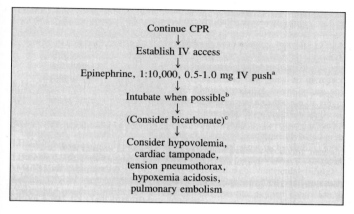

Continue CPR
↓
Establish IV access
↓
Epinephrine, 1:10,000, 0.5-1.0 mg IV push[a]
↓
Intubate when possible[b]
↓
(Consider bicarbonate)[c]
↓
Consider hypovolemia,
cardiac tamponade,
tension pneumothorax,
hypoxemia acidosis,
pulmonary embolism

This sequence was developed to assist in teaching how to treat a broad range of patients with electromechanical dissociation. Some patients may require care not specified herein. This algorithm should not be construed to prohibit such flexibility. Flow of algorithm presumes that electromechanical dissociation is continuing. CPR indicates cardiopulmonary resuscitation; IV, intravenous.

[a]Epinephrine should be repeated every 5 minutes.

[b]Intubation is preferable. If it can be accomplished simultaneously with other techniques, then the earlier the better. However, epinephrine is more important initially if the patient can be ventilated without intubation.

[c]Value of sodium bicarbonate is questionable during cardiac arrest, and it is not recommended for routine cardiac arrest sequence. Consideration of its use in a dose of 1 mEq/kg is appropriate at this point. Half of original dose may be repeated every 10 minutes if it is used.

Index

When you publish a book, it's the world's book. The world edits it.

—PHILIP ROTH

our favorite books

A journal designed for the book club discussion leader (or the book club "secretary," if your group is that organized) and to be passed around at book club gatherings.

date started:

our book club history

book club name

founding member(s)

date of first meeting

reason for forming group

methods/reasons for choosing books

topics and themes we like discussing

"extras" at our gatherings (i.e., drinks and snacks)

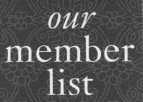

our
member
list

**A handy list of
contact information
for everyone
in the group**

*It is with a good book
as it is with good company.*

—RALPH WALDO EMERSON

name

address

phone (HOME)

(WORK)

(MOBILE)

e-mail

name

address

phone (HOME)

(WORK)

(MOBILE)

e-mail

name

address

phone (HOME)

(WORK)

(MOBILE)

e-mail

name

address

phone (HOME)

(WORK)

(MOBILE)

e-mail

name

address

phone (HOME)

(WORK)

(MOBILE)

e-mail

name

address

phone (HOME)

(WORK)

(MOBILE)

e-mail

name

address

phone (HOME)

(WORK)

(MOBILE)

e-mail

name

address

phone (HOME)

(WORK)

(MOBILE)

e-mail

name

address

phone (HOME)

(WORK)

(MOBILE)

e-mail

name

address

phone (HOME)

(WORK)

(MOBILE)

e-mail

name

address

phone (HOME)

(WORK)

(MOBILE)

e-mail

name

address

phone (HOME)

(WORK)

(MOBILE)

e-mail

name

address

phone (HOME)

(WORK)

(MOBILE)

e-mail

name

address

phone (HOME)

(WORK)

(MOBILE)

e-mail

name

address

phone (HOME)

(WORK)

(MOBILE)

e-mail

name

address

phone (HOME)

(WORK)

(MOBILE)

e-mail

name

address

phone (HOME)

(WORK)

(MOBILE)

e-mail

name

address

phone (HOME)

(WORK)

(MOBILE)

e-mail

name

address

phone (HOME)

(WORK)

(MOBILE)

e-mail

name

address

phone (HOME)

(WORK)

(MOBILE)

e-mail

name

address

phone (HOME)

(WORK)

(MOBILE)

e-mail

name

address

phone (HOME)

(WORK)

(MOBILE)

e-mail

name

address

phone (HOME)

(WORK)

(MOBILE)

e-mail

name

address

phone (HOME)

(WORK)

(MOBILE)

e-mail

name

address

phone (HOME)

(WORK)

(MOBILE)

e-mail

name

address

phone (HOME)

(WORK)

(MOBILE)

e-mail

name

address

phone (HOME)

(WORK)

(MOBILE)

e-mail

name

address

phone (HOME)

(WORK)

(MOBILE)

e-mail

name

address

phone (HOME)

(WORK)

(MOBILE)

e-mail

name

address

phone (HOME)

(WORK)

(MOBILE)

e-mail

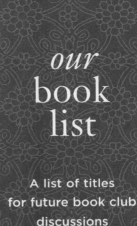

our
book
list

**A list of titles
for future book club
discussions**

*Every book teaches a lesson,
even if the lesson is only that
one has chosen the wrong book.*

—MASON COOLEY

title	title
author	author
RECOMMENDED BY	RECOMMENDED BY

title	title
author	author
RECOMMENDED BY	RECOMMENDED BY

title	title
author	author
RECOMMENDED BY	RECOMMENDED BY

title	title
author	author
RECOMMENDED BY	RECOMMENDED BY

title	title
author	author
RECOMMENDED BY	RECOMMENDED BY

title	title
author	author
RECOMMENDED BY	RECOMMENDED BY

title	title
author	author
RECOMMENDED BY	RECOMMENDED BY

title

author

RECOMMENDED BY

title

author

RECOMMENDED BY

title

author

RECOMMENDED BY

title

author

RECOMMENDED BY

title

author

RECOMMENDED BY

title

author

RECOMMENDED BY

title

author

RECOMMENDED BY

title

author

RECOMMENDED BY

title

author

RECOMMENDED BY

title

author

RECOMMENDED BY

title

author

RECOMMENDED BY

title

author

RECOMMENDED BY

title

author

RECOMMENDED BY

title

author

RECOMMENDED BY

title

author

RECOMMENDED BY

title

author

RECOMMENDED BY

title

author

RECOMMENDED BY

title

author

RECOMMENDED BY

title

author

RECOMMENDED BY

title

author

RECOMMENDED BY

title

author

RECOMMENDED BY

title

author

RECOMMENDED BY

title

author

RECOMMENDED BY

title

author

RECOMMENDED BY

title

author

RECOMMENDED BY

title

author

RECOMMENDED BY

title

author

RECOMMENDED BY

title

author

RECOMMENDED BY

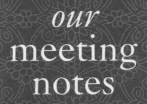

*To produce a mighty book,
you must choose a mighty theme.
No great and enduring volume can
ever be written on the flea, though
many there be who have tried it.*

—HERMAN MELVILLE

plot (plot), *n.* 1. the main story of a literary or dramatic work. *v.i.* 2. to devise the plot of a literary work.

date _____ time _____

meeting location _____
_____
_____

discussion leader _____

attendees _____
_____
_____
_____

title _____

author _____

publisher/date _____

category FICTION

MEMOIR

BIOGRAPHY

HISTORY

OTHER NONFICTION

recommended by _____

questions or topics prepared by the discussion leader

HIGHLIGHTS OF OUR CONVERSATION

reactions to the discussion topics, memorable debates, passionate exchanges

our favorite characters

our favorite quotes

ratings (TALLY UP THE MEMBER VOTES IN THE FOLLOWING AREAS)

FOR FICTION/MEMOIR

character development: A ___ B+ ___ B ___ C ___ F ___

development of setting: A ___ B+ ___ B ___ C ___ F ___

pace: A ___ B+ ___ B ___ C ___ F ___

writing style: A ___ B+ ___ B ___ C ___ F ___

Total average grade ____

FOR NONFICTION

depth of research: A ___ B+ ___ B ___ C ___ F ___

interest level of topic: A ___ B+ ___ B ___ C ___ F ___

pace: A ___ B+ ___ B ___ C ___ F ___

writing style: A ___ B+ ___ B ___ C ___ F ___

Total average grade ____

OTHER ESSENTIALS

book club beverages
_____

_____

book club snacks
_____

_____

_____

expenses to divide
_____

_____

date

time

meeting location

discussion leader

attendees

title

author

publisher/date

category FICTION

MEMOIR

BIOGRAPHY

HISTORY

OTHER NONFICTION

recommended by

questions or topics prepared by the discussion leader

HIGHLIGHTS OF OUR CONVERSATION
reactions to the discussion topics, memorable debates, passionate exchanges

our favorite characters

our favorite quotes

ratings

FOR FICTION/MEMOIR

character development: A ____ B+ ____ B ____ C ____ F ____

development of setting: A ____ B+ ____ B ____ C ____ F ____

pace: A ____ B+ ____ B ____ C ____ F ____

writing style: A ____ B+ ____ B ____ C ____ F ____

Total average grade ____

FOR NONFICTION

depth of research: A ____ B+ ____ B ____ C ____ F ____

interest level of topic: A ____ B+ ____ B ____ C ____F ____

pace: A ____ B+ ____ B ____ C ____F ____

writing style: A ____ B+ ____ B ____ C ____F ____

Total average grade ____

OTHER ESSENTIALS

book club beverages
_____

_____

book club snacks
_____

_____

expenses to divide
_____

_____

date   time

meeting location

discussion leader

attendees

title

author

publisher/date

category   FICTION

            MEMOIR

            BIOGRAPHY

            HISTORY

            OTHER NONFICTION

recommended by

questions or topics prepared by the discussion leader

HIGHLIGHTS OF OUR CONVERSATION

reactions to the discussion topics, memorable debates, passionate exchanges

our favorite characters

our favorite quotes

ratings (TALLY UP THE MEMBER VOTES IN THE FOLLOWING AREAS)

FOR FICTION/MEMOIR

character development: A ＿＿ B+ ＿＿ B ＿＿ C ＿＿ F ＿＿

development of setting: A ＿＿ B+ ＿＿ B ＿＿ C ＿＿ F ＿＿

pace: A ＿＿ B+ ＿＿ B ＿＿ C ＿＿ F ＿＿

writing style: A ＿＿ B+ ＿＿ B ＿＿ C ＿＿ F ＿＿

Total average grade ＿＿＿

FOR NONFICTION

depth of research: A ＿＿ B+ ＿＿ B ＿＿ C ＿＿ F ＿＿

interest level of topic: A ＿＿ B+ ＿＿ B ＿＿ C ＿＿ F ＿＿

pace: A ＿＿ B+ ＿＿ B ＿＿ C ＿＿ F ＿＿

writing style: A ＿＿ B+ ＿＿ B ＿＿ C ＿＿ F ＿＿

Total average grade ＿＿＿

OTHER ESSENTIALS

book club beverages

book club snacks

expenses to divide

nar•ra•tive (narʹə tive), *n.* 1. a story or account of events, experiences, or the like, whether true or fictitious. 2. the art, technique, or process of narrating. *adj.* 3. consisting of or being a narrative: *narrative poetry.*

A great book should leave you with many experiences, and slightly exhausted at the end. You live several lives while reading it.

—WILLIAM STYRON

date _____   time _____

meeting location _____
_____
_____

discussion leader _____

attendees _____
_____
_____
_____
_____

title _____

author _____

publisher/date _____

category   FICTION

MEMOIR

BIOGRAPHY

HISTORY

OTHER NONFICTION

recommended by _____

questions or topics prepared by the discussion leader

_____

_____

_____

_____

_____

_____

_____

_____

_____

_____

_____

HIGHLIGHTS OF OUR CONVERSATION

reactions to the discussion topics, memorable debates, passionate exchanges

_____

_____

_____

_____

_____

_____

_____

_____

_____

our favorite characters

our favorite quotes

ratings

FOR FICTION/MEMOIR

character development: A ___ B+ ___ B ___ C ___ F ___

development of setting: A ___ B+ ___ B ___ C ___ F ___

pace: A ___ B+ ___ B ___ C ___ F ___

writing style: A ___ B+ ___ B ___ C ___ F ___

Total average grade _____

FOR NONFICTION

depth of research: A ___ B+ ___ B ___ C ___ F ___

interest level of topic: A ___ B+ ___ B ___ C ___F ___

pace: A ___ B+ ___ B ___ C ___F ___

writing style: A ___ B+ ___ B ___ C ___F ___

Total average grade _____

OTHER ESSENTIALS

book club beverages
_____

_____

book club snacks
_____

_____

expenses to divide
_____

_____

date _____ time _____

meeting location _____

_____

_____

discussion leader _____

attendees _____

_____

_____

_____

_____

title _____

author _____

publisher/date _____

category FICTION

MEMOIR

BIOGRAPHY

HISTORY

OTHER NONFICTION

recommended by _____

questions or topics prepared by the discussion leader

HIGHLIGHTS OF OUR CONVERSATION
reactions to the discussion topics, memorable debates, passionate exchanges

our favorite characters

our favorite quotes

ratings (TALLY UP THE MEMBER VOTES IN THE FOLLOWING AREAS)

FOR FICTION/MEMOIR

character development: A ___ B+ ___ B ___ C ___ F ___

development of setting: A ___ B+ ___ B ___ C ___ F ___

pace: A ___ B+ ___ B ___ C ___ F ___

writing style: A ___ B+ ___ B ___ C ___ F ___

Total average grade ____

FOR NONFICTION

depth of research: A ___ B+ ___ B ___ C ___ F ___

interest level of topic: A ___ B+ ___ B ___ C ___ F ___

pace: A ___ B+ ___ B ___ C ___ F ___

writing style: A ___ B+ ___ B ___ C ___ F ___

Total average grade ____

OTHER ESSENTIALS

book club beverages _____

_____

book club snacks _____

_____

_____

expenses to divide _____

_____

date _____ time _____

meeting location _____

_____

_____

discussion leader _____

attendees _____

_____

_____

_____

title _____

author _____

publisher/date _____

category   FICTION

          MEMOIR

          BIOGRAPHY

          HISTORY

          OTHER NONFICTION

recommended by _____

questions or topics prepared by the discussion leader

HIGHLIGHTS OF OUR CONVERSATION

reactions to the discussion topics, memorable debates, passionate exchanges

our favorite characters

our favorite quotes

ratings

FOR FICTION/MEMOIR

character development: A ___ B+ ___ B ___ C ___ F ___

development of setting: A ___ B+ ___ B ___ C ___ F ___

pace: A ___ B+ ___ B ___ C ___ F ___

writing style: A ___ B+ ___ B ___ C ___ F ___

Total average grade ____

FOR NONFICTION

depth of research: A ___ B+ ___ B ___ C ___ F ___

interest level of topic: A ___ B+ ___ B ___ C ___F ___

pace: A ___ B+ ___ B ___ C ___F ___

writing style: A ___ B+ ___ B ___ C ___F ___

Total average grade ____

OTHER ESSENTIALS

book club beverages _____

_____

book club snacks _____

_____

_____

expenses to divide _____

_____

char•ac•ter (karˈik tər), *n.*
1. the aggregate of features and traits that form the individual nature of a person or thing.
2. a person represented in a drama, story, etc.

A classic is a book that has never finished saying what it has to say.

—ITALO CALVINO

A classic is a book that doesn't have to be written again.

—CARL VAN DOREN

"Classic." A book which people praise and don't read.

—MARK TWAIN

date

time

meeting location

discussion leader

attendees

title

author

publisher/date

category   FICTION

MEMOIR

BIOGRAPHY

HISTORY

OTHER NONFICTION

recommended by

questions or topics prepared by the discussion leader

HIGHLIGHTS OF OUR CONVERSATION

reactions to the discussion topics, memorable debates, passionate exchanges

our favorite characters

our favorite quotes

ratings (TALLY UP THE MEMBER VOTES IN THE FOLLOWING AREAS)

FOR FICTION/MEMOIR

character development: A ____ B+ ____ B ____ C ____ F ____

development of setting: A ____ B+ ____ B ____ C ____ F ____

pace: A ____ B+ ____ B ____ C ____ F ____

writing style: A ____ B+ ____ B ____ C ____ F ____

Total average grade ____

FOR NONFICTION

depth of research: A ____ B+ ____ B ____ C ____ F ____

interest level of topic: A ____ B+ ____ B ____ C ____ F ____

pace: A ____ B+ ____ B ____ C ____ F ____

writing style: A ____ B+ ____ B ____ C ____ F ____

Total average grade ____

OTHER ESSENTIALS

book club beverages

book club snacks

expenses to divide

date _____   time _____

meeting location _____

_____

_____

discussion leader _____

attendees _____

_____

_____

_____

title _____

author _____

publisher/date _____

category FICTION

MEMOIR

BIOGRAPHY

HISTORY

OTHER NONFICTION

recommended by _____

questions or topics prepared by the discussion leader

HIGHLIGHTS OF OUR CONVERSATION
reactions to the discussion topics, memorable debates, passionate exchanges

our favorite characters

our favorite quotes

ratings

FOR FICTION/MEMOIR

character development: A ___ B+ ___ B ___ C ___ F ___

development of setting: A ___ B+ ___ B ___ C ___ F ___

pace: A ___ B+ ___ B ___ C ___ F ___

writing style: A ___ B+ ___ B ___ C ___ F ___

Total average grade _____

FOR NONFICTION

depth of research: A ___ B+ ___ B ___ C ___ F ___

interest level of topic: A ___ B+ ___ B ___ C ___F ___

pace: A ___ B+ ___ B ___ C ___F ___

writing style: A ___ B+ ___ B ___ C ___F ___

Total average grade _____

OTHER ESSENTIALS

book club beverages
_____

_____

book club snacks
_____

_____

_____

expenses to divide
_____

_____

date

time

meeting location

discussion leader

attendees

title

author

publisher/date

category FICTION

MEMOIR

BIOGRAPHY

HISTORY

OTHER NONFICTION

recommended by

questions or topics prepared by the discussion leader

HIGHLIGHTS OF OUR CONVERSATION
reactions to the discussion topics, memorable debates, passionate exchanges

our favorite characters

our favorite quotes

ratings (TALLY UP THE MEMBER VOTES IN THE FOLLOWING AREAS)

FOR FICTION/MEMOIR

character development: A ____ B+ ____ B ____ C ____ F ____

development of setting: A ____ B+ ____ B ____ C ____ F ____

pace: A ____ B+ ____ B ____ C ____ F ____

writing style: A ____ B+ ____ B ____ C ____ F ____

Total average grade ____

FOR NONFICTION

depth of research: A ____ B+ ____ B ____ C ____ F ____

interest level of topic: A ____ B+ ____ B ____ C ____ F ____

pace: A ____ B+ ____ B ____ C ____ F ____

writing style: A ____ B+ ____ B ____ C ____ F ____

Total average grade ____

OTHER ESSENTIALS

book club beverages
_____

_____

book club snacks
_____

_____

_____

expenses to divide
_____

_____

sym•bol (simˈbəl), *n.* 1. something used for or regarded as representing something else, esp. a material object representing something immaterial; emblem or sign. 2. *psychoanal.* any object or idea that represents or disguises a repressed wish or impulse.

The more I like a book, the more reluctant I am to turn the page. Lovers, even book lovers, tend to cling. No one-night stands or "reads" for them.

—ANATOLE BROYARD

date   time

meeting location

discussion leader

attendees

title

author

publisher/date

category   FICTION

MEMOIR

BIOGRAPHY

HISTORY

OTHER NONFICTION

recommended by

questions or topics prepared by the discussion leader

_____

_____

_____

_____

_____

_____

_____

_____

_____

_____

HIGHLIGHTS OF OUR CONVERSATION

reactions to the discussion topics, memorable debates, passionate exchanges

_____

_____

_____

_____

_____

_____

_____

_____

our favorite characters

our favorite quotes

ratings

FOR FICTION/MEMOIR

character development: A ___ B+ ___ B ___ C ___ F ___

development of setting: A ___ B+ ___ B ___ C ___ F ___

pace: A ___ B+ ___ B ___ C ___ F ___

writing style: A ___ B+ ___ B ___ C ___ F ___

Total average grade ____

FOR NONFICTION

depth of research: A ___ B+ ___ B ___ C ___ F ___

interest level of topic: A ___ B+ ___ B ___ C ___F ___

pace: A ___ B+ ___ B ___ C ___F ___

writing style: A ___ B+ ___ B ___ C ___F ___

Total average grade ____

OTHER ESSENTIALS

book club beverages
_____

_____

book club snacks
_____

_____

expenses to divide
_____

_____

date

time

meeting location

discussion leader

attendees

title

author

publisher/date

category   FICTION

MEMOIR

BIOGRAPHY

HISTORY

OTHER NONFICTION

recommended by

questions or topics prepared by the discussion leader

HIGHLIGHTS OF OUR CONVERSATION

reactions to the discussion topics, memorable debates, passionate exchanges

our favorite characters

our favorite quotes

ratings (TALLY UP THE MEMBER VOTES IN THE FOLLOWING AREAS)

FOR FICTION/MEMOIR

character development: A ___ B+ ___ B ___ C ___ F ___

development of setting: A ___ B+ ___ B ___ C ___ F ___

pace: A ___ B+ ___ B ___ C ___ F ___

writing style: A ___ B+ ___ B ___ C ___ F ___

Total average grade ____

FOR NONFICTION

depth of research: A ___ B+ ___ B ___ C ___ F ___

interest level of topic: A ___ B+ ___ B ___ C ___ F ___

pace: A ___ B+ ___ B ___ C ___ F ___

writing style: A ___ B+ ___ B ___ C ___ F ___

Total average grade ____

OTHER ESSENTIALS

book club beverages

book club snacks

expenses to divide

date

time

meeting location

discussion leader

attendees

title

author

publisher/date

category   FICTION

MEMOIR

BIOGRAPHY

HISTORY

OTHER NONFICTION

recommended by

questions or topics prepared by the discussion leader

HIGHLIGHTS OF OUR CONVERSATION
reactions to the discussion topics, memorable debates, passionate exchanges

our favorite characters

our favorite quotes

ratings (TALLY UP THE MEMBER VOTES IN THE FOLLOWING AREAS)

FOR FICTION/MEMOIR

character development: A ___ B+ ___ B ___ C ___ F ___

development of setting: A ___ B+ ___ B ___ C ___ F ___

pace: A ___ B+ ___ B ___ C ___ F ___

writing style: A ___ B+ ___ B ___ C ___ F ___

Total average grade ____

FOR NONFICTION

depth of research: A ___ B+ ___ B ___ C ___ F ___

interest level of topic: A ___ B+ ___ B ___ C ___F ___

pace: A ___ B+ ___ B ___ C ___F ___

writing style: A ___ B+ ___ B ___ C ___F ___

Total average grade ____

OTHER ESSENTIALS

book club beverages

book club snacks

expenses to divide

fore•shad•ow (fôr shad′ō), *v.*
to show or indicate beforehand;
prefigure.

*The covers of this book
are too far apart.*

—AMBROSE BIERCE

date _____ time _____

meeting location _____

_____

_____

discussion leader _____

attendees _____

_____

_____

_____

_____

title _____

author _____

publisher/date _____

category   FICTION

MEMOIR

BIOGRAPHY

HISTORY

OTHER NONFICTION

recommended by _____

questions or topics prepared by the discussion leader

reactions to the discussion topics, memorable debates, passionate exchanges

our favorite characters

our favorite quotes

ratings <small>(TALLY UP THE MEMBER VOTES IN THE FOLLOWING AREAS)</small>

FOR FICTION/MEMOIR

character development: A ___ B+ ___ B ___ C ___ F ___

development of setting: A ___ B+ ___ B ___ C ___ F ___

pace: A ___ B+ ___ B ___ C ___ F ___

writing style: A ___ B+ ___ B ___ C ___ F ___

Total average grade ____

FOR NONFICTION

depth of research: A ___ B+ ___ B ___ C ___ F ___

interest level of topic: A ___ B+ ___ B ___ C ___ F ___

pace: A ___ B+ ___ B ___ C ___ F ___

writing style: A ___ B+ ___ B ___ C ___ F ___

Total average grade ____

OTHER ESSENTIALS

book club beverages

book club snacks

expenses to divide

date

time

meeting location

discussion leader

attendees

title

author

publisher/date

category FICTION

MEMOIR

BIOGRAPHY

HISTORY

OTHER NONFICTION

recommended by

questions or topics prepared by the discussion leader

HIGHLIGHTS OF OUR CONVERSATION
reactions to the discussion topics, memorable debates, passionate exchanges

our favorite characters

our favorite quotes

ratings

FOR FICTION/MEMOIR

character development: A ___ B+ ___ B ___ C ___ F ___

development of setting: A ___ B+ ___ B ___ C ___ F ___

pace: A ___ B+ ___ B ___ C ___ F ___

writing style: A ___ B+ ___ B ___ C ___ F ___

Total average grade ____

FOR NONFICTION

depth of research: A ___ B+ ___ B ___ C ___ F ___

interest level of topic: A ___ B+ ___ B ___ C ___F ___

pace: A ___ B+ ___ B ___ C ___F ___

writing style: A ___ B+ ___ B ___ C ___F ___

Total average grade ____

OTHER ESSENTIALS

book club beverages

book club snacks

expenses to divide

date   time

meeting location

discussion leader

attendees

title

author

publisher/date

category   FICTION

            MEMOIR

            BIOGRAPHY

            HISTORY

            OTHER NONFICTION

recommended by

questions or topics prepared by the discussion leader

HIGHLIGHTS OF OUR CONVERSATION
reactions to the discussion topics, memorable debates, passionate exchanges

our favorite characters

our favorite quotes

ratings (TALLY UP THE MEMBER VOTES IN THE FOLLOWING AREAS)

FOR FICTION/MEMOIR

character development: A ___ B+ ___ B ___ C ___ F ___

development of setting: A ___ B+ ___ B ___ C ___ F ___

pace: A ___ B+ ___ B ___ C ___ F ___

writing style: A ___ B+ ___ B ___ C ___ F ___

Total average grade ____

FOR NONFICTION

depth of research: A ___ B+ ___ B ___ C ___ F ___

interest level of topic: A ___ B+ ___ B ___ C ___ F ___

pace: A ___ B+ ___ B ___ C ___ F ___

writing style: A ___ B+ ___ B ___ C ___ F ___

Total average grade ____

OTHER ESSENTIALS

book club beverages

book club snacks

expenses to divide

pa•thet•ic fal•la•cy
(pə thet′ik fal′ə sē), *n.* the
endowment of nature, inanimate
objects, etc., with human traits
and feelings, as in *the smiling sky.*

'Tis the good reader that makes the good book; a good head cannot read amiss: in every book he finds passages which seem confidences or asides hidden from all else and unmistakably meant for his ear.

—RALPH WALDO EMERSON

date   time

meeting location

discussion leader

attendees

title

author

publisher/date

category   FICTION

            MEMOIR

            BIOGRAPHY

            HISTORY

            OTHER NONFICTION

recommended by

questions or topics prepared by the discussion leader

_____

_____

_____

_____

_____

_____

_____

_____

_____

_____

HIGHLIGHTS OF OUR CONVERSATION
reactions to the discussion topics, memorable debates, passionate exchanges

_____

_____

_____

_____

_____

_____

_____

_____

_____

our favorite characters

our favorite quotes

ratings (TALLY UP THE MEMBER VOTES IN THE FOLLOWING AREAS)

FOR FICTION/MEMOIR

character development: A ___ B+ ___ B ___ C ___ F ___

development of setting: A ___ B+ ___ B ___ C ___ F ___

pace: A ___ B+ ___ B ___ C ___ F ___

writing style: A ___ B+ ___ B ___ C ___ F ___

Total average grade ____

FOR NONFICTION

depth of research: A ___ B+ ___ B ___ C ___ F ___

interest level of topic: A ___ B+ ___ B ___ C ___F ___

pace: A ___ B+ ___ B ___ C ___F ___

writing style: A ___ B+ ___ B ___ C ___F ___

Total average grade ____

OTHER ESSENTIALS

book club beverages
_____

_____

book club snacks
_____

_____

expenses to divide
_____

_____

date _____ time _____

meeting location _____

_____

_____

discussion leader _____

attendees _____

_____

_____

_____

_____

title _____

author _____

publisher/date _____

category   FICTION

MEMOIR

BIOGRAPHY

HISTORY

OTHER NONFICTION

recommended by _____

questions or topics prepared by the discussion leader

HIGHLIGHTS OF OUR CONVERSATION

reactions to the discussion topics, memorable debates, passionate exchanges

our favorite characters

our favorite quotes

ratings (TALLY UP THE MEMBER VOTES IN THE FOLLOWING AREAS)

FOR FICTION/MEMOIR

character development: A ___ B+ ___ B ___ C ___ F ___

development of setting: A ___ B+ ___ B ___ C ___ F ___

pace: A ___ B+ ___ B ___ C ___ F ___

writing style: A ___ B+ ___ B ___ C ___ F ___

Total average grade ____

FOR NONFICTION

depth of research: A ___ B+ ___ B ___ C ___ F ___

interest level of topic: A ___ B+ ___ B ___ C ___F ___

pace: A ___ B+ ___ B ___ C ___F ___

writing style: A ___ B+ ___ B ___ C ___F ___

Total average grade ____

OTHER ESSENTIALS

book club beverages
_____
_____

book club snacks
_____
_____
_____

expenses to divide
_____

date

time

meeting location

discussion leader

attendees

title

author

publisher/date

category   FICTION

MEMOIR

BIOGRAPHY

HISTORY

OTHER NONFICTION

recommended by

questions or topics prepared by the discussion leader

HIGHLIGHTS OF OUR CONVERSATION
reactions to the discussion topics, memorable debates, passionate exchanges

our favorite characters

our favorite quotes

ratings (TALLY UP THE MEMBER VOTES IN THE FOLLOWING AREAS)

FOR FICTION/MEMOIR

character development: A ___ B+ ___ B ___ C ___ F ___

development of setting: A ___ B+ ___ B ___ C ___ F ___

pace: A ___ B+ ___ B ___ C ___ F ___

writing style: A ___ B+ ___ B ___ C ___ F ___

Total average grade ___

FOR NONFICTION

depth of research: A ___ B+ ___ B ___ C ___ F ___

interest level of topic: A ___ B+ ___ B ___ C ___ F ___

pace: A ___ B+ ___ B ___ C ___ F ___

writing style: A ___ B+ ___ B ___ C ___ F ___

Total average grade ___

OTHER ESSENTIALS

book club beverages _____

_____

book club snacks _____

_____

expenses to divide _____

_____

flash•back (flash′bak′), *n.*
the insertion of an earlier
event into the chronological
structure of a novel, motion
picture, play, etc., or the scene
so inserted.

A book is a version of the world.
If you do not like it, ignore it;
or offer your own version in return.

—SALMAN RUSHDIE

date _____ time _____

meeting location _____

_____

_____

discussion leader _____

attendees _____

_____

_____

_____

_____

title _____

author _____

publisher/date _____

category FICTION

MEMOIR

BIOGRAPHY

HISTORY

OTHER NONFICTION

recommended by _____

questions or topics prepared by the discussion leader

HIGHLIGHTS OF OUR CONVERSATION
reactions to the discussion topics, memorable debates, passionate exchanges

our favorite characters

our favorite quotes

ratings (tally up the member votes in the following areas)

FOR FICTION/MEMOIR

    character development: A ___ B+ ___ B ___ C ___ F ___

    development of setting: A ___ B+ ___ B ___ C ___ F ___

    pace: A ___ B+ ___ B ___ C ___ F ___

    writing style: A ___ B+ ___ B ___ C ___ F ___

Total average grade ____

FOR NONFICTION

    depth of research: A ___ B+ ___ B ___ C ___ F ___

    interest level of topic: A ___ B+ ___ B ___ C ___F ___

    pace: A ___ B+ ___ B ___ C ___F ___

    writing style: A ___ B+ ___ B ___ C ___F ___

Total average grade ____

OTHER ESSENTIALS

book club beverages _____

_____

book club snacks _____

_____

_____

expenses to divide _____

_____

date   time

meeting location

discussion leader

attendees

title

author

publisher/date

category   FICTION

           MEMOIR

           BIOGRAPHY

           HISTORY

           OTHER NONFICTION

recommended by

questions or topics prepared by the discussion leader

HIGHLIGHTS OF OUR CONVERSATION

reactions to the discussion topics, memorable debates, passionate exchanges

our favorite characters

our favorite quotes

ratings (TALLY UP THE MEMBER VOTES IN THE FOLLOWING AREAS)

FOR FICTION/MEMOIR

character development: A ___ B+ ___ B ___ C ___ F ___

development of setting: A ___ B+ ___ B ___ C ___ F ___

pace: A ___ B+ ___ B ___ C ___ F ___

writing style: A ___ B+ ___ B ___ C ___ F ___

Total average grade ____

FOR NONFICTION

depth of research: A ___ B+ ___ B ___ C ___ F ___

interest level of topic: A ___ B+ ___ B ___ C ___F ___

pace: A ___ B+ ___ B ___ C ___F ___

writing style: A ___ B+ ___ B ___ C ___F ___

Total average grade ____

OTHER ESSENTIALS

book club beverages
_____

_____

book club snacks
_____

_____

_____

expenses to divide
_____

_____

date _____ time _____

meeting location _____

_____

_____

discussion leader _____

attendees _____

_____

_____

_____

_____

title _____

author _____

publisher/date _____

category FICTION

      MEMOIR

      BIOGRAPHY

      HISTORY

      OTHER NONFICTION

recommended by _____

questions or topics prepared by the discussion leader

HIGHLIGHTS OF OUR CONVERSATION

reactions to the discussion topics, memorable debates, passionate exchanges

our favorite characters

our favorite quotes

ratings (TALLY UP THE MEMBER VOTES IN THE FOLLOWING AREAS)

FOR FICTION/MEMOIR

character development: A ___ B+ ___ B ___ C ___ F ___

development of setting: A ___ B+ ___ B ___ C ___ F ___

pace: A ___ B+ ___ B ___ C ___ F ___

writing style: A ___ B+ ___ B ___ C ___ F ___

Total average grade ____

FOR NONFICTION

depth of research: A ___ B+ ___ B ___ C ___ F ___

interest level of topic: A ___ B+ ___ B ___ C ___F ___

pace: A ___ B+ ___ B ___ C ___F ___

writing style: A ___ B+ ___ B ___ C ___F ___

Total average grade ____

OTHER ESSENTIALS

book club beverages
_____

_____

book club snacks
_____

_____

expenses to divide
_____

set•ting (set′ing), *n.* the locale or period in which the action of a novel, play, film, etc., takes place.

Reading is equivalent to thinking with someone else's head instead of with one's own.

—ARTHUR SCHOPENHAUER

date

time

meeting location

discussion leader

attendees

title

author

publisher/date

category   FICTION

MEMOIR

BIOGRAPHY

HISTORY

OTHER NONFICTION

recommended by

questions or topics prepared by the discussion leader

HIGHLIGHTS OF OUR CONVERSATION
reactions to the discussion topics, memorable debates, passionate exchanges

our favorite characters

our favorite quotes

ratings (TALLY UP THE MEMBER VOTES IN THE FOLLOWING AREAS)

FOR FICTION/MEMOIR

character development: A ___ B+ ___ B ___ C ___ F ___

development of setting: A ___ B+ ___ B ___ C ___ F ___

pace: A ___ B+ ___ B ___ C ___ F ___

writing style: A ___ B+ ___ B ___ C ___ F ___

Total average grade ___

FOR NONFICTION

depth of research: A ___ B+ ___ B ___ C ___ F ___

interest level of topic: A ___ B+ ___ B ___ C ___F ___

pace: A ___ B+ ___ B ___ C ___F ___

writing style: A ___ B+ ___ B ___ C ___F ___

Total average grade ___

OTHER ESSENTIALS

book club beverages

book club snacks

expenses to divide

date _____ time _____

meeting location _____

_____

_____

discussion leader _____

attendees _____

_____

_____

_____

_____

title _____

author _____

publisher/date _____

category FICTION

MEMOIR

BIOGRAPHY

HISTORY

OTHER NONFICTION

recommended by _____

questions or topics prepared by the discussion leader

HIGHLIGHTS OF OUR CONVERSATION
reactions to the discussion topics, memorable debates, passionate exchanges

our favorite characters

our favorite quotes

ratings (TALLY UP THE MEMBER VOTES IN THE FOLLOWING AREAS)

FOR FICTION/MEMOIR

character development: A ___ B+ ___ B ___ C ___ F ___

development of setting: A ___ B+ ___ B ___ C ___ F ___

pace: A ___ B+ ___ B ___ C ___ F ___

writing style: A ___ B+ ___ B ___ C ___ F ___

Total average grade ____

FOR NONFICTION

depth of research: A ___ B+ ___ B ___ C ___ F ___

interest level of topic: A ___ B+ ___ B ___ C ___ F ___

pace: A ___ B+ ___ B ___ C ___ F ___

writing style: A ___ B+ ___ B ___ C ___ F ___

Total average grade ____

OTHER ESSENTIALS

book club beverages
_____

_____

book club snacks
_____

_____

_____

expenses to divide
_____

_____

date   time

meeting location

discussion leader

attendees

title

author

publisher/date

category   FICTION

            MEMOIR

            BIOGRAPHY

            HISTORY

            OTHER NONFICTION

recommended by

questions or topics prepared by the discussion leader

HIGHLIGHTS OF OUR CONVERSATION

reactions to the discussion topics, memorable debates, passionate exchanges

our favorite characters

our favorite quotes

ratings

FOR FICTION/MEMOIR

character development: A ____ B+ ____ B ____ C ____ F ____

development of setting: A ____ B+ ____ B ____ C ____ F ____

pace: A ____ B+ ____ B ____ C ____ F ____

writing style: A ____ B+ ____ B ____ C ____ F ____

Total average grade ____

FOR NONFICTION

depth of research: A ____ B+ ____ B ____ C ____ F ____

interest level of topic: A ____ B+ ____ B ____ C ____F ____

pace: A ____ B+ ____ B ____ C ____F ____

writing style: A ____ B+ ____ B ____ C ____F ____

Total average grade ____

OTHER ESSENTIALS

book club beverages
_____

_____

book club snacks
_____

_____

expenses to divide
_____

_____

fic•tion (fik′shən), **n.** 1. the class of literature comprising works of imaginative narration, esp. in prose form. 2. works of this class, as novels or short stories.

*To feel most beautifully alive
means to be reading something
beautiful, ready always to apprehend
in the flow of language the sudden
flash of poetry.*

—GASTON BACHELARD

date _____ time _____

meeting location _____

_____

_____

discussion leader _____

attendees _____

_____

_____

_____

_____

title _____

author _____

publisher/date _____

category   FICTION

        MEMOIR

        BIOGRAPHY

        HISTORY

        OTHER NONFICTION

recommended by _____

questions or topics prepared by the discussion leader

HIGHLIGHTS OF OUR CONVERSATION
reactions to the discussion topics, memorable debates, passionate exchanges

our favorite characters

our favorite quotes

ratings (TALLY UP THE MEMBER VOTES IN THE FOLLOWING AREAS)

FOR FICTION/MEMOIR

character development: A ___ B+ ___ B ___ C ___ F ___

development of setting: A ___ B+ ___ B ___ C ___ F ___

pace: A ___ B+ ___ B ___ C ___ F ___

writing style: A ___ B+ ___ B ___ C ___ F ___

Total average grade ____

FOR NONFICTION

depth of research: A ___ B+ ___ B ___ C ___ F ___

interest level of topic: A ___ B+ ___ B ___ C ___ F ___

pace: A ___ B+ ___ B ___ C ___ F ___

writing style: A ___ B+ ___ B ___ C ___ F ___

Total average grade ____

OTHER ESSENTIALS

book club beverages

_____

book club snacks

_____

_____

expenses to divide

_____

date   time

meeting location

discussion leader

attendees

title

author

publisher/date

category   FICTION

                 MEMOIR

                 BIOGRAPHY

                 HISTORY

                 OTHER NONFICTION

recommended by

questions or topics prepared by the discussion leader

HIGHLIGHTS OF OUR CONVERSATION
reactions to the discussion topics, memorable debates, passionate exchanges

our favorite characters

our favorite quotes

ratings (TALLY UP THE MEMBER VOTES IN THE FOLLOWING AREAS)

FOR FICTION/MEMOIR

character development: A ___ B+ ___ B ___ C ___ F ___

development of setting: A ___ B+ ___ B ___ C ___ F ___

pace: A ___ B+ ___ B ___ C ___ F ___

writing style: A ___ B+ ___ B ___ C ___ F ___

Total average grade ____

FOR NONFICTION

depth of research: A ___ B+ ___ B ___ C ___ F ___

interest level of topic: A ___ B+ ___ B ___ C ___F ___

pace: A ___ B+ ___ B ___ C ___F ___

writing style: A ___ B+ ___ B ___ C ___F ___

Total average grade ____

OTHER ESSENTIALS

book club beverages

book club snacks

expenses to divide

date   time

meeting location

discussion leader

attendees

title

author

publisher/date

category   FICTION

             MEMOIR

             BIOGRAPHY

             HISTORY

             OTHER NONFICTION

recommended by

questions or topics prepared by the discussion leader

HIGHLIGHTS OF OUR CONVERSATION

reactions to the discussion topics, memorable debates, passionate exchanges

our favorite characters

our favorite quotes

ratings (TALLY UP THE MEMBER VOTES IN THE FOLLOWING AREAS)

FOR FICTION/MEMOIR

character development: A ___ B+ ___ B ___ C ___ F ___

development of setting: A ___ B+ ___ B ___ C ___ F ___

pace: A ___ B+ ___ B ___ C ___ F ___

writing style: A ___ B+ ___ B ___ C ___ F ___

Total average grade _____

FOR NONFICTION

depth of research: A ___ B+ ___ B ___ C ___ F ___

interest level of topic: A ___ B+ ___ B ___ C ___F ___

pace: A ___ B+ ___ B ___ C ___F ___

writing style: A ___ B+ ___ B ___ C ___F ___

Total average grade _____

OTHER ESSENTIALS

book club beverages
_____

_____

book club snacks
_____

_____

_____

expenses to divide
_____

_____

chap•ter (chap′ter), *n.* a main division of a book, treatise, or the like, usu. bearing a number or title.

Promiscuity is like never reading past the first page. Monogamy is like reading the same book over and over.

—MASON COOLEY

date

time

meeting location

discussion leader

attendees

title

author

publisher/date

category   FICTION

MEMOIR

BIOGRAPHY

HISTORY

OTHER NONFICTION

recommended by

questions or topics prepared by the discussion leader

HIGHLIGHTS OF OUR CONVERSATION
reactions to the discussion topics, memorable debates, passionate exchanges

our favorite characters

our favorite quotes

ratings (TALLY UP THE MEMBER VOTES IN THE FOLLOWING AREAS)

FOR FICTION/MEMOIR

character development: A ____ B+ ____ B ____ C ____ F ____

development of setting: A ____ B+ ____ B ____ C ____ F ____

pace: A ____ B+ ____ B ____ C ____ F ____

writing style: A ____ B+ ____ B ____ C ____ F ____

Total average grade ____

FOR NONFICTION

depth of research: A ____ B+ ____ B ____ C ____ F ____

interest level of topic: A ____ B+ ____ B ____ C ____F ____

pace: A ____ B+ ____ B ____ C ____F ____

writing style: A ____ B+ ____ B ____ C ____F ____

Total average grade ____

OTHER ESSENTIALS

book club beverages
_____

_____

book club snacks
_____

_____

_____

expenses to divide
_____

_____

date _____ time _____

meeting location _____

_____

_____

discussion leader _____

attendees _____

_____

_____

_____

_____

title _____

author _____

publisher/date _____

category   FICTION

            MEMOIR

            BIOGRAPHY

            HISTORY

            OTHER NONFICTION

recommended by _____

questions or topics prepared by the discussion leader

HIGHLIGHTS OF OUR CONVERSATION
reactions to the discussion topics, memorable debates, passionate exchanges

our favorite characters

our favorite quotes

ratings (TALLY UP THE MEMBER VOTES IN THE FOLLOWING AREAS)

FOR FICTION/MEMOIR

character development: A ___ B+ ___ B ___ C ___ F ___

development of setting: A ___ B+ ___ B ___ C ___ F ___

pace: A ___ B+ ___ B ___ C ___ F ___

writing style: A ___ B+ ___ B ___ C ___ F ___

Total average grade ____

FOR NONFICTION

depth of research: A ___ B+ ___ B ___ C ___ F ___

interest level of topic: A ___ B+ ___ B ___ C ___ F ___

pace: A ___ B+ ___ B ___ C ___ F ___

writing style: A ___ B+ ___ B ___ C ___ F ___

Total average grade ____

OTHER ESSENTIALS

book club beverages _____

_____

book club snacks _____

_____

_____

expenses to divide _____

_____

our
book club recipes

Books give us
food for thought,
and thinking makes
us hungry.
Here's the best of our
book club dishes.

*A book does not make bad jokes,
drink too much or eat more than
you can afford to pay for.*

—KENNETH TURAN

our
favorite
book-
stores

A list of wonderful
booksellers in our
own town and in
places that we've
visited.

*A good book is the best of friends,
the same today and for ever.*

—MARTIN TUPPER

our
bookstores